TABLE OF CONTENTS

VOLUME TWO (Continued)

PART IV. SURGERY OF THE BREAST AND CHEST

Chapter 25.—Breast
Chapter 26.—Bronchi
Chapter 27.—Pleuræ and Lungs
Chapter 28.—Pulmonary Artery
Chapter 29.—Mediastinum
Chapter 30.—Esophagus
Chapter 31.—Heart and Pericardium

VOLUME THREE

PART V. SURGERY OF THE ABDOMEN

Chapter 32.—Opening and Closing the Abdomen
Chapter 33.—Stomach
Chapter 34.—Intestines
Chapter 35.—Liver and Biliary Passages
Chapter 36.—Pancreas
Chapter 37.—Spleen
Chapter 38.—Hernia

PART VI. SURGERY OF THE PELVIC REGION

Chapter 39.—Gynecologic Operations
Chapter 40.—Genito-Urinary Organs

MODERN SURGICAL TECHNIC

BY

MAX THOREK, M.D., K.L.H.(France); K.C.(Italy)

PROF. CLINICAL SURGERY, COOK COUNTY GRADUATE SCHOOL OF MEDICINE; ATTENDING SURGEON, COOK COUNTY HOSPITAL; SURGEON-IN-CHIEF, THE AMERICAN HOSPITAL; CONSULTING SURGEON, MUNICIPAL TUBERCULOSIS SANITARIUM; CORRESPONDING MEMBER, SOCIÉTÉ DES CHIRURGIENS DE PARIS, FRANCE; ROYAL ACADEMY OF MEDICINE, TORINO, ITALY; SURGICAL SOCIETY, MADRID, SPAIN; SOCIEDADE DAS SCIENCIAS MEDICAS, LISBON, PORTUGAL; FELLOW INTERNATIONAL COLLEGE OF SURGEONS; FELLOW NATIONAL ACADEMY OF MEDICINE, COLOMBIA, SOUTH AMERICA; SURGICAL ACADEMY, MEXICO; HONORARY FELLOW, BULGARIAN SURGICAL SOCIETY; HON. FELLOW EGYPTIAN MEDICAL ASSOCIATION, CAIRO, EGYPT; FELLOW, INTERNATIONAL COLLEGE OF ANESTHETISTS; ETC., ETC.

COMPLETE IN THREE VOLUMES

WITH 2174 ILLUSTRATIONS, ORIGINALS PRINCIPALLY BY W. C. SHEPARD

WITH A FOREWORD BY

DONALD C. BALFOUR, M.B., M.D. (Tor.) LL.D., F.A.C.S., F.R.A.C.S.

HEAD OF SECTION IN DIVISION OF SURGERY, THE MAYO CLINIC; DIRECTOR AND PROFESSOR OF SURGERY, THE MAYO FOUNDATION FOR MEDICAL EDUCATION AND RESEARCH, GRADUATE SCHOOL, UNIVERSITY OF MINNESOTA, ETC., ETC.

VOLUME ONE

GENERAL OPERATIVE CONSIDERATIONS
SURGERY OF THE HEAD AND NECK
AND PLASTIC SURGERY

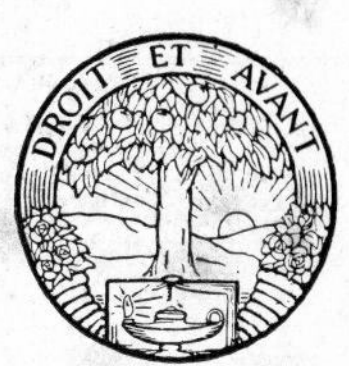

PHILADELPHIA LONDON MONTREAL NEW YORK

J. B. LIPPINCOTT COMPANY

PRINTED IN THE UNITED STATES OF AMERICA

TO AN INEXHAUSTIBLE SOURCE OF CONSTANT INSPIRATION

MY WIFE

AND

MY SON, DR. PHIL THOREK

This volume is affectionately dedicated by
the Author

PREFACE

There is no lack of excellent treatises covering the field of operative surgery. But the available works fall, generally, into two categories: voluminous systems which, while containing a wealth of material, offer such a multiplicity of procedures as to prove confounding, and single volumes which are too abridged to afford detailed information sufficient for the student and general surgeon—a sort of plethora in one, and an obvious deficiency in the other.

It is for this reason that the author felt there existed a genuine need for a succinct work on surgical operations, up-to-date as regards important advances in surgical technic and including, in order to be practical, a sufficiently detailed description of each procedure in all commonly performed operations. The aim of this book is to supply this need. It is intended particularly for students, for general surgeons and for those general practitioners who are occasionally called upon to perform emergency operations.

There is always a certain feeling of diffidence in presenting a new book to one's professional colleagues. The author's personal experience of over thirty years in the daily practice of general surgery, in observing the methods of master surgeons at home and abroad and in teaching surgical technic must be his excuse for presuming to present the surgical profession with a practical book of this kind, one which he believes contains the most important facts for those for whom it is intended.

There are those who think that whatever is new is the best. This is not always so. A multitude of standard surgical procedures of today are not new, but improvements of cruder methods which had their inception in the mists of antiquity. Indeed, many old operations are still modern, and in many respects surgeons of today do not excel in, perhaps they do not equal, the technic of their predecessors. Sentiment and justice demand that we should not forget those who pioneered for us, and, although no attempt is made to delve thoroughly into the history of surgery, yet some historical notes are included and credit given to those who have developed particular surgical procedures.

Surgical technic is no one's prerogative and no man has ever lived who has excelled in every field of surgery. Highly technical procedures of an elective type, not commonly performed, have only been sketched for completeness' sake. Emergency operations which any surgeon may have to perform have been included in the general scheme.

I have considered it important to give the high-lights of surgical anatomy preceding operative procedures. Unfortunately, many text-books of surgical technic of today allot little space to such important subjects as amputations, ligation of blood vessels, fractures, dislocations, etc., etc.; of this I took cognizance and I have included them in this work. In describing operations I have adopted the step-by-step method, for the benefit of the student and of the inexpert operator to whom methodical procedures are essential until he has become proficient. Some of the operative procedures are original methods, but for the most part they are the standard procedures whose value has been confirmed by time.

On the principle that, as the Chinese say, "one picture is worth a thousand words," extensive illustration has been employed. Not only do illustrations spare lengthy descriptions, but they give a much clearer idea of what the author intends to convey. In this connection, I wish to extend my warmest acknowledgment to Mr. W. C. Shepard. He is an outstanding artist who has combined his remarkable ability for graphic illustration with his profound knowledge of surgical anatomy in bringing out the salient points pertaining to the various operations.

My sincere thanks and grateful acknowledgments go to the many authors who have kindly granted me permission to reproduce original illustrations; to the authors of treatises from which descriptions of certain standard operations have been borrowed; to Dr. Harry L. Pollock who graciously read the manuscript on surgery of the ear, nose and throat; to Dr. Oscar B. Nugent for suggestions on surgery of the eye; to Dr. Raymond W. McNeally from whose contributions on the surgery of the vascular system I have liberally borrowed, and for his critical and painstaking editing of the chapter on vascular surgery; and to Dr. Donald L. Dickerson for some of the sketches made from life and for proofreading parts of the manuscript; to Misses Angela Bartenbach and Hebilly-Magda West for supplementary illustrations, to Dr. Horace E. Turner for careful proofreading and suggestions in the chapter on Orthopedics, as well as to Miss Leona Tanner for the careful typing of the manuscript—a nerve-taxing task.

Lastly, special gratitude is expressed to the publishers for their unfailing courtesy, untiring and boundless cooperation regardless of expense, invaluable advice and general help in the production of this book.

If this work meets with the same kind reception as did my last, "Surgical Errors and Safeguards," the forgone vacations and the intensive effort which has been put forth in the years just passed to accomplish this task will appear infinitesimal as compared with the gratification of the author.

Max Thorek

The American Hospital of Chicago
1938

FOREWORD

The remarkable advances in the scope and quality of surgery during the past fifty years have been studied from many different viewpoints. The scope of surgery has been enormously expanded by remarkable results effected in established as well as in new fields, by scientific and safe approach to every part of the body, by the willingness to discard apparently well-established major surgical procedures for simpler methods, and by the consequent great and rapid increase in the number of practicing surgeons. During this period, surgery also can be credited with giving impetus to clinical and laboratory methods of identifying lesions in early stages of their evolution and with the attempt to control, ameliorate, abort and prevent those conditions which are known to be dependent on disturbed physiologic processes, so that in all surgical fields the approach to sound surgical treatment is more and more made through research being carried out in clinical and experimental laboratories. The factors contributing to these great advances in surgery, therefore, have come from every field of medicine, and have been applied chiefly in stressing the basis on which successful treatment may be founded, namely, accurate diagnosis.

The necessary application of the great increase in knowledge in the basic sciences, particularly in physiology, pathology and biochemistry, to the practice of surgery, and the emphasis which has been given their importance, are likely to obscure the fact that surgical results always will be directly dependent upon the technical skill and judgment with which such knowledge is applied. A profound knowledge of fundamental fields without good judgment, technical skill and experience usually means unsatisfactory surgery. Further advances in surgery, therefore, will depend, to a considerable extent, on the capacity of man to improve in such technical pursuits, and any contribution which may aid in this advance is important.

When such a contribution has the intent of presenting a general picture of surgical technic in the various fields, it represents a vast undertaking because of the enormous number of surgical procedures which must be evaluated and from which selections must be made so as to give a comprehensive, clear, and authoritative picture of the status of modern surgical technic. In this primary purpose this work has succeeded admirably and should be an invaluable reference for all general surgeons and for those who are limiting their surgical practice to particular fields. The text and illustrations are designed to facilitate the application of these methods, and since the avoidance of errors in technic is often dependent on whether or not the surgeon knows what should be done and how it should be done, the volume should be indispensable to those who have the responsibility of the surgery in their communities.

Donald C. Balfour, M.D.

Mayo Clinic,
Rochester, Minn.

CONTENTS

VOLUME I

PART ONE

GENERAL OPERATIVE CONSIDERATIONS

CHAPTER PAGE

1. The Surgeon and His Art ... 3
2. The Surgeon and the Patient ... 6
   - History Taking ... 6
   - Pre-operative Care ... 7
   - Mental Attitude of Patient and Surgeon ... 9
3. Postoperative Considerations ... 11
   - Immediate Sequelae ... 11
     - Shock ... 11
     - Hemorrhage ... 13
     - Infection ... 13
   - Postoperative Care and Late Complications ... 14
     - Thirst ... 14
     - Catharsis ... 14
     - Diet ... 16
   - Postoperative Pain ... 17
4. Operating Pavilions and the Operation in General ... 18
   - Operating Pavilions ... 18
   - The Operating Room ... 21
   - The Operation in General ... 25
   - Surgical Instruments ... 38
   - Electrosurgery ... 44
5. Sterilization of Surgical Supplies ... 46
   - Preparation of Materials ... 47
6. Anesthesia ... 54
   - General Anesthesia ... 54
     - Preparation of Patient ... 54
     - Induction ... 54
     - Ether ... 57
     - Chloroform ... 75
     - Mixtures ... 75
     - Ethyl Chloride ... 75
     - Nitrous Oxide ... 76
     - Basal Anesthetics ... 76
     - Ether-Colonic Anesthesia ... 81
   - Regional Anesthesia ... 84
     - Spinal Anesthesia ... 84
     - Sacral Anesthesia ... 89
     - Parasacral Nerve Block ... 90
     - Trans-sacral Nerve Block ... 91
     - Paravertebral and Splanchnic Anesthesia ... 93
   - Local Anesthesia ... 100

PART TWO

SURGERY OF THE HEAD AND NECK AND PLASTIC SURGERY

CHAPTER PAGE

7. Surgery of the Scalp and Pericranium ... 107
   - Injuries ... 107
     - Wounds ... 107
     - Avulsion ... 107
   - Tumors ... 107
     - Meningocele and Encephalocele ... 107
     - Sebaceous Cysts ... 108
     - Angioma ... 109
     - Cirsoid Aneurysm ... 109
   - Malignant Tumors ... 111

8. Surgery of the Skull and Brain ... 113
   - Injuries of the Cranial Vault ... 113
     - Scalp Wound with Possible Fracture ... 113
     - Simple Fracture with Depressed Bone ... 113
     - Compound Comminuted Fracture ... 114
     - Penetrating Wounds of the Brain ... 117
     - Concussion of the Brain ... 118
     - Methods of Reducing Intracranial Tension ... 118
     - Fractures of the Base of the Skull ... 119
     - Intracranial Bleeding ... 119
     - Brain Abscess ... 121
   - Operations on the Skull and Brain (General) ... 122
     - Craniocerebral Topography ... 124
     - Anesthesia ... 126
     - Form of Bone Flap ... 127
     - Control of Hemorrhage ... 127
     - Methods of Opening the Skull ... 131
     - Subtemporal Decompression ... 148
     - Closure of Cranial Defects ... 150
   - General Principles Underlying the Removal of Tumor of the Brain ... 155
     - Exposure of the Brain ... 156
     - Tumors of the Convexity of the Hemispheres ... 159
     - Tumors of the Frontal Lobes ... 159
     - Tumors of the Temporal, Parietal and Occipital Regions ... 160
     - Subtentorial Tumors ... 160
     - Angiomas of the Cerebral Hemispheres ... 162
     - Cysts and Cystic Collections of Fluid in the Brain ... 162
     - Epilepsy ... 166
   - Diagnostic Puncture of the Brain Ventricles and Cisternae ... 168
     - Ventricular Puncture ... 168
     - Ventriculography ... 170
     - Hydrocephalus ... 172

9. Surgery of the Ears and Adjacent Structures ... 178
   - Operations on the External Ear ... 178
     - Hematoma Auris ... 178
     - Cauliflower Ear ... 178
     - Prominent Ears ... 178
     - Macrotia ... 179
     - Removal of Foreign Bodies from Auditory Canal ... 179
     - Furuncle of Auditory Canal ... 180
     - Removal of Polypi from Auditory Canal ... 181

CHAPTER PAGE

Removal of Exostoses of the Auditory Canal 181
Operations for Infections of the Middle Ear and Intracranial Complications 181
Myringotomy 181
Mastoiditis 183
Extradural Abscess 192
Temporosphenoidal Abscess 192
Sinus Thrombosis 193
Ligation and Resection of the Internal Jugular Vein 195

10. Surgery of the Face 197
Infections 197
Carbuncle of the Face 197
Actinomycosis of the Face 198
Tumors of the Face 199
Meloplasty 199
Defects without Cicatrical Maxillary Occlusion 199
Defects with Cicatrical Maxillary Occlusion 203
Injuries to the Bones of the Face 204
Fracture of the Upper Jaw 204
Fracture of the Malar Bone 204
Fracture of the Zygoma 205
Operations on the Divisions of the Trigeminal Nerve and the Gasserian Ganglion 205
Trigeminal Neuralgia 205
Removal of the Gasserian Ganglion 217
Neurectomy 222

11. Surgery of the Sinuses and Tonsils 224
Operations on the Sinuses 224
Frontal Sinus 224
Maxillary Sinus 225
Ethmoid Sinus 229
Sphenoid Sinus 229
Operations on the Tonsils 231
Tonsillectomy 231
Removal of Pharyngeal Adenoids 238
Infections 241
Peritonsillar Abscess 241
Operations for Retropharyngeal Abscess 241

12. Surgery of the Lips, Tongue and Lymph Nodes 243
Surgery of the Lip 243
Plastic Surgery of the Lower Lip 243
Carcinoma of the Lower Lip 243
Operations on the Tongue 250
Removal of Angioma of the Tongue 250
Acute Abscess of the Tongue 250
Ranula 251
Removal of Foreign Bodies from the Tongue 252
Tongue-Tie 252
Excision of the Tongue 253
Macroglossia 254
Chronic Glossitis 254
Excision of the Cervical Lymph Nodes, Submaxillary Glands and Fascial Structures of the Neck in Connection with Operations for Carcinoma of the Tongue and Floor of the Mouth 265

13. Surgery of the Salivary Glands 267
Injuries 267

CHAPTER PAGE

Acute Infections 267
Sublingual Gland 267
Submaxillary Gland 267
Parotid Gland 267
Calculus of the Salivary Glands and Ducts 267
Sublingual Duct 267
Wharton's (Submaxillary) Duct 268
Calculus of the Parotid Duct 269
Tumors of the Parotid Gland 270
Benign Tumors 270
Salivary Fistulas 276
Fistulas of Stensen's Duct 276

14. Surgery of the Jaws, Upper Lip and Cheek 281
Operations on the Upper Jaw 281
Excision of the Upper Jaw 281
Operations on the Lower Jaw 284
Temporo-maxillary Ankylosis 285
Dislocation of the Jaw 289
Subluxation of the Jaw 290
Resection of Alveolar Process 293
Partial Resection of the Horizontal Ramus of Lower Jaw 293
Resection and Exarticulation of Lower Jaw 294
Nerve Anastomosis for Facial Paralysis 297
Surgery of the Upper Lip 305
Harelip and Cleft Palate 305
Operations for Cleft Palate 312

15. Surgery of the Orbit and Eye 320
Operations on the Orbit 320
Incision for Orbital Cellulitis 320
Osteoplastic Resection of the Outer Wall of the Orbit 320
Operations on the Eye 321
Anesthesia 325
Removal of Foreign Bodies 325
Operation on the Conjunctiva 327
Operations on the Eyelids 328
Operations on the Cornea 339
Keratectomy 340
Operations on the Sclera 341
Operations on the Iris 342
Operations on the Ocular Muscles 346

16. Surgery of the Nose 352
Rhinoplastics 352
Local Anesthesia 352
Tampon of Nasal Cavities for Nasal Hemorrhage 353
Total Rhinoplasty 354
Subtotal Rhinoplasty 363
Simple Rhinoplasty 365
Submucous Resection of the Nasal Septum 368
Abscess of the Nasal Septum 370
Tumors of the Nose 371
Foreign Bodies in the Nose 372

17. Surgery of the Neck and Cervical Endocrine Glands 375
Injuries of the Neck 375
Cut Throat 375
Fractures of the Larynx and Trachea 376

CHAPTER PAGE

Rupture of the Trachea with Retraction of Lower End 377
Foreign Bodies in the Pharynx and Esophagus 377
Burns and Scars 377
Infections of the Neck 378
Furuncles and Carbuncles of the Neck 378
Cellulitis and Lymphodenitis 379
Ludwig's Angina 380
Peri-esophageal Suppuration and Mediastinitis 383
Diagnostic Operations on the Neck 383
Laryngoscopy 383
Esophagoscopy 386
Operations on the Neck 387
Intercricoid Laryngotomy 387
Tracheotomy 387
Intubation 395
Pharyngotomy 398
External Esophagotomy 402
Laryngectomy 405
Excision of Cervical Ribs 408
Removal of the Cervical Sympathetic 412
Torticollis 415
Spasmodic Torticollis 416
Cysts and Tumors of the Neck 422
Removal of Tumors of the Neck in General 422
Tumors of the Carotid Body 432
Operations on the Thyroid Gland 435
Thyroidectomy 441
Ligation of the Thyroid Arteries 462
Complications Following Thyroidectomy 467
Transplantation of Thyroid Tissue 468
Ancillary Thyroid Operations 468
Operations on the Parathyroid Gland 471
Parathyroidectomy 472
Operations on the Thymus 480
Thymectomy 480
Tumors of the Thymus 482

18. Principles of Plastic Surgery and Skin Grafting 484
Reconstructive and Aesthetic Plastic Surgery 484
Two Main Principles of Plastic Repair 485
Methods of Plastic Repair 485
Reverdin Grafts 507
Thiersch Grafts 512
Wolfe-Krause Method 514
Sieve Graft 516
Skin Periosteum Bone Grafts 520
Mucous Membrane 520
Grafting in X-Ray Burns 522
Treatment of Burns 523

VOLUME ONE

Part I

GENERAL OPERATIVE CONSIDERATIONS

CHAPTER	PAGE
1. The Surgeon and His Art	3
2. The Surgeon and His Patient	6
3. Postoperative Considerations	11
4. Operating Pavilions and the Operation in General	18
5. Sterilization of Surgical Instruments	46
6. Anesthesia	54

ORIENTATION

In this section of the work, general subjects are discussed. While operative surgery has made tremendous strides in the last decades, the marvel of the recuperative powers of the human body are as baffling today as they were centuries ago and even the most experienced surgeon must acknowledge his indebtedness to it. Both the potentialities of the Vis Medicatrix Naturae and the degree of skill of the surgeon decide the outcome of the particular surgical problem. There is much in what Ambroise Paré (1510-1590), the greatest surgeon of his time, has said in relation to the healing powers of Nature which is summed up in the famous inscription on his statue "Je le pansay, Dieu le guarit." Nevertheless, the more competent the surgeon, the kinder nature seems to serve him; ignorance and surgical transgressions are resented by her.

The importance of the relationship between the surgeon and patient and the psychic attitude of each to one another are stressed. The responsibility of the surgeon does not cease when the patient is wheeled out of the operating room. It is then when the responsibility of proper postoperative care falls on his shoulders. This phase is discussed in Chapter 3 and, while the arrangement and equipment of operating pavilions and the conduct of the operation in general is subject to the taste and opinions of various surgeons, a general outline and the essentials of these has been described in Chapter 4.

Of utmost importance, of course, is the surgeon's armamentarium but no matter how skillfully fabricated, his instruments may become dangerous weapons if not subjected to proper sterilization. This has been described in Chapter 5. Part I concludes with "Anesthesia" in all its modern phases of practice. It is refreshing to observe the present-day trend of specialization in this important field. While volumes have been written on the subject and there is still much to be learned, the successful administration of an anesthetic is based upon a thorough understanding of the physiologic principles involved, of the mode of action of the anesthetic used, etc. Much research remains to be done here. Hewitt summarizes the question of the action of anesthetics as follows: "All that we can say is, that general anesthesia is probably brought about by some change of physico-chemical character within the protoplasm of the nerve cells; that the most delicate and vulnerable of the nervous elements, those which give to the organs their characteristics, peculiarities, attributes and functions, are first affected, and that finally, the most resistant centers upon which life is dependent are attacked. Whether the change is due to the local effect of the anesthetic itself, upon the cell contents, or whether some alteration in the blood produced by the anesthetic is the immediate cause of such change is at present impossible to say."

The discussion of the various types of anesthesia begins with the history of anesthesia and includes an evaluation of all methods in use today. Local (infiltration) or block anesthesia of various operations is described preceding the description of the respective operation.

MODERN SURGICAL TECHNIC

CHAPTER 1

THE SURGEON AND HIS ART

"Surgery is not only a matter of operating skillfully. It must engage in its service qualities of mind and of heart that raise it to the very highest pinnacle of human endeavor. A patient can offer you no higher tribute than to entrust you with his life and his health, and by implication, with the happiness of all his family. To be worthy of this trust we must submit for a lifetime to the constant discipline of unwearied effort in the search of knowledge, and of most reverent devotion to every detail in every operation that we perform." (Lord Moynihan.)

There is no human calling which demands from those who follow it a greater endowment of the best human qualities and the highest developments of technical knowledge and skill than the art of surgery. In major surgical work, and often, indeed, in lesser, the stake at issue is human life; the surgeon stands between the patient and death. On the one hand, the surgeon's judgment, knowledge and skill may save a life otherwise doomed; on the other hand, erroneous or careless surgical procedures may and often do bring either death or life-long misery to a patient who has had a comparatively easily corrected condition. The surgeon's responsibility is, therefore, a sacred one, for he is often an arbiter of life and death and responsible only to his own conscience.

He who wishes to become a true surgeon must possess many virtues and much skill. His virtues must be sympathy, patience, self-denial and self-disinterestedness. By this last, I mean that the object of his work must always be the good of his patient rather than the enhancement of his own reputation or personal aggrandizement.

The safety of the patient upon whom a surgical operation is being performed must always be the prime objective; every other surgical consideration is secondary. Therefore, brilliancy of technic should never be permitted to eclipse safety. In the past, too many surgeons were obsessed with the illusion of brilliant operating; the patient was considered merely a vehicle through which they could exhibit their rapidity of manipulation and technical skill. Of such surgeons it could truly be said that "the operation was successful but the patient died." Today, fortunately, the successful surgeon is the safe surgeon; one who reduces surgical interference to the absolutely necessary minimum and yet accomplishes the objects of surgery. These objects are to relieve pain, save life and restore physiological function.

In connection with the foregoing, I might cite the celebrated French surgeon Doyen, who said:

"Surgery is one of the noblest arts; too many of its practitioners have made it a trade. Its operations were, at the beginning of the last century, the appanage of a few, and surgeons regarded the accomplishments and reputation of being a brilliant operator as the highest attainable honor. . . . The surgeon should be an artist, not a manipulator. . . . It is high time that the fact should be recognized that any one cannot improvise himself a surgeon, and that it does not suffice, in order to constitute an operator, to be able to manipulate some dozens of hemostatic forceps more or less adroitly."

The name of "surgeon" is merited only by one who is a profound and accomplished clinician and at the same time a prudent and skillful operator.

At the present time the increase of surgical operative work by general practitioners, owing to the increased facilities offered by the many small hospitals throughout the country, tends to make ambitious young men undertake major surgical operations for which neither their training, experience nor resources render them fit. I do not refer to emergency surgery which must be done even in the face of known risks, but to elective surgery which should be done only by the competent. As Kocher says: "The more surgery has become the common property of medical men the more it is incumbent upon any one who intends to devote himself to the practice of surgery to take every opportunity of improving his technique."

The medical profession justly complains that unwarranted operations are often undertaken by men of little experience. Unfortunately, warranted operations are also often undertaken by men of the same type.

What steps are necessary, therefore, in order that one should merit the dignified title of surgeon? First, a long apprenticeship under masters of the surgical art in order to obtain a profound knowledge not alone of diagnosis but also of the indications for any operative procedure. Second, a thorough knowledge of anatomical structures and physiological functions with special references to the manner in which these may be affected by surgical operative manipulations. Third, in so far as possible, a skilled technic in the actual performance of operations not only on the cadaver but on the living subject; and one must know every detail in the management of these cases in the pre- and postoperative phases under normal and abnormal circumstances. Fourth, understanding of the constitution of different types of patients, to be able to decide on operability and on the best time to operate as well as on the best type of operation for a given case. As Watson truly says:

"For every operation there is really only one good method and the surgeon must act according to the findings, as his experience and judgment tell him and he must perform his work simply and well. Every surgeon worthy of the name should not only be conscious of his sagacity and aptitude but be more particularly conscious of his limitations so that he is really fit to judge what he is capable of undertaking and performing for the ultimate cure of his patient."

While the ultimate cure of the patient is always the prime object of surgical interference, the preservation of physiologic function, if at all possible, is also an essential. A good surgeon, while always ready to perform heroic surgery if actually demanded, will refrain as long as possible from removing or excising a necessary limb or organ and in every operative procedure there must be method. Every extirpation, resection or reconstructive operation must be planned and executed on strictly anatomical and physiological lines.

When we consider the seriousness of a major surgical operation, the necessity for painstaking examination and clinical observation of a patient by the surgeon before he arrives at a definite diagnosis is at once seen. Today, diagnostic procedures are better than at any period of surgical history. Yet, if sins of surgical commission based on hasty and erroneous diagnosis are recorded anywhere, there must be a very large number of such records.

Lastly, as regards technic: it is a matter of constant practice. Manual dexterity is not picked up from books or by observing others. Knowledge of the best methods of doing any kind of surgical work is acquired only by experience and by keeping one's self acquainted with new methods as they appear and practicing them. Practice alone makes perfect but there is no use in being perfect in what itself is faulty. Technic distinguishes the surgical artist from the mere manipulator.

Taking into consideration the surgeon as a whole, Lord Moynihan aptly said, "He must have an eagle's eye, a lady's hand and a lion's heart" to which I would add a personality that inspires hope and confidence; his attitude towards his patients must be one of sympathy and gentle commiseration with an ever watchful solicitude for their care and safety.

CHAPTER 2

THE SURGEON AND THE PATIENT

"One essential matter is that he (the observer) must have seen the patient and elicited the symptoms from the patient. He must have watched the patient and noted the progress of the disease and the manifestations that accompany its progress, and have correlated the signs during life with those found at operation or death." *Sir James Mackenzie.*

In an emergency surgical operation there is, of course, no time for study, but in most other conditions there is sufficient time before operation for the surgeon to become more or less thoroughly acquainted with his patient. If possible, every surgical operation should be preceded by a period of complete physical and mental rest during which the constitutional peculiarities and the resistance power of the patient should be noted.

The surgeon can learn a good deal from the patient at his preliminary interviews. The trained eye may frequently observe constitutional and other peculiarities; but it is only after complete history taking and diagnostic procedures that a definite decision can be reached as to the true nature of the patient's trouble and as to the necessity for a surgical operation, as well as to the patient's capacity to undergo such operation as may be decided upon. There should be no failure as regards carelessness or want of thoroughness in respect to the **preoperative investigation** of a patient. The diagnostic paraphernalia is now vastly extended and all essential and unusual facts can be recorded and correlated with symptoms.

HISTORY TAKING

The complete history taking of the patient comprises many subdivisions and entails much care. Such important work should never be delegated to nurses or other subordinates; it demands the careful attention of the surgeon himself. He must personally verify the findings of the particular complaint to which the patient has called attention.

A patient was referred to me with a diagnosis of a possible malignancy of the descending colon (loss of weight, pain in the left colon region and somewhat suggestive x-ray findings). Pain was elicited while examining the patient's abdomen and palpating the left colon. During the course of the examination, I discovered the man was wearing a suspensory bandage. He said that he occasionally had a dragging sensation in the left testicle. Upon inspection, after removal of the suspensory bandage, it was discovered that the man had a malignancy of the testicle and that the pains along the left colon were in all probability due to retroperitoneal metastases from the testicular tumor.

The simplest complete record of every patient operated upon should contain:

1. A concisely written statement of the condition of the patient; his history, as stated and elicited.
2. A short orderly account of a general systematic examination noting particularly any abnormal findings.
3. The diagnosis, tentative or otherwise.

4. A short note on the treatment and an epitome of the surgical operation and findings disclosed.
5. Reference to any complications.
6. A note of the final results.

As regards the examination, the heart, lungs and kidneys should always be investigated with special care, no matter what the nature of the surgical procedure might be. In operations on any part of the intestinal tract, the mouth and teeth should receive special care and all foci of infection should be removed to obviate postoperative parotitis and postoperative pneumonia. Matters which should interest the surgeon are: any tendency to hemophilia or to acidosis, obesity, alcoholism and constitutional peculiarities.

PREOPERATIVE CARE

Patients are admitted to the hospital for elective operations at least by 3 o'clock on the afternoon on the day preceding the operation. Wherever possible the patient should be observed for a day or two prior to the operation. On admission the patient is given a tub bath. The presence of skin eruptions or anything unnatural about the patient is reported by the nurse to her superior.

A preoperative diet should furnish a high percentage of nutritive value in small bulk, should be readily and rapidly assimilated and should leave a minimum amount of intestinal residue. The diet on the day or two preceding an operation should be light. After midnight preceding the morning of the operation fluids are restricted or withheld unless specifically ordered otherwise.

In emergency operations, if food has been taken within six hours of operation, the stomach should be emptied before operation by lavage with plain warm water or with the addition of a small amount of sodium bicarbonate.

Catharsis. As a general rule it is considered unwise to disturb a patient's rest on the night before operation by giving him cathartics. Normal intestinal movements and functions are disturbed and it is possible that there may be an increase in absorption of intestinal toxins and a greater permeability of the intestine to bacteria. A mild purgative may, however, be given.

In the average case no special preparation is needed prior to the afternoon of the day preceding operation. A tub bath is given then and the entire field of operation cleansed thoroughly with green soap and water. The umbilical pit receives particular attention if it will be in the field of operation.

The entire field of operation is shaved. In abdominal operations this includes up to the nipple line, and posteriorly to the midaxillary line; the entire pubic region is thoroughly shaved. It is important that this area be shaved closely so that the finest hair is removed. To neglect this invites skin infections. Avoid injuring the skin with a razor. In gynecologic operations, it is well to do a complete vaginal preparation, unless contraindicated (virgo intacta). In hernia operations, the scrotum and contiguous areas are also surgically prepared.

After shaving, the entire abdomen is scrubbed thoroughly with green soap and water for three minutes; the field is now dried and treated with ether and 70 per cent alcohol. A sterile towel is placed over the field and kept in place with adhesive straps.

Unless there is some specific reason, all patients to whom an anesthetic is given receive a hypodermic injection of one-fourth grain of morphine sulphate with 1/150 grain of atropin sulphate three-quarters of an hour before going to surgery. After the injection has been given, the patient is kept quiet.

The patient's hair must be in order and free from hairpins. False teeth must be removed. The patient's bladder should be emptied and a record of the quantity of urine before the operation made; the large bowel is emptied by enema. If the patient does not void the interne or surgeon must be notified. If necessary, the patient should be catheterized. The patient should don a fresh gown and leggings. He or she is not to receive relatives and should be left in a

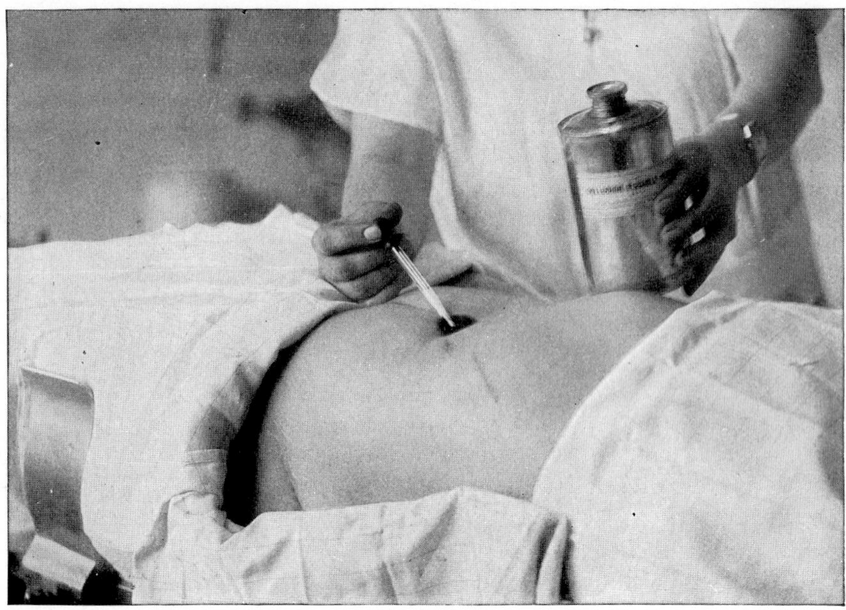

FIG. 1. After thorough preparation with iodine the umbilical pit is sealed with collodion, as shown in this illustration.

darkened, quiet room after the hypodermic injection is given. In all elective abdominal operations and where not contraindicated, I administer routinely before the operation an ampule of pitressin. It has served me well.

No patient is admitted to the operating suite unless accompanied by a complete history and physical examination, complete blood, urine and other special analyses, or if no preoperative diagnosis is recorded on the chart.

The patient is brought to surgery twenty minutes before operating schedule time and placed in proper position on the operating table. After the patient has been anesthetized, the entire field of operation and abdomen is exposed by removing the sterile towel. With a sterile sponge on a forceps the entire area is again gone over with ether. In case of the abdomen, the ether is permitted to drip into the umbilical pit but the sponge is never allowed to touch it. With this sponge, first cleanse over the site of the proposed incision. Always work away from the proposed line of incision until the entire field is cleansed. Discard the sponge. With a fresh sponge cleanse the umbilicus and again discard the sponge used. Following the preparation with ether, the same procedure is repeated with a 3½ per cent iodine solution and again a final preparation with 70 per cent alcohol.

Carefully remove all iodine, thus preventing burns. Seal the umbilical pit with collodion (Fig. 1). Drape the patient with a heavy sterile towel and remove him or her to the operating room for final draping.

Male herniotomy patients are subjected to a complete scrotal and penis preparation with tincture of merthiolate 1:1000 (Mo. 99).

MENTAL ATTITUDE OF PATIENT AND SURGEON

It is most desirable that the patient should go to surgery in as calm a state of mind as possible. Newer methods of preparing a patient include pre-anesthetic medication so that the patient is in a semi-conscious state before being anesthetized. This will be fully discussed in the chapter on General Anesthesia, page 54.

Every surgeon has observed that the cheerful, optimistic type of patient makes good progress while the nervous, overstrained, morbid and depressed one fails to make headway. Crile has pointed out that fear and apprehension lead to exhaustion of the bodily reserve and deplete the adrenal reserve. The only preventive is to try, before the operation, and after it, to calm the neurotic patient in every possible way and to induce him to take a cheerful outlook. All suggestive influences which tend to raise the patient's spirits and remove dread and fear are warranted even though the outlook is grave. Surgeons and their personnel should never betray any form of anxiety or apprehension in the presence of the patient, or by their actions or glances lead him to suspect that he is facing a serious crisis. Even life-saving measures should as far as possible be done in a matter-of-fact way as if they were routine.

No patient who shows an apathetic, fatalistic attitude towards an operation should be operated upon while in that frame of mind. My personal experience has been that a patient who is convinced that he will not recover from an operation or does not wish to recover not infrequently has his wish fulfilled. I have, therefore, made it a practice to try to change such a mental attitude of the patient. A hopeful, confident frame of mind is frequently a most important factor toward a favorable surgical prognosis.

The mental attitude of the patient very often depends on the mental attitude of the surgeon and plays a most important rôle from many points of view. Cheerful surroundings, a cheerful surgeon, a pleasant nursing staff and a form of suggestive therapy accomplished by the conduct of the surgeon are essentials for success. Personally, if I were ill, I would not permit a surgeon whose demeanor recalls the mortuary or the embalmer to minister to my physical needs. Apprehensive patients gain much, though they be seriously ill, by the warranted influences suggested by the surgeon. Of course, the relatives of the patient should at all times know the truth of the existing condition.

Two young women were scheduled to be operated on by the author for simple "interval" removal of the appendix. They occupied adjoining beds. Both were in splendid condition except that one of the patients, a young woman of nineteen, made the statement to the nurses that "she feels confident that she will never leave the hospital alive." This form of comment she indulged in rather frequently. It was, however, not looked upon by the attendants as a matter of importance. Both patients were operated on in the same forenoon. There were no complications or difficulties of any sort during the operative procedure. Both were returned to bed in excellent condition. The first post-operative day nothing unusual was observed. On the second day, the patient referred to began to have visual hallucinations of "churches," "funerals," "joining her mother in heaven," etc. She sang and muttered almost incessantly about the visions in the skies, etc. Her general physical condition was excellent. On the third day sedatives were used. On the fourth day during an attack of violent temper she tore her dressings off, became almost unmanageable and had to be restrained. The visual hallucinations became worse and with all resources at command to alleviate the condition it was all in vain. Death ensued on the eighth day following a "simple appendectomy." A remarkable sidelight of the case is that the second patient, referred to above, occupying the next bed, seeing the dilemma of her friend with whom she had been discussing religious topics prior to the operation, went into a cataleptic state which lasted about two days from which state she finally emerged following sedation, suggestion, etc. Thus, it is wise not to operate on a patient whose mind is set, at the outset, that he or she will not recover. An attempt is made to dissuade the individual and convince them, by every means possible (sustained suggestion), that a hopeful attitude is justified and that there surely is no need for apprehension. In predisposed individuals the psychic trauma may precipitate an acute mental upset.

In the postoperative period constant watchfulness of the patient by the surgeon himself is as important as the technical operation per se and is as much a part of the surgeon's personal duty as is the operation. His experience will enable him to observe the first symptoms of any approaching complication which, in many instances, he may be able to avert. The surgeon's neglect of the aforesaid may end in fatality.

CHAPTER 3

POSTOPERATIVE CONSIDERATIONS

IMMEDIATE SEQUELAE

In every major operation, especially those involving vital organs, all or some of certain sequelae may eventuate to a greater or lesser degree. These are shock, hemorrhage, infection, obstruction and embolism. With clean aseptic surgery, regard for hemostasis, gentle manipulation and careful preparation of the patient, these may be reduced to a minimum and clinical manifestations may be very slight, but some degree of shock and pain may always be expected.

Shock

Shock is the result of many causes. The best definition is perhaps that it is a reflex depression of the vital functions owing to bodily injury whether traumatic or operative. The one common finding in shock is the persistently low blood pressure. The symptoms of internal hemorrhage may be confused with those of shock, but while shock may be present without hemorrhage, considerable hemorrhage is always accompanied by some shock. In shock from any cause, should the systolic blood pressure register 90 mm. of mercury or less, restorative measures are immediately called for: oxygen, glucose and sodium bicarbonate; external and internal heat; blood transfusion, etc. Tranfusion is the specific remedy for shock due to hemorrhage. The fall in blood pressure may be temporarily combated by intravenous infusions of saline.

The operative prophylaxis of surgical shock is provided for by Crile in the special technic which he devised and named anoci-association—a technic which can be utilized to advantage in most major operations. It minimizes physical and psychic factors concerned in the production of operative shock and at the same time attempts to reduce postoperative pain and discomfort. The idea is to prevent harmful or painful impulses reaching the central nervous system following irritation of the sensory nerves, whether owing to division or to pull upon the various sensory nerves that may be involved in the area of the operation. The essential step in Crile's method is to block the nerves supplying the operative field by regional or infiltration analgesia using a solution of ½ to 1 per cent novocaine to which adrenalin is added.

When a patient who has been subjected to a long and exhausting operation is returned to his bed, external heat should be applied (not by means of hot water bottles) under careful supervision, and such other restoratives as may be indicated.

In so far as they may be considered nervous phenomena, postoperative vomiting and hiccough are partly the result of shock.

Vomiting, of course, is also associated with the after-results of anesthesia. The important point in connection with excessive postoperative vomiting is that the patient may become so weak that he is unable to expel the vomitus. This may be drawn into the larynx or sucked into the lung by inspiration causing aspiration pneumonia. If no mechanical means suffice to bring up the vomitus, resort to gastric lavage or Levine tube aspiration (Fig. 2). Generally when postoperative vomiting persists for six hours (or for a shorter period if copious),

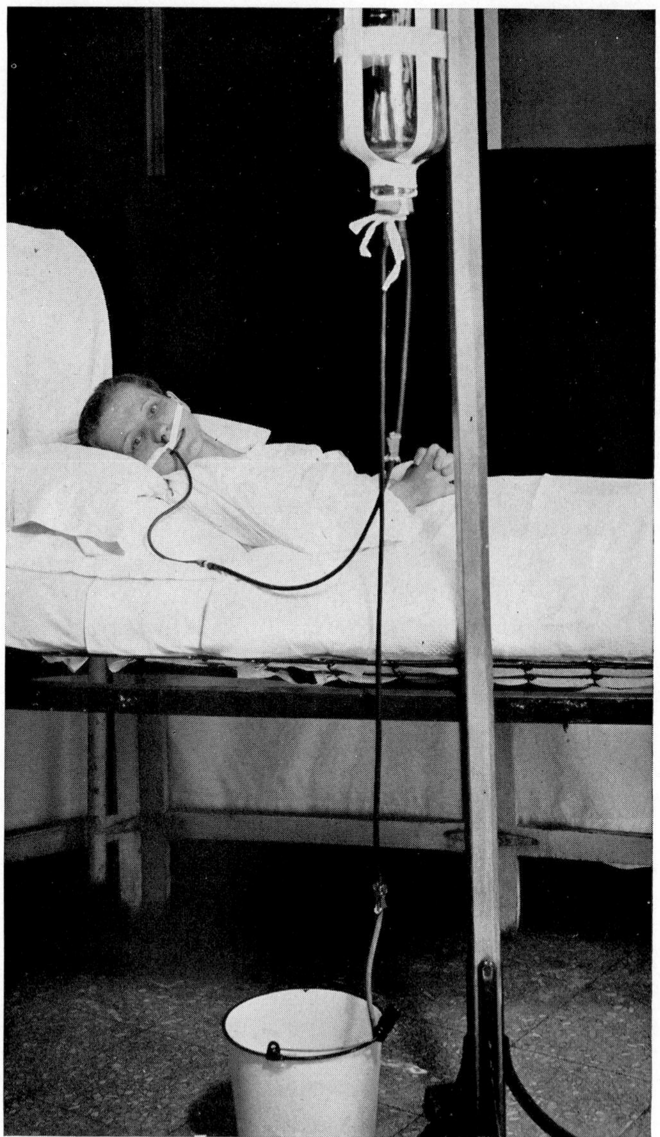

FIG. 2. Wangensteen suction with Levine tube in patient with acute dilation of the stomach following appendectomy. Intravenous saline transfusion. Recovery. (Authors Surgical Service, Cook County Hospital.)

the condition should be met by gastric lavage with hot water to which 2 drams of sodium bicarbonate has been added to the quart of water; the stomach is filled and then the fluid siphoned off several times.

Hiccough is more frequently observed after upper abdominal operations.

It is said to be due to an irregular spasmodic contraction of the diaphragm caused by irritation of the pneumogastric nerve. It is probably one of the effects of surgical shock. There are no known certain means of relief, but among those that are commonly practised, compression of the diaphragm is one of the best.

Before leaving the subject of operative shock it may be reiterated that much of extra-vigorous surgery, such as the rough use of retractors, the picking up of small vessels with powerful clamps, the roughness of unnecessary haste, the forceful and harmful use of swabs and packs should be entirely dispensed with. Such practices devitalize and impair the power of repair of the tissues. The maintenance of a gentle and careful technic not only minimizes shock, but it makes all the difference between a good and bad operative result.

HEMORRHAGE

The surgeon should carefully examine all bleeding points before terminating an operation: oozing is best controlled by gauze packs wrung out of hot saline solution; larger vessels should be located and ligated. It is superfluous to reiterate that during an operation the operative field should be kept as bloodless as possible. The surgeon will soon learn that he can control hemorrhage in the vast majority of cases by good light and exposure of the part and prompt action. There should be no excitement in the presence of a copious hemorrhage. The necessary steps must be undertaken with calmness, method and expedition. The more pronounced the surgeon's sang-froid under such circumstances, the better.

Postoperative hemorrhage may become manifest up to the fifth or sixth day following operation and even much later when owing to erosion of a blood vessel, to the spread of infection or to the pressure of a drainage tube or tight pack. The detachment of clots, slipping of ligatures and cutting through of blood vessels usually give rise to postoperative bleeding. The only treatment is to expose the blood vessel promptly and control hemorrhage. If the loss of blood is severe, restorative measures will be called for as well.

INFECTION

Even with the most rigorous aseptic technic no surgeon can feel absolutely sure that postoperative infection in some degree will not appear. Sometimes operative wounds show signs of slight infection along the suture line, the so-called stitch abscess, manifested by redness, swelling and pain with a rise in temperature. If small and localized, one or two sutures may be removed and a hot moist antiseptic dressing applied. But if more extensive the wound may require opening up and the insertion of a small drain tube. Stitch abscesses may, perhaps, be best avoided by observing meticulous asepsis, avoiding dead spaces, approximation without strangulation and careful hemostasis. It is asserted that positive cultures of infective microorganisms can be obtained in over 50 per cent! of fresh surgical wounds. The phagocytic powers of the tissues can, however, dispose of most of those. The surgical field may become infected in the course of an operation when a hollow viscus is opened; in such cases drainage is imperative.

POSTOPERATIVE CARE AND LATE COMPLICATIONS

The surgical operation is only one phase in the treatment of some definite disease and if the surgeon has undertaken the complete treatment of the patient his responsibility does not end with the operation but continues until the patient is finally discharged as recovered. The postoperative care of a patient must not be indiscriminately left to subordinates; many complications may arise and in this period the surgeon must prove himself also a physician, and the early recognition of the signs of impending complications may be detected by his experienced eye rather than be left to the observation of those with less mature judgment.

The number of complications which may follow as a direct or indirect result of surgical operations is very large depending upon the constitution of the patient, his preoperative condition, the type of operation and unforeseen accidents. An incomplete list of such complications includes postoperative backache, gastric dilatation, intestinal distention and obstruction, postoperative bronchitis and pneumonia, thrombophlebitis, pylephlebitis, pulmonary infarction and embolism, urinary retention, renal complications, acidosis, parotitis, postoperative paralysis, intestinal obstruction, etc.

While any one or more of these may occur as a sequel to an otherwise carefully executed operation, yet it would not be good surgical judgment unduly to alarm a patient by informing him of their possibility as the chances are greatly in favor of no serious complication occurring.

Vigilance, constant vigilance, is the proper attitude of the surgeon until the period in which the development of a complication might occur has passed. The modern practice of thorough preoperative preparation of the patient, when the operation is an elective one, has obviated many of the possible complications, but some still strike like a bolt from the blue.

Some of the first considerations that will arise in the immediate postoperative period are those of thirst, catharsis, nutrition and postoperative pain.

THIRST

If the patient can drink and there is no contra-indication inherent in the type of operation, water may be given if the patient desires it. Preferably the water should be hot, not lukewarm, with a little bicarbonate of soda added; or, weak tea may be given. Ice sucking is not desirable since it tends to increase the thirst. Proctoclysis is, however, the best method of relieving thirst. The rate of flow should be about 8 ounces per hour for rectal absorption. Continuous subcutaneous absorption (hypodermoclysis) (Fig. 3) may also be employed using freshly distilled sterile water heated to 110° or 115° F. There is a considerable loss of body fluids following anesthesia and during operation which, coupled with the fact that the postoperative intake of fluid is much limited for a time, makes it very necessary that the patient's tissues should obtain fluid by some other means. (Fig. 4.)

CATHARSIS

While postoperative catharsis should be avoided as far as possible, yet the surgeon should carefully watch the postoperative action of the bowels and relieve them if necessary by other means. In the average case a disturbance of the normal action of bowel movement, which may have been quite regular preoperatively, may, on account of the general organic upset consequent upon operation, last one or two days until the organism has regained its equilibrium. If the general improvement in the patient is satisfactory a simple enema after the second day will add to the patient's comfort. If, however, reaction is delayed, following prolonged surgical manipulations or other cause then nature must be assisted by medication. Calomel or a saline cathartic may be used.

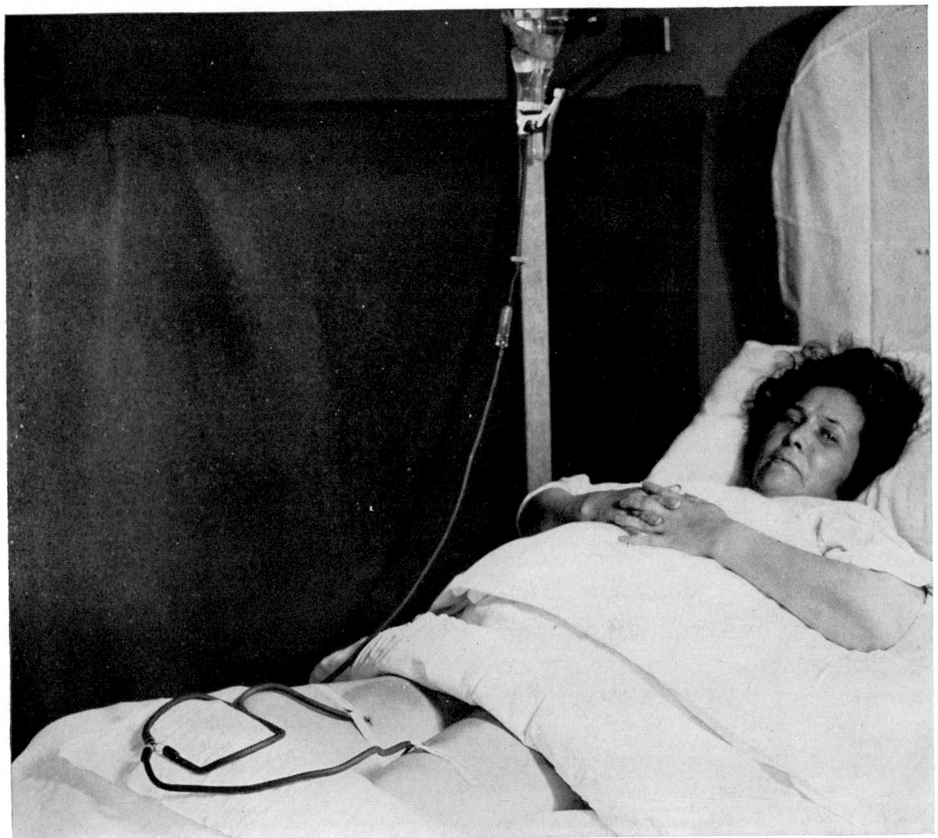

Fig. 3. Method of administering hypodermoclysis of salt solution in the thighs.

Opium is said to aid the central nervous system in regaining control of the mechanism of defecation. As a general rule very active cathartics, when given early following operation, irritate the stomach and intestine. This is especially true when purgatives have been used preoperatively, as they bring about a violent and unnatural action leaving the intestine in a condition of marked disturbance, causing gas pains.

The inconveniences of preoperative purgation are on the whole greater than the advantages, especially when we remember that the functions of the liver and kidneys are also not only disturbed but rendered less resistant to the intoxication of the anesthetic. The intestine itself is in a state of hypotonicity and dehydration. Soap and water enemas, prior to operation, seem to be better than purgatives and conduce to a better postoperative action of the bowels; if purgatives must be given preoperatively they should be administered two or three days before the operation.

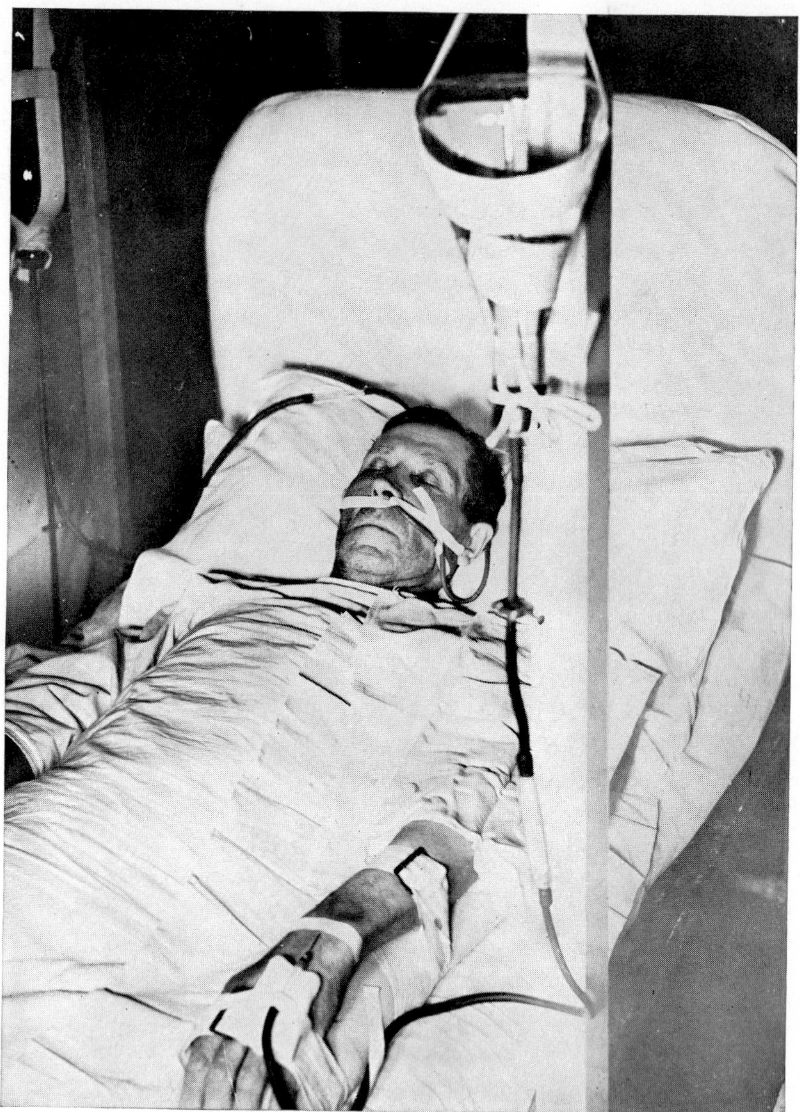

FIG. 4. Continuous duodenal suction and intravenous administration of sodium chloride and glucose.

DIET

In major surgical operations which vary in their influence on nutrition and disturb the physiologic factors concerned in metabolism, there is a varying time during which feeding of the patient must be strictly limited, that is to say, until the normal physiologic functions have been more or less restored. Long experience has shown that the resumption of normal dietaries must be gradual and depend upon the patient's desires and his reactions to food.

POSTOPERATIVE PAIN

Much of the postoperative pain and discomfort of a patient is the result of putting him in a strained or cramped position either during the operation or in the immediate postoperative period. Other causes are too tight bandages, especially following the reduction of fractures. In such cases the limb often swells and gangrene may result.

The position of a patient following an abdominal operation is particularly important; correct position hastens recovery; faulty positions invite complications. A slightly modified Trendelenberg position is said to help in the prevention of postoperative thrombosis.

The postoperative use of morphine is perhaps open to question. But, apart from the alleviation of severe pain, it is said that morphine slows respiration thus diminishing lymph flow. Recent work has shown that morphine definitely increases peristalsis of the small bowels.

CHAPTER 4

OPERATING PAVILIONS AND THE OPERATION IN GENERAL

OPERATING PAVILIONS

While a good surgeon with able assistance may be able to accomplish excellent work under the most adverse physical conditions, it is generally agreed that it is to the advantage of all concerned to have the surgical pavilion so designed that approved technic may be facilitated, functional efficiency assured and technical equipment made readily available.

Because of the differences of technic and requirements of different groups of surgeons, it has never been found possible to design a single surgical pavilion which will suit all hospitals, and so it is imperative, when the planning of such a unit is under consideration, to study carefully the specific requirements of that institution, incorporating therein such local variants as may be necessary to meet the requirements of those who are to work therein.

I am indebted to Dr. Wm. H. Walsh, hospital consultant of Chicago, for the following suggestions germane to the question under discussion. He was kind enough to prepare for this work two sketches of operating pavilions, one for a hospital with from 100 to 200 surgical beds, and another designed for an institution with from 400 to 500 surgical beds. No attempt has been made to show the layout of the surgical operating facilities required for a small general hospital for the reason that because of the restricted space therein available many of the facilities provided in the larger institution must be omitted. The sketches shown, however, may serve as an excellent guide to those who are obliged for lack of space, to work in more restricted quarters. A description of the sketches follows:

This drawing (Fig. 5) attempts to show an ideal layout for the surgical operating pavilion of a hospital with from 100 to 200 surgical beds. This section of the hospital should preferably be located on the top floor of a building of sufficient height and area to accommodate the number of beds for which it is designed.

1. This space is provided for the storage of a special urological or fracture table while one or the other is in use. Thus, room #3 may be used for a double purpose by simply changing tables. 2. Major operating rooms, when possible, are planned in pairs and between them provision is made for water and utensil sterilization and surgeons' wash-up sinks. This arrangement provides ready accessibility of hot and cold sterile water, permits the sterilization of instruments and sutures with the least possible delay, and gives the surgeons direct access to operating rooms after scrubbing up. 3. As elsewhere noted, it is desirable to provide the facilities for x-ray examination in the operating section and these are usually so located as to be accessible to two separate operating rooms. In this instance the x-ray generator is in space #14, thus making it available for genito-urinary and orthopedic work in #3 and any other use desired in the minor operating room #7.

4. In this sterilizing room provision is made only for sterile water and instruments, and autoclaves are located adjacent to the nurses' workroom for reasons elsewhere explained. 5. The surgeons' scrub-up sinks usually located between two operating rooms, are convenient to the surgeons and are so arranged as to obviate the necessity of the surgeon with clean hands passing through the corridor. 6. This util-

ity room is slightly different from the same room designed for patients floors, but is equally necessary to an operating suite. 7. Minor operating rooms are, like those for major work, usually arranged in pairs with the same facilities between them. 8. On either side of the doctors' room are toilet and shower bath facilities which were designed in this instance to meet a situation where men and women surgeons operate at the same time. 9. Elevators of special size and design. 10. A reserve supply of sterile dressings should always be on hand and this room is provided for that purpose. 11. For the convenience of the surgeons in the recording of their work, space is provided either for dictaphones or a stenographer. 12. A suitable place is necessary for the storage of surgical instruments and this is placed adjacent to the sterile supply room. 13. This is the doctors' rest and dressing room and should be equipped with lockers. 14. Supplementary x-ray apparatus already mentioned. 15. Anesthetizing rooms have a sub-corridor for the elimination of noise.

16. For the immediate examination of tissue it is considered desirable to place

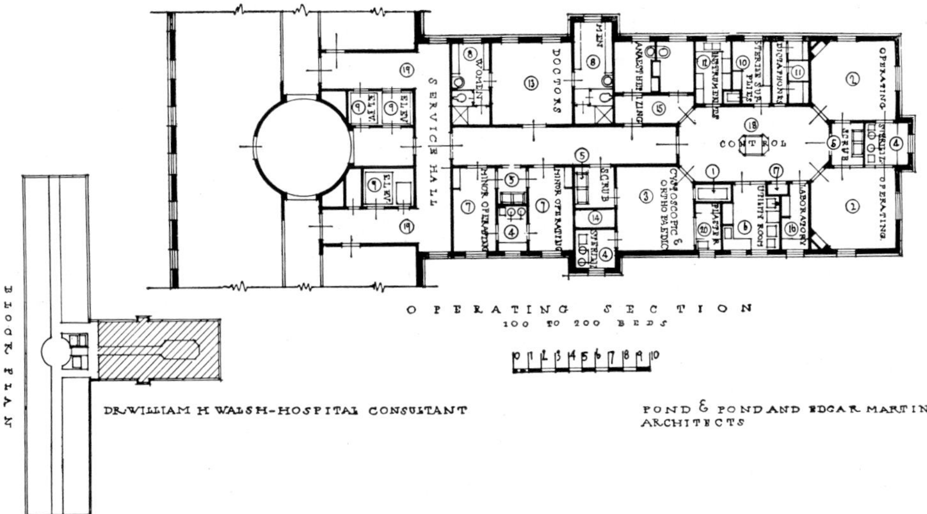

FIG. 5. Surgical operating pavilion for hospital with 100-200 beds.

facilities in the operating suite for that purpose. Equipment for freezing, slicing and microscopic examination of tissues is required here. 17. Warming cabinets are for the storage of blankets to be used on patients immediately after operation. 18. This control desk is intended to coordinate all activities of the section and a well-trained nurse is required constantly on duty. All communications to the various parts of the hospital are transmitted through this center. Orders to start anesthetization of waiting patients, and routing of patients to the various operating rooms is controlled here. The use of this system saves the time of all concerned, assures the full usage of all facilities and obviates the necessity of supervisors running around from one place to another in order to keep things moving smoothly. Special telephone and signal systems are required to perfect this system.

19. Service halls adjacent to the elevators give privacy and keep the patient traffic away from all other. 20. The plaster room is for the storage and preparation of plaster used for bone fractures and thus is located adjacent to the orthopedic room.

The absence of a nurses' workroom in this sketch will be noted. This omission is due to the fact that in the institution for which this design was intended there is an obstetrical pavilion on the floor immediately below and the facilities therein provided are adequate for both pavilions. A small lift in room #10 brings the sterile supplies from the floor below.

This sketch (Fig. 6) closely approximates the ideal for a surgical section of a hospital of from 400 to 600 beds. It is located on the top floor of a vertical type building which would have at least twelve stories. Above this floor there may be arranged a gallery for medical students so that all operating rooms may be visible from above. In this sketch a gallery extends down into one major operating room so as to bring observers close to the field of operation.

1. The foyer or general lobby for the surgical floor. 2. Four general operating rooms are shown, one of which has the gallery extending into it. 3. Cystoscopic and orthopedic operating rooms with water and instrument sterilizers between. 4. and 5. Also scrub-up sinks for doctors and nurses. 6. Utility room for the major surgical section and another for the minor surgical section. 7. The surgical floor is designed so as to separate the minor and major sections as far as possible and the various minor operating rooms here can be used for surgical dressings, infected cases or other purposes. 8. Toilet, shower bath and locker rooms for male and female surgeons adjoining the doctors' lounging and dressing room. 9. There are four elevators intended for the entire building but only two of them, as shown, extend up to this floor and, when the surgical floor is in operation these two elevators may be reserved for

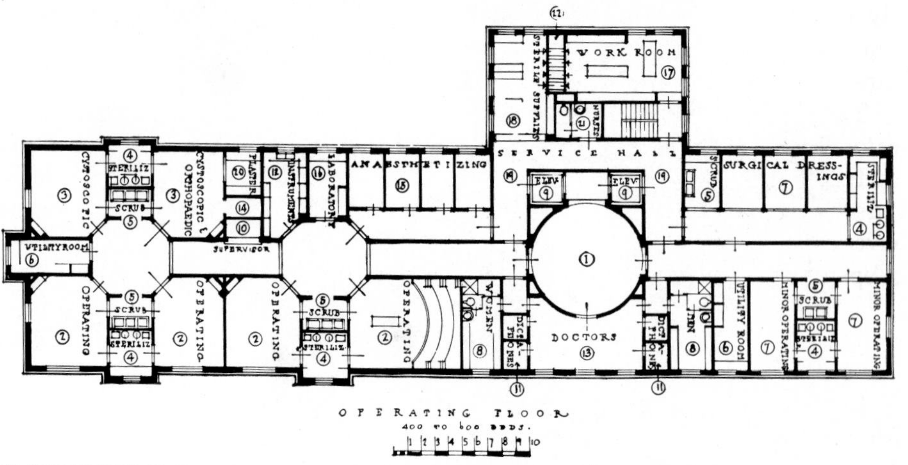

FIG. 6. Surgical section of a hospital of from 400-600 beds.

that exclusive use. These elevators open into the service hall for patients and also into the main foyer for doctors, nurses, visitors and students. 10. Station for nursing supervisor in charge of traffic and communications, especially equipped with telephone connections and signals. 11. Cubicles for the convenience of surgeons in dictating surgical notes either to a clerk or into a dictaphone, to be transcribed in the clinical record office. These are a part of the surgeons' suite. 12. Surgical instrument room. 13. The surgeons' lounging and dressing room. 14. Space for supplementary x-ray apparatus adjoining orthopedic, urological and gynecological operating rooms. 15. Four separate compartments within a sub-corridor for anesthetizing. 16. Small laboratory for emergency and tissue examinations. 17. Nurses' workroom for the preparation of all surgical dressings which are sterilized in autoclaves and stored in 18 until required in the operating rooms or elsewhere in the hospital. 19. Service halls already mentioned and designed to prevent surgical cases from passing through the main foyer. 20. The plaster room for the storage and preparation of dressings for orthopedic cases, adjoining the operating room intended for this specialty. 21. Toilet and wash room for female nurses. 22. Autoclaves for the sterilization of dressings which are prepared and inserted from the nurses' workroom and removed on the other side into the room intended for their storage and distribution.

In hospitals of 50 beds or thereabouts, it is rarely possible to provide space for more than one room for operative surgery. Correlated facilities must needs be curtailed here. In every instance, however, it is absolutely essential to provide a surgeon's scrub-up sink, the necessary equipment for the sterilization of instruments, water and dressings. These are preferably to be located outside of the operating room. However small the hospital, a nurses' workroom is an indispensable necessity. Here dressings are prepared for sterilization, the various solutions made, surgical trays set up, etc. In very small hospitals, this room will not only supply the needs of the operating room but will serve for other surgical functions.

No matter how small a hospital is, a dressing room for the surgeon is a necessity. It should be located close to the operating room. Wherever possible, shower and toilet facilities should be provided.

Where only one operating room must be used for all classes of surgical operations, the need for sanitation and cleaning the room is imperative, particularly if being used for pus cases. Such hospitals should have in this operating room, tile walls and floors with a suitable drain in the floor to facilitate complete cleansing at frequent intervals.

There is a tendency in the small hospital, because of limited personnel, to locate the delivery room either immediately adjoining the operating room or closely adjacent thereto. As far as practical, this tendency should be discouraged because of the danger of cross infection. Thus wherever possible, the delivery room should be located on a different floor from the operating room and the operating room supervisor should not function in both places.

THE OPERATING ROOM

Every surgeon has his own pet idea about the "ideal operating room." Some wish the walls of their operating rooms painted gray, others green and still others black. My own preference is for white—it urges vigilance for cleanliness and is in harmony with the spirit of the activities (Fig. 7). The important general principle agreed upon by all surgeons are:

ILLUMINATION

Good Light. Too much fuss is made about where the windows should be placed. Is it not a fact that most of us operate by some sort of artificial light, no matter how bright the sun may be shining? It is not the high cost or complicated construction of the apparatus that matters but how efficient a source of light it is. It should be remembered that no matter how fine an electric illuminating equipment may be, provision should be made for an accessory (emergency) source of light in case the former ceases to function. Gas or a battery light may be resorted to.

The most important requirement for an efficient operating room light is that it give a maximum of light with a minimum of heat. This is obtained from the American Luminare (Fig. 8). The degree of light is under absolute control and may be adjusted to the visual requirements of the surgeon for either superficial or deep light penetration since it has a range of 1000 to 3000 foot candle intensity. It is practically shadowless and permits the surgeon to operate with comfort. Its optical system eliminates glare.

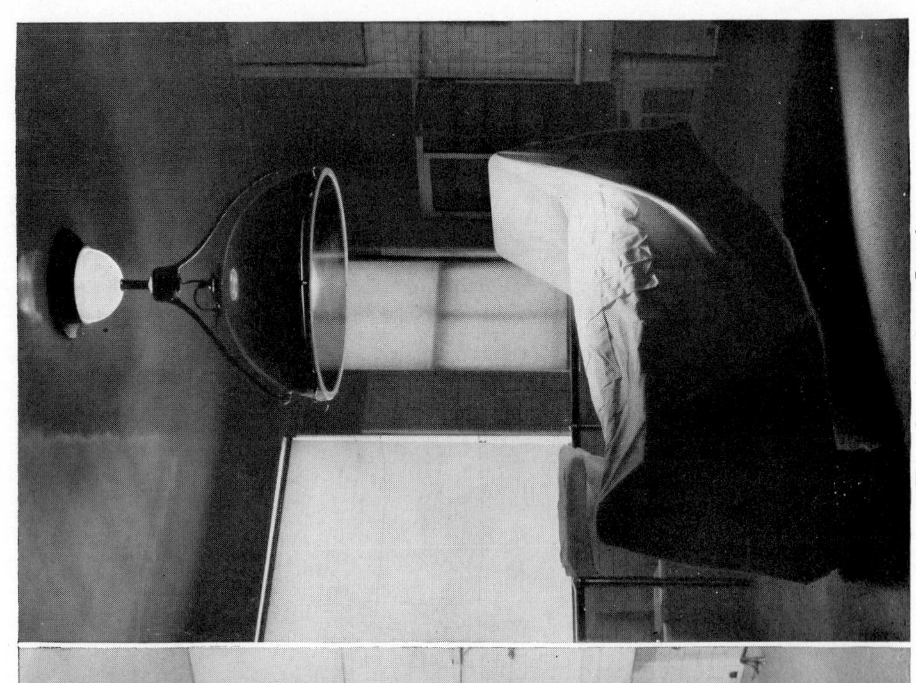

Fig. 7. Operating Room, American Hospital, Chicago.

Fig. 8. American Luminare.

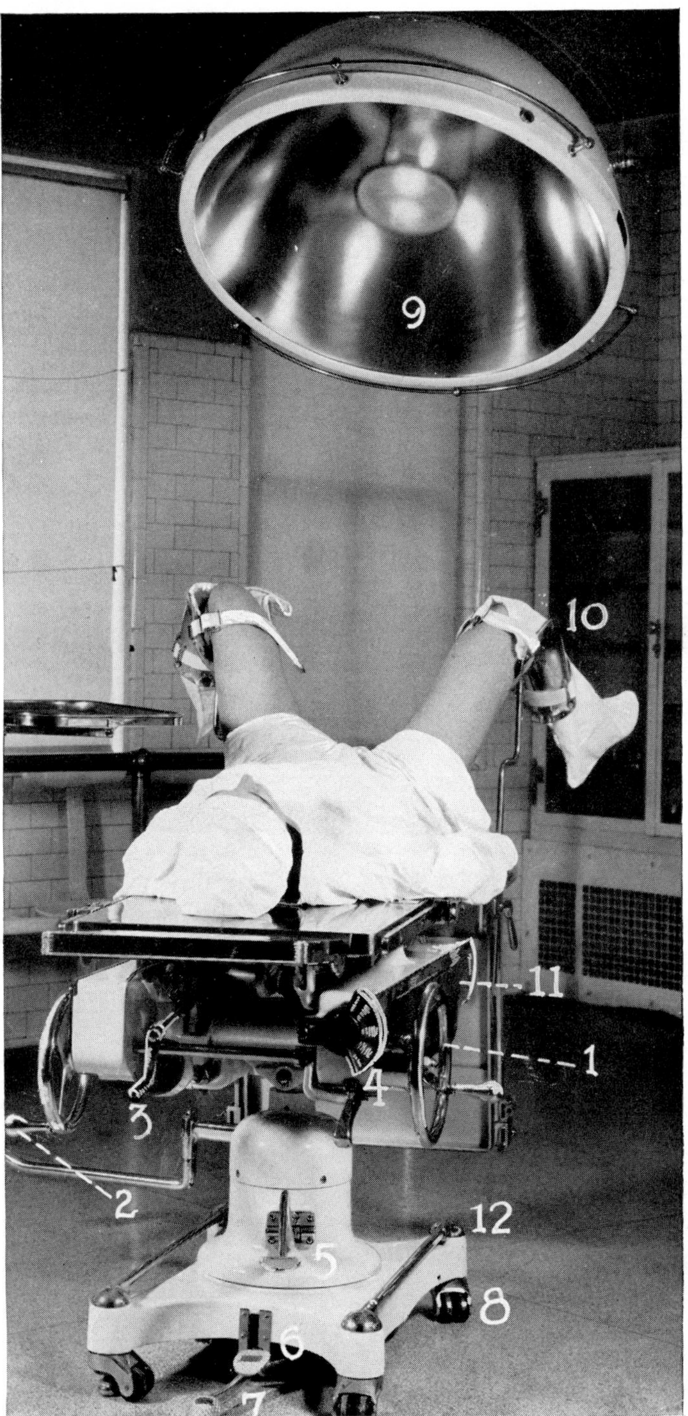

FIG. 9. Head end controlled operating table (American Kny-Scheerer): 1. This wheel controls all positions during the manifold operations with the exception of the Trendelenburg positions, 2. Trendelenburg control, 3. kidney bridge control, 4. tiltometer and lateral tilt and controlled dial, 5. elevating pedal, 6. base block pedal, 7. floor lock pedal, 8. stabilizing feet, 9. luminare, 10. Bierhoff knee crutches, 11. concealed gear encasement, 12. surgeon's foot rail.

VENTILATION

Above all, the patient must be protected from **draughts**; many postoperative pneumonias result from disregard of this precaution. In abdominal operations particularly, the temperature should be warm (between 70° and 75° F.) yet well-ventilated.

EFFICIENT OPERATING ROOM EQUIPMENT

Operating Table. There are numerous good operating tables at the disposal of the surgeon. A table that promptly responds to the needs of change of

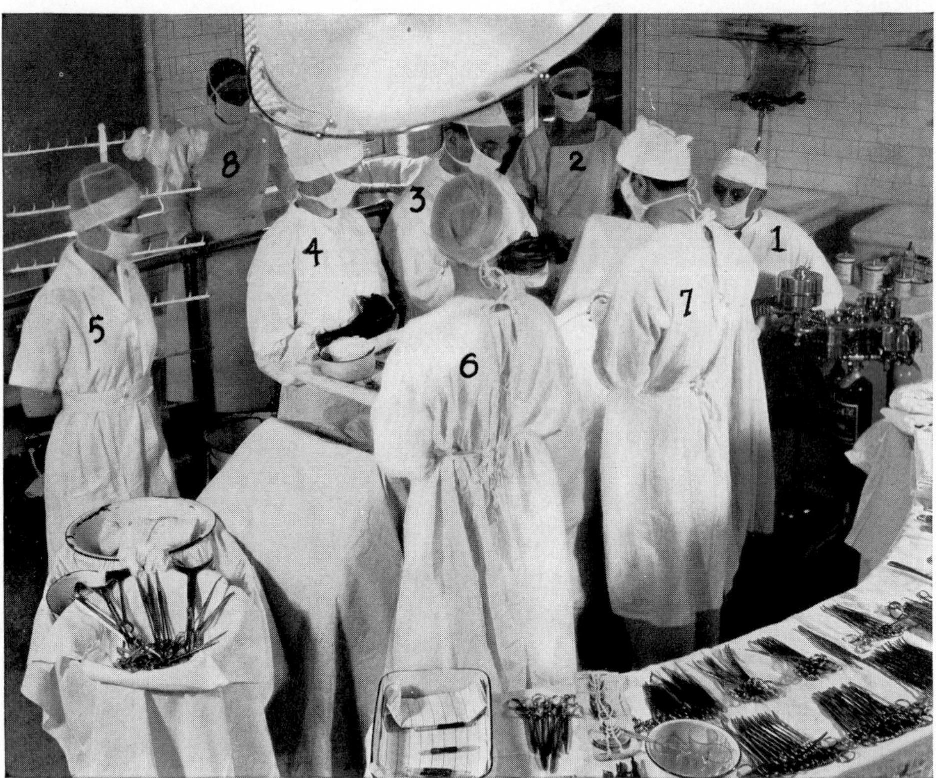

FIG. 10. General "set-up" for operation: 1. anesthetist, 2. circulating nurse, 3. operating surgeon, 4. second assistant, 5. surgical supervisor, 6. surgical nurse, 7. first assistant, 8. spectator.

position without disturbing the patient and discomfiting the operating team is of great value. The author derives much comfort from a "Head End" Control Operating Table which permits the anesthetist, without moving from his seat, to control without disturbance and with precision every operating position required by the surgeon. (Fig. 9.) It is an extremely versatile instrument of precision in meeting emergencies and in obtaining required precise positions so necessary in operative procedures.

The placement of the operating room equipment is best seen in the appended diagram (Fig. 10). I have basins on either side, one for rinsing the hands, the other as a receptacle for soiled sponges and instruments. Dropping these on the floor is both unsurgical and unesthetic. The assistant has a similar arrangement on the other side.

The position of the patient on the operating table will be discussed when describing the particular operation.

Strict decorum in the operating room should be insisted upon. Loud conversations between assistants and nurses should not be tolerated.

THE OPERATION IN GENERAL

In the actual conduct of any surgical operation, the surgeon of limited experience cannot afford to take any risk but must proceed methodically, step by step, in an orderly manner, not omitting any step in strict asepsis and operative technic that established standard procedure has recognized as essential. In the case of an experienced surgeon, who by constant practice has become thoroughly familiar with all technical details, a certain amount of latitude may be allowed in omitting or varying steps in the technic, when he is perfectly confident of the end to be attained and the means of reaching it. While time is often the essence of success in surgical work, yet the nicest judgment is required to discriminate between hurry and deliberate, calculated rapidity in doing what is actually necessary. Any surgical operation, especially a major one, is a serious matter for the patient; if it must be done so as to accomplish a definite purpose for which it is justified, then the quicker it can be correctly executed the better.

Clean, deliberate, purposeful, but still rapidly executed, sure work should be the aim of every surgeon; but to boast of being able to do an operation in a very short time, merely for the sake of rapidity alone, is a confession of surgical weakness. Note the following aphorism.

"There are surgeons who operate upon the 'canine' principle of savage attack, and the biting and tearing of tissues are terrible to witness. There are they who operate with one eye upon the clock and who judge the beauty of any procedure by the fewness of the minutes it has taken to complete. There are other surgeons who believe in the 'light hand', who use the utmost gentleness, and who deal lovingly with every tissue they touch." (Moynihan.)

PERSONNEL

Planned rapidity in execution is greatly enhanced by good team work. A surgeon works best with those who are accustomed to his personal methods and who are perfectly trained to do what is necessary with the least amount of direction from the operating surgeon. Such a personnel in an operating room anticipates every step in the surgical ritual and each is ready to do his or her part at the right moment. They facilitate the conduct of an operation and in an emergency they can be relied upon to act with calmness and judgment.

Assistants, not how many but how well-trained, should be the slogan. Some surgeons have too many assistants; others go to the other extreme—like Kümmel who picks out his own instruments and threads his own needles. I concur with Eugene St. Jacques who says, "few but well-trained hands are the desideratum."

ASEPTIC TECHNIC

At present surgical technic has evolved into the aseptic method and there are certain general principles governing this method which should be thoroughly understood by all who attempt either manipulative or cutting operations. It is known that when the edges of a surgically clean wound are carefully coapted and kept at rest prompt healing by first intention will ensue, unless the wound is invaded by certain species of bacteria (the pyogenic group). When such are present to any extent, inflammatory signs will be manifest which delay and prevent healing. Living tissues possess a natural power of resistance to infection depending on the individual's general resistance, and it is a part of surgery to strengthen this natural defense as much as possible. Prevention of wound infection further demands that everything used in the performance of an operation must be germ-free and that the field of operation should be protected from contamination by the operating personnel who come in contact with the patient. The thoroughness of sterilization, the care exercised by the operating surgeon and his assistants must be to a great extent a matter of surgical conscience and personal responsibility. The care of the surgical armamentarium can be reduced to a routine, mechanical process; there are various methods to accomplish this. The method of sterilization of instruments, etc., will be described in a separate chapter on Sterilization, p. 46.

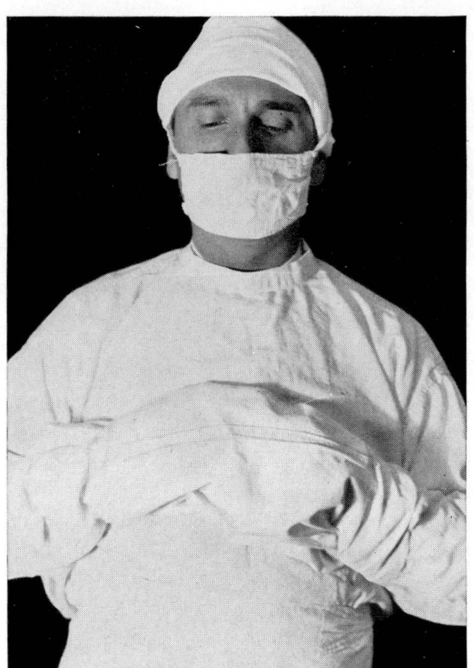

FIG. 11. Surgeon's attire in operating room. Cap made of stockinette which tends to adhere to the forehead absorbing perspiration. Gloved hands are protected by "muff."

The maintenance of strict asepsis from the bacteriologic point of view is one of the chief aims in formulating the steps of modern surgical technic. Not only should steps be taken to prevent the introduction of micro-organisms into a surgical wound but attempts should also be directed to control the spreading of any infective foci which already exist in the living tissues. Regarding the surgeon and his assistants who have necessarily to come in contact with organs and tissues, the use of sterilized rubber gloves is imperative. Though there is no known method of keeping the hands absolutely sterile, the use of rubber gloves must not prevent the fullest and most detailed preparation of the hands before they are thrust into gloves.

The method for skin preparation I have used for a couple of decades and am still partial to is as follows:

Technic of Scrubbing the Hands of Surgeon and Assistants

Before entering the scrubroom, surgeons, assistants and nurses shall don the customary operating attire. Under no circumstances shall this operating outfit be worn over street clothes.

Anyone having an abrasion on the forearms, hands or fingers or who has recently had contact with contagious diseases or postmortem or septic material shall not participate in an operation before having cleansed himself thoroughly (antiseptic tub bath).

Shoes worn on the street must be changed to operating room shoes (tennis or special rubber shoes).

Cap and Mask. Before scrubbing is begun an operating cap and mask should be donned. Special care must be taken to cover all of one's hair and have the mask cover the nose as well as the mouth (Fig. 11).

The finger nails shall be free from all foreign matter, such as liquid polish, nail white, etc., and should be trimmed short.

CLEANSING IS DONE AS FOLLOWS

Liquid green soap is supplied from an automatic container, or, if bar soap is used, it is kept in the hand lying on top of the brush when not in use. For many years, I have used a hard, alkaline surgical soap containing a minute quantity of powdered pumice and found it very effective in removing superficial impurities. Wash the hands with warm, running water, delivered by means of an automatic knee or foot pedal. Never use water in a wash basin because it simply represents a solution of dirt.

Wash the hands and arms four inches above the elbow with soap and hot water to loosen the dirt. Remove all subungual dirt with an orange wood stick or file.

Begin scrubbing with a medium soft, sterile brush. Start with the thumb of the left hand, follow to the index, middle, third and little fingers in succession. Scrub the palm of the hand, across the nails, up to and including the wrist. Rinse thoroughly and frequently during this process and use a fresh supply of soap. Repeat the same procedure on the right hand, wrist and forearm. Consider that each finger has four sides; brush each side, scrub between the fingers and go on to the next digit. Scrubbing in a haphazard manner is to be avoided. The forearms are scrubbed up and including at least two inches above the elbows.

Keep the arms flexed permitting the water or solution to drip from the elbows, not from the finger tips. Particular attention should be paid to the numerous corners and crevices about the nails and fingers; they are difficult to cleanse thoroughly. Allow a minimum of five minutes for the cleansing of one hand. Time the complete scrub period at a minimum of about fifteen minutes. This accomplished, rinse the hands in cold water to contract the pores. Some surgeons accomplish more in ten minutes of thorough, systematic scrubbing than others in half an hour of haphazard "fiddling." Also "too thorough" scrubbing does more harm than good. Besides injuring the skin, remember that the Staphylococcus epidermidis albus cannot entirely be "scrubbed off" no matter how prolonged and vigorous one's efforts may be. Fortunately, this coccus is non-pathogenic; yet, under certain circumstances and favorable conditions many non-pathogenic micro-organisms may become pathogenic.

Keep the hands and arms flexed and away from the sides of the body and scrub again in a 1 per cent Lysol solution, sterile water and a 50 per cent alcohol solution. The solution basins have a sterile glass label indicating the solution. At least one minute should be allowed for the hands to remain in each solution. Finally, the fingers are dipped into a cup containing 1:1000 Metaphen Solution.

Don a sterile gown held by the "scrub" nurse (Figs. 12-13).

Dry the hands in a sterile towel.

Put on sterile gloves. (Fig. 14.) I have devised and used for many years a "glove muff" over the gloved hands and forearms as shown in Fig. 11. This is good insurance against undesirable contact.

After all is said and done the most important factor in preparing the hands for a surgical operation is not the type of antiseptic used but how well the surgeon knows to take advantage of the proper use of soap and water.

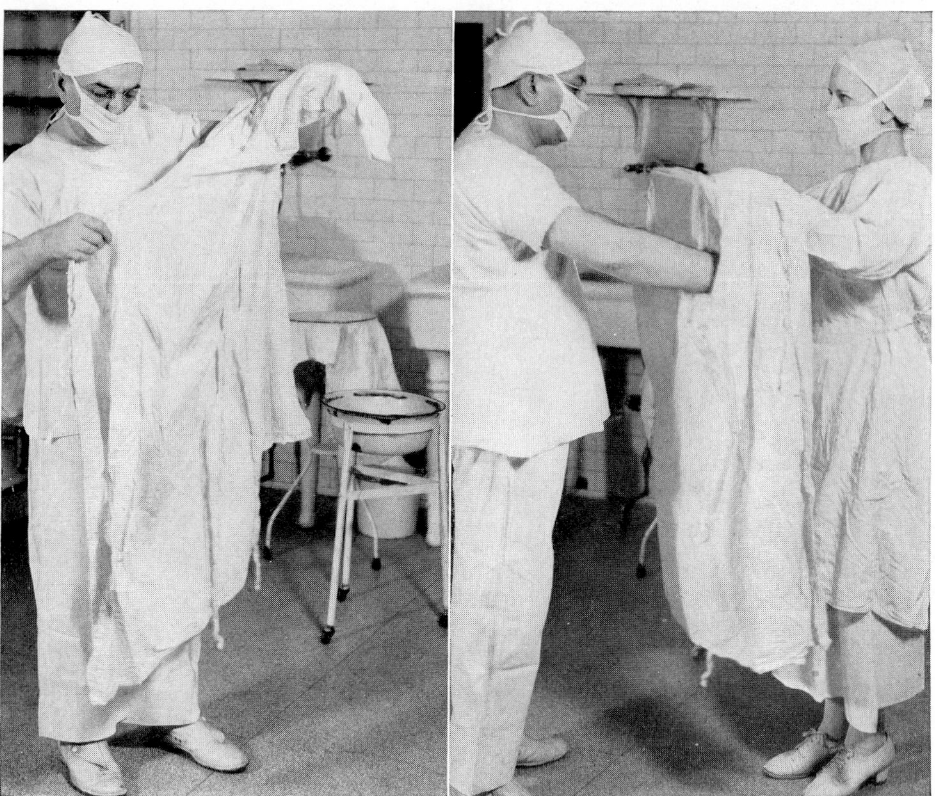

FIG. 12. Wrong method of putting on operating gown.

FIG. 13. Proper method of putting on operating gown.

The surgeon and his personnel should never relax vigilance regarding the completeness of all aseptic precautions. His own habits of personal cleanliness go without saying.

Frequently washing of hands is resorted to in such manner that the bar of soap held by the surgeon is placed on the shelf, picked up again to be redeposited on the shelf innumerable times during the scrubbing procedure. It can readily be seen that contamination of the bar of soap and the hands is quite likely under such circumstances.

This is obviated by the various soap dispensing devices on the market of which the Midland (Lohador) Foot Pedal Liquid Soap Dispenser is an excellent example (Fig. 15). The soap container is large, not requiring frequent refills and the pedestal as well as the pedal of sturdy construction. The dispensing nozzle may be swung into a complete arc for the convenience of a number of individuals who may use it for scrubbing. A simple piston arrangement in the soap pump delivers the soap equally. The amount of soap to be delivered at one stroke of the piston may be regulated to the individual requirements.

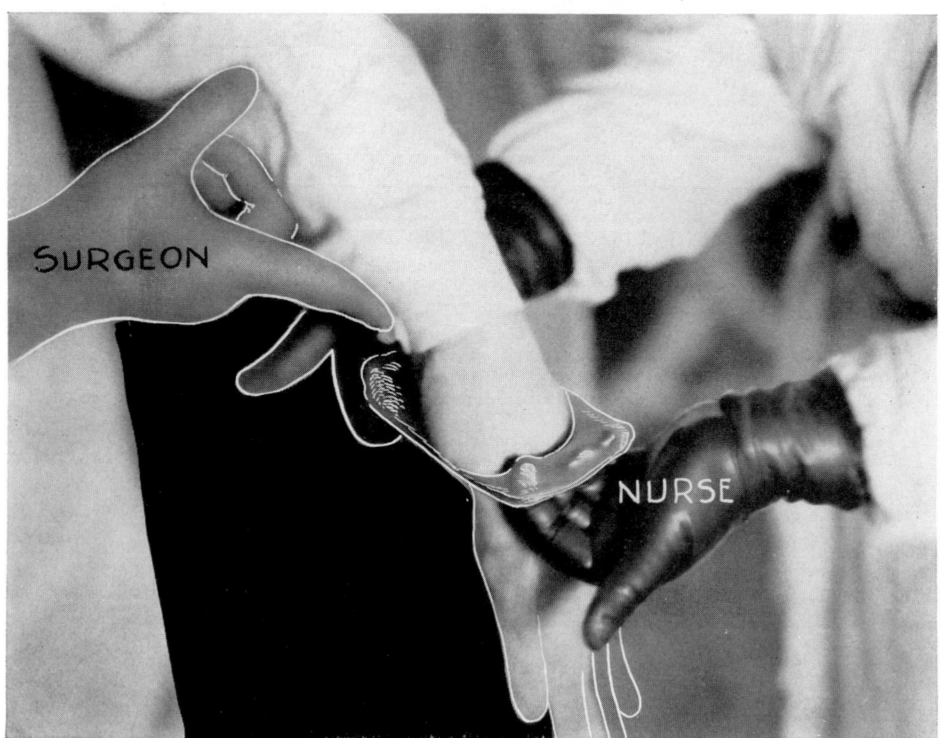

FIG. 14. Proper way of donning gloves by the surgeon. The nurse holds the glove and the surgeon plunges his hand into it as depicted.

Air Sterilization

Very recently, aseptic technic has been extended to the sterilization of the operating-room air by the use of radiant energy having bactericidal properties (light in the ultra-violet spectrum, less than 2600 Angstroms wave length, with high bactericidal and low erythemal effect). Such irradiation has reduced almost to extinction those infections, usually staphylococcic, which arise from that general air infection which exists even in hospitals equipped with air filters. While all the air of the operating room is not sterilized, the lamps are powerful enough to kill any bacteria floating in from outside the operating field. Impermeable masks prevent bacteria being blown into the wound whence they may locate in spots protected from the lamp.

The advantages of such sterilization are: ability to reopen wounds without fear of lighting up buried infection; postoperative elevations of temperature are lower and of shorter duration and postoperative pain is reduced; the general systemic reaction has been less severe; healing has been more satisfactory and recovery more rapid.

Tubes (Fig. 16) emitting such light are placed over the operating table and the various instrument sections. Oiled silk masks, from which the air is removed by suction are worn to prevent all possibility of droplet infection and to protect the operating-room personnel from the light. This, even if elevated as far as possible above the table is still very close to their heads, especially considering continuous exposure. Such masks have the additional advantage of necessitating less rebreathing than the ordinary ones.

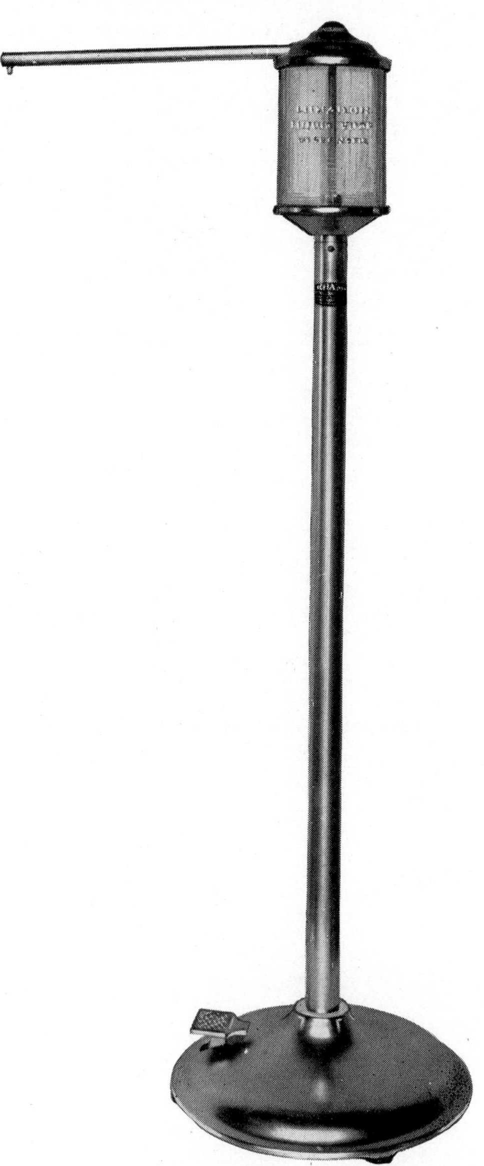

FIG. 15. Foot-pedal liquid soap dispenser.

ANESTHETIZED PATIENT

After all aseptic precautions have been attended to, the steps to be taken after the anesthetized patient has reached the operating room are generally as follows:

1. Arranging the patient in the correct position on the operating table.
2. Exposure of the operative field and adequate protection of other parts of the body.
3. Final preparation of the skin, if necessary.
4. Draping with sterile sheets.
5. Arrangements of accessory tables, stands and sponge racks.

These duties are allocated to definite members of the operating-room personnel. The patient should be placed in that position which is most convenient to the surgeon for the particular operation, which does not unduly interfere with the functions of the anesthetist and which will not in any way contribute to pain (Fig. 17) or later disability of the patient. It must be remembered that the patient is unable to call attention to or complain of a continuously uncomfortable or painful position which in some cases may involve nerves and ligaments to a degree that leads to temporary paralysis. The hands and arms of the patient should generally be placed in full extension along the sides of the trunk. No constriction on any part of the body should interfere with free circulation unless such is a part of the surgical technic. I have seen cases where the neglect of such precautions, even in first class hospitals, have led to serious postoperative accidents to patients (Fig. 18).

In manipulative surgery, such as orthopedic procedures, the skin of the affected area should be surgically prepared just as in the case of a cutting operation because it may become necessary to incise if the manipulative procedures fail.

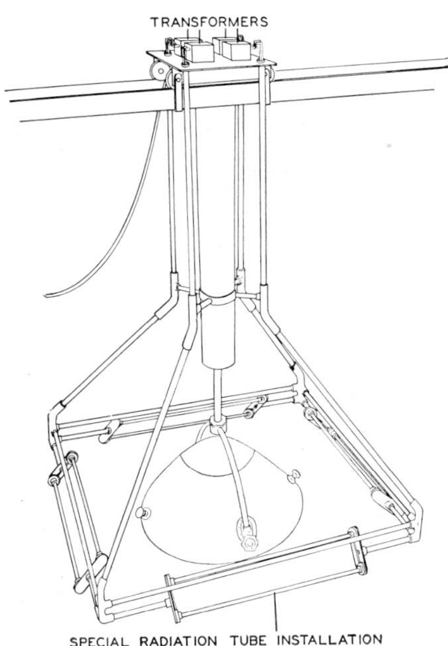

Fig. 16. Bactericidal radiation unit as used in experiments and operations. The radiation is in the ultraviolet range of the spectrum, predominantly below 2,600 angstroms and has a high bactericidal action and a relatively low erythemal effect. The eight tubes are mounted to form a square with opposite tubes five feet apart, the center of the cluster four feet above the operative incision which was approximately five feet from the center of the individual tubes. The supply and instrument tables are within the effective range of this radiation. This arrangement was made with the idea of sterilizing the air of the entire room if possible so no reflectors are used. More effective radiation can be obtained by bringing this cluster of tubes closer together, and having in addition a unit with a reflector to place directly over the instrument and supply tables. The air in the entire room is not sterilized but it is thought that the barrage of radiation will kill any organisms before they can float into the center of the field and settle in the wound. All supply tables must be stacked within the effective range of this radiation and must be covered when not protected by the radiation. All members of the operating team who are directly over the wound should wear an impermeable mask over the nose and mouth so that organisms cannot be blown directly into the wound without a period of exposure sufficiently long to cause their death. Once in the wound they may fall in a location where they are protected from the radiation. (Designed by Westinghouse Lamp Co.) From Hart and Gardner, Trans. South. Surg. Asso., 49:376, 1937.)

In open operations, no viscus or vital organ should be allowed to come into contact with the skin. Of course, there must be necessarily a good many exceptions to this general rule, but some surgeons go so far as to lift up all tissues with forceps and to thread needles and fix ligatures in the same way. The point is that traumatism and the possibility of infection should be obviated as far as possible. For the same reason before opening any hollow viscus every precaution should be taken to isolate it. In abdominal work the intestines should be kept protected in the abdominal cavity, except the particular portion demanding surgical attention. Such protection is best accomplished by the use of hot saline compresses; the same remark applies when operations, such as the removal of a breast for carcinoma calls for the opening up of extensive areas. When packing viscera away from infected or suspected areas, to protect them from contamination, dry packs should never be used as they stick to the surface of the viscus and, in the case of the bowel especially, when pulled away they undoubtedly injure the delicate serous membrane and invite formation of adhesions.

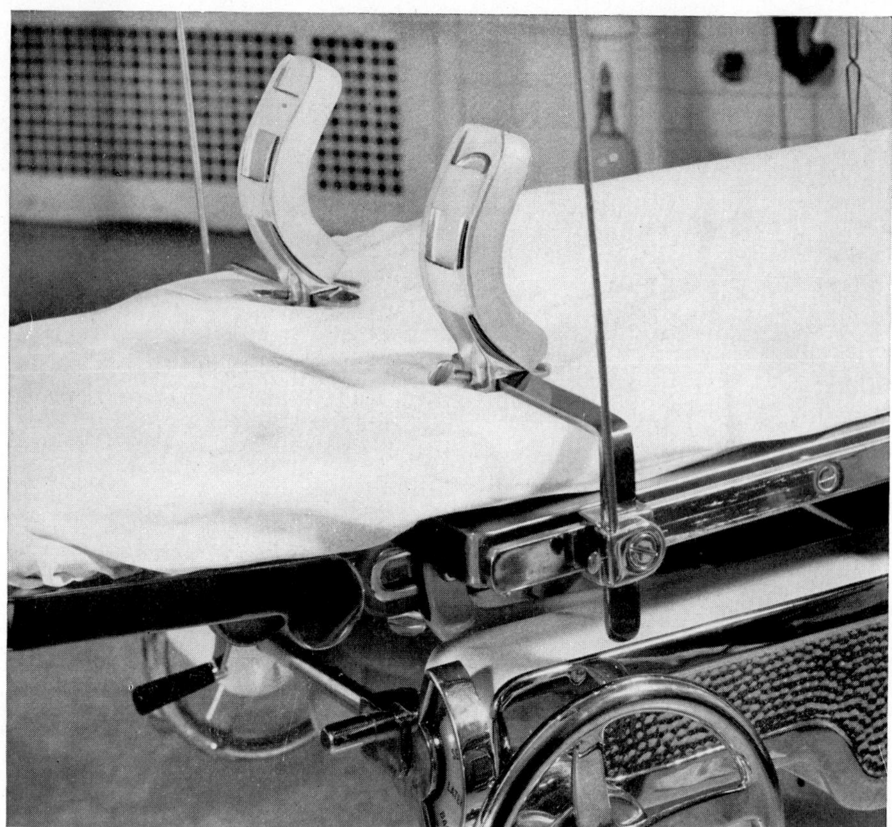

FIG. 17. Comfortable shoulder brace attachment to support the patient. (American-Kny-Scheerer Co.)

INCISION

In regard to incisions, the general rule is to use that incision which will permit good exposure of the underlying parts without inflicting injury to any important structures, so that there can be complete restoration of the anatomic relations and preservation of function of the parts. Other things being equal, for all operations, long incisions are much preferable to short ones; less force is necessitated in retracting wound edges with less consequent traumatism to the patient. Under aseptic conditions, the long incision will heal just as quickly as a short one. "Button-hole" incisions, so favored by some surgeons are to be deprecated; there is no justification in working in the dark as injuries may be inflicted to some organ without the surgeon being aware of it.

For any operation, the incision should be sufficiently large to give easy access to the site of disease; it should preserve all nerves; it should avoid all unnecessary trauma to muscles; and it should preserve the vascular supply.

Although a separate chapter is devoted to surgical incisions yet the importance of abdominal incisions deserves a special word said here, since there is much controversy regarding the relative value of vertical, oblique and transverse incisions. Kocher said that the only incisions in the abdomen which can be regarded as normal are the median and the transverse in the upper abdomen and the oblique passing from above downward and inward, in the lower part of the abdomen, for these incisions do not damage the nerves supplying the muscles of the abdominal wall. In certain cases, such as gallbladder surgery, a combination of these incisions may be used.

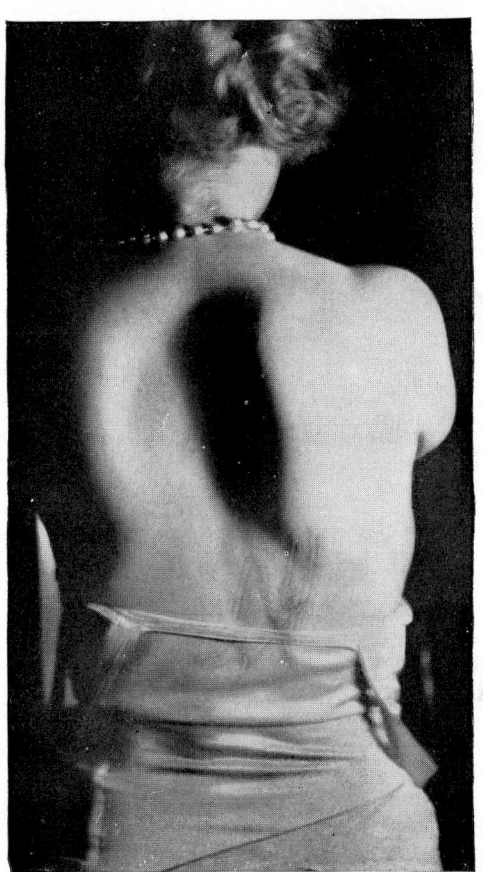

FIG. 18. Compression paralysis of the long thoracic nerve due to faulty position of the patient on operating table. "Winged scapula."

An extensive abdominal incision, apart from the median, paramedian or transverse, will more or less damage the nerve supply. The main objection to the median incision is the possibility of the occurrence of postoperative ventral hernia, and the statistics of the Mayo Clinic show that 2 per cent of the abdominal operations performed there were for ventral hernia following previous abdominal section. Kocher attributes this complication to imperfect asepsis and improper suturing, and recommends Lenander's incision to obtain good exposure and increased firmness along the line of suturing. This incision now goes under the name of paramedian and is made about one inch lateral to the midline. The anterior wall of the rectus sheath is divided in the line of the cutaneous incision and the inner leaf of the sheath dissected free, medially. The rectus is then drawn outward and the abdomen opened through the posterior layer of the sheath more or less in line with the anterior sheath incision. At the conclusion of the operation, the posterior layer, consisting of the peritoneum and transversalis fascia, is sutured with catgut, every care being taken that the raw edges are everted. Ventral hernia rarely follows a paramedian incision.

The transverse incision is advocated mainly because it is considered to be more anatomically and physiologically correct than others. The surgeon must decide, according to his experience and judgment and the nature of the operation, what incisions or combination of incisions he will employ. In a general way, it may be said that it is of no great surgical consequence which way the muscles are divided, especially the rectus abdominis, provided the re-suturing is correctly performed.

Adhesions are a common postoperative sequela, caused primarily by faulty surgical technic such as unnecessary irritation of delicate tissues, prolonged exposure, pulling and tearing of tissues, chemical irritation and forcible packing with large quantities of dry gauze. In the peritoneal cavity especially, all surfaces should be treated with the maximum of gentleness and at the end of the operation some surgeons use a bland solution such as sodium citrate or sterile olive oil in addition to omentization of any injured surfaces.

Foreign Bodies. With the perfection of technic arrived at in present day surgery, it would seem almost impossible that there would be any risk of leaving behind in an opened cavity any surgical instrument. Nevertheless the fact remains that it happens from time to time even with most careful surgeons.

In **emergency surgery,** as in industrial accidents and in severe traumatisms, such as compound fractures, where there is little time for preoperative treatment the wound should be freely opened up and cleansed thoroughly. Infected and devitalized tissues, including doubtful muscle tissue, should be removed with a sharp knife and all debris removed. As elsewhere, gentleness of manipulation should be the keynote of treatment. All bleeding points should be secured and clots removed. Then, if the Carrel-Dakin method of wound irrigation is employed, the instillation tubes should be introduced in such a way that the whole wound field is thoroughly irrigated with the antiseptic fluid. Gauze compresses and packs may be employed but must not interfere with the action of the tubes. Dakin's Solution is a combination of chlorinated lime with bicarbonate of soda. It was used extensively in the World War and in civil surgery.

INFECTION

It is my impression, gained from a series of experiments on animals and from hospital work, that in most instances wound infections may be avoided by careful technic.

Most wound infections are caused by large quantities of catgut becoming imbedded in the abdominal wall. It is small wonder that the absorptive powers of the system become overburdened when it is recalled the amount of catgut used in ligating vessels and closing wounds in abdominal operations.

I often limit myself to a single catgut suture in closing the peritoneum. An occasional bleeding vessel is ligated, but forcipressure and torsion is usually depended upon for hemostasis. The remainder of the wound is closed with one dermal suture, or a suture of silkworm gut or silk. The type of suture material is not of so much importance as is its sterility and nonabsorbability and the fact that it holds in its grip the fasciae, panniculus adiposus and skin.

Following the study of 3000 abdominal wounds, in the Women's Hospital of New York, Goff states that, "With all other factors remaining constant, the adoption of the silk sutures had, in the work of all surgeons who used them, invariably resulted in a very decided reduction in the incidence of faulty union. The total average incidence of faulty union in clean abdominal incisions from all causes, was 12.1 per cent in wounds closed by absorbable sutures, while with non-absorbable sutures it was only 4.3 per cent!"

Injury to the abdominal wall during operation may be avoided by retracting the wound very gently and for short periods of time and by avoiding mass ligatures of the subcutaneous tissues, devitalization of fat, fascia, muscle and skin by artery forceps and by the use of laparotomy sponges that are too hot.

Figure (19 A-B) depict my single suture method which tends to eliminate dead spaces in the wound. Forcipressure is also very helpful.

Observance of these suggestions in combination with thorough preoperative preparation of the patient has given us very satisfactory primary union in our work.

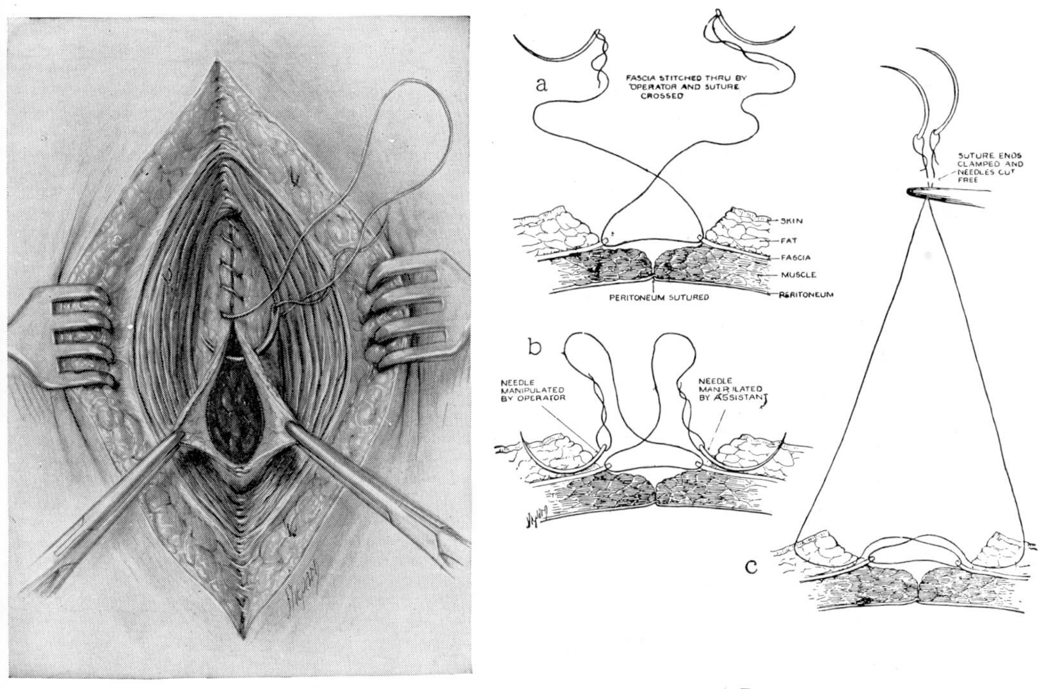

FIG. 19. A. Author's method of closure of abdominal wound. Peritoneum is closed with continuous catgut suture; B. author's method of wound closure: a. fascia stitched through and suture crossed, peritoneum sutured, b. one needle is manipulated by the operator and the other by assistant, c. suture ends clamped and needles cut free.

However, infections have been known to follow the most rigid asepsis and painstaking technic. Leaky or faulty sterilizers, insufficient scrubbing of the surgeon's hands, especially of the thumb, index and middle fingers of the right hand, torn gloves and the repeated use of the same alcohol for soaking the hands may all be sources of infection.

In injuries to the extremities it is much better to dress the limb with antiseptic dressing and delay operating for a day or so, to a time when there will be much less danger of shock and not infrequently a way may even be seen where the limb may be saved.

It is frequently desirable to leave an antiseptic dressing on an open wound for at least twenty-four hours before suturing it.

In the surgery of special regions, such as in the terminal portions of the ileum and colon, which swarm with infectious organisms, extraordinary precautions must be taken. If the bowel is divided, swab the ends to be reunited with iodine or still better, use the diatherm knife.

In certain infections, some surgeons still irrigate the peritoneal cavity. One or two pints of saline is poured in slowly through a funnel and tube before the peritoneum is sutured. After some years' experience with peritoneal irrigations, I discontinued its use.

It may be remarked that catgut is often blamed for postoperative infections when in effect rough handling and poor surgery is the cause.

DRAINAGE

Finally, to drain or not to drain? The opinions of surgeons on this question are still at variance. The safe rule appears to be: that drainage is unnecessary when a surgical operation has been conducted aseptically and there has been no indication or manifestation of sepsis, but when there is any doubt in the surgeon's mind, the operative field should be drained. It should be remembered that drainage in itself is a necessary evil; the drain is always a foreign body which irritates and opens up an avenue for the entrance of infection.

Drainage is indicated:

1. When doubt exists as to the complete and efficient removal of infectious matter.
2. When complete hemostasis has not been obtained.
3. When some necrosis may be expected owing to severe lacerations or contusions.
4. When it is impossible to avoid an actual or potential cavity in the deeper layers of a wound in which serum, blood or pus may collect.

When they can be employed, gravity drains are the best. But drainage may also be effected against gravity and then depends upon reversal of the circulation in the local lymphatics. A drain or gauze pack invites an increased flow of lymph in an effort to extrude the foreign body. This flow of lymph flushes out the cavity. Suction and aspiration drainage, depending upon some external motor arrangement, or siphonage may be resorted to in some cases when the usual modes of drainage cannot be applied (Fig. 20).

Occasionally the removal of a drainage tube is followed by pyrexia, to the discomfiture of the surgeon. This need cause no alarm, for, as a rule, the fever is of a transient nature and without bad prognostic significance.

When drainage tubes should be removed is a question that must be decided by the indications in each individual case. Too prolonged retention of drainage tubes, as already pointed out, often proves disastrous, and sometimes results in intestinal obstruction and fecal fistula from pressure necrosis. While this is so, I still find it difficult to be divorced from the dictum—"When in doubt always drain." Numerous incidents in my experience have stressed the value of keeping this dictum inviolate, although I am fully aware that many experienced and competent surgeons hold the opposite view. For myself: "experientia docet."

While much condemnation is directed against gauze drains, their judicious use often proves beneficial. Common sense as to quality and quantity of drainage material will yield good results. In our work we use rubber drains, cigarette

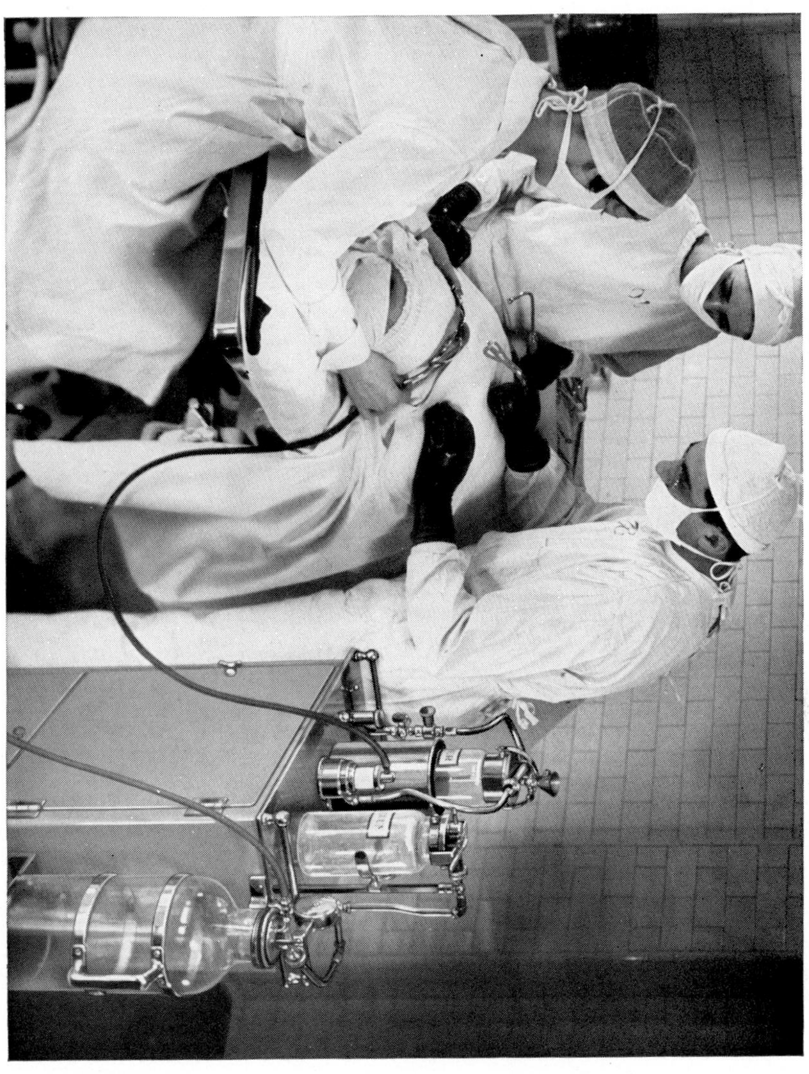

FIG. 20. Suction pump in use. (Courtesy, V. Mueller & Co.)

drains and gauze packs. The Mikulicz pack also has a distinct and valuable place in the armamentarium of the surgeon.

There are various methods by which drainage can be instituted, depending upon the nature, the quantity and the surroundings of the fluid which is to be drained. The types in most common use are the capillary, tubular, combined capillary and tubular, and absorbable drains. Of the capillary drains, several small lengths of catgut or silkworm gut placed together makes a suitable method of draining small amounts of serous exudates. A piece of gauze or wick may be used, but should be removed as soon as possible to prevent coagulation of the fluids in the drain. Another form of capillary drain is made by placing a piece of thin rubber tissue around a strip of gauze. This is known as the cigarette drain and has proved to be more efficient than the individual gauze drain.

There are several varieties of **tubular** drains. Ordinary rubber tubes about ½ inch in diameter are frequently used. The tube is perforated on its sides and at its distal end. A safety pin or suture may be used to keep the tube from slipping.

The rubber tubes are occasionally split longitudinally with resultant decreased rigidity.

Another type of tubular drain is the dressed drain, a rubber tube covered by several layers of iodoform gauze around which is placed a thin sheet of rubber tissue. It is very often used in surgery of the abdomen.

Wetherill's drain made out of rubber tubing is sometimes employed. Rigid tubes made from glass, celluloid or hard rubber are occasionally used. A rubber collar may be applied around the tube to which a safety pin or suture can be attached to prevent slipping of the tube.

The combined capillary and tubal drain is made by placing an ordinary rubber tube around a group of capillary drains.

Absorbable drains consist of the decalcified bone drain which was suggested by Neuber and the chicken-bone drain presented by Macewen. The chicken-bone drain is prepared as follows: denude the tibiae and femora of the chicken. Place in 20 per cent HCl until the bones are soft. Cut off the ends of the bone with a scissors. Elevate the endosteum at one end and push it through to the other end together with its contents. Boil in a saturated solution of ammonium sulphate to sterilize. Wash with sterile water or an antiseptic solution. Preserve in alcohol or iodoform in alcohol solution. The durability of the tube in the tissues is about eight days. Durability may be enhanced by placing the bone in a sterile solution of chromic acid.

SURGICAL INSTRUMENTS

The importance of the quality and adaptability of surgical instruments should not be overlooked by the surgeon. Since the welfare of the patient may be endangered, it would seem fitting to require of the manufacturer an ethical responsibility equal to that of the surgeon who must rely so much upon the dependability of the instruments used.

If an instrument fails to qualify or seems inadequate to meet the requirements for which it was intended, the manufacturer should be held morally or ethically responsible. It has been advocated that the name of the manufacturer in such a case be made known so that other surgeons may be duly warned. A case has been reported where an operating table collapsed during an operation owing to defective construction.

It would seem a good idea for authoritative bodies to formulate some form of protection as a means of aiding the surgeon in the purchase of dependable instruments; that is, establishing a standard which manufacturers should be obliged to adhere to and which should serve as a guide to surgeons in choosing their equipment.

It might be well to mention here that a fellowship of the Mellon Institute of the University of Pittsburgh has for its very laudable objective the study of surgical supplies. Slayton has published an article outlining the scope of this work. Among other things, this fellowship is to determine the definite needs of surgeons and other specialists and to standardize products such as gauze, bandage materials, sutures, instruments, etc., from a scientific, rather than a commercial standpoint.

Manufacturers to whom the surgeon must turn for equipment to be used where life and future usefulness are in the balance, should be governed by the high ethical standards of the medical profession rather than by the tenets of commercialism.

The assurance of perfect instruments does much to inspire confidence and assurance to the operator, while an accident occurring during an operation may be so upsetting to the surgeon as to endanger the life of the patient.

There would seem to be a modern tendency toward elevating the price and lowering the quality, fostered chiefly by ideas of carelessness and indifference. There is no shortage of either materials or craftsmen in this country, so there would appear to be no reasonable excuse for putting anything but superior instruments on the market.

Figure 21 shows a defective tonsil-snare; its appearance does not betray the defect. In use it either did not produce the desired tension on the loop or it fell completely apart. This instrument repeated this performance several times before being discarded.

In Figure 22 (A, B and C) three trephines are shown which broke during one operation. The skull to which they were applied was of ordinary density. "A" had never been used before; observe the turned edge; "B" was considered an old and trustworthy instrument; it broke also. The third trephine "C" was brought into service but was discarded after a few turns on account of a broken guard. The fourth instrument served to complete the operation which was performed under an intense mental strain lest another accident occur.

Figures 23, 24, and 25 depict a varied collection of broken needles, forceps, scalpels, mallet, etc. They speak for themselves except to say that such is an almost daily occurrence with many surgeons.

According to Jackson and Jackson,[1] defects appearing in faulty surgical instruments may be due to (a) the use of poor or improper material, (b) defective design, or (c) improper tempering of steel instruments.

Nonoxidizable steel, vanadium steel and other alloys generally do not pos-

[1] Archives of Otolaryngology, Sept. 1935, Vol. 22, pp. 293-303.

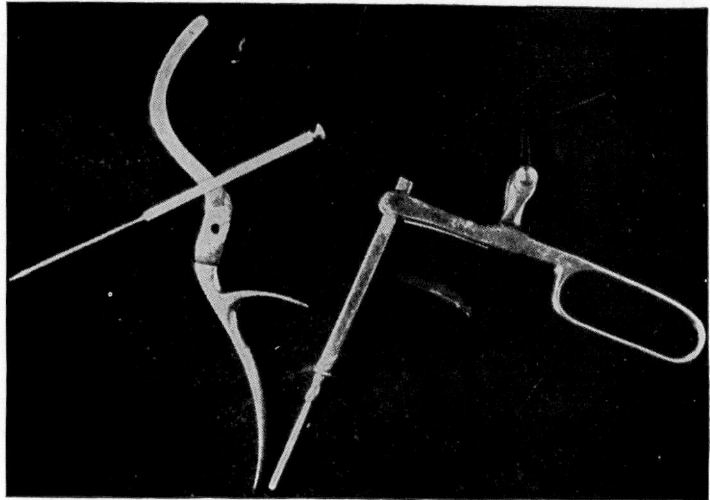

FIG. 21. Tonsil snare, broken during an operation.

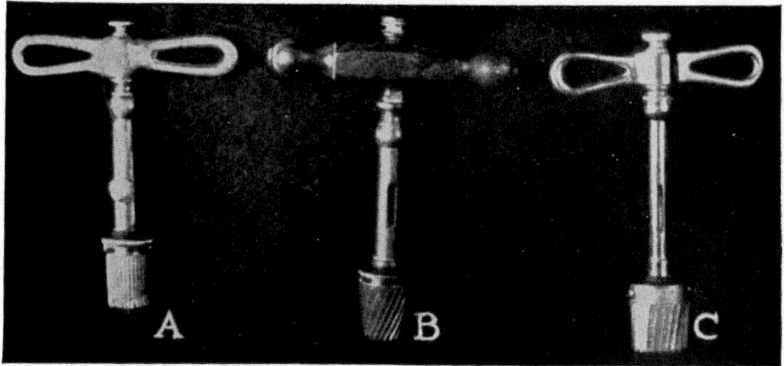

FIG. 22. Three trephines, broken during a single operation. The metal was too soft to resist the hardness of the bone.

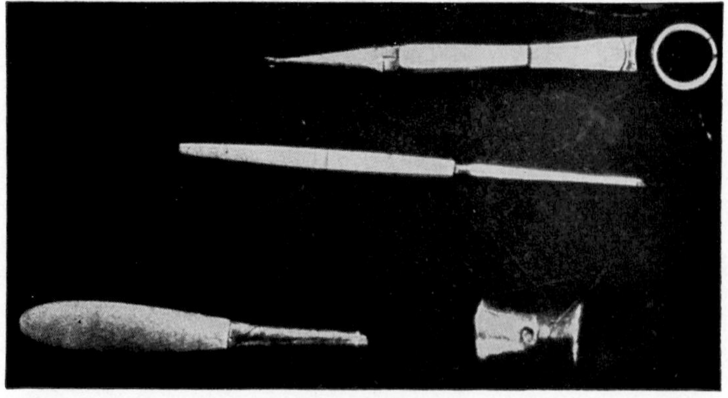

FIG. 23. Instruments broken during operation.

sess the reliable qualities necessary for delicate surgical instruments. All instruments which require an elastic action: saws, rasps, rongeurs, knives, shears, scissors, and cutting instruments generally, should be made of the best tool steel. In manufacture, hand-forging followed by hand filing, tempering, grinding and

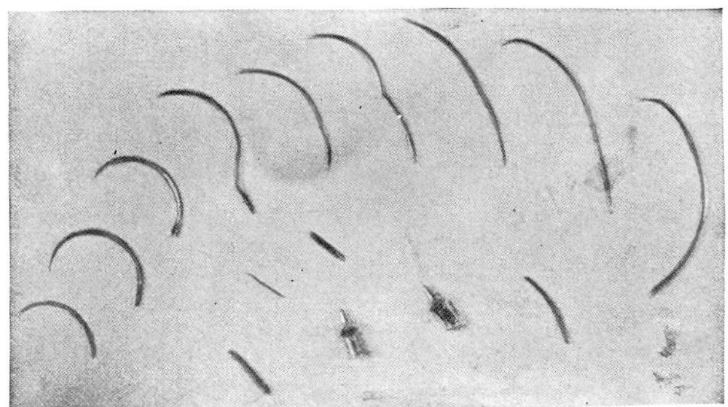

FIG. 24. Broken needles.

sharpening by skilled workmen is necessary. At the most a few instruments may need to be glass-hard at the cutting edge and far enough back for resharpening; for the rest, tempering which will draw the hardness and permit of bending is necessary. Because rasps look like files (which have to be glass hard for

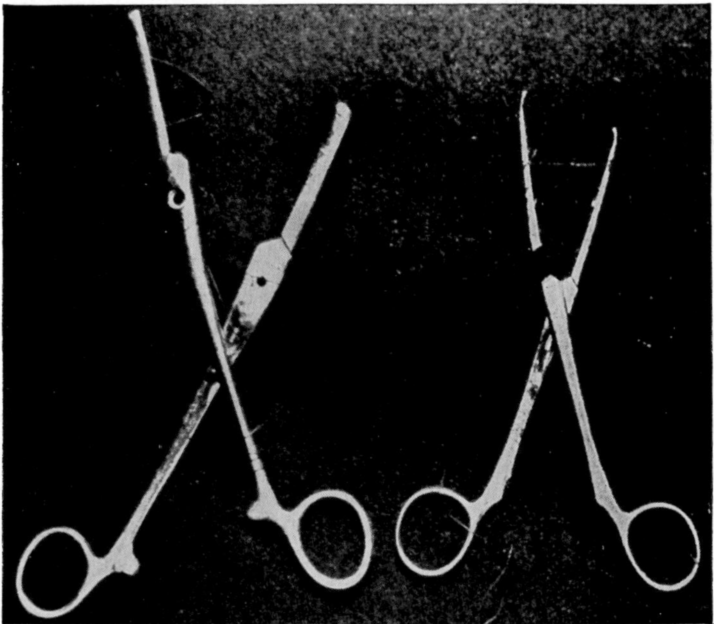

FIG. 25. Artery forceps that could not withstand the strain of service.

use on metal) such instruments are usually made glass-hard, accounting for broken nasal rasps, etc. Temper can be tested with a file which will bite if the steel is tempered, and slide off if glass-hard. Since springs must have a good elastic action and be hard to a degree approximating the limit at which it will break before it will retain a bent position, they are unreliable—the more so because of the severe treatment which they receive. Any instrument which is to be bent back and forth must have all the hardening removed by annealing.

All surgical instruments should be cleaned immediately after use and stored in a dry place. The chlorine and acidity of city water will corrode them unless

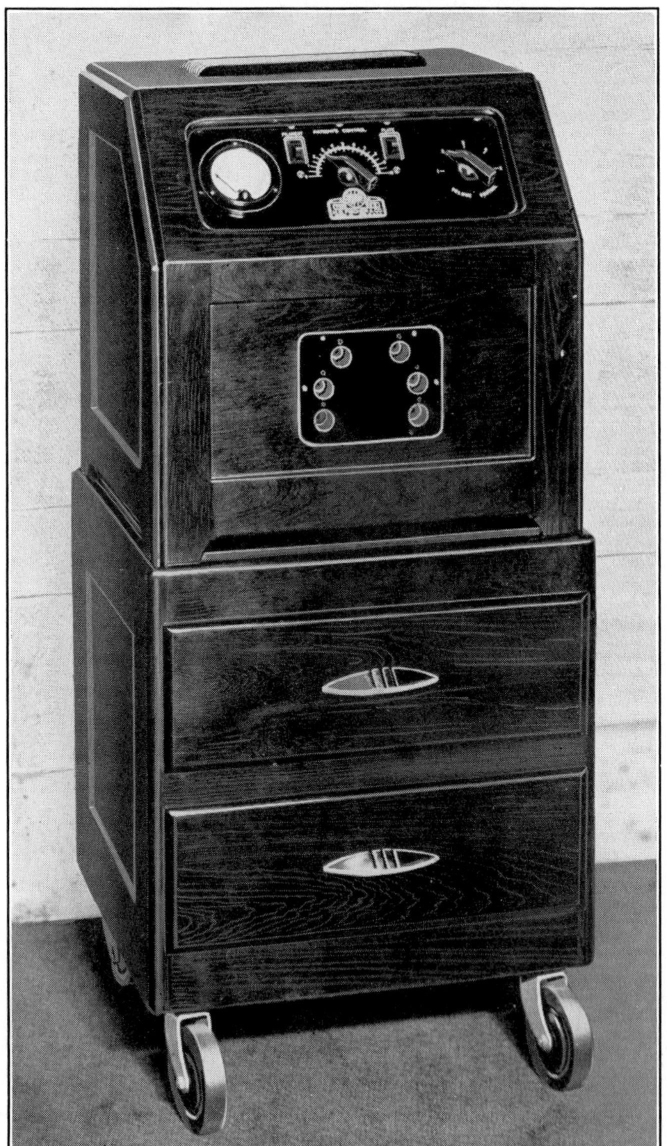

FIG. 26. Fischer short wave apparatus (12 meters).

neutralized by sodium bicarbonate; sterilization by alcohol may ruin them because of the denaturing substances. In sterilizing steel instruments it is well to remember that high temperatures often affect the temper of the steel and make it more brittle, hence it snaps, bends or breaks easily. Needles are rendered less elastic and knives do not take such a keen edge. Instruments which have been subjected to heat or chemical sterilization should be retested before use.

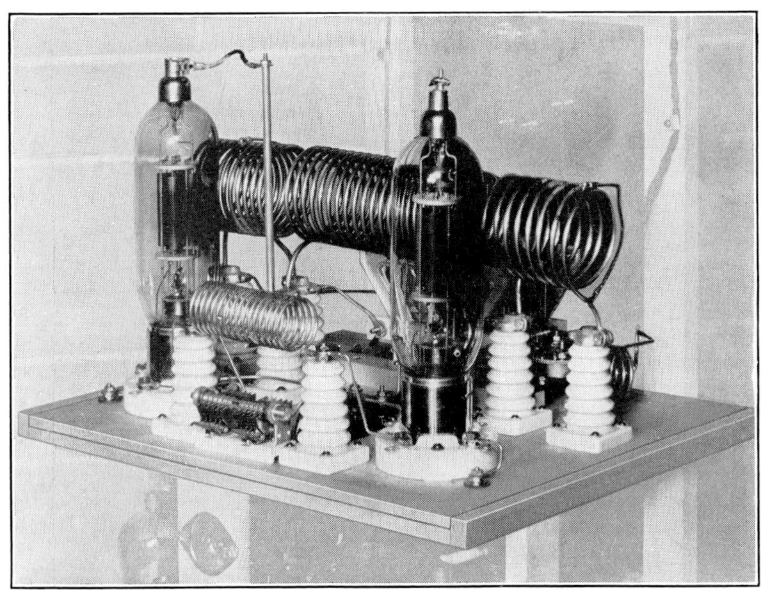

Fig. 27. Interior view of the apparatus depicted in Fig. 26 showing the construction of power oscillators (on upper platform) and mounted power transformer controls and rectifying tubes (on lower platform).

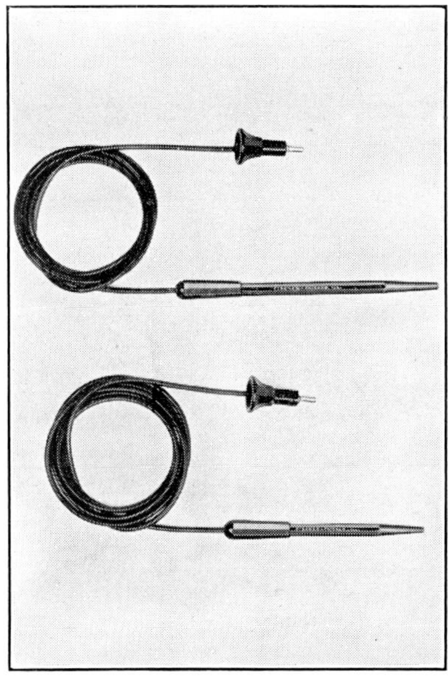

Fig. 28. Fischer's surgical handles.

Specific surgical instruments will be alluded to in conjunction with the operation in which they are used.

ELECTROSURGERY

In modern operating rooms many surgeons resort to electric currents for hemostasis, division of tissues and for destruction of neoplasms. The apparatus used for this purpose by the author is shown in Figures 26 and 27.

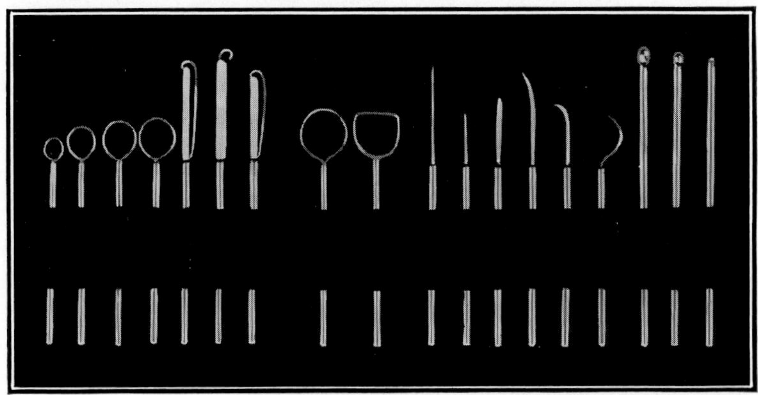

FIG. 29. Knives, reamers, electrodes and loops used in electrosurgery.

Space does not permit a thorough discussion of the subject; suffice it to say that the surgeon should possess at least a rudimentary knowledge of the physical properties of electric currents and their effects upon living tissues. A properly constructed diathermy apparatus may be used, but the short wave

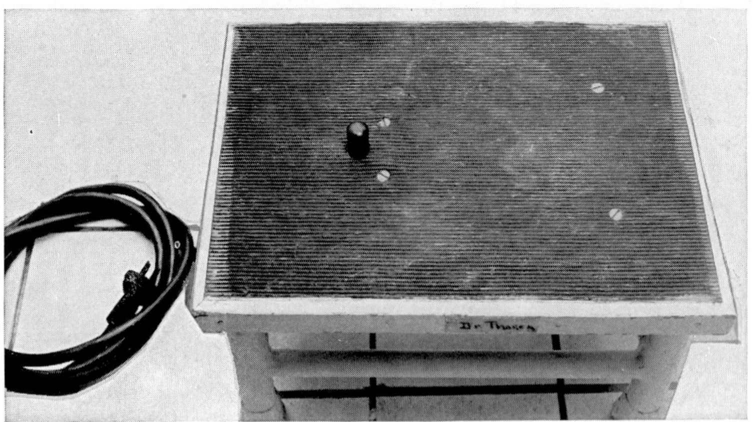

FIG. 30. Author's foot-switch.

machines obviate insulating the patient thereby avoiding burns and permitting efficient work.

Accessories used in the short wave apparatus are a handle (Figs. 28-29) and a variety of loops, knife blades, needle points, reamers and coagulating ball electrodes to suit a given purpose.

For electrosurgical obliteration of the gallbladder (see author's operation) a special electrode is used.

I have found a good deal of inconvenience with the time-honored foot switch which tends to move about on the floor of the operating room. To steady it, I have incorporated the switch in a substantial operating room stool which assures steadiness and comfort (Fig. 30).

The beginner will do well to become thoroughly acquainted with the technic of cutting and electrocoagulation. This is best accomplished by practicing on a

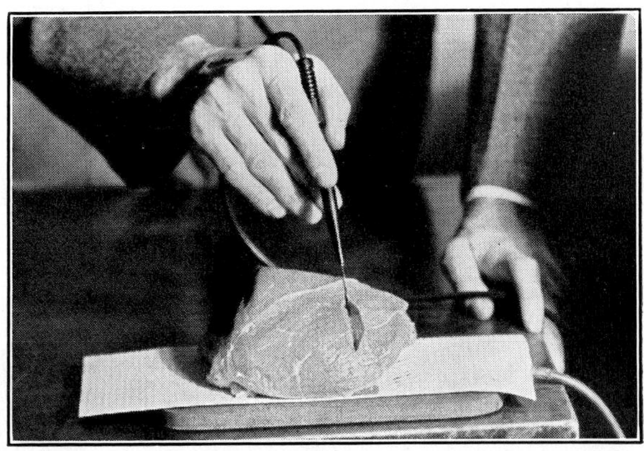

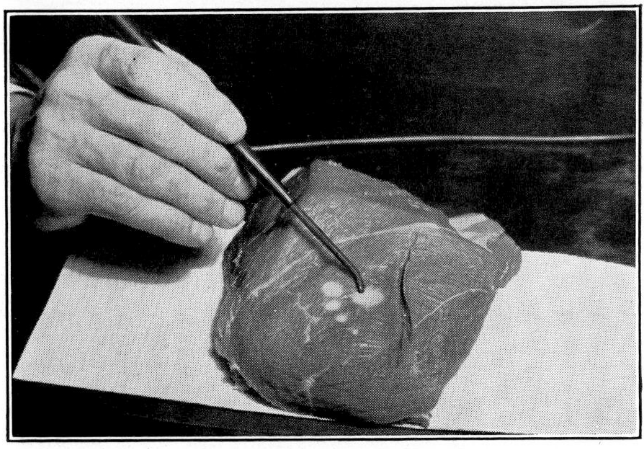

FIGS. 31 and 32. Practicing on raw beef. Electrocutting and coagulation.

piece of raw beef. Dexterity soon is acquired (Figs. 31-32). An acquaintance with the terminology now extant will prove of value (see chapter on gallbladder surgery).

Wm. A. Gross found that the coagulated areas produced by sharp electrodes are pyramidal when using the long wave apparatus. When using the blunt electrode with the short wave apparatus the coagulated area is round and conforms more or less to the outline of the electrode. A cross section of the electrocoagulated tissue also shows that the depth of action of the current depends upon the amount of pressure used against the point of contact.

CHAPTER 5

STERILIZATION OF SURGICAL SUPPLIES

Paul Muni's picture—"The Story of Louis Pasteur"—brought to mind certain facts with which every surgeon will do well to refresh his memory from time to time. It is no exaggeration to state that in most surgeries, when things have been running smoothly for a long time, there is a tendency to relax from close observation of high standards—a state of mind that surely invites trouble.

In our modern hospitals with all the elaborate equipment now considered necessary, it seems a far cry to those days when anyone would seriously question the need for precise methods of sterilizing. But it is just sixty years since

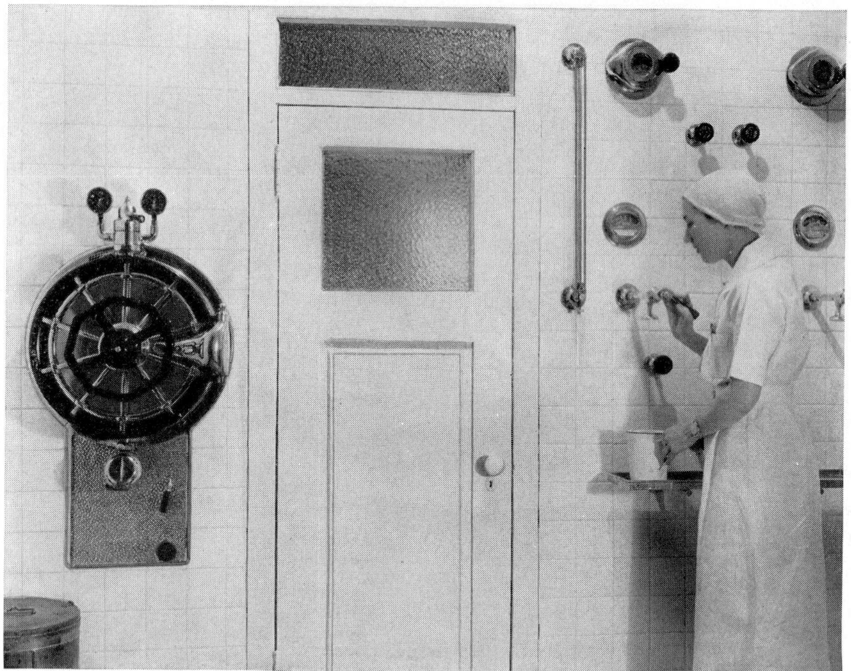

Fig. 33. Built in sterilizer unit, American Hospital, Chicago. (Courtesy American Sterilizer Company.)

Robert Koch isolated the first known disease-producing organism—anthrax. During this period, the 1870's, Lister was proving that his antiseptic methods did avoid infections, and his only sterilizing agency was carbolic acid, and an infinitely painstaking personal attention to detail. Pasteur at that time was still trying to convince scientists that microbes do not spring into existence spontaneously.

The average surgeon is not called upon to supervise sterilization of his supplies, has in fact no voice (as he should) in the conduct of the surgery beyond the immediate field in which his work is done. He accepts the materials given him to work with on the supposition that someone else has subjected them to proper sterilization. In a well conducted hospital, usually nothing goes very seriously wrong that could be charged to lax sterilization. Still, there are few surgeons who have not experienced difficulties with infections, grave or otherwise, that have been hard to explain.

I am convinced that a large percentage of these infections might be avoided and that imperfect sterilization or perhaps improper methods of handling sterile supplies accounts for too many of them. I am aware that surgeons have neither the time nor inclination to become sterilization experts, nor do I suggest that. They might advantageously inform themselves fundamentally about certain modern procedures that are of paramount importance to the end that they are able to assist at least in an advisory capacity in the selection of suitable equipment, and in the establishment of systems of technic that are above criticism (Fig. 33).

The institution's sterilizing equipment need not be new to be thoroughly modern, certainly in so far as performance is concerned. Some of the most accurately performing apparatus I know of has been in use for many years. It is important to keep old sterilizers up to date, for at least two of the most outstanding developments applicable to sterilizers have been brought out in very recent years.

PREPARATION OF MATERIALS AND METHODS OF STERILIZATION

I shall not attempt to go deeply into this detail other than to suggest that there is grave need for the standardization of methods in accordance with plans which have been worked out scientifically. At the present every hospital establishes its own standards, more or less, too frequently from the standpoint of expediency, and with insufficient thought about results. To cite a typical example: The surgical supervisor in a prominent hospital in her effort to protect hypodermic syringes from injury, placed them individually in small test tubes, and closed the open ends with tight fitting corks. Of course there was no sterilizing effect at all because steam could not enter the tube. In another hospital a new method of sterilizing rubber gloves was invented—a system of formaldehyde sterilization about the equivalent of the metal boxes used in barber shops marked "Sterilizer." This system was used until a series of postoperative infections resulted in an overhauling of sterilizing procedures, and the return to the steam method.

The interested reader will find much worthwhile information in condensed form in Weeden B. Underwood's "A Textbook of Sterilization." This little volume of about one hundred pages is brim full with essentials germane to the subject of sterilization. It condenses the principles of the substratum upon which the important subject of sterilization is built in a most admirable and comprehensive manner. Particularly, the surgeon who must "read and run" will find it of inestimable value.

INSTRUMENTS AND UTENSILS

Boiling. No one can seriously criticize the old system of thorough boiling for instruments and utensils, preferably in water containing 1% sodium carbonate. The period of boiling, however, is important and is too often cut short. Normally, the period should be from 15 to 20 minutes with instruments or

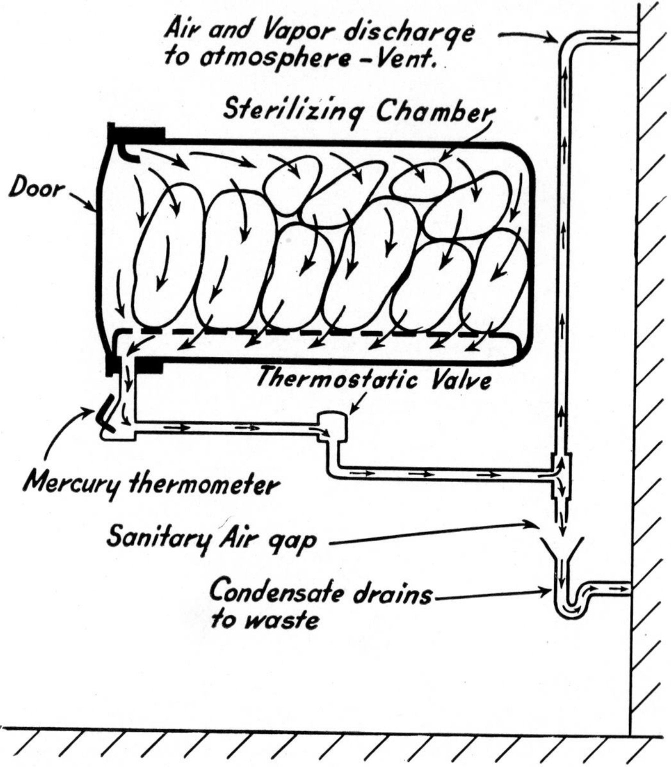

FIG. 34. This diagram illustrates the scientifically correct method of sterilizing surgical supplies in the pressure steam sterilizer. The basic principles are easily applicable to any sterilizer and surgeons are perfectly justified in demanding the adoption of the system which has become the recognized standard with reputable manufacturers of sterilizers.

Faulty elimination of air is the cause of practically all sterilization failures. This system provides for complete drainage of both air and condensate from the chamber, and it measures in unquestionably correct terms the character of the steam applied to the load and its temperature, regardless of the pressure applied.

The principle is beautifully simple. When steam is admitted to the chamber, the air being more than twice heavier than steam will gravitate unfailingly to the lower areas. Arrows indicate the movement of steam and air during the evacuation process. Air will continue to flow from the bottom exit, through the thermometer chamber and the thermostatic valve to the vent, until hot steam finally follows the air and causes the thermostatic valve to close. Thereafter the thermostatic valve will open briefly, only to discharge cooler condensate and air pockets as they gradually gravitate from the load to it.

The thermometer serves a dual purpose. (The mercury thermometer is recommended rather than any of the vapor tension types because of its known permanent qualities of reliability.) First, it serves as a detector of any interruption to the free discharge of air from the chamber. This is vitally important because the discharge piping is constantly subject to clogging with sediment. If for any reason the discharge of air is impeded or interrupted, the temperature will rise slowly or not at all—if the line is altogether closed. It cannot indicate sterilizing temperature until the chamber is filled with steam of the character indicated by the temperature.

Second, it (rather than pressure) is the gauge of sterilization upon which the operator depends. One cannot time the exposure until the temperature has risen to an amply safe range. It safeguards against the thing that is responsible for nearly all failures, the attempt to sterilize with adequate pressure but with inadequate temperature.

Finally, the air and condensate discharge from the chamber takes place through a piping system protected by a sanitary air gap. There is no close connection to the waste through which sewer gas or worse might be conducted to the sterilizer. Critical inspectors will insist upon such protection but far too frequently inspection is lax and many sterilizers are in use in which there is no such protection.

utensils entirely covered with water. Under no circumstances should the period of boiling be reduced below 15 minutes except with the expressed approval of the surgeon, perhaps in pressing emergency, when the period may be reduced to 10 minutes.

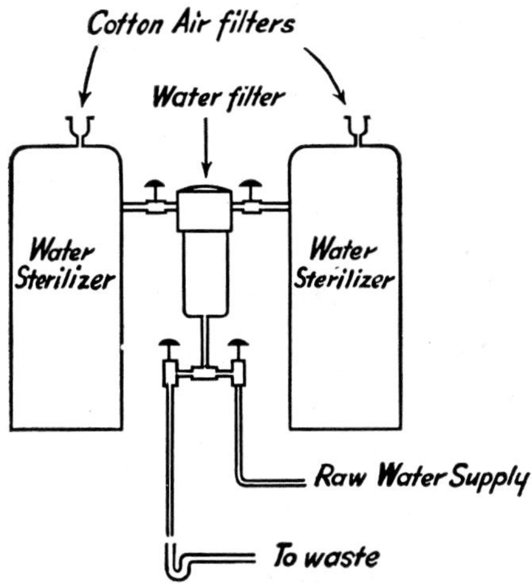

FIG. 35. This diagram illustrates an obsolete system of water filtration still in common use. The opportunities for pollution are so numerous and obvious that explanations do not seem necessary. However, very few surgeons ever take the trouble to analyze the piping on existing equipment and are thus not aware of the hazards constantly presented.

There is a valved direct cross connection between the water supply and the waste which no sanitary inspector would ever approve if his attention were called to it. In most communities there are rules which specifically forbid such connections, because under certain adverse conditions the contents of the waste would surely be drawn into the water supply line. The much discussed World's Fair epidemic was traced to similar faulty connections.

The water filter has four valved connections leading respectively to the two sterile water tanks, to the raw water supply and to the waste. Every one of these valves is constantly subject to leakage and slow leakage (the kind from which highly dangerous pollution originates) cannot be detected by the operator.

Leaky valves permit sometimes a constant slow flow of raw water through the (polluted) filter to either or both tanks. Under other conditions back pressure in the waste (a far from uncommon condition) will conduct sewage to the filter and thence to the sterile tanks.

Every water sterilizer in the process of cooling down after sterilization, is subject to high degrees of vacuum—20″ or more. If there is a leaky connection to the filter, nothing can prevent the intake of the contents of the filter, which in this type is always foul, because it collects the solids from all water passing through it in filtering thousands of gallons of raw water, and cannot be sterilized at all.

Sterile water pollution from air contacts is one of the real sources of trouble. Many water sterilizers provide no means at all for filtering incoming air as water is withdrawn, while others furnish the ridiculous cotton filtering apparatus shown by the diagram. During sterilization steam escapes through the air filtering cup, wets the cotton and leaves behind some condensate which serves to wash down the dust polluted walls. The unsterile condensate filled with dust is then conducted by gravity direct to the sterile product and begins another slow process of contamination, the results of which can be measured by examination of the water after a few hours' standing—and after half or more of the water has been drawn out.

Steam Pressure. In many hospitals both utensils and instruments are now being sterilized by steam pressure and special sterilizers are constructed for the purpose. The method is desirable because it undoubtedly adds to the safety factor, and requires no greater period of time—10 to 15 minutes being ample.

One marked advantage in this system is that it eliminates the formation of lime or scale on the instruments or utensils, which is highly objectionable in localities where the raw water contains impurities which deposit in this way.

Oil Sterilization. The use of oil sterilizers for delicate cutting instruments, I believe, should be discouraged. It is questionable whether the temperature normally developed in such apparatus is sufficiently high to insure sterilization, at least, of resistant organisms, in the brief interval of exposure designated. The recommended period is 10 to 15 minutes at about 300° F., or slightly higher. The performance is strictly dry heat sterilization since no moisture is present and according to all authorities on this subject, the temperature should be very much higher and the period longer. One investigator, Dr. E. E. Ecker of the University Hospitals of Cleveland, thinks that the temperature should be at least 350°-360° F. and the period not less than 15 minutes. At this higher

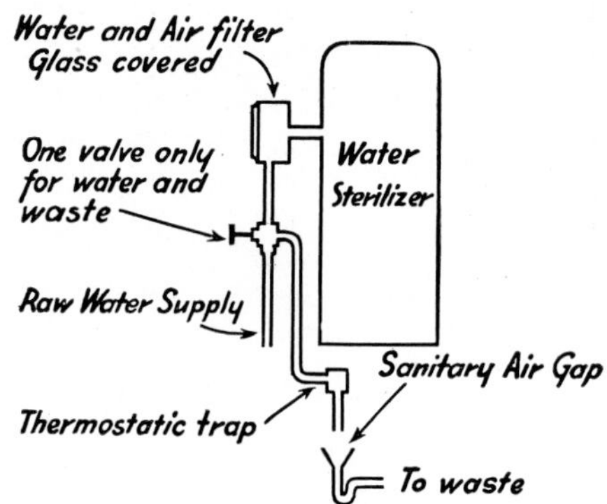

FIG. 36. The system of water and air filtration and the piping illustrated in this diagram is recommended because of its simplicity and because it protects against the sources of pollution common to the older system shown by Fig. 35.

There is a separate water and air filter for each tank and each filter has a glass cover so that the operator can see the flow of water to check performance. Each filter is controlled by just one double acting valve instead of four valves as used on the old system. When this valve is closed against the flow of water, a secondary opening conducts leakage to the waste instead of the tank. This provides positive protection against pollution from leaky valves.

When water is sterilized, steam from the dome of the tank is conducted through the water and air filter and through the thermostatic trap to the air gap protected waste. When the trap becomes heated by steam it closes and holds the steam under pressure for thorough sterilization of the filter. The system is entirely automatic in this respect.

All air taken in as water cools or is withdrawn is required to pass through the (sterilized) filter which removes all dust.

These features of protection fortunately can be applied to old equipment—and they or their equivalent should be required in every surgery.

range of temperature the oil is inclined to disintegrate and certainly the fumes given off are most objectionable. I am inclined to believe also, that the removal of oil from instruments following sterilization by this method may offer further opportunity for reinfection.

SOLUTIONS

This subject is of tremendous importance and it is much misunderstood. Like sterile water, solutions in the process of sterilizing and cooling breathe in a manner which subjects them to contamination. When the sterilized flask is removed from the sterilizer it begins immediately to cool and to draw in air. If the flask is not well protected the intaken air will certainly contaminate. This necessitates a method of stoppering which will effectually filter all dust from the air taken in.

Stoppering. There are so many methods in use that it is difficult to separate the good ones from the bad ones, but many that are in use are distinctly open to criticism. It is probable that the most effective system involves the use of fluted paper caps which are now available, made from fairly stiff, smooth coated paper, shaped to fit the commonly used sizes of flasks. This paper cap is bound on with cotton tape very compactly against the neck of the flask, preferably covered with two or three thicknesses of muslin also bound on into a neat cover. The use of gauze, cotton or muslin for the inner cover of the flask, next to the solution, is objectionable because of the probability that shreds of lint will find their way into the solution.

Exhaustion of Sterilizer. Careless methods of sterilizing, however, will render useless the most elaborately planned system of stoppering. If the sterilizer pressure is exhausted rapidly following sterilization, there will be very rapid ebullition of the liquid which will saturate the stopper and cause a considerable part of the solution to boil over into the sterilizer. Once saturated, no stopper can properly protect the solution. To avoid this sort of thing, solutions should always be sterilized by themselves, and following sterilization, heat should be turned off and the entire sterilizer permitted to cool as slowly as possible. In this way, provided the flasks have not been filled more than about two-thirds full, there will be a minimum loss of solution from the flasks due to evaporation and no rapid ebullition which will saturate the stoppers.

PROTECTION OF STERILIZED WATER

This detail I consider to be of sufficient importance to justify considerable thought. Water is very easily rendered sterile but it is subject to radical contaminating influences as I shall attempt to show.

Multiple Valve, Stone Filter Systems. The older system of filtering water as it is delivered from the supply line to the two sterilizing reservoirs, makes use of a single stone filter having valved connections to the raw water supply, to the drainage system, and to each of the two reservoirs. It is a physical impossibility to guard against leakage of valves and with this multiplicity of valves there is far too much opportunity for undetected pollution of the sterile supply. In addition stone filters cannot be sterilized at all—they collect filth from the water passing through them for weeks, or perhaps months, before they are cleaned at all—become excellent breeding grounds for bacteria which adds further to the possibility for pollution.

Similarly the method of filtering the air taken into water sterilizers as water is withdrawn, by drawing it through cotton filled cups, has been proved to be totally ineffective. Many water sterilizers make no provision whatever for the filtration of air.

Water in the process of sterilizing and cooling actually breathes, and this fact accentuates the opportunity for pollution from raw water or air. When heated as in sterilizing, steam forms and pressure is created and some steam will escape from various openings. Then when the water is cooled the condensation of steam causes a high degree of vacuum which will draw in impurities, either water or air, through any unprotected opening that exists. This detail is of far more importance than appears on the surface. These dangerous sources of contamination are most difficult to detect because the intake of polluted matter cannot be observed by the operator. If the water filtering system contains a leaky connection to the drain, the intake will come directly from the sewage system. In one test case of which I am aware, colonies of colon bacilli were found on the surface of a stone filter 6″ from the sterile water reservoir with no protection between, except one leaky valve.

This sort of thing has no place in modern surgery—should not be tolerated. Frequent tests of sterile water after it has cooled to room temperature and after two-thirds or more of the capacity of the tank has been exhausted, and after the water has been standing several hours will be indicative of its purity. Tests made immediately after sterilization are useless because the infection drawn in commonly must be given an opportunity to mix with the water in the reservoir, part of which is of course sterile.

Single Valve System. One manufacturer has appreciated the common faults of our older system of filtering air and water and has developed protective features of infinite value. Each reservoir has an individual water and air filter combined with but one valve controlling it. That one valve serves a dual purpose. When opened it delivers filtered water to the reservoir and the flow of water is visible to the operator through a glass cover. When this valve is closed against the flow of water, a secondary outlet is opened up through which any leakage of raw water through the valve is conducted directly to an open funnel waste, rather than to the water reservoir. The open funnel disposes of any possibility of contamination from the waste system, a most important detail.

There is no opening to the sterile water reservoir through which air is drawn except through the filtering system which is so constructed that it effectually removes the dust from intaken air. The entire filter is automatically sterilized by steam pressure each time the water is sterilized, leaving it free from contaminating organisms which otherwise might find their way into the sterilizer.

TEMPERATURE CONTROL OF PRESSURE STEAM STERILIZERS

Steam sterilization of surgical supplies is the most critical of all surgical sterilization procedures—most subject to failure. The older method as followed in most hospitals today, provides the operator no gauge of the true sterilizing function of the machine other than the pressure, whereas the one factor in which we are interested (temperature) is not measured at all. Pressure, of course, is necessary in order to secure the higher temperatures required, but it by no means follows that adequate temperatures are secured merely by the application of pressure. On the contrary, sterilizer load temperatures can and do vary under the pressure controlled system all the way from slightly higher than room temperatures up to the full possible temperature of the steam. To this fact—the blind use of pressure gauges with no measured regard for temperatures—must be charged many sterilization failures.

We need no longer be handicapped by this obviously faulty system. Modern sterilizers can be made to include provision for measuring the temperature of the applied steam—at the coolest part of the sterilizing chamber. The apparatus to which I refer provides a mercury thermometer, as reliable as our clinical thermometers, in the lower outlet from the chamber in which position it has the marked advantage of indicating the temperature at the coolest location—is thus protective against false indications. This is an important feature because when sterilizers are air clogged—the common cause of failure—variations within the chamber may be very great. The discharge outlet is the coolest point because any air within the chamber will gravitate unfailingly to that point and, of course, reduce the temperature.

This feature is quite easily applicable to old sterilizers and every surgeon is perfectly justified in insisting that this safeguarding feature be provided. It ranks perhaps as the most outstanding improvement in sterilizer design since Pasteur's time.

CHAPTER 6

ANESTHESIA

GENERAL ANESTHESIA

Although at the present time, at least in all hospitals of any size, general anesthesia is induced by specially trained assistants or professional anesthetists—as it should be—it must, nevertheless, be remembered that the surgeon who undertakes to perform an operation is responsible for every phase of it, including the administration and maintenance of anesthesia; also that the emergencies of general surgical practice may demand the carrying out of such procedures by the surgeon himself. Hence, it is necessary and expedient that the surgeon should be thoroughly acquainted with most of the methods of anesthesia in actual practice and be familiar with the practical application of them.

The first and most important question in connection with anesthesia is the safety of the patient, and although there is no known method of inducing general anesthesia that is entirely free from danger, yet the danger differs in degree according to the anesthetic agent used, the amount used and the mode in which it is administered as well as the condition and adaptability of the particular patient. In some diseased conditions certain anesthetic agents are entirely proscribed; in others they must be given with watchfulness; in all cases circumspection and care must be employed, not only because of the physiologic action of the drug used, but because the carrying out of a surgical operation may profoundly change the tolerance of a patient to the action of the drug as well as to anesthesia itself. The actual effect of many drugs used for anesthesia on diseased and healthy tissues is not too well known and although experience may reasonably be relied upon in anticipating results, yet no absolutely definite prediction may be given in any particular case.

PREPARATION OF PATIENT

The respiratory system should be carefully checked in the preparation of the patient for anesthetization. Also, kidney function should be normal because some anesthetics particularly affect the kidneys. Purgatives should be avoided; a mild laxative may be given. Salines dehydrate the patient. Glucose is valuable and helps to combat postoperative acid intoxication.

No solid food should be given for six hours prior to the administration of a general anesthetic. The mouth and throat should be washed out with an antiseptic solution and all foreign substances, such as dental plates, removed. The bladder should be emptied either voluntarily or by catheter. In the case of an emergency operation, the stomach contents may be washed out, if necessary.

INDUCTION

General anesthesia may be induced by the inhalation of gaseous vapor or by the introduction of the anesthetizing agent into the rectum or the vascular system.

The chemical agents commonly used are ether, nitrous oxide, ethyl chloride, ethyl bromide, chloroform (rarely used in America), and the barbiturates. A few other substances have been tried but their use has for various reasons not become general.

The variety of agents and the diversity of methods have made it possible to induce general anesthesia without especially severe danger in almost any condition. For instance, compensated cardiac cases do not contraindicate general anesthesia, particularly if nitrous oxide and oxygen or ethylene be used.

There are four phases or stages in inducing general anesthesia:

1. The first stage ends at the loss of volitional self-control; the higher cortical centers lose their activity; pain sense is lost; the conjunctival reflex is partly abolished.
2. The second stage of anesthesia ends with loss of consciousness.
3. The third stage, or deep anesthesia, ends with muscular relaxation. This is the stage required for major surgical operations.
4. There is a fourth stage to be feared —that of respiratory paralysis, generally due to an overdose of the anesthetic agent.

The pupillary reaction is the most reliable guide to the depth of anesthesia.

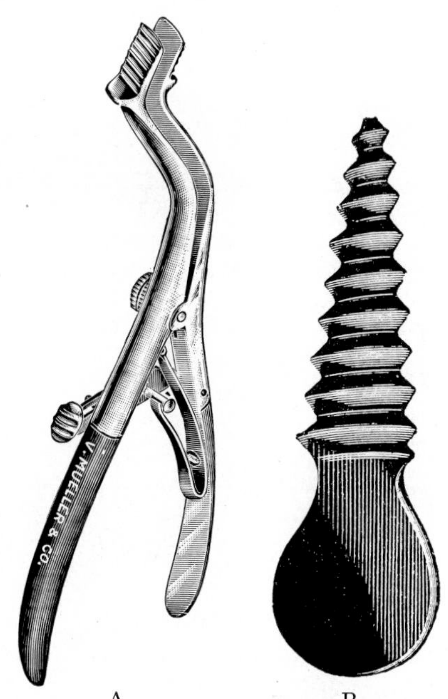

FIG. 37. A. Roser's mouth gag modified by Ream and Bosworth. Large anterior ledge prevents wedge from slipping into mouth; B. oral screw.

Obstruction of the airways may result from:

1. The falling back of the tongue, obstructing the pharynx.
2. The presence of a large amount of saliva, mucus or vomitus in the air passages and back of the throat.
3. Closure of the lips when the nostrils are blocked.
4. Spasm of the larynx,

and this may be remedied by:

1. Forcible opening of the mouth (Fig. 37 [a & b], Fig. 38)
2. Pulling the tongue forward
3. The use of a wire breathing tube (Fig. 39, [a & b]) and
4. Removal of secretions with gauze swabs on forceps. (Fig. 40.)

Cardiac failure may occur as a result of overdosage of the anesthetic used or it may sometimes supervene in the first or excitement phase of light anesthesia, particulary if chloroform is the anesthetic used. Such an emergency is usually associated with (a) a fall in blood pressure, (b) irregular and rapid pulse and (c) pallor. The symptoms are those of impeded or arrested circulation; the jaw drops, the face becomes ashen, the lips are livid, the pupils dilate, there is gasping and finally cessation of respiration. The treatment is:

1. Prompt artificial respiration (Figs. 41, 42, 43, 44, 45),

2. Massage of the heart (Fig. 46) and

3. Intracardiac injection of adrenalin (see chapter on "Surgery of the Chest").

Generally speaking, the patient is under better control in the case of

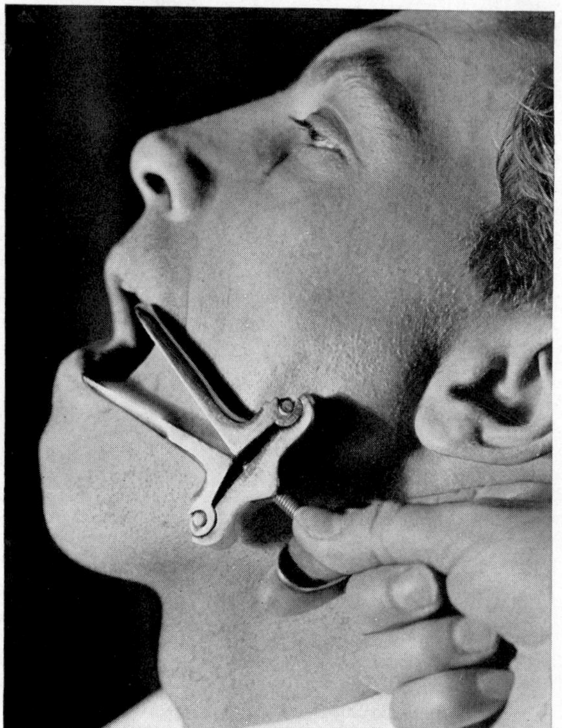

FIG. 38. Forcible opening of mouth with Heister's mouth-gag.

respiratory or cardiac failure with inhalation anesthesia than with rectal anesthesia. Inhalation anesthesia with nitrous oxide or ether is easier to control than chloroform. (In India and other tropical countries chloroform is still used because of the excessive volatility of ether).

All **types of breathing** may be observed during anesthesia from the deep respirations of the strong patient to the feeble breathing of the fragile child.

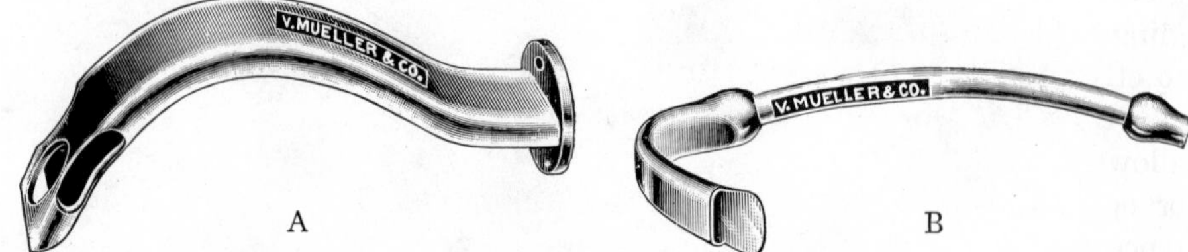

FIG. 39. A. Breathing tube and tongue controller; B. ether vapor tube.

1. Rapid breathing is usually due to nervousness or to the need for more oxygen.

2. Deep breathing usually indicates surgical anesthesia, but if muscular twitching is also present it may denote the presence of asphyxia.

3. Shallow breathing is usually noted when consciousness is lost under light

anesthesia. In deep anesthesia, it may indicate the approach of respiratory paralysis.

Irregular breathing is generally considered to denote impending central respiratory paralysis.

An anesthesia record should be kept and recording done during the operation. Untoward manifestations during anesthesia should be reported to the surgeon at once. The anesthetist should maintain a quiet, cheerful, and confident attitude at all times and should be concerned with nothing but the administration of the anesthetic and the effect thereof on the patient.

Anesthesia may be induced in almost any posture of the patient required by the surgeon, but care should be taken to avoid pressure on nerves as this may result in a pressure-paralysis. This refers particularly to abduction of the arm and unusual positions of the legs; such nerve pressure paralyses are sometimes very painful and persistent.

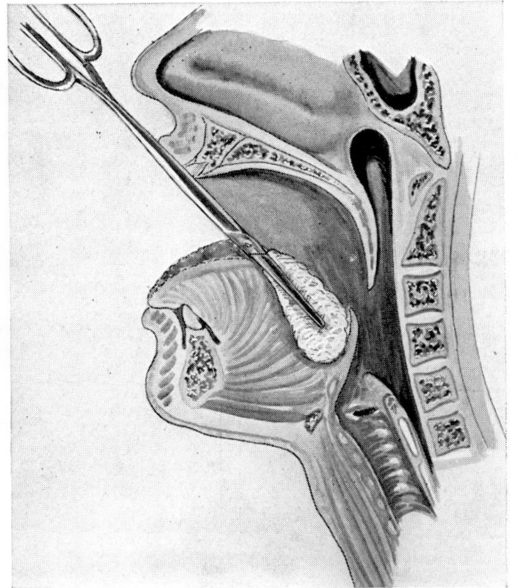

FIG. 40. To relieve obstruction in respiration during anesthesia, Gantermann's manipulation which consists of pressing the base of the tongue forward with a sponge held in the grasp of a forceps is a simple and effectual measure.

ETHER

Ether still is, when expertly administered, and in the absence of contra-indications, the anesthetic par excellence, although in hot climates climatological conditions often force the surgeon to use chloroform.

Ether is less powerful in its anesthetic effects than chloroform but more so than nitrous oxide. It is, therefore, used mostly for a great number of operative procedures. Ether stimulates the heart, the respiratory and circulatory systems. It causes excitation in the first stage, coughing and a great increase in the secretion of saliva and mucus. It does not, so far as is known, give rise to primary heart failure. Aside from the initial excitation and struggling caused in some patients of a nervous disposition, the only serious drawback to ether as a general anesthetic is the fact that its vapor is explosive.

Ether may be administered either by the open or closed method. The first allows the patient plenty of air; the second is a rebreathing method. The first or open method allows an even administration and helps to prevent the occurrence of the so-called ether pneumonia. Prolonged ether administration should be avoided in poor risks (it causes a rise in arterial pressure), in septic cases and in operations upon damaged kidneys.

In operations about the head, the nature of which prevents the use of a cone over the nose and mouth, the intrapharyngeal or intratracheal method of administering, or rather maintaining, ether anesthesia is employed. The initial induction is by the usual inhalation method; a rubber tube is then passed into

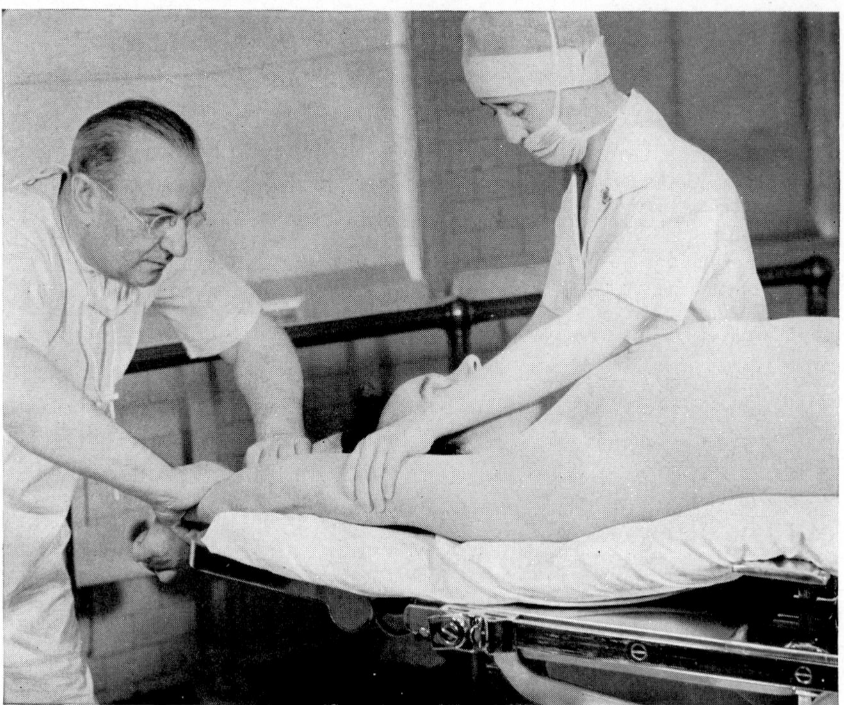

FIG. 41. Sylvester's method of artificial respiration, first movement.

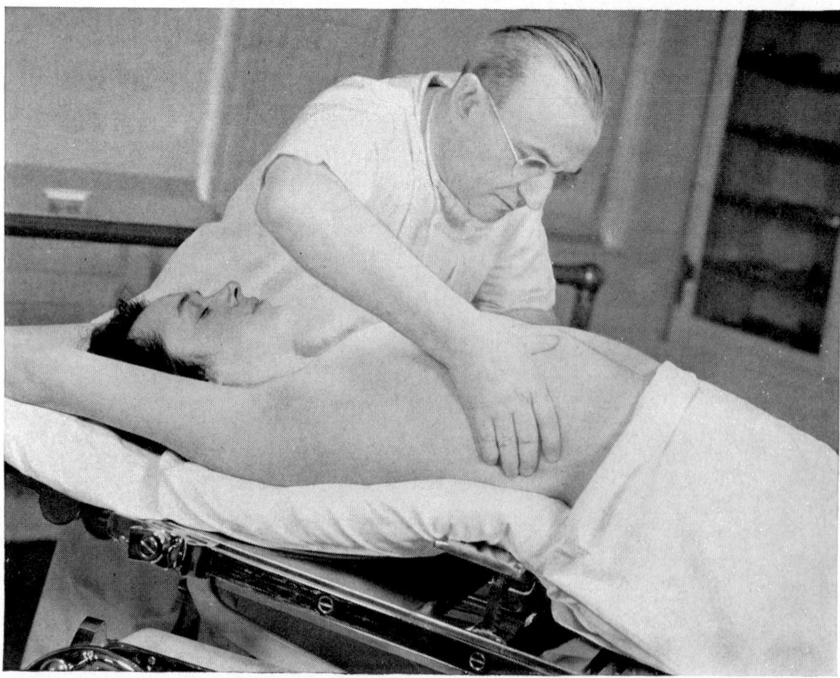

FIG. 42. Sylvester's method of artificial respiration, second movement.

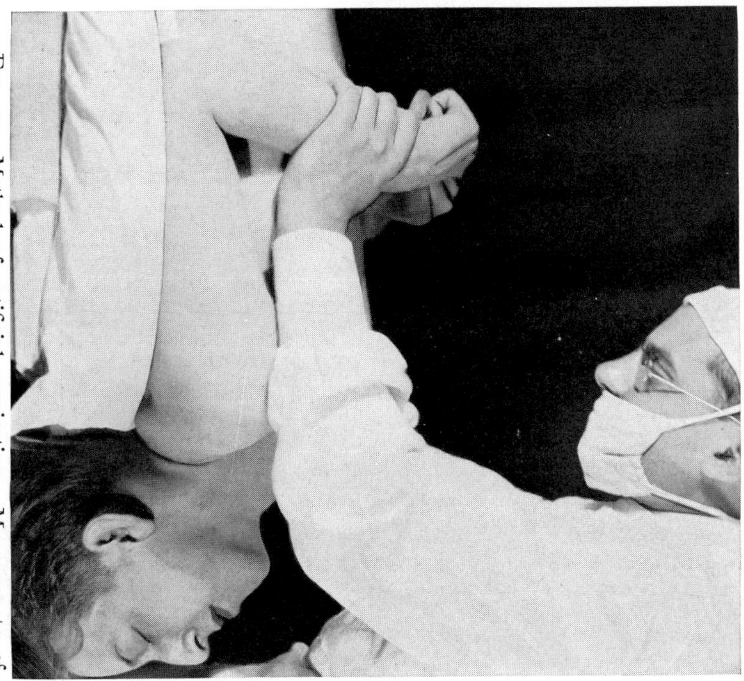

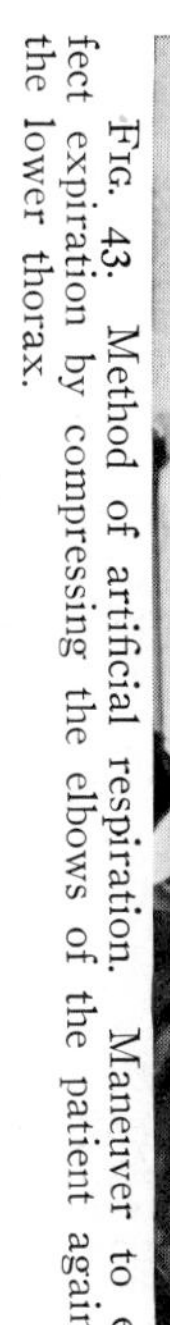

Fig. 43. Method of artificial respiration. Maneuver to effect expiration by compressing the elbows of the patient against the lower thorax.

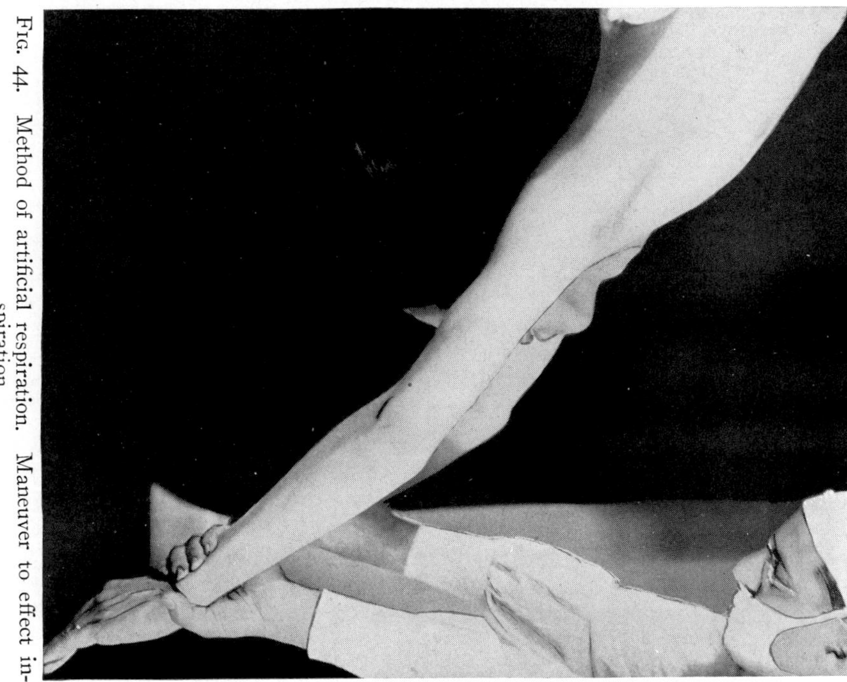

Fig. 44. Method of artificial respiration. Maneuver to effect inspiration.

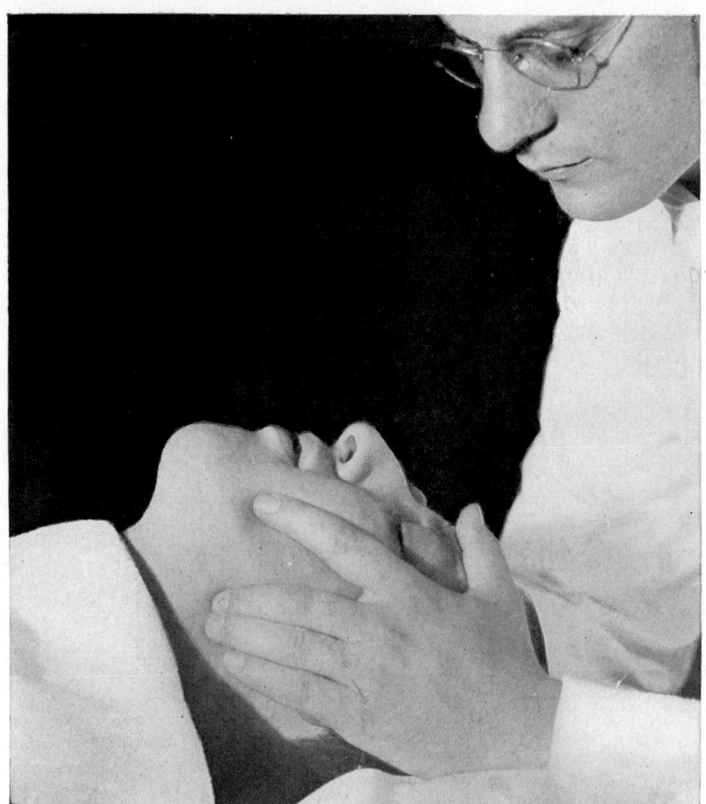

FIG. 45. Method of bringing the jaw forward and with it the base of the tongue when the latter tends to obstruct the air passages during profound anesthesia.

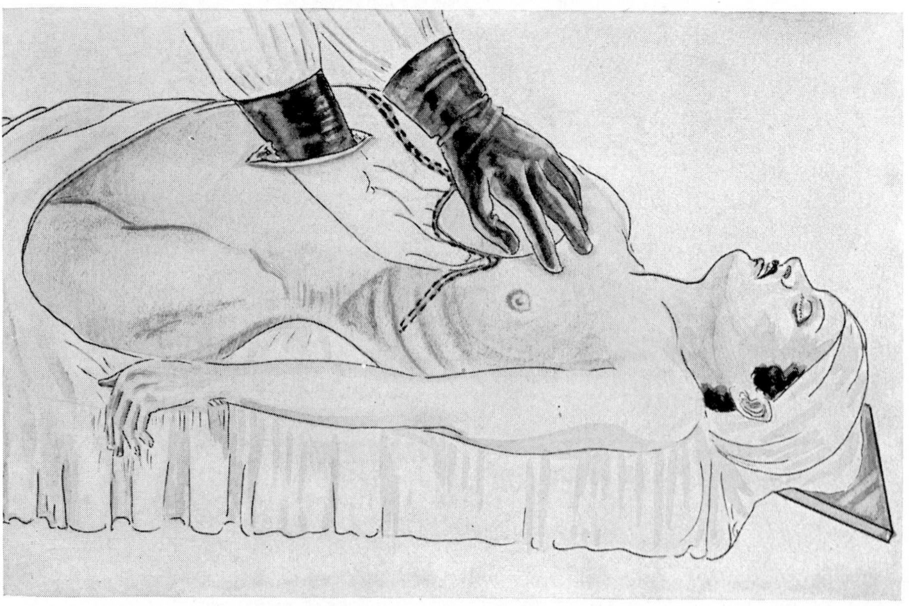

FIG. 46. Bimanual massage of the heart with the hand introduced into the abdomen. The heart is palpated through the diaphragm and pushed upward into the region of the palm of the left hand which is resting on the chest. Rhythmical pressure exerted against the anterior chest wall in cooperation with the hand in the abdomen exerts the necessary movements of massage in the endeavor to bring the heart back to function.

the posterior pharynx or directly into the trachea and the delivery of the ether continued by this means.

The inhalation of ether for surgical anesthesia may thus be accomplished by the

1. Open Method:
   a. Drop Method (a continuous dropping of ether onto gauze stretched over an open mask).
   b. Open Cone Method (pouring small quantities onto an open cone, intermittently).
2. Closed Method: (The vapor is caught in a closed bag when exhaled and rebreathed partially or completely).
3. Vapor Method: (The liquid ether may be converted into vapor and administered into the pharynx or trachea by nasal, mouth, pharyngeal, or intratracheal insufflation).

The necessary paraphernalia for administering ether via the open method consists of a large wire mask (Fig. 47) covered with 10 to 12 layers of gauze. (The several thicknesses of gauze are necessary for the vaporization of ether; if the gauze becomes cold and moist, proper vapor tension cannot be maintained from a small surface.)

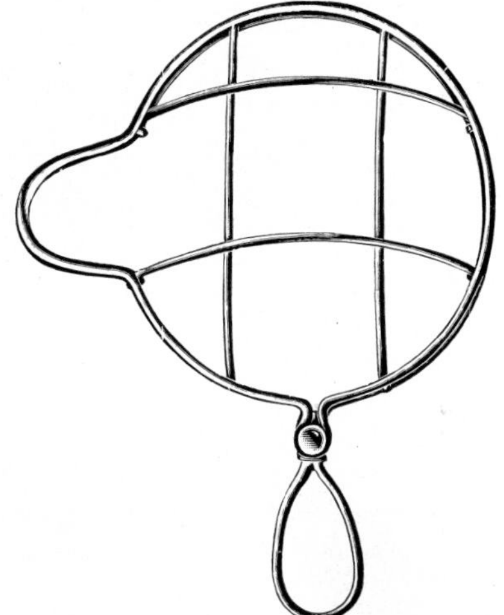

FIG. 47. Ochsner's inhaling mask.

Open Methods of Administering Ether

DROP METHOD

Step 1. Cover the patient's eyes with a pad dampened in boric acid solution and protected by a strip of gutta-percha tissue. Hold the mask loosely in front of the face of the patient and drop a little ether on it so that the patient may become accustomed to the odor. Any pleasant odor which will at first overpower that of ether is advantageous, e.g., such as is obtained by adding a few drops of essence of orange (Gwathmey). (Fig. 48.)

Step 2. Increase the ether dropping gradually (from 1 to 2 drops per second).

Step 3. Place the mask securely against the patient's face. Respirations are noted and the ether dosage governed accordingly; the latter may be gradually increased to 4 drops per second if breathing is smooth and regular. Gradually, after a few minutes the patient passes into a subconscious state.

Step 4. Keep the mask thoroughly saturated with ether.

Comment: Difficulty is likely to be experienced if the early dosage is irritating (coughing, light breathing, or holding of the breath). When the peak of administration is reached, the dosage of ether should be decreased. Just sufficient dropping should be maintained to carry the patient to complete surgical anesthesia for as long as necessary. The level of anesthesia maintained should be neither too light nor too profound.

When administering ether by the drop method to children, the anesthetist should begin with enough dosage to accomplish a state of unconsciousness quickly. Impregnate the mask with ether and place it on the face immediately. The forcible inspirations thus produced will enhance the unconscious state. Encouragement, kindness, but firmness, when needed, are essentials. If the tension becomes marked, lessen the dosage, remove the mask and permit a breath of fresh air. The younger the child the quicker anesthesia will ensue. Obviously, the danger of overdosage is greater in children than in adults.

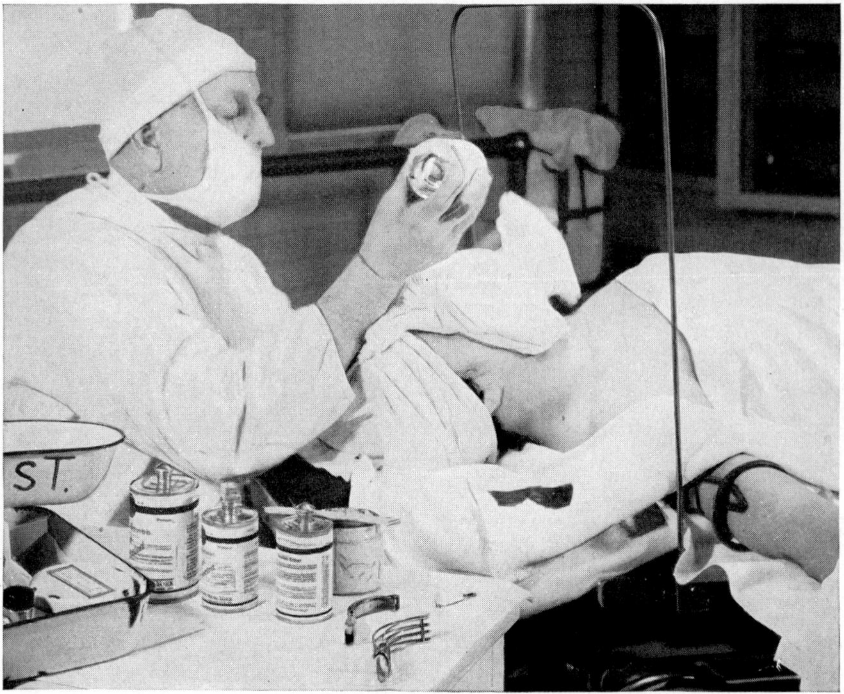

FIG. 48. Drop method of ether.

CONE METHOD

This is usually resorted to in out-of-the-hospital practice.

Step 1. Pour onto the gauze a few drops of ether, then a dram and after about 3 minutes keep the gauze saturated at all times (supplying 2 to 4 drams at a time).

Step 2. Gradually decrease the ether until there is a 5-minute interval between the 2- to 4-dram doses.

Comment: The cone used in this case may be made of folded newspaper, a cuff, or of metal. As a rule, a mask is made of a newspaper cone covered with a towel into which is packed a half-yard of gauze which acts as an ether reservoir. This method is generally used for short emergency operations (reducing fractures, etc.). Its chief disadvantages are where prolonged operation becomes necessary and because irregularity of the state of anesthesia is maintained.

Closed Methods of Administering Ether

A special apparatus is necessary for administering this type of anesthesia.

Step 1. If ether is used alone, partially inflate the breathing bag and pour a few drops of ether into the reservoir.

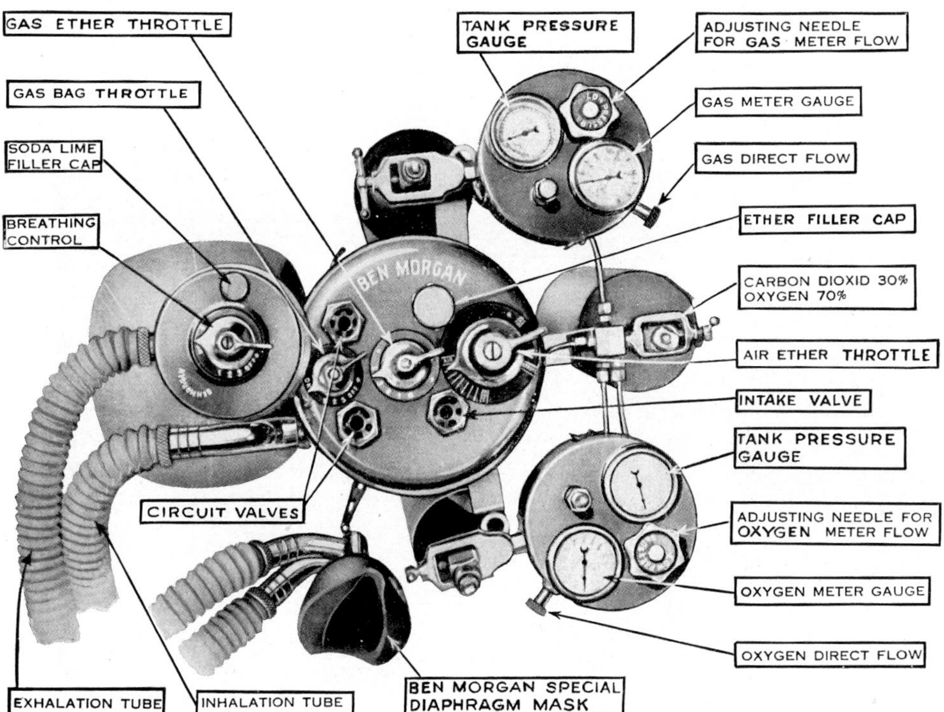

FIG. 49. *Breathing control:* Canister contains soda lime (4-8 mesh) for the removal of the excess carbon dioxide. *Soda lime filler cap:* For emptying and refilling with fresh soda lime. *Gas bag throttle:* Cut-off for gas bag. Controls rebreathing when air-ether is used by turning to numbers 1 for large patients, 2 for medium and 3 for children. Closes or opens the passage to the gas bag and is set at position "ON" during gas or gas-ether anesthesia. *Gas-ether throttle:* When turned to position "E" admits strong ether-vapor into the gas. *Tank pressure gauge:* Indicates amount of gas in tank. *Adjusting needle for gas meter flow:* Wheel when turned to right shows gas meter gauge flow. *Gas meter gauge:* Low pressure indicator. *Gas direct flow:* For adding large quantity of gas when needed. *Ether filler cap:* Remove to pour in ether. *Note:* Ether is removed through stopcock underneath apparatus. *Carbon dioxide 30%—70%:* For stimulating respirations. *Air-ether throttle:* Carburetor control of air-ether dosage. *Intake Valve:* Admits air-ether. Prevents exhaling back through the source of supply. *Tank pressure gauge:* Indicates amount of gas in tank. *Adjusting needle for oxygen meter flow:* Wheel when turned to right shows oxygen meter gauge flow. *Oxygen meter gauge:* Low pressure indicates oxygen flow at gallons per hour. *Oxygen direct flow:* Emergency flow oxygen. *Ben Morgan special diaphragm mask:* The diaphragm lends itself to the contour of the face. *Inhalation tube—exhalation tube—circuit valves*—Circuit breathing necessary when filter method is used.

Step 2. Place the mask on the face lightly and increase the dosage by pouring small quantities of ether at intervals.

Step 3. After a minute or two, open the air vent so that exhaled gases may be renewed. Thus air is refreshed and ether controlled.

Comment: This is the least desirable of any method. The anesthetist must be highly skilled to avoid asphyxia, respiratory difficulties and aspiration of retained mucus and saliva in refractory subjects.

The Ben Morgan Apparatus (Figs. 49, 50, 51) embodies all of the features of modern gas anesthesia apparatus in which gas is given through a soda lime filter entailing a minimal consumption of gas. The gas (ethylene, nitrous oxide or cyclopropane) may be combined with ether in any quantity desired. Carbon dioxide is available and under control of the anesthetist (Figs. 52-53). In addition, the apparatus enables the anesthetist to avail himself of the open drop method through the time-honored mask. The "drop method" thus resorted to definitely controls ether dosage and is controlled by the carburetor principle. Rebreathing is controlled by a cut-off on the rebreathing bag.

VAPOR METHODS

(Intrapharyngeal and Intratracheal Insufflation)

The particular advantages of this procedure are that the dosage of the anesthetic used is more easily controlled and is more uniform than in the methods of administration described. A great deal of body-heat may be saved by moistening the vapor, and most important of all, the bulk of air-vapor mixture may be administered, for instance, into the pharynx, satisfying air needs and relieving respiratory strain, thus preventing partial asphyxia which so often accompanies the usual methods of administration of ether.

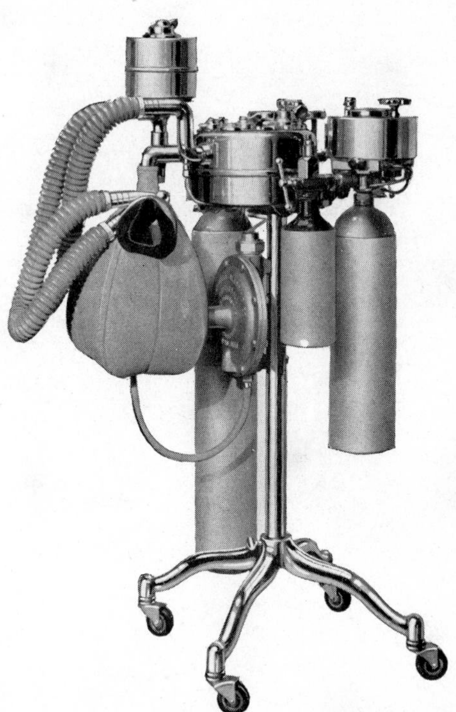

Fig. 50. Ben Morgan anesthesia apparatus, Model K-30.

The unique characteristic of these procedures is that air or oxygen is forced into the lungs or an anesthetic and, if the intratracheal method is used, it is administered intermittently. Care must be taken to avoid overdistension of the lungs causing ruptured air vesicles; pressure should not exceed 30 mm. Hg. An electric vaporizer or foot bellows may be used to deliver air or oxygen into the lungs. Intratracheal insufflation is accomplished with more speed and facility but, unless the anesthetist is skilled, valuable time may be lost while the catheter is being inserted into the trachea; however, its chief objection lies in the fact that air or oxygen is permitted to escape through the mouth or nose or enter the stomach. Adhesive plaster may be used to seal the lips; pressure, together with the nasal tubes, will prevent air escaping in that direction.

BRANOWER'S INTRAPHARYNGEAL INSUFFLATION ANESTHESIA

(Fig. 54)

The expensive, complicated and rather cumbersome negative and positive pressure chambers of Sauerbruch and Meyer have been largely supplanted by the

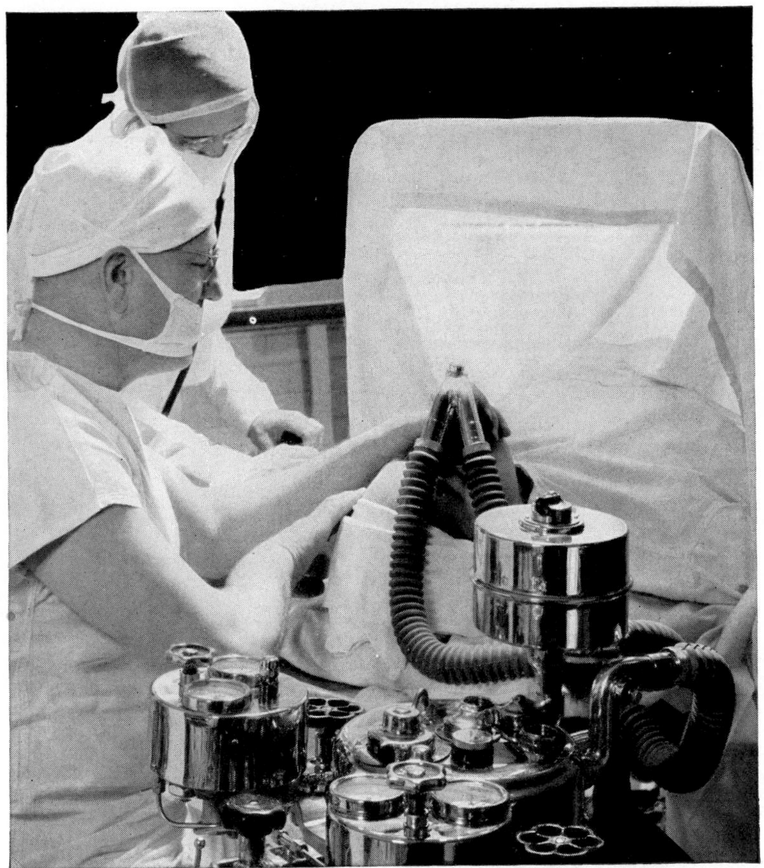

Fig. 51. Ben Morgan apparatus in use.

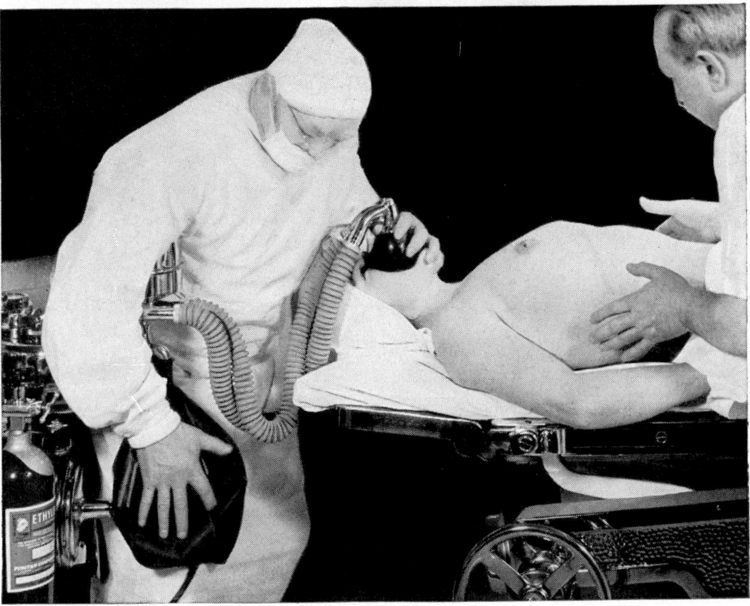

Fig. 52. Method of administering carbon dioxide. Step 1. Inhalation.

simpler forms of apparatus for maintaining a constant positive pressure either by intratracheal or intrapharyngeal means. The Meltzer-Auer method of intratracheal insufflation was one of the outstanding achievements in the steady progress of thoracic surgery. One of the drawbacks to this form of maintaining pressure is that it inflates not only the lung on the operative side, but also the normal lung and, therefore, is prone to cause embarrassment to the surgeon by crowding the mediastinum and the operative field. Pharyngeal pressure assures a constant supply of air at a low pressure which results in quiet breathing

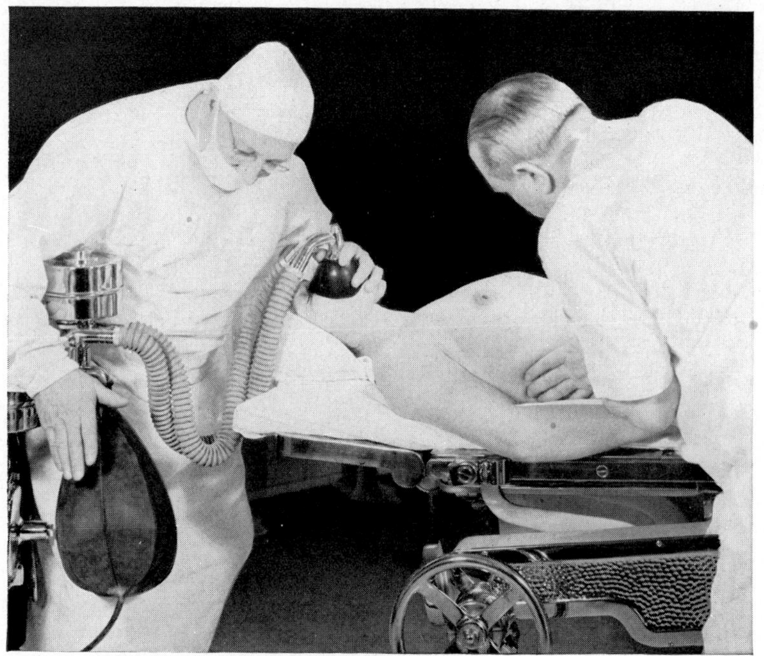

FIG. 53. Method of administering carbon dioxide. Step 2. Exhalation aided by compression of the lower thorax.

throughout the operation but which in addition, enables the anesthetist to increase or decrease the pressure at will, according to the requirements of the moment. The Branower method requires no mask and allows the anesthetist to observe the face of the patient at all times. The equipment consists essentially of the following:

1. A foot bellows, which provides a sufficient supply of air which is conducted through a tube into a rubber reservoir where the pressure is equalized. From the reservoir the air flows directly into the tube leading to an air filter.
2. The air filter is composed of many layers of moist gauze through which the air flows to
3. A three-way valve which is constructed in a way which permits the anesthetist to insufflate any volume of air combined with the anesthetic or air not combined with the anesthetic or to deflate the lungs by diverting all air from the patient.

4. The ether bottle connected on one side to the air filter and on the other to the
5. Metal nasal tube consisting of a piece of brass tubing 4 inches long having a lumen 3/16 inch in diameter. This tube is connected by its distal end with a piece of rubber tubing, the lumen of which varies 3/16 to 1/8 inch in diameter, depending upon the requirements of the patient.

Technic.

Step 1. Induce anesthesia by the ordinary inhalation method.

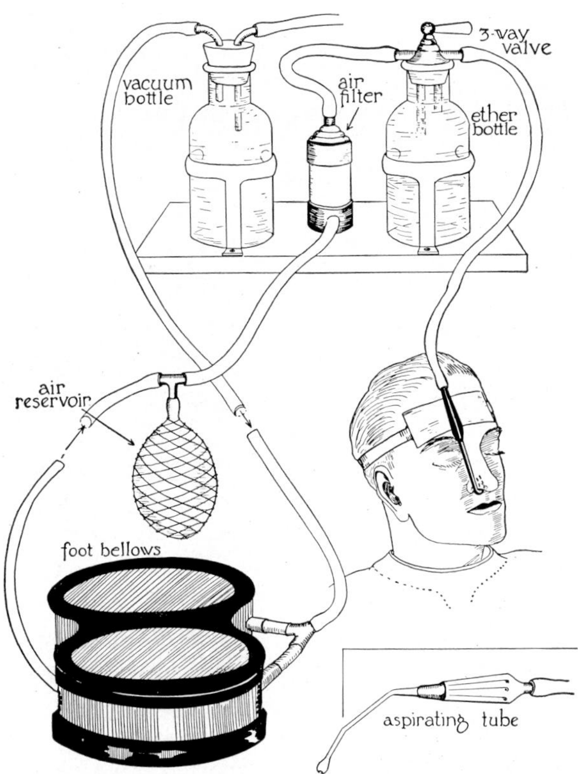

Fig. 54. Branower's intrapharyngeal insufflation anesthesia.

Step 2. Apply vaseline to the free end of the rubber nasal tube and insert it through a nostril into the pharynx.

Step 3. Connect the proximal end of the rubber tube with the metal nasal tube which connects the former with the insufflation apparatus. Insufflation is begun by using the foot bellows. Continue pumping-motions of the foot at the rate of 60 to 90 per minute.

Step 4. Where it is desirable to inflate the lung, increase the pumping motions and occlude the free nostril. Be careful to see that the three-way valve is placed so as to permit the entrance of air only.

PHARYNGEAL INSUFFLATION ANESTHESIA

This method is practically on a par with endotracheal insufflation and is considered superior to face mask delivery of ether. Its chief advantages are the same as those of endotracheal insufflation, viz., existing obstruction of the upper air passages is overcome by a tidal bulk which is delivered behind and below the base of the tongue; mucus, saliva and blood is thrust outward by an air stream, thus minimizing "ether pneumonia"; and the anesthesia is even and full.

Technic. Use the same air pressure and vapor apparatus as for endotracheal insufflation. A metallic Y-forked tube, shaped to fit the nose and forehead, is used as a delivery device. Each fork is equipped with an Nr. 18 F. soft rubber catheter about 13 cm. long with double or multiple eyelets. (Fig. 55.)

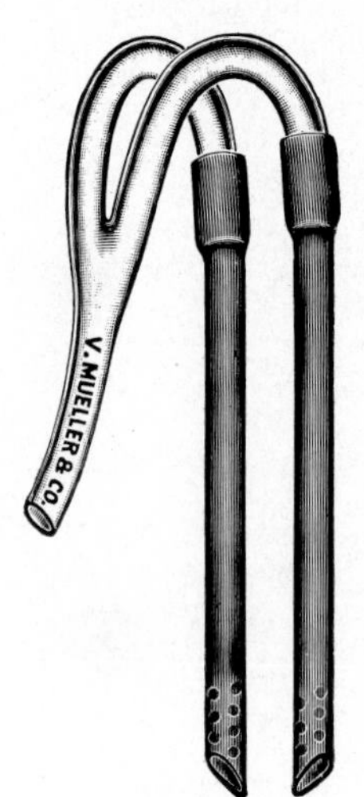

Fig. 55. Israel's double suction tube for use through the nose.

Step 1. Induce anesthesia in the usual way; if ether is employed insufflation is not started for 9 or 12 minutes.

Step 2. Lubricate the catheters. Tilt the nose upward and introduce a catheter into each nostril along the inferior strait of the nasal chamber directing the catheter toward the pharynx. If one nostril is obstructed introduce both catheters in the other; if both are obstructed, introduce the catheters into the mouth. Insertion is continued until the eyelet of the catheter lies at the level of the epiglottis (about 12 cm.).

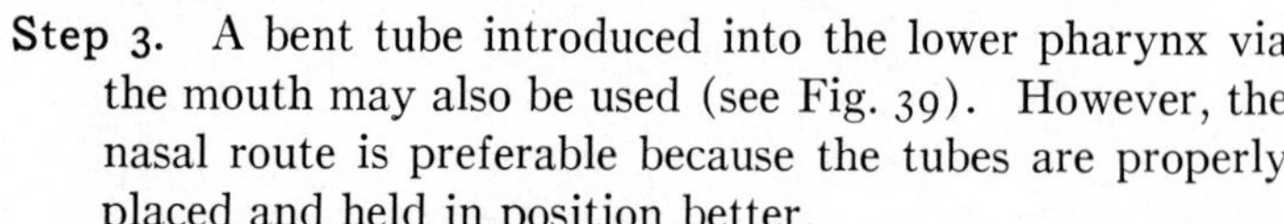

Step 3. A bent tube introduced into the lower pharynx via the mouth may also be used (see Fig. 39). However, the nasal route is preferable because the tubes are properly placed and held in position better.

The amount of anesthetic agent administered should be sufficient to meet the needs of each inspiration without extraneous dilution. Insufflation of about 18 liters per minute usually suffices though it may be lowered or raised according to the needs of the patient.

INTRATRACHEAL INSUFFLATION

Intratracheal insufflation consists of the introduction of ether vapor into the trachea at a point close to its bifurcation. One long tube is used to deliver the ether past the vocal cords and upper air passages where respiratory obstruction is most likely to take place.

Inspiration is made easy for the patient by the introduction of the vapor under pressure directly into the trachea. A tube, of much smaller diameter than the glottis, provides for expiration and for the escape of any excess vapor. "Instead[1] of concentrated ether vapor, diluted with atmospheric air, a volume of vapor sufficient for all the respiratory needs of the patient is given. This volume, under sufficient pressure, is such that even during the inspiration, with the glottis but partially obstructed by the tube, no atmospheric air will enter; there will be no inward flow at any time into the trachea along the sides of the tube. On the contrary, there should be a constant flow to the outside. This flow will naturally be less at the time of inspiration but it will never altogether cease except when the delivery is cut off. Since the lungs do contract at regular intervals during normal respiration, this action should be stimulated by frequently releasing the positive pressure."

[1] Flagg, Palul, Anesthesia, J. B. Lippincott Co., 1932.

The necessary apparatus consists of Connell's anesthetometer, an intratracheal catheter, a laryngoscope and mouth prop. (Figs. 56, 57, 58, 59.)

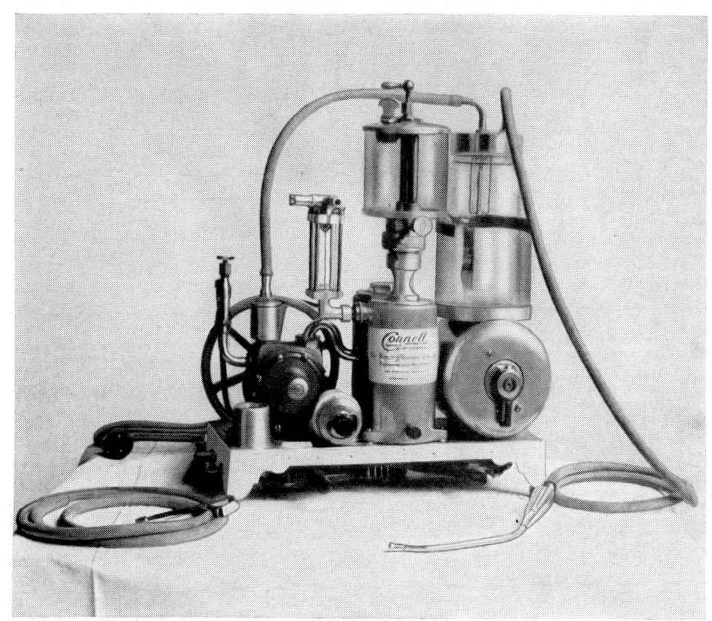

FIG. 56. The Connell insufflation suction apparatus. (Flagg's Anesthesia, J. B. Lippincott Company.)

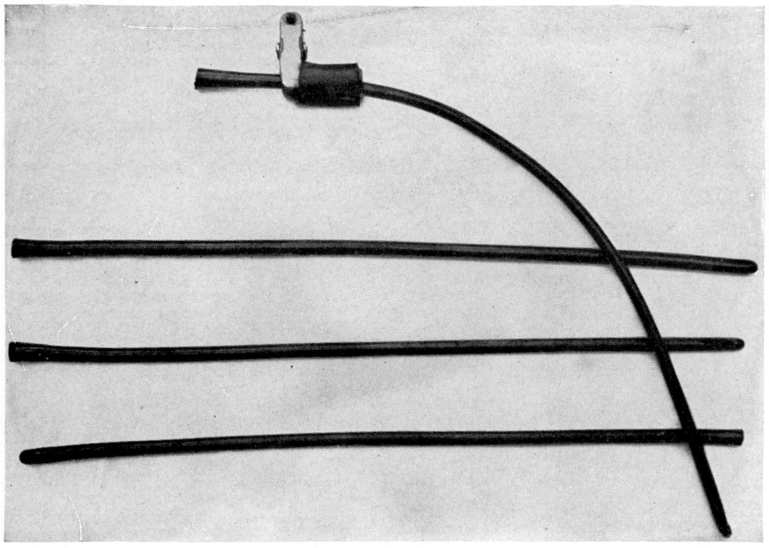

FIG. 57. Intratracheal catheter and special mouth prop. (Flagg's Anesthesia, J. B. Lippincott Company.)

Technic

Step 1. Place 6 silk-wound urethral catheters marked off 10½ inches from the tip, in a container of ice-water.

Step 2. Make sure that the anesthetometer is delivering 50 mm. of vapor ten-

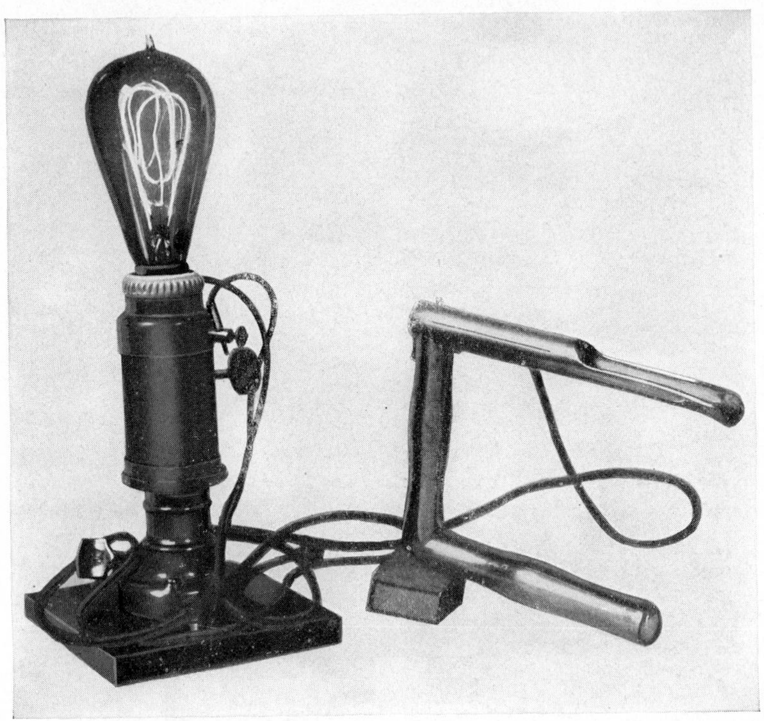

FIG. 58. Jackson laryngoscope and rheostat. (Flagg's Anesthesia, J. B. Lippincott Company.)

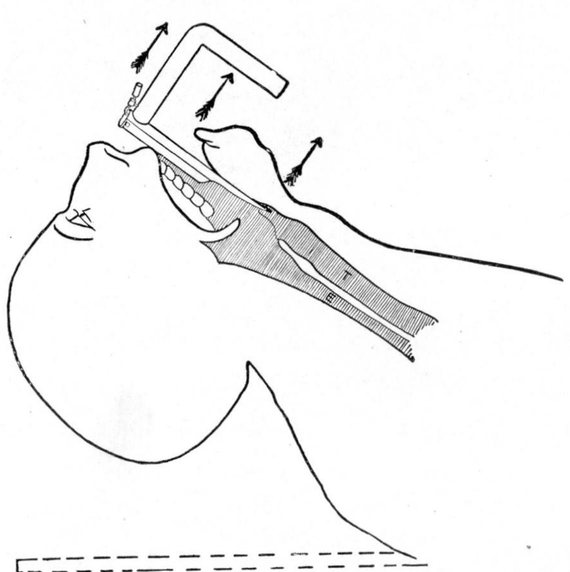

FIG. 59. Schema illustrating the most important point in the exposure of the larynx with the direct laryngoscope, namely, the lifting of the patient's head off the table with the instrument, in the direction of the three darts. The usual fault is prying with the upper teeth as a fulcrum instead of lifting. (Flagg's Anesthesia, J. B. Lippincott Company.)

sion, that the emergency gauge is working and regulate the pressure so that it remains between 18 and 20 mm. of mercury. Have the foot bellows at hand and see that the light in the laryngoscope is working.

Step 3. Induce anesthesia either by the semi-open or closed drop method. Do not attempt intubation before anesthetizing the larynx.

Step 4. After the patient is anesthetized and reclining flat on his back, grasp the head, extending it so that the chin forms almost a straight line with the sternum and neck. Grasp the laryngoscope in the left hand and slip it over the upper part of the tongue exposing the epiglottis. Slip the lip of the instrument over the epiglottis and raise the tongue and attached muscles (Fig. 59).

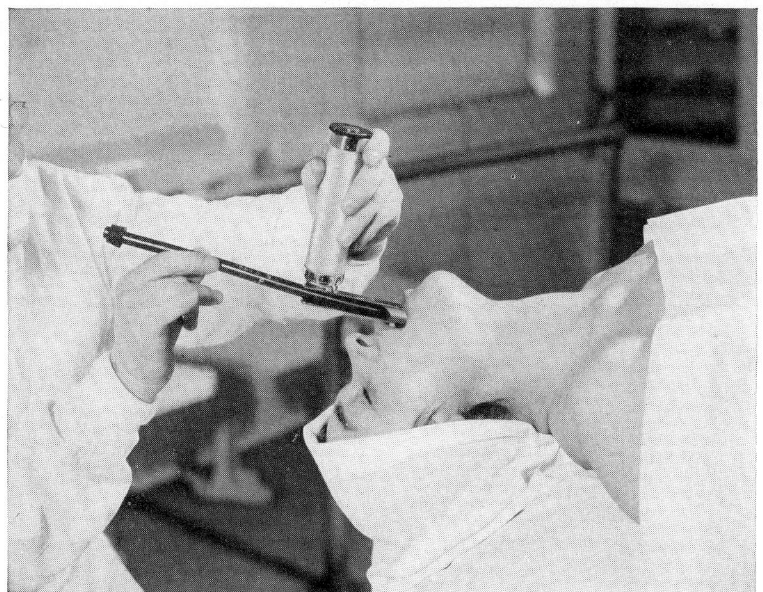

Fig. 60. Intratracheal insufflation anesthesia.

Step 5. While holding the laryngoscope in the left hand, grasp a proper-sized catheter in the right hand and slip it through the laryngoscope into the glottis up to the 10½ inch mark. Hissing of air will follow and the patient may cough; however, normal breathing is quickly resumed. A hissing sound emitted when the catheter is placed in position assures the surgeon that it has been properly placed. If it is not heard, it is likely that the tube has slipped into the esophagus.

Step 6. Place the mouth prop in position, insert the delivery tube and connect the machine. From this point the procedure is much the same as that followed during intrapharyngeal anesthesia except that the flow is interrupted two, three or four times a minute by pinching the tube. Maintenance is ideal, if the agent is properly administered.

Step 7. Quick recovery takes place when the valve is turned to pure air, thus expelling all ether from the lungs. Detach the tube, permitting the patient to breathe through the catheter for a few minutes thus preventing a slight acapnia. Postoperative illness is very rare; the vocal cords are seldom injured by the catheters. There is no need to worry over pulmonary complications.

IMPROVED TECHNIC FOR INTRATRACHEAL ANESTHESIA

The apparatus for the administration of intratracheal anesthesia has been improved greatly during recent years. **Flagg** states that when Magill of London introduced his two-way catheter holder it occurred to him that one tube which would enable the patient to breathe easily would be a welcome innovation.

Three different sizes of inhalation tubes are now furnished with Flagg's intratracheal inhalation apparatus (Fig. 60-61) which are designed to fit men, women and infants. By using this instrument the surgeon is able to apply the principles of bronchoscopy and is assisted by the relaxation and control of the reflexes.

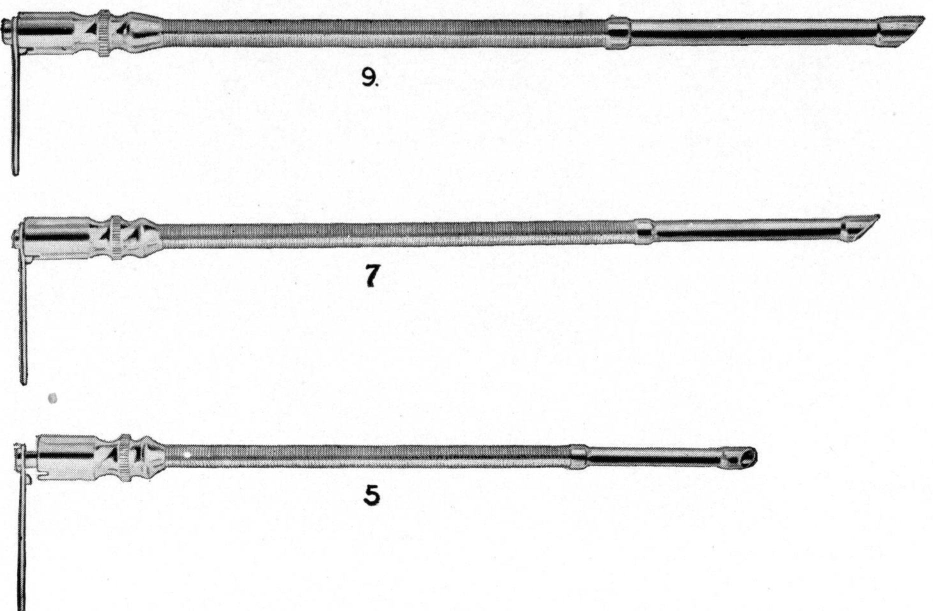

FIG. 61. Flagg intratracheal inhalation tube. (Flagg's Anesthesia, J. B. Lippincott Company.)

The **Flagg apparatus** is composed of a rigid and a flexible portion. The rigid part is long enough so that the tube is self-retaining when the patient's head is bent; it may be extubated by extending the head. The instrument is chrome-plated with a non-rusting spring. The flexible section is protected by Penrose tubing which is replaced when necessary. The tube may be utilized in administering ether from the container or nitrous oxide with oxygen and ethylene from a gas machine.

At the same time that Flagg was improving the intratracheal inhalation tube, he was also working on a laryngoscope which was composed of a blade, a hollow handle and dry batteries (Fig. 62). The lights are durable and the dry batteries may be easily replenished; thus the flashlight idea replaced the insufflation and inhalation technic, except in chest surgery. The apparatus is easily transported, tends to improve the relaxation of the patient and gives a better view of the glottis in the absence of morphine and atropine. Suction should be instituted preceding, during and succeeding intubation and extubation. A No. 14 French catheter is of aid here.

Intubation Technic.

Step 1. Administer gas or ether until the patient is completely relaxed. Have the intratracheal tube, connecting tube and laryngoscope, all sterilized, at hand.

Step 2. Remove the inhaler and pharyngeal tube. Practice suction of the pharynx. Extend the patient's head. Grasp the laryngoscope in the left hand.

Step 3. Separate the lips and teeth of the patient with the fingers and direct the laryngoscope over the tongue. Expose the epiglottis. Insert the tip of the laryngoscope beyond the epiglottis, lift up the tongue and expose the larynx.

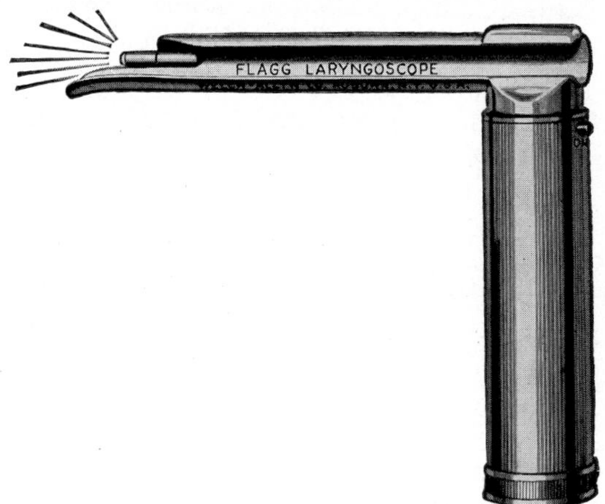

FIG. 62. Flagg laryngoscope. (Flagg's Anesthesia, J. B. Lippincott Company.)

Step 4. Carefully introduce the intratracheal tube between the vocal cords; inhalation will separate the cords in case of spasm. Remove the stylet from the intratracheal tube, remove the laryngoscope and bend the patient's head. The patient will now breathe easily through the tube. Connect a tube to the anesthesia container.

Step 5. If the operation does not include the mouth, pack a strip of gauze saturated with albolene into the pharynx. The use of a mouth-gag and a lubricant on the tip of the tube often facilitates the procedure.

Comment: The larynx is less likely to be injured when exposed under anesthesia than while the patient is conscious. The muscular relaxation which follows permits one size of the instrument to be used on all patients. The use of an anesthetic permits the surgeon to be more deliberate in the steps of intubation and thus serves as a safety measure. An intratracheal tube which fits easily into the larynx is more satisfactory than one which fits too snugly.

Blood, mucus or fluid passing down the sides of the tube are soon detected by the respiratory sounds. Full etherization will prevent respiratory spasm. The following practical hints have been garnered from Flagg's excellent work on anesthesia.

Increase the depth of the anesthesia if continued spasm of the vocal cords ensues. Respiratory spasm may be due to the heat of the freshly sterilized instruments or to other causes but is not alarming if the color and pulse of the patient are satisfactory. Breathing or blowing oxygen through the intratracheal tube may relieve spasm.

Removable dentures should not be left in place during this procedure. The laryngoscope is likely to break porcelain crowns as well as caps. To prevent postoperative tenderness of the pharynx, apply oiled gauze over the tongue and take plenty of time to pack the dry gauze.

If the patient coughs persistently, withdraw the tube one or two inches. In some instances the airways may be obstructed even though the tube is apparently properly placed. In such cases it may be withdrawn too far with the patient's head extended or the rubber covering may have split permitting air to escape from the side of the tube. If the patient seems to be breathing through the mouth while the tube is in place, it is an indication that the tube is too small and that a larger one should be substituted.

If the trachea emits a quantity of blood or mucus upon suction, the tube is probably too small and the pack in the pharynx displaced. This may also be caused by a defect in the rubber cover or to the catheter having been left in the tube too long.

If extubation is difficult, administer anesthesia.

The tube is in the esophagus if the patient breathes quietly with little air coming through the tube. A dry tube introduced during spasm of the vocal cords is likely to result in injury to the mucous membrane. Extubation should be aided by lifting the rigid portion of the instrument upward with the finger tips, out of the mouth.

Intratracheal anesthesia eliminates the necessity for apparatus designed to warm and heat the anesthetic vapor. It keeps the field of operation free from exsufflated vapor, as well as anesthetic.

Normal respiration is maintained and the carbon dioxide supply is conserved; blood and foreign matter are excluded. Light anesthesia may be employed and artificial respiration controlled by simple methods. It makes possible the anesthetization through the nose and throat by ether, gas, oxygen, ethylene, etc. The trachea is protected from external pressure. A light ether anesthesia makes possible a field of operation similar to that produced by chloroform and protects against blood aspiration. It also affords an aseptic field for plastic operations on the face.

The chief advantages of this method are: it prevents lung collapse during intrathoracic operations; it is specifically indicated for intra-oral operations (excision of the tongue, lower jaw and cleft palate operations); for operations on the head, neck, trachea and larynx; in emergency operations for intestinal obstructions where vomitus may collect in the upper air passages, etc. The return flow of air causes blood, clots, secretions and infectious material to be expelled thus diminishing the danger from pulmonary infections.

On the other hand, the disadvantages are: a special, detailed knowledge of the technic is absolutely essential; expensive and complex equipment is necessary; deep anesthesia must be induced before introduction of the tube by the novice; intubation by direct vision is necessary; and the intratracheal tube is present in the mouth.

CHLOROFORM

Any degree of anesthesia from analgesia to deep narcosis may be produced by the inhalation of chloroform. It has the advantage that it is easily administered, requires no elaborate apparatus, does not carry with it the danger of explosion and is perhaps the pleasantest method for the patient. On the other hand, deep narcosis by chloroform may have severe effects on the system, namely, chloroform poisoning, expressed particularly by edema and necrosis of the liver with dilatation and diminution of the power of the heart. Unlike ether, chloroform does not irritate the respiratory passages. Its use should not be forced in the case of struggling children. It is contra-indicated in the case of patients in shock or when shock is likely to be produced by the operation; also in alcoholics or in patients with septic intoxication or in acetonuria. Chloroform is not as suitable for very lengthy operations as are other anesthetic agents.

ANESTHETIC MIXTURES

The so-called "A. C. E." mixtures which consist of one part alcohol, two parts chloroform and three parts ether, or some modification of this formula, have been very popular in Europe, the object being to counteract any tendency to circulatory depression from a too-concentrated chloroform vapor. The chief objection to this mixture is that the ingredients do not vaporize at the same rate, the more volatile agent vaporizing first. The results of this method are similar to those of chloroform.

Although perhaps less dangerous than chloroform alone, the accidents attributed to the use of these mixtures are numerous and they are less safe than ether alone. Grégoire is partial to Schleich's inhalation anesthetic mixture administered through an Ombrédanne apparatus.

ETHYL CHLORIDE

The inhalation of ethyl chloride causes a very rapid loss of consciousness without excitation. Hence, it may be used on account of its rapid effect before the induction of general anesthesia by ether and this perhaps is its greatest indication. It is only suitable for short operations because the margin of safety between the stage of surgical anesthesia and a lethal dose is rather small. It depresses the circulation; the patient's color does not change, as a rule, hence there is no warning sign of approaching danger.

Many surgeons believe that the use of ethyl chloride is as dangerous as that of chloroform and its mortality rate is high. Death from this anesthetic agent is due to respiratory failure which precedes cardiac failure. In any case, its use is likely to be followed by headache, nausea and vomiting to an excessive degree, in some cases.

Ethyl bromide has the same physical effects as ethyl chloride and is used as an anesthetic agent to a limited degree. Many believe it to be more objectionable than the chloride. **Both the chloride and bromide are inflammable.**

NITROUS OXIDE

Nitrous oxide gas, with or without oxygen, is the anesthetic of choice for short surgical operations which necessitate general anesthesia. It has all the advantages but fewer disadvantages than ethyl chloride. There is rapid loss of consciousness and rapid reawakening with fewer after effects. It is not very suitable for children but it can be used for cardiac patients or for patients suffering from acute infections. It does not give as much muscular relaxation as ether and when this is necessary its use may have to be supplemented by ether vapor. Patients whose respiration is not too good or whose cardiac action is affected should get plenty of oxygen with the nitrous oxide. The objection to nitrous oxide and oxygen anesthesia is that it requires a cumbersome apparatus and generally must be administered by one specially trained in its technic, yet it is worth the expense and trouble. Its use is coming gradually but surely to the fore in major surgical procedures.

The special features of gas anesthesia are the steady deepening of respirations and the dusky cyanosed look of the face; the pupils dilate, the eyeballs roll, and the conjunctival reflex is lost.

In the hands of an expert anesthetist, I prefer nitrous oxide-oxygen for goiter operations and other procedures about the head and neck. In surgery of the thorax and abdomen, ethylene anesthesia, properly administered, has served me well.

Many patients have an exaggerated dread of anesthesia and the anticipation of passing through the ordeal fills them with fear, restlessness and anxiety which very often interferes with the easy induction of anesthesia. Within recent years many methods have been devised to overcome this condition by the use of medicaments termed pre-anesthetics. These generally are alkaloidal sedatives which allay the apprehension of nervous patients, make induction of anesthesia easier and make it possible to maintain anesthesia with a smaller amount of the anesthetizing agent than is ordinarily employed. The patient is in a semi-conscious condition when the anesthetic is administered and since the drowsy effect of the pre-anesthetic lasts much longer than that of the anesthetic, the patient remains asleep much longer than usual. The disadvantages of pre-anesthetics are generally that their use abolishes certain eye reflexes which inform the surgeon or anesthetist of the progress of anesthesia. The safety of the patient, which has already been mentioned, is the first requisite of anesthesia. Postoperative nausea and vomiting are frequently increased. Yet, in selected cases I am very partial to scopolamine-morphine administered about an hour before the patient is taken to the operating room (see scopolamine-morphine anesthesia, p. 80).

BASAL ANESTHETICS

Hypnotics derived from urea and alcohol which are used for pre-operative medication as well as the anesthetic agent per se are termed basal anesthetics.

Salts of barbituric acid are the most important urea derivatives in popular use. Phenobarbital, allonal and barbital are used mostly as sedatives. Sodium amytal is considered useful as a hypnotic, analgesic and anesthetic. The intravenous injection of the barbiturates disturbs the colloidal equilibrium of the blood; they should be administered orally. The only advantage of the intravenous injection over the oral use is rapidity of action.

The barbiturates do not affect the heart and liver; they produce little toxicity, but they may be responsible for a mild form of hysteria. The special advantages gained from using barbiturates are that induction of anesthesia is rather smooth, relaxation of the patient may be obtained sooner, gas anesthesia is more effective and the patient may be prepared sooner. The chief objections to their use are that reflex excitability is increased; respiratory interference is likely to accompany their use; complete anesthesia is almost impossible to attain and the interval during which it is effective is too brief for satisfactory surgery. There seems to be no satisfactory antidote to use in case of an overdose. It is not reliable unless used in conjunction with scopolamine or morphine. For surgery, therefore, its use is limited.

Sodium Amytal

This is marketed in three-grain capsules. One capsule is usually given to the patient the night before the operation and two or three capsules are given a couple of hours preceding the time for which the operation is scheduled. The patient goes to the operating room in a somnolent condition offering no resistance to the anesthesia.

Pernocton

Pernocton is slower in action than sodium amytal; its effects last longer. Large doses of pernocton are not free from danger; it is recommended only for hypnosis; the amount required to produce this effect is quite safe.

Avertin

Avertin (tribromethyl alcohol) is used quite extensively as a basal anesthetic. It was introduced by Willstaetter and Duisberg of Germany in 1928.

Avertin is packed in 25 and 100 cc. containers after it has been dissolved in amylene hydrate. It crystallizes in distilled water at a low temperature. At 104° F. it decomposes into hydrobromic acid and dibromacetaldehyde; the latter is an irritant which may cause necrosis of the bowel. The dose varies from .06 to 0.1 cc. (60 to 100 mg.) to a kilogram; the maximum dose as a basal anesthetic is 0.1 cc. per kilo (2.2 lbs.) of body weight.

The equipment necessary for administering this drug consists of an empty container with a stopper which will hold 500 cc., a container of distilled water, a thermometer, a pipette marked in ccs., a small rectal tube equipped with a funnel, lubricant, avertin solution, Congo red, a dropper and a glass receptacle for testing purposes.

Step 1. Weigh the patient and determine the dosage by calculating his weight in relation to the drug.

Step 2. Heat the distilled water to 40° C., add the avertin solution; shake well.

Step 3. Test one or two cc. with Congo red; a satisfactory solution is indicated by an orange color.

Step 4. Inject the solution slowly while the patient is lying on the left side. Note the blood pressure and time of injection.

The usual reaction from the patient takes place in 5 to 10 minutes after the drug has been administered. Usually, a feeling of drowsiness is quickly followed by a deep sleep (in rare instances the patient becomes excited during the administration of avertin necessitating the prompt administration of a general anesthetic). Complete relaxation now follows; a pharyngeal tube may be inserted and in some instances an exposure of the larynx may be obtained. The patient is prepared and if no response is elicited when the towel clamps are applied, the incision may be made. Nitrous oxide or ether may now be administered to complete the anesthesia. The surgeon should always be prepared to do a laryngoscopy and intubation.

After several hours the patient regains consciousness in a very satisfactory manner but until then should be watched for symptoms of approaching asphyxiation.

The use of avertin is not advisable in operations which involve the airways owing to the possibility of postoperative obstruction. Killian reports that avertin does more injury to the respiratory center than either chloroform or ether and that it affects the liver in the same manner as does chloroform.

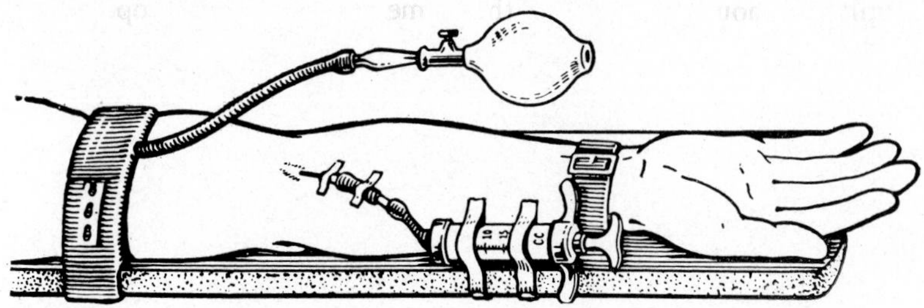

FIG. 63. Dickson Wright's splint for use in evipan anesthesia and other intravenous injections. (Hamilton Bailey, Emergency Surgery, John Wright and Sons, Ltd., Bristol.)

The chief advantages of this drug lie in the fact that it reduces mental shock as well as irritation to the respiratory passages. It does not cause as much vomiting as do ether or chloroform and makes postoperative medication unnecessary due to the extended period of unconsciousness.

The chief objections to its use are its high mortality, depression of the respiratory and circulatory centers, acidosis, muscular rigidity, the necessity of constant watchful nursing until the patient regains consciousness and the usual disadvantages of synergistic anesthesia.

Comment. It is a matter of controversy whether or not the reduced quantity of gas-oxygen or ether necessary when used in conjunction with avertin compensates for the disadvantages offered by the drug. Its power to induce anesthesia without the knowledge of the patient as well as its use in acute pulmonary conditions which do not involve the airways are very valuable.

The routine use of avertin or the barbiturates as a preanesthetic is not advocated. Their inconstant action renders their use unsafe in many operations.

Evipan Anesthesia

Evipan sodium is a preparation of barbituric acid which disintegrates speedily after it is administered. It is marketed in powder form in ampules which are accompanied by ampules of distilled water in which the powder is dissolved preparatory to injection. It is injected in the arm of the patient as shown in Figs. 63, 64 at the rate of 1 cc. in fifteen seconds; about 3 cc. is usually sufficient for a dose. The judgment of the anesthetist must dictate the dose required for a given case. Dickson Wright's splint is of value in administering this anesthetic.

Comment: Evipan anesthesia induces a short, safe period of analgesia which is very desirable in brief operations such as reducing fractures, opening abscesses, etc.

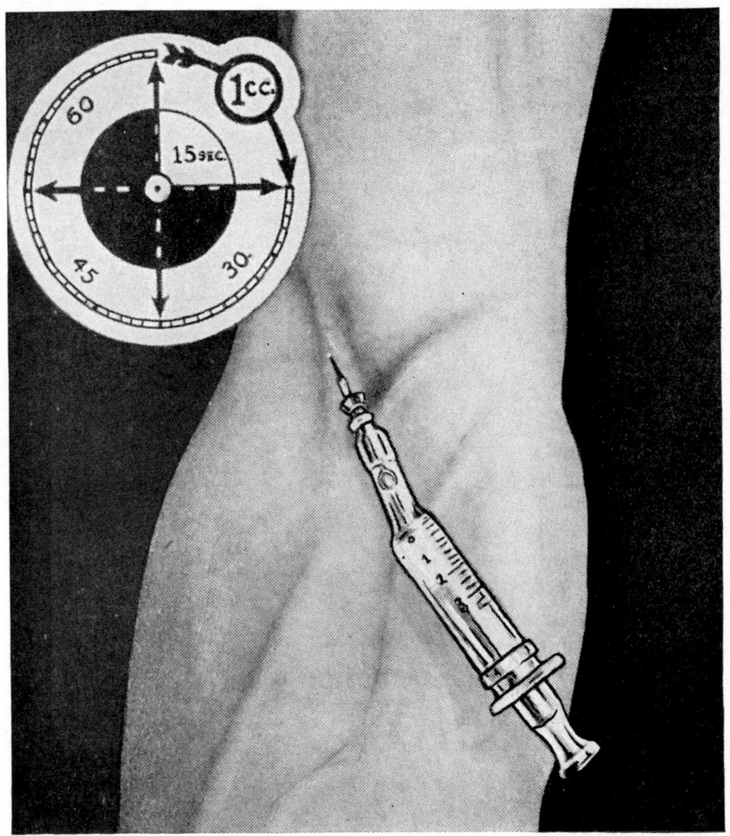

FIG. 64. Three or 4 cc. of evipan sodium is injected at 1 cc. per 15 seconds. The remainder of the appropriate dose is injected somewhat more quickly. (Hamilton Bailey, Emergency Surgery, John Wright & Sons, Ltd., Bristol.)

It is not recommended in operations requiring more than 15 minutes. No premedication is used and the use of any form of barbiturates is strictly contraindicated. In the case of abdominal operations, however, where muscular relaxation is desired, Jarman and Abel recommend a Hoffman-la Roche preparation containing omnopon, gr. 2/3, and scopolamine, gr. 1/150 which may be given an hour before the operation to patients between the ages of 16 and 70.

Evipan anesthesia is contraindicated in patients who have low blood pressure or defective functions of the kidneys or liver.

When an overdose of evipan has been given, strychnine injected intravenously is of value.

Commenting on evipan anesthesia, Jentzer, Oltamare, Poncet[1] conclude as follows:

The advantages of evipan are:

1. Total absence of excitement at the beginning of anesthesia. The patient goes to sleep physiologically without the fear of the inhalation mask and suffocation.
2. Abolition of headaches; nausea is much less marked than after ether and vomiting is rare.
3. Abolition of the mask affords an opportunity to operate on the face and mouth with no difficulty.
4. Complete postoperative amnesia, thus entirely eliminating psychic shock. This is particularly valuable when the anesthetic must be repeated for a number of sittings.

With reference to its advantages over avertin the following may be included:

1. Minimal drop of blood pressure.
2. No increased vascularity in the parenchymatous organs.
3. Simplicity of administration; better asepsis may be practiced. It is less distressing and affords an opportunity to inject fractional doses.
4. More prompt awakening as compared with ether.
5. Complete anesthesia without preliminary medication.

Scopolamine-Morphine Analgesia

My experiences with so-called "twilight sleep anesthesia"[2] (hyoscine-morphine analgesia) have convinced me that its judicious use is to be preferred and certainly is followed by better results than with basal anesthetics thus far used.

The anesthetic action here arises from the synergistic effect of scopolamine and morphine. The patients are carefully examined particularly with reference to the cardiovascular and renal apparatus. They are prepared the day before operation and are kept in a darkened room with absolute quiet enforced. The external auditory canal is plugged with cotton.

Step 1. Three hours before operation a dose of 1/100 gr. scopolamine and 1/6 gr. morphine are injected subcutaneously.

Step 2. The dose is repeated 1 hour before the operation.

This dosage is used in patients between the age of fifteen and sixty years. The dose is decreased according to the age of the patient. In those of seventy and over, 1/200 gr. of scopolamine is used—not more than two doses. Those patients who have not reached the age of fifteen are not given scopolamine. This form of anesthesia is supplemented by nitrous oxide-oxygen or ether, or a mixture of both, depending upon the type of the case and indications or contraindications in the respective patients. Chloroform is banished from our work. The method is not used in obstetrical surgery.

To obviate postoperative acidosis and relieve the dryness of the oral membranes and thirst as well as to replenish the vascular system with fluid, the

[1] Presse Medicale No. 33-25, April, 1934.

[2] Max Thorek: Clinical study of one thousand cases of scopolamine-morphine anesthesia. *Ill. Med. Jour.* June, 1921.

patient is given, directly before he is put to bed, an enteroclysis of 3 quarts of tap water at about 100 degrees F. to which 4 drachms of sodium bicarbonate have been added; in shock, the addition of some brandy is advisable. It goes without saying that when operations are done about the vagina, rectum and perineum, as well as in cases of perforative appendicitis and extensive resection of the lower bowel, enteroclysis is omitted and venoclysis substituted. To avoid excessive distention the colon tube should never be introduced higher than 3 inches in the lower bowel. This is imperative.

Comment. Scopolamine-hydrobromide-morphine anesthesia, supplemented by gas or ether, as required, is a distinct advance in narcosis, and with experienced supervision, perfectly safe.

The failures of earlier observers were due to reliance on scopolamine exclusively as a means of inducing narcosis. Therein lies the danger; and, recognizing the danger it can be forestalled. Chloroform should never be used as an adjunct to scopolamine; nitrous oxide and ether should be given preference.

The advantages of this method of anesthesia are:

1. Suppression of operative fear in the patient.
2. Absolute loss of consciousness.
3. Amnesia as to preparation, etc., incident to the operative procedure.
4. Continuation of sleep four to eight hours after the operation is completed.
5. Elimination of postoperative nausea, vomiting and the harmful straining incident to it.
6. Complete relaxation of the viscera and minimizing the incidence of such unpleasant complications as pneumonia and shock.

The method should never be entrusted to the untrained and the surgeon should supervise and direct the procedure. Occasionally the respirations will be found to drop to six or even four per minute; but, inasmuch as the scopolamine is rapidly eliminated by the kidneys, no ill results will follow if the glottis is prevented from obstructing respirations during the period of complete anesthesia. No complications were observed in our series of about 1000 cases, and the method was found to be a most excellent one. It is our belief that as an adjunct this method possesses a great many advantages over the usual methods which are practiced today.

ETHER-COLONIC ANESTHESIA

This procedure was suggested by Pirogoff in Russia. J. T. Gwathmey popularized and improved the method in this country.

Complete surgical anesthesia may be obtained by placing a mixture of ether, oil and paraldehyde in the rectum of the patient one hour before operation. This form of anesthesia is indicated in operations about the head. A chloretone suppository and hypodermic injection of morphine should precede the administration of this anesthetic mixture.

Gwathmey's Technic. The patient's bowels are kept at rest for 36 hours preceding the operation. The night preceding the operation the patient may be allowed tea and toast for supper. An enema is given two hours later, followed by two tap-water enemas 20 minutes apart. Complete colonic irrigation is essential. Two hours prior to the operation, a low, clear water enema is given. Wherever possible walking is encouraged. The ears of the patient are plugged with cotton, the face covered with a towel and the room darkened.

Step 1. Place the patient in the Sims' position one hour before operation.

Step 2. Exclude the air from the rubber tubing and catheter to be used, by filling them with warm oil to the funnel.

Step 3. Insert the catheter 6 to 8 inches in the rectum. Permit any fluid or fecal matter to drain out by lowering the funnel. Refill the funnel with oil and exclude all air.

Step 4. Raise the funnel and pour in the retention enema mixture (warm) consisting of:

	Ether	*Oil*	*Paraldehyde*
	1. 4 ounces (120 cc.)	2 ounces (60 cc.)	2 drams (8 cc.)
	2. 5 " (150 cc.)	2½ " (75 cc.)	2 " (8 cc.)
or	3. 6 " (180 cc.)	3 " (90 cc.)	2 " (8 cc.)

This step should consume from 15 to 20 minutes.

Step 5. Now clamp the catheter below the glass connection so that no air escapes. Exert pressure on the perineum with a towel for 15 minutes.

Gwathmey admonishes that great gentleness should be observed in all manipulations and care should be taken to keep the patient quiet at all times. Because this procedure is more of the type of an analgesia than anesthesia, a few drops of ether, nitrous oxide or ethylene may be used to quiet the patient where necessary—never to induce anesthesia.

Danger Signals. Slight cyanosis, dulled lid-reflex and stertor. Upon their appearance, support the lower jaw or insert a breathing tube. An important feature is the ability to distinguish between analgesia with unconsciousness (usually associated with colonic anesthesia) and surgical inhalation anesthesia with automatic respiration. The superimposition of a third stage inhalation anesthesia on a light colonic anesthesia will result in the patient passing into the fourth or danger zone promptly.

After the patient is returned to bed, siphon off any residue in the rectum. Flush the colon with warm water thoroughly. Following this, 3 to 6 ounces of warm black coffee are instilled and the tube is withdrawn. No nausea, vomiting or pain accompanies the final awakening since analgesia continues for some time after consciousness has returned.

Hazleton's technic utilizes very little ether, anesthesia being brought about chiefly by morphine and magnesium sulphate.

Prepare the patient the same as above. An hour before operation, inject intramuscularly 1 ampule of

Magnesium sulphate, C.P.	gr. xv (1 Gm.)
Morphine sulphate	gr. 1/6 (0.0108 Gm.)
Novocaine	gr. 5/6 (0.05 Gm.)
Aq. dist.	ad mxxxij (2 cc.)

to be repeated twice at 15-minute intervals (Gwathmey).

After the last injection, start a Murphy drip of 8 ounces (240 cc.) of a 6 per cent glucose solution with 4 drams (16 cc.) of ether (25 to 30 drops per min.).

When the operation is over, this solution is discontinued and 1,000 cc. of a 6 per cent glucose with 1 dram Lugol solution is begun and carried on until it is all used.

The chief advantages of the method are:

1. It is not depressing.
2. It is easier; it is not necessary to flush the colon afterwards.
3. Less ether is employed.
4. The patient receives stimulation throughout the operation.
5. The anesthetic state continues longer than when 4 to 6 ounces of ether are used.

THREATENING DEATH UNDER GENERAL ANESTHESIA

A competent anesthetist manages to have within easy reach at all times, an emergency kit containing (1) adrenalin solution, (2) alpha-lobeline (1/6 gr.), (3) a Ricord syringe with hypodermic needles and (4) cardiac puncture needles 3¼ in. in length.

Emergency resuscitation is resorted to in asphyxia:

1. The result of respiratory failure (blue asphyxia).
2. That due to cardiac failure (white asphyxia).

Type 1 is comparatively simple to overcome.

(1) Clear the airways.
(2) Pull the tongue forward.
(3) Administer oxygen; resort to
(4) Artificial respiration and finally administer
(5) An intravenous injection of alpha-lobeline.

This is usually followed by the desired result.

Stretching of the anal sphincter is often used in these cases if they do not readily respond to other methods.

Type 2 is a serious complication requiring prompt, competent aid. Treatment consists of

(1) Artificial respiration (Figs. 6-7-8-9-10).
(2) Hot packs about the precordium.
(3) Intracardiac injection of adrenalin and
(4) Cardiac massage.

carried out in the order given for fully twenty minutes after the heart has apparently failed to function.

Comment: Fundamental to any effort to avoid impending asphyxia, is the elimination of the deadly lingual check valve, formed when the tongue drops back into the throat: then air can be expired, but all efforts to inspire drive the valve more firmly into its seat.

The best way to eliminate it is by direct laryngoscopy (Fig. 65).

With the patient on his back the direct laryngoscope is inserted backward until it touches the back wall beyond the tongue. Then by a lifting motion the head of the patient is hung up on the cylindric part of the instrument. This brings the tongue away from the back wall of the throat, allows air to get down back of the tongue into the larynx, and eliminates the deadly lingual check valve.

The bronchoscope is introduced into the larynx and trachea through the laryngoscope. Do not connect the oxygen tube to the bronchoscope until after the oxygen pressure has been regulated, in order to avoid a heavy discharge of oxygen.

Aspiration of secretions through the laryngoscope or bronchoscope prevents the patient drowning in his own secretions.

If means for direct laryngoscopy are not at hand, artificial respiration is the alternative. The best method being the prone-pressure method but

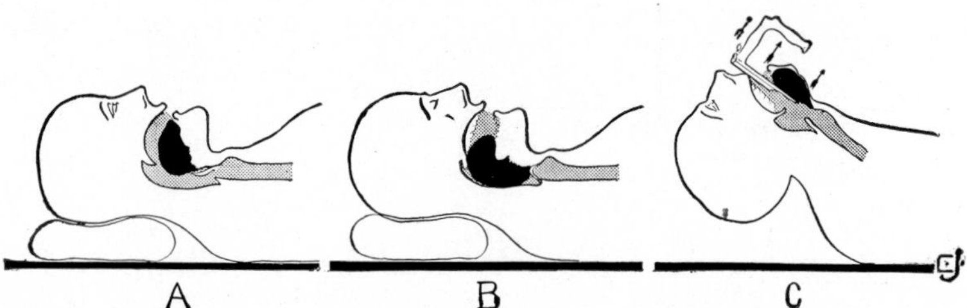

FIG. 65. The death zone. A. Normal position of the tongue, B. in the relaxation of the impending asphyxia the tongue drops backward obstructing the ingress of air. If artificial respiration is started with the tongue in this position, the patient will be killed by the pumping of air out of the lung on the compression stroke while no air can enter on the inspiratory stroke; the tongue forms a check valve permitting passage in one direction only. For artificial respiration the tongue should be drawn forward with tongue forceps or the fingers covered with a handkerchief or gauze, but the best way to open up this death zone is with the direct laryngoscope as shown at C. Oxygen and carbon dioxide can then be insufflated. Every ambulance and every accident ward should be equipped with a direct laryngoscope, a 5 mm. bronchoscope, and a tank of oxygen with 5 per cent carbon dioxide. An aspirator for secretions would be useful, but in an emergency, gauze, or even a handkerchief, can be used to clear secretions out of the death zone. (Courtesy of Jackson and Jackson.)

regardless of the method used, it is necessary to see that the tongue is drawn out and held out.

The necessary equipment for the prevention of asphyxial death that should be in every ambulance and every accident ward is: 1 direct laryngoscope; 1 bronchoscope, 5 mm. by 30 cm. of full lumen aspirating pattern; 1 tank filled with oxygen containing a 5 per cent mixture of carbon dioxide; 1 piece rubber tubing, about 4 ft. long attached to the tank outlet.

REGIONAL ANESTHESIA

SPINAL ANESTHESIA

Spinal anesthesia is a form of regional anesthesia used especially for operations upon the lower abdomen and lower extremities in patients who are for any reason unsuitable subjects for general anesthesia. This method affords complete freedom from pain but not from pressure sensation in the operative field; the tissues are absolutely relaxed; the intestines are contracted and do not obtrude upon the abdominal incision; expulsion of flatus or other content of the bowel is strongly stimulated; there is no toxic action from the anesthetic substance on the brain, liver, kidneys, or lungs and there is no irritation of the respiratory tract.

Although these advantages are great and conceded in the hands of those thoroughly competent and familiar with the technic of its administration, it must be remembered that the administration of spinal anesthesia requires an accurate and very precise technic for uniform results. Accidents in the application of the technic or of the physiologic actions involved, are less capable of being remedied than in other methods of inducing anesthesia, and are more likely to be the cause of a fatality. The surgeon performing the operation, who must accept responsibility for the anesthesia, is more likely to be blamed for a fatality when spinal anesthesia is being used than when anything goes wrong under general inhalation anesthesia. It is said that in a very small percentage of cases, spinal anesthesia has been followed by more or less permanent **paralysis** of the lower limbs, of the bladder or of the anus. This I cannot substantiate as being quite correct from a rather large series of personally observed cases (our last series, 350 cases). More or less unpleasant bladder symptoms have followed the use of tropacocaine-hydrochloride in my hands and in those of Dr. Phil Thorek, but these were of transitory nature. One death resulted at my hands from the use of spinocaine.

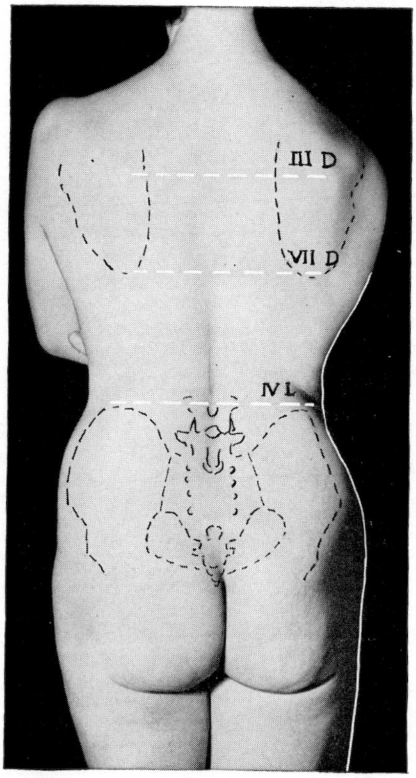

Fig. 66. Spinal anesthesia. It is essential that one is oriented as to the positions of the anatomical structures concerned in spinal anesthesia. The upper transverse white lines correspond to the spines of the scapulae and consequently to the third dorsal vertebra. The middle white dotted line corresponds to the angles of the scapula, therefore, to the 7th dorsal vertebra. The crest of the ilia are represented by the lowest dotted white line, therefore, the 4th lumbar interspace (after Dogliotti).

After an orgy of trial with all substances recommended for spinal anesthesia, I have returned to novocaine or one of its refined allies (procaine crystals or neocaine).

Spinal anesthesia may be employed in the case of patients with high blood pressure or for those who have renal insufficiency; but it is not suitable for those with low blood pressure or who are in a state of shock. Neither should it be employed for those with sepsis or those who are running a high temperature, in the case of restless children, nervous individuals or those afflicted with cerebrospinal lues.

Although, theoretically, high spinal anesthesia may be employed, yet the possibility of cerebral, cardiac and respiratory complications contraindicate such attempts. (Fig. 66).

The most convenient place for injecting the dural sac is generally through the space between the third and fourth lumbar vertebrae. I rarely inject higher than the second lumbar interspace. Gravitation plays a very important part in the movement of the fluid within the subarachnoid space. A fluid of light or heavy specific gravity may be employed according to the circumstances, and its diffusion in the spinal canal fairly well controlled. Supposing the canal empty, the solution will run downward and collect distally in the sacral region when the patient is placed in the dorsal position.

The armamentarium needed for the induction of spinal anesthesia includes a spinal trocar and cannula (Fig. 67) with a sharp point, a glass syringe of 5 cc. capacity to fit the cannula, a hypodermic syringe with a fine needle, the selected anesthetizing fluid and a small quantity of ½ per cent novocaine for cutaneous anesthetization.

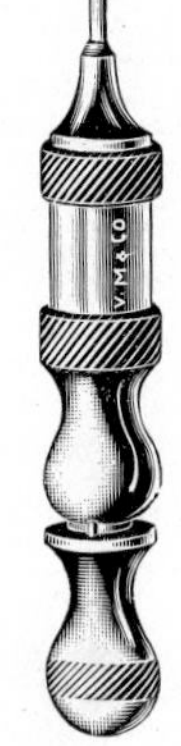

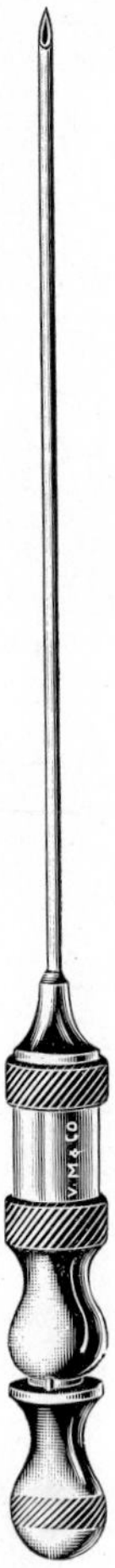

FIG. 67. Needle for spinal anesthesia.

Commenting on Spinal Anesthesia Complicated by the Breaking of the Spinal Puncture Needle, Ernest R. Anderson concludes[1] that

"Semiflexible needles made of a good quality steel should be used. The needles should be properly cared for to keep them from rusting. All needles, before their introduction, should be tested with the stylets removed. Care should be taken to prevent any movement of the patient when the needle is **in situ.**

"When a spinal puncture needle breaks, leaving a segment embedded, the site of the puncture should be localized. The patient should be informed of the breakage and the broken needle removed. The localization and the removal of the segment are aided by passing a second spinal puncture needle and by taking anteroposterior and lateral X-rays."

(a) For operations in the upper abdomen, the second lumbar interspace is selected;

(b) For lower abdominal operations and the lower extremities the second or third lumbar interspace;

(c) For the genital region, the third or fourth lumbar interspace is best.

Failure to obtain anesthesia occurs in from 2 to 4 per cent of cases. This may be due to failure to enter the spinal canal or to imperfect entrance, to too rapid injection, to insufficient diffusion of the anesthetizing fluid or to obstruction of the spinal canal by a tumor, etc.

The danger signals in spinal anesthesia are gulping and nausea, which precede a precipitate fall in blood pressure; this is usually due to cerebral anemia and should be combated by lowering the head and chest. Respiratory distress is denoted by cyanosis and shallow breathing; it should be combated by respiratory stimulation methods. Regurgitation vomiting may drown the patient. Cessation of heart action is always fatal if it exceeds 7 minutes in duration; if it occurs, it calls for cardiac massage, intracardiac injection of adrenalin, or both.

Technic. (Figs. 68, 69, 70). The night before the operation sodium amytal is administered. On the morning prior to taking the patient to the operating room, administer hypodermically 1/100 grain of hyoscine hydrobromide and ¼ grain of morphine sulphate. Half an hour before the operation administer ¾ grain of ephedrine subcutaneously and immediately after the injection of the

[1] The Journal-Lancet, Minneapolis, Nov. 15, 1935.

anesthetizing fluid into the subarachnoid space inject (subcutaneously) seven and one-half grains of caffeine sodium benzoate. In children, the enfeebled and in those suffering from shock preoperation sedatives should be omitted.

Step 1. The patient is made to sit upon the side of the operating table well back from the edge with his elbows at his side and the forearms crossed in front of the abdomen. The head is then tilted forward until the chin touches the chest. The patient is held by the assistant's left arm which passes around the patient's abdomen.

Step 2. The patient's back is now prepared with iodine and thoroughly neutralized with alcohol. A horizontal line connecting both iliac crests will transect the spinous process of the fourth lumbar vertebra. The usual point of injection is just above this line.

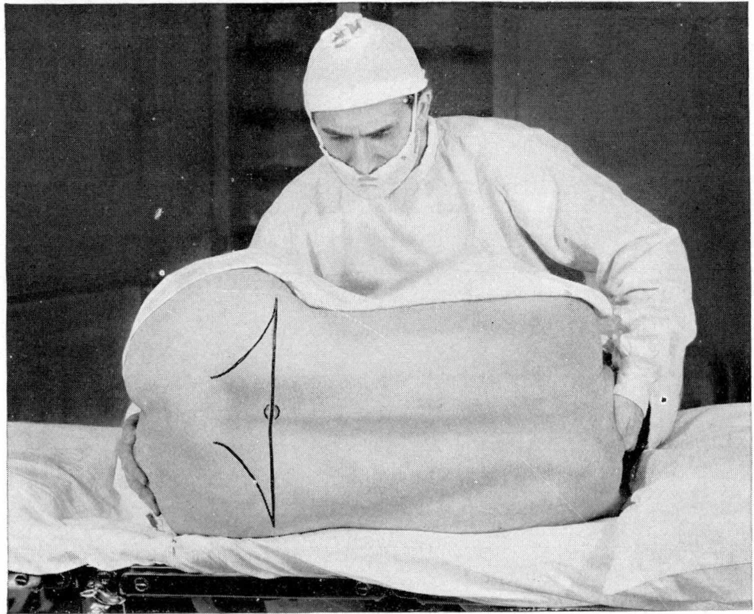

FIG. 68. Proper position in which the assistant places patient for administering spinal anesthesia or lumbar puncture. The vertical line connects the anterior superior spinous processes. The ring denotes the interspace between the third and fourth lumbar vertebrae.

Step 3. The syringe, piston and the needle which have been sterilized by boiling for ten minutes in distilled water without alkali are made ready for use. While the needle is being introduced a certain sense of resistance is felt which is followed by a sudden "pop" indicating that the needle has entered the subarachnoid space.

Step 4. About 15 drops of cerebrospinal fluid are permitted to escape into the ampule containing procaine or novocaine crystals. These are dissolved and aspirated from the ampule into the barrel of the syringe and thence transferred via the needle resting **in situ** into the subarachnoid space. The greater the pressure at which the solution is introduced the higher will be the level of anesthesia. By **barbotage** is meant the aspiration and reintroduction of the anesthetizing fluid into the subarachnoid space. This may be repeated two or three times; the oftener it is repeated the greater the diffusion of the anesthetic fluid, hence the higher the level of anesthesia.

Step 5. The instant the needle is withdrawn, the puncture aperture is dabbed with a little iodine and the puncture point covered with a small square of adhesive plaster or collodion. The patient is now placed in position for operation. The table is quickly tilted so as to lower the shoulders 2 inches below the level of the hips.

Comment: A great source of satisfaction is experienced by the surgeon who has an experienced anesthetist at the head of the table to supervise

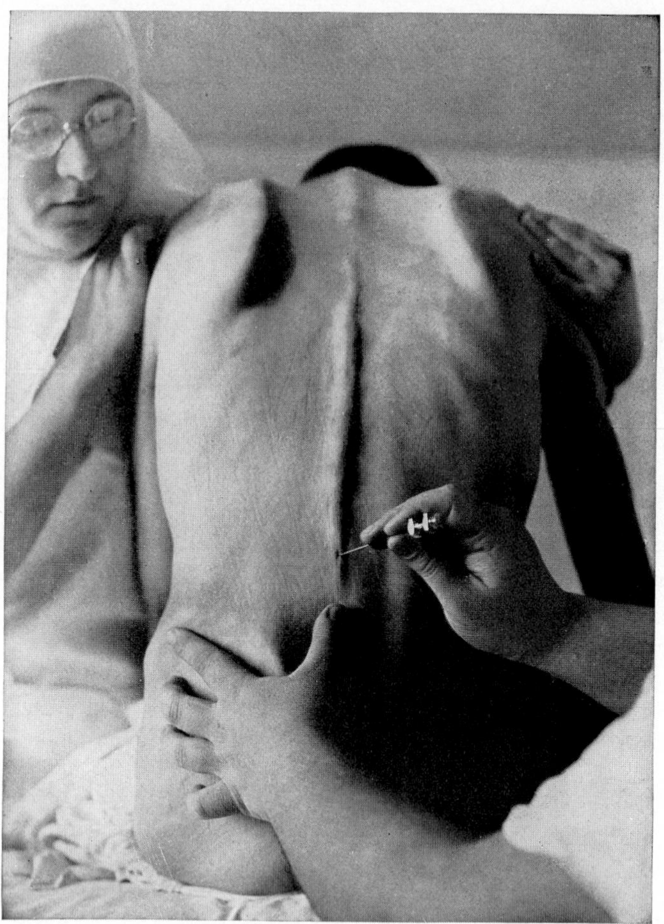

FIG. 69. Correct position of patient.

the pulse, respirations and color of the face. Let the anesthetist converse with and encourage the patient and never ask the patient whether he experiences pain; if such be the case he will apprize you quickly enough. Besides, such questions as, "Do you feel this?" or "What do you feel?" will fix the patient's attention to the operation. This is wrong. Instead, blood pressure readings should be taken frequently and thus the patient's attention diverted. When trained assistants are available, I like to supply slowly a 5 per cent solution of glucose intravenously while the operation is in progress. Bystanders and operating room personnel must not speak

above a whisper. Wherever possible, I refrain from informing the patient as to when the operation is to be performed.

The danger period of spinal anesthesia is from five to twenty-five minutes after the injection.

Danger signals are, as already stated: marked fall in blood pressure, cyanosis, or respiratory depression (irregularity or embarrassment). Premonitory signs are nausea or vomiting. If these persist, lower the patient's head further and give 8 to 12 drops of adrenalin or 1 grain of ephedrine subcutaneously. In a young, vigorous individual a drop in the systolic blood pressure to 30 mg.

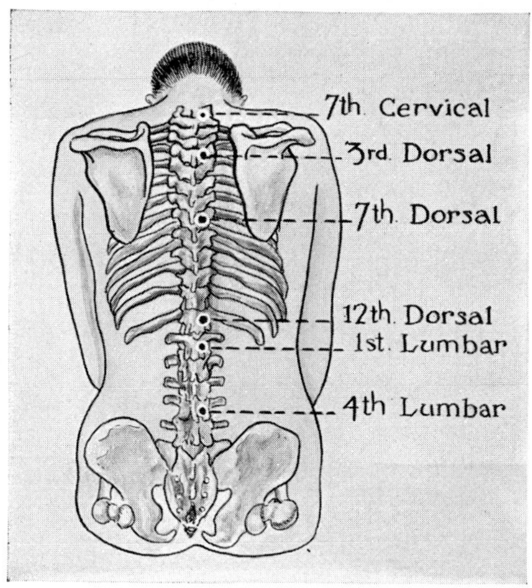

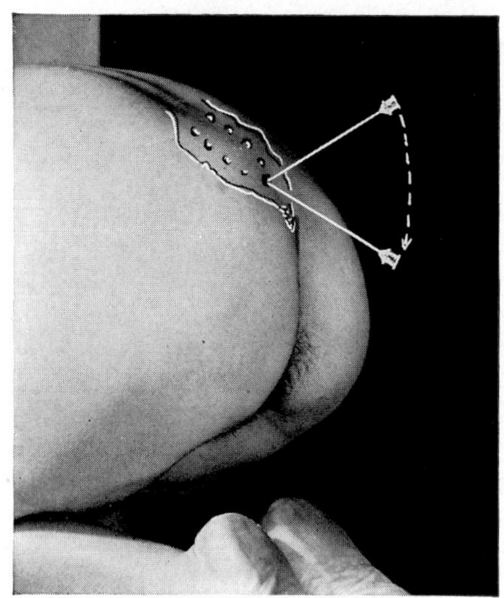

FIG. 70 FIG. 71

FIG. 70. Localization of spinous interspaces.

FIG. 71. Sacral anesthesia, patient in the elbow position. The upper needle shows the first movement in entering the hiatus of the sacrum. The arrow points to the second step which consists in directing the needle downward, then upward into the hiatus where the injection is to be made.

may cause no apprehension while a fall to 50 mg. in an obese, weakened or aged individual should be immediately counteracted.

Loss of voice is an early sign of respiratory failure. In impending respiratory failure give alpha-lobeline hypodermically. Respiratory depression may also be combated by rebreathing of oxygen.

We prefer to leave the patient for 12 to 24 hours after operation in the Trendelenburg position and watch for possible untoward symptoms which are combated as they arise.

Headache will sometimes follow the withdrawal of cerebrospinal fluid.

SACRAL ANESTHESIA

Blocking the sacral nerves within the sacrum produces a very efficient surgical anesthesia of the structures these nerves supply. It is highly recommended by surgeons and urologists who have used it.

This type of anesthesia may be induced by injecting the anesthetic solution into (a) the sacral canal; (b) by paraneural injection of the nerve trunks at their terminals and (c) by paraneural injections into the posterior sacral foramina. It should be remembered at all times that the fluid is outside the meninges of the spine, consequently this should not be confused with spinal anesthesia.

The apparatus necessary for administering sacral anesthesia consists only of a proper supply of needles and a syringe. The needles should be as fine as stability will permit thus lessening the pain and injury caused by their frequent introduction into the soft tissues. An assortment of needles of different lengths is necessary; they should be made of a high grade flexible steel and have a sharp cutting edge. A small spinal puncture needle which will bend but will not break is used for injecting the sacral canal.

A satisfactory solution consists of 1 per cent novocaine solution with 5 drops of adrenalin added to 100 cc. just before using.

Technic. Sterilize the skin surface the same as for other surgical procedures. Place the patient on his abdomen with a cushion under the hips thus raising the buttocks and accentuating bony prominences.

Step 1. With the index finger of the left hand follow the posterior surface of the coccyx upward until the sacral cornua are palpated on each side. The fourth sacral spine may be felt a little higher; this forms the apex of the isosceles triangle which guards the entrance to the sacral canal.

Step 2. Make a dermal wheal within this triangle and infiltrate the subcutaneous tissues and sacrococcygeal membrane.

Step 3. Introduce a fine spinal puncture needle through the skin with bevel upward at a 25-degree angle; after puncturing a membrane and striking the bone of the front wall, it is slightly withdrawn, depressed still further until it is almost parallel to the sacral canal; then direct it slightly upward for a short distance (4 to 5 cm.). If blood or spinal fluid escapes, withdraw the needle or change its position until this stops. (Figs. 71-72.)

Step 4. Slowly and carefully inject 25 to 30 cc. of the solution mentioned above. There is no resistance if the needle is properly placed. After half of the amount has been injected, slowly withdraw the needle so that at the conclusion its point is just inside the sacrococcygeal membrane.

If carried out correctly, anesthesia of the pelvic floor and viscera usually requires about 20 minutes.

PARASACRAL NERVE BLOCK

Place the patient in the lithotomy position.

Step 1. Make two dermal wheals at the sacrococcygeal articulation about 1½ to 2 cm. from the median line.

Step 2. Introduce a longer needle past the edge of the sacrum anteriorly, parallel to the median line and extending to the second sacral foramen. Twenty cc. of ½ per cent novocaine-adrenalin solution is used.

Step 3. Withdraw and direct the needle at an angle anteriorly toward the innominate bone. Thrust the needle deeper until it contacts the promontory of the sacrum near the first sacral foramen. Inject 10 to 20 cc. here. Repeat the procedure on the opposite side. Make a final injection of 5 cc. between the coccyx and rectum.

A guiding finger in the rectum is of great assistance in governing the direction of the needle.

Comment: Parasacral nerve block is a painstaking and difficult procedure which does not always result so successfully as other methods. There is also the danger of puncturing other tissues when injecting the perineum and of spreading an infection when a septic area is crossed.

TRANS-SACRAL NERVE BLOCK

Step 1. Place a dermal wheal laterally and below the sacral cornu. This determines the position of the sacral notch on the lower border of the sacrum where the fifth sacral nerve lies.

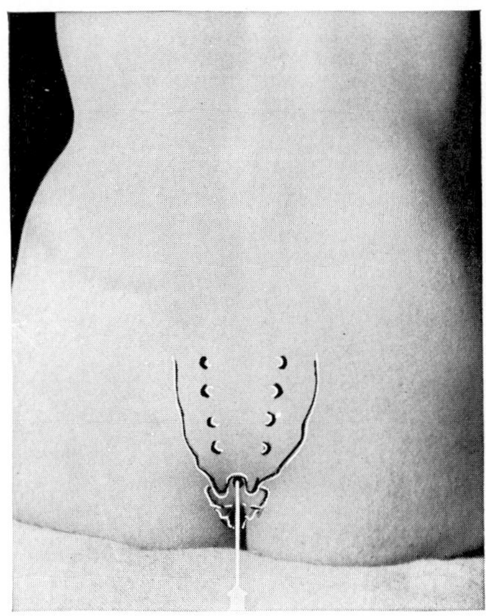

FIG. 72

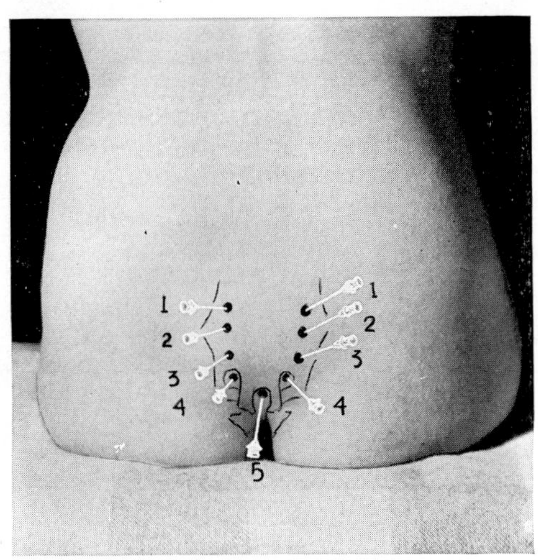

FIG. 73

FIG. 72. Sacral anesthesia in the sitting position.

FIG. 73. Trans-sacral anesthesia (blocking of the sacral nerves as they emerge from the sacral foramina). The five sacral branches are usually infiltrated. Wheals are made overlying the proposed points of puncture. One appears above the second sacral foramen while another wheal appears just below and lateral to the corun of the sacrum (above the fifth foramen). All foramina are equally treated. The method may be useful as an adjunct to high sacral and pre-sacral anesthesia.

Step 2. Ascertain the most prominent point of the posterior iliac spines by palpation and place another dermal wheal 2½ cm. medial and ½ cm. dorsal; this indicates the position of the second sacral foramen. Place two more wheals between the two first made. Place a fifth one above the second at the first sacral foramen. (Fig. 73.)

Step 3. Determine the position of the foramina by inserting the needle downward and slightly inward perpendicular to the tangent of the sacrum. Bone is likely to be struck during the first efforts and thus the distance from the skin to the posterior surface of the sacrum is estimated. When the needle has seemed to penetrate a membrane but by further penetration does not contact bone, the foramen has been entered. On account of the downward curvature of the sacrum and greater thickness of the overlying soft tissues, the needle should be inclined more in locating the higher foramina. The foramina and nerve trunks decrease in size from above downward making it necessary to inject larger amounts of solution in the higher foramina.

Low caudal injection combined with trans-sacral block of the upper four sacral nerves gives a very satisfactory anesthesia lasting two to three hours. It is especially efficacious in operations for prolapsed rectum, plastic operations on rectal sphincters, etc.

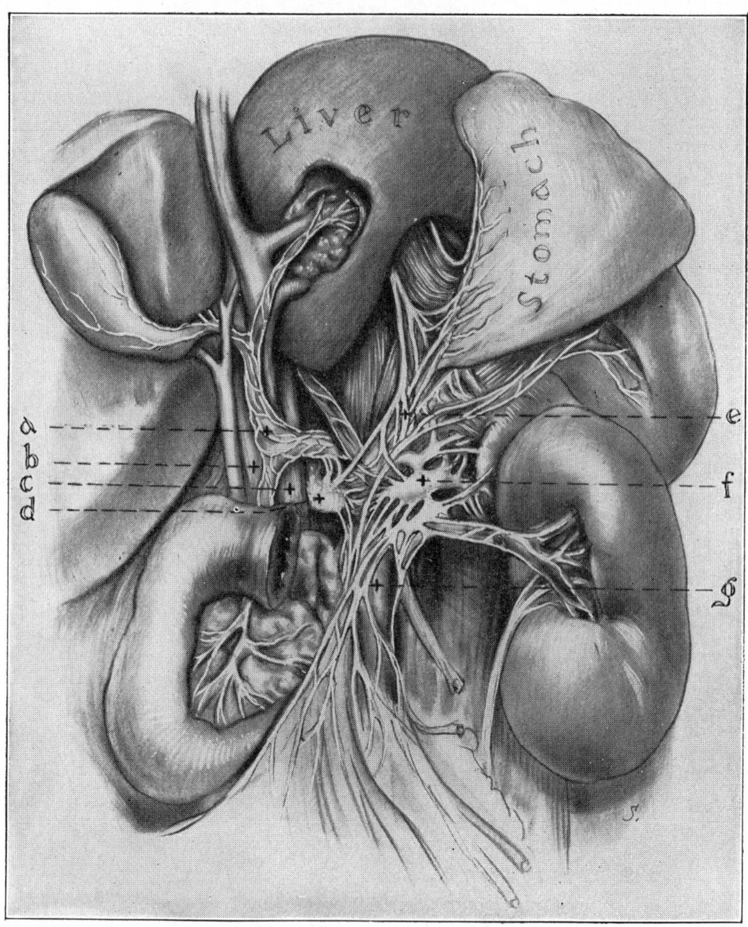

FIG. 74. a. Hepatic plexus, b. portal vein, c. inferior vena cava, d. semilunar ganglion, e. splenic and gastric plexuses, f. semilunar ganglion, g. abdominal aorta. (Hertzler's Local Anesthesia, 5th edition, C. V. Mosby.)

Comment: Difficulties following sacral nerve block are mild, if the procedure has been correctly carried out; caudal injection is different. The after-effects are dependent upon the strength, amount and adrenalin content of the solution injected. Palpitation of the heart and a rise in pulse rate often follow. In the more severe cases respiration is increased, dyspnea, pallor, perspiration and a giddy feeling are observed. Injections should be delayed until these conditions are corrected; as a rule, however, these sequelae are not serious.

Therapeutic Application

In some instances caudal injection has been used therapeutically where the sacral nerves were involved. It has been found useful in treating sciatica, lumbago, tabes, sexual neuroses, and intractable pruritus ani and vulvae.

PARAVERTEBRAL AND SPLANCHNIC ANESTHESIA

It is the objective of splanchnic anesthesia to infiltrate a small concealed region at the level of the first lumbar vertebra, posterior to the large vessels in the prevertebral space. A vast system of sympathetic fibers course along the blood-vessels here to combine in forming the celiac plexus which generally appears as two rather irregular semilunar ganglia. On the aorta and its main branches, inferior plexuses continue caudalward. The major and lesser splanchnic nerves enter into this network proximally; the major splanchnic nerve is formed by fibers from the sixth, seventh, eighth and ninth thoracic sympathetic ganglia and enters the abdomen at the 12th rib to join the celiac plexus. The lesser splanchnic nerve generally begins with two branches from the tenth and eleventh thoracic ganglia. It runs parallel with the major splanchnic nerve on a more dorsal plane and partly the celiac plexus but mostly the renal and suprarenal plexuses.

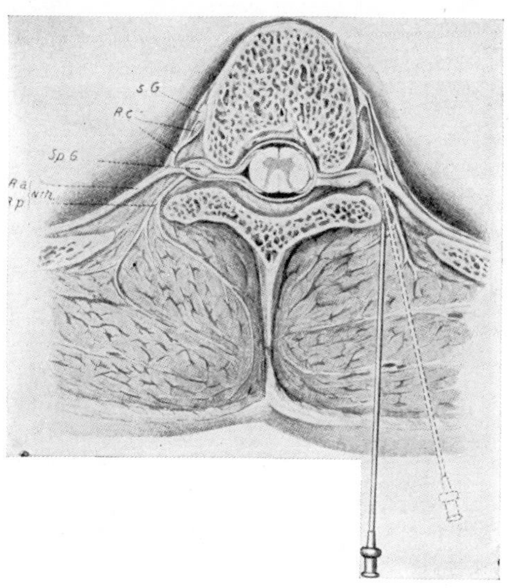

Fig. 75. Technic of paravertebral anesthesia. Cross section at the level of the thoracic spine. Needles depict their course in injecting anesthetizing fluid. S.G. Sympathetic ganglion, R.c. Rami communicantes, Sp.G. Spinal ganglion, R.a. Ramus anterior of the N. thoracalis, R.p. Ramus posterior of the N. thoracalis (after Felix Mandl.)

In this country, spinal anesthesia has superseded splanchnic and paravertebral anesthesia as a method of choice. In Europe, Dogliotti advocates paravertebral anesthesia while Finsterer is one of the strongest protagonists of splanchnic anesthesia. In most clinics, it is used only in cases where spinal or inhalation anesthesia are for one reason or another contraindicated. Generally, it is difficult to introduce a needle accurately and deeply into the tissues; to be effective, it must be about 18 to 20 caliber; thinner needles deflect too much. Considerable injury may be done if a needle of this size penetrates a large vessel.

In the posterior approach for splanchnic anesthesia the powerful muscles of the back must be penetrated. These differ greatly in different individuals, thus measurements are of little value; a landmark should be established in the deeper tissues and the needle re-directed from this point. One can never be sure that the needle has reached its objective.

PARAVERTEBRAL ANESTHESIA

Blocking the spinal nerves at their point of exit at the intervertebral foramina would be ideal were it not for the difficulties mentioned above as well as the added one that so large a number of separate injections are required in this method. Since the approach to the nerve is always approximate, the quantity of fluid must be increased proportionately. The amount of novocaine in the solution varies between 15 and 30 grains; a preanesthetic consisting of ¼ to ½ grain of morphine or its equivalent is always administered before this, so it will be readily seen that no weak patient should be subjected to this ordeal. It should be considered an occasional and not a routine method of administering anesthesia. Theoretically, it may be indicated in operations on the thorax or

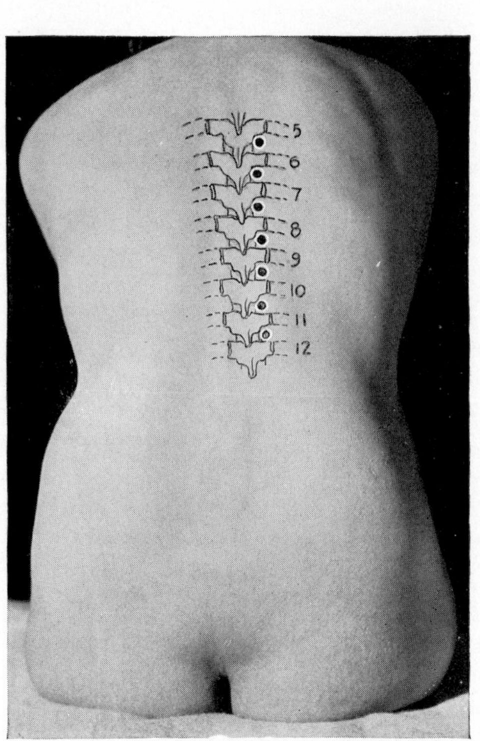

Fig. 76

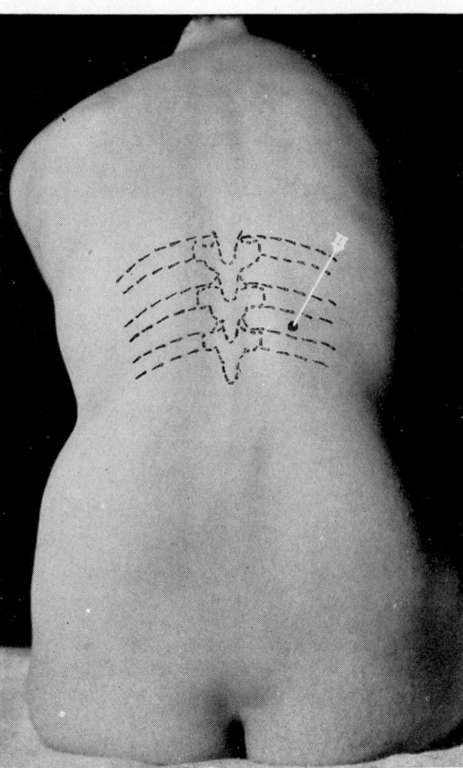

Fig. 77

Fig. 76. Paravertebral intercostal nerve block.

Fig. 77. Paravertebral anesthesia, showing sites of injection. The number of nerves selected varies between two and four. The last rib is the most convenient guide for localizing the desired nerve. A point 4 to 5 cm. lateral to the spinous process is usually selected. Pass the needle directly to the transverse process of the respective rib. Mark the point on the needle where it emerges from the skin (clamp with an artery forceps). Mark a cm. nearer to the base and pass the needle to this depth directing the point of the needle mesially. Inject about 10 cc. of anesthetizing fluid.

in serious abdominal lesions such as infections of the gallbladder, cecum, colon, pelvis or kidneys. In operations on the thoracic esophagus, it is the sovereign anesthetic. When practised as outlined by Dogliotti[1] it is an excellent procedure.

Technic. The patient is placed on his side; some surgeons advocate a sitting position (Frönig-Siegel). From two to four nerves are usually injected. (Figs. 75, 76, 77.)

Step 1. The 12th rib is a convenient guide for locating the desired point of puncture. Locate a point 4 to 5 cm. lateral to the spinous processes.

Step 2. Direct the needle inward to the rib of the respective transverse process.

[1] A. Mario Dogliotti: Trattato di Anestesia Torino. Un. Tip. Edit Torino 1935.

Place an artery clamp at the point of exit of the needle. Mark a point a cm. nearer the base and insert the needle to this depth while the point is directed medially. Inject from 10 to 15 cc. of the anesthetizing solution at this site.

Comment: If the condition of the patient seems to indicate it, quinine-urea hydrochloride may be used for skin infiltrations; novocaine should be reserved for perineural injections. It is advisable to infiltrate the abdominal wall in conjunction with paravertebral blocking.

SPLANCHNIC ANESTHESIA

Posterior Route (Kappis)

One advantage of the posterior route is that the injection is made prior to the incision of the abdomen, one or two injections by this method showing the same results as many injections do via the paravertebral method.

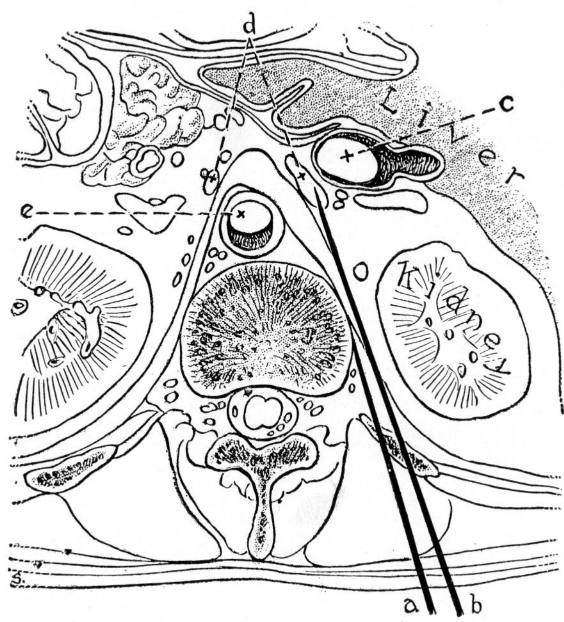

FIG. 78. *a.* Needle passes obliquely inward and medially, striking surface of the vertebra, *b.* the needle is partly withdrawn and then directed more deeply to the semilunar ganglion, *c.* portal vein, *d.* semilunar ganglia, *e.* aorta. (Hertzler's Local Anesthesia, 5th Edition, C. V. Mosby.)

Step 1. Place the patient on his side and locate the 12th rib and the first lumbar spine by means of a finger and thumb.

Step 2. Insert the needle at a point 4 finger-breadths from the midline of the spine and direct it inward and toward the midline. (Figs. 78, 79, 80.)

Step 3. Partially withdraw the needle and introduce it again more laterally so that it passes along the side of the vertebral body. Labat advises that the needle should not pass more than 1 cm. deeper than when impinged against the side of the vertebral body. This is sound advice but the ganglion will not be reached at this depth. There is a fatty resistance around the ganglia which raises them from the bone. It is permissible to go a centimeter deeper if care is exercised and the piston of the syringe is drawn; if blood appears in the syringe a vessel is punctured.

Step 4. After the needle has reached the desired depth, inject the novocaine solution (the amount used varies from 25 to 40 cc. of a 1 per cent solution).

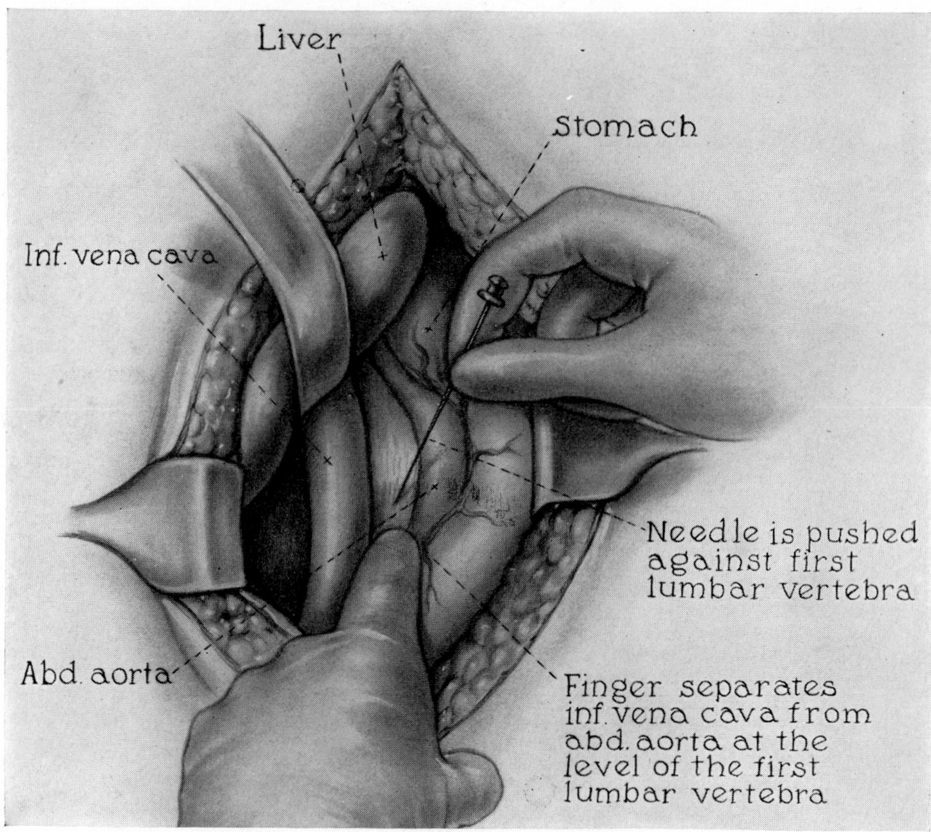

FIG. 79. Method of doing splanchnic anesthesia by the anterior route. (Hertzler's Local Anesthesia. C. V. Mosby.)

Anterior Route

If there is no pathology to interfere with entering the abdominal parietes, this is easier to perform than the posterior route. An objectionable feature of this method is that the injection is made after the abdomen has been opened.

Step 1. After the stomach and lesser omentum have been exposed, push the stomach to the left with the index finger until the vertebral body is felt.

Step 2. Palpate the aorta and push it to one side so that a needle may pass. Inject the solution at the lateral border of the vertebra. Injection is made below the celiac axis.

Step 3. Palpate the space between the pancreas and the hepatic artery on the right side and inject the solution here.

Comment: Braun uses 50 cc. of a ½ per cent solution while Pauchet used 20 to 40 cc. of a 1 per cent solution. Another objectionable feature of this procedure, besides the one mentioned above, is that the viscera must be displaced before the injections are begun. If the general condition of the patient contraindicates general anesthesia it seems there would be likely to be pathologic changes in the common duct making the point of

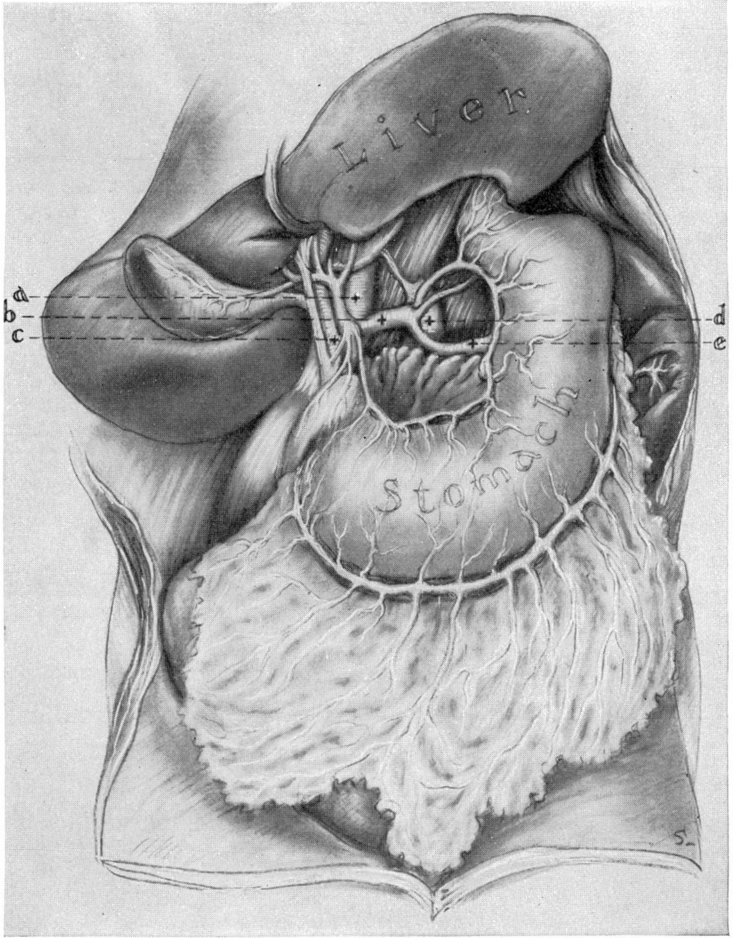

Fig. 80. a. Inferior vena cava, b. hepatic artery, c. portal vein, d. abdominal aorta, e. splenic artery. (Hertzler's Local Anesthesia, 5th edition, C. V. Mosby.)

injection inaccessible. This procedure is not recommended for the beginner in surgery. Meeker has reported 42 cases where splanchnic anesthesia was administered and in 18 of these cases a general anesthetic had to be resorted to. Thus it will be noted that the results are not encouraging even in the hands of some experts; others remain enthusiasts of the method.

Charles Harrison Arnold (Lincoln, Nebraska) points out the details of the technic of anterior splanchnic anesthesia:

Step 1. Anesthetize the abdominal wall in the usual way with 1 per cent novocaine solution to which has been added 3 minims of adrenalin solution to each ounce of novocaine solution. The anesthetized area should extend from the ensiform cartilage to the umbilicus.

Step 2. Make the midline incision through the abdominal wall into the peritoneal cavity. Handle the structures very gently and carefully. Anesthetize the peritoneum for an area of one and one-half to two inches from the cut margin all around the incision. This obviates the pain which might result when retractors are placed on the peritoneum.

Step 3. After anesthetization and hemostasis have been completed, insert the left hand (if right-handed) and pull the stomach gently downward until the gastrohepatic ligament, or lesser omentum comes into view; then make an injection into this structure of the same solution used in the abdominal wall. Make this with the ordinary hypodermic needle infiltrating an area of perhaps three inches in diameter.

Step 4. Exert gentle pressure with the forefinger of the left hand down onto the gastrohepatic ligament until one meets the abdominal aorta. Slide the aorta gently over to the left, push the pancreas downward causing the finger to meet with the anterior bodies of the first or second lumbar vertebra, bringing it to rest between the abdominal aorta and the vena cava in the region of the celiac axis in the midst of the celiac plexus.

Step 5. Grasp a large Finsterer splanchnic needle, which is about seven inches long, with a short bevel point, with the right hand, insert it, guiding it with the forefinger of the left hand until it meets or contacts the anterior body of the vertebra upon which the forefinger is resting. If there is any bleeding, withdraw the needle and re-insert it, but if care is exercised in sliding the abdominal aorta over toward the left and keeping the finger pressed firmly on the vertebra, the surgeon will experience no difficulty whatsoever in introducing the needle as above stated.

Step 6. When the point of the needle rests firmly on the anterior body of the vertebra, hold it in position with the right hand while withdrawing the left hand from the abdominal cavity, and from 75 to 100 cc. of ½ per cent solution of novocaine with the usual amount of adrenalin is introduced into the retroperitoneal space which floods the same and produces anesthesia of all the upper abdominal viscera.

Comment: In using the finger as a guide, Finsterer removes his glove for this purpose, but from his experience, Arnold did not find this necessary, probably because the gloves used in America are of much finer quality and thinner in structure, therefore not interfering with one's sense of touch, as do the heavier gloves used in Vienna.

Anesthesia begins within three to five minutes and lasts for two and one-half to three hours.

With the patient in the semi-sitting position the administration of splanchnic anesthesia would be facilitated because it would require less pulling downward of the stomach and pancreas before injecting the splanchnic nerve plexus.

For his first patient, the surgeon should select, if possible, a thin individual because in such a case, the anesthetization of the splanchnics is

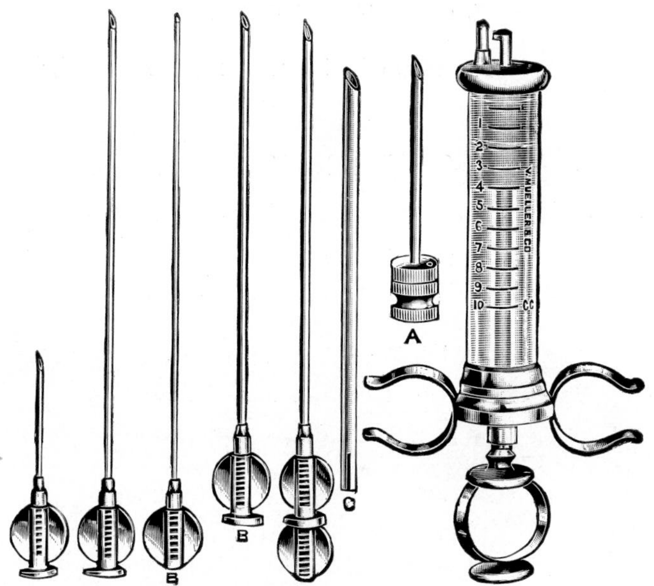

FIG. 81. Syringe for local anesthesia.

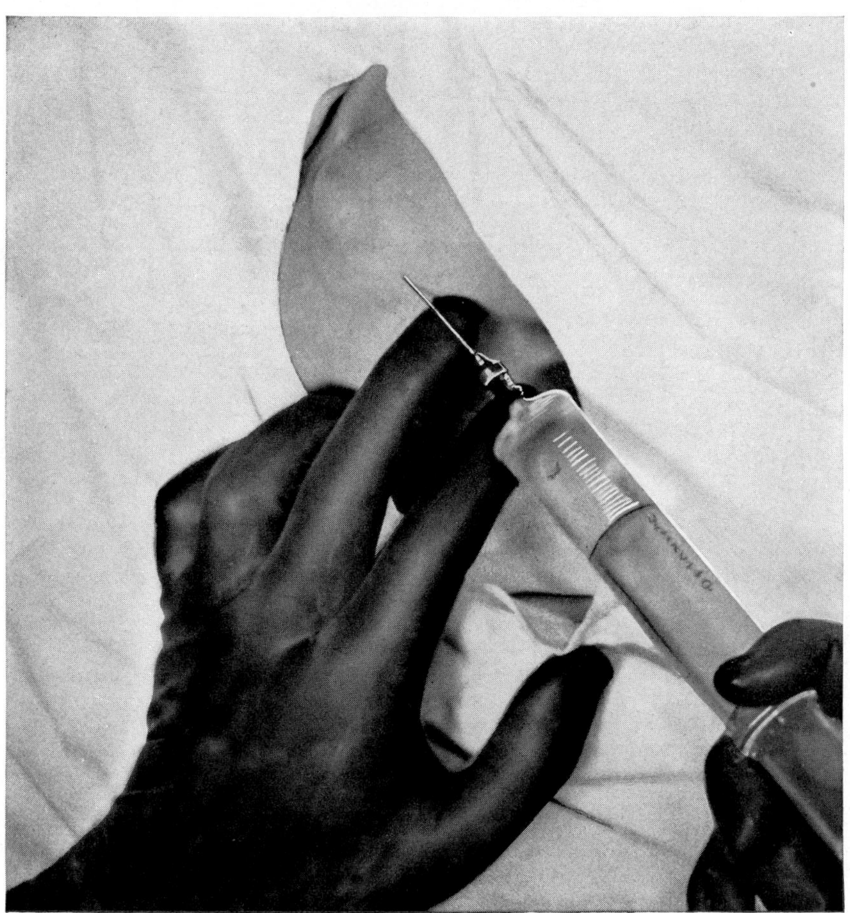

FIG. 82. Local anesthesia. Removal of lipoma under local anesthesia. Infiltration of skin over fatty tumor.

rather simple, while in the case of a large obese individual, it obviously becomes more difficult.

LOCAL ANESTHESIA

Novocaine, known in America as procaine, is the agent most generally used for inducing local anesthesia. It is safer and less toxic than cocaine.

Procaine may be boiled in normal salt solution and adrenalin, adrenin or epinephrin added after it has cooled to body temperature. Or, sterilize a medicine glass and dropper with the instruments. Have a supply of sterile water at hand. Before the operation is begun, drop as many (2 to 4 two-grain) procaine

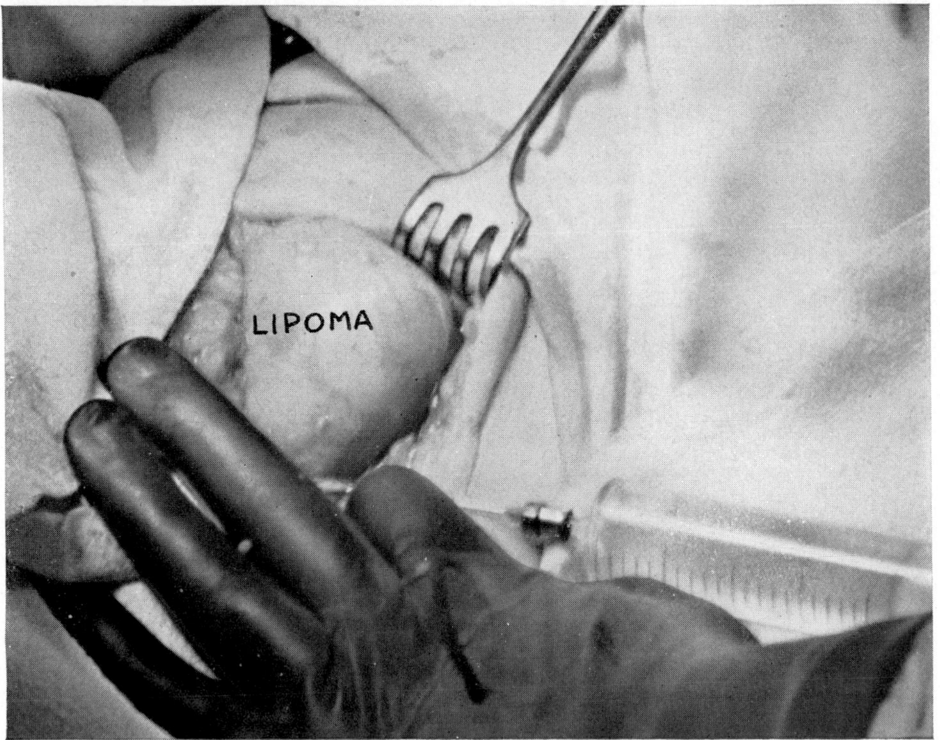

FIG. 83. Exposure of tumor after skin and subcutaneous tissues have been infiltrated.

tablets as previously calculated to be needed for the operation into a medicine glass. Crush the tablets and fill the glass with sterile water. Add the desired amount of adrenalin to the solution. Mix thoroughly. A fresh solution is thus always readily obtainable. The following formula recommended by **Fisher** is satisfactory:

Procaine	1.5
Sodium Chloride	0.92
Thymol	0.025
Distilled Water	100.0

This makes a 1½ per cent procaine solution in normal salt solution plus 1/3 gr. of thymol added as a preservative. This solution may be boiled and

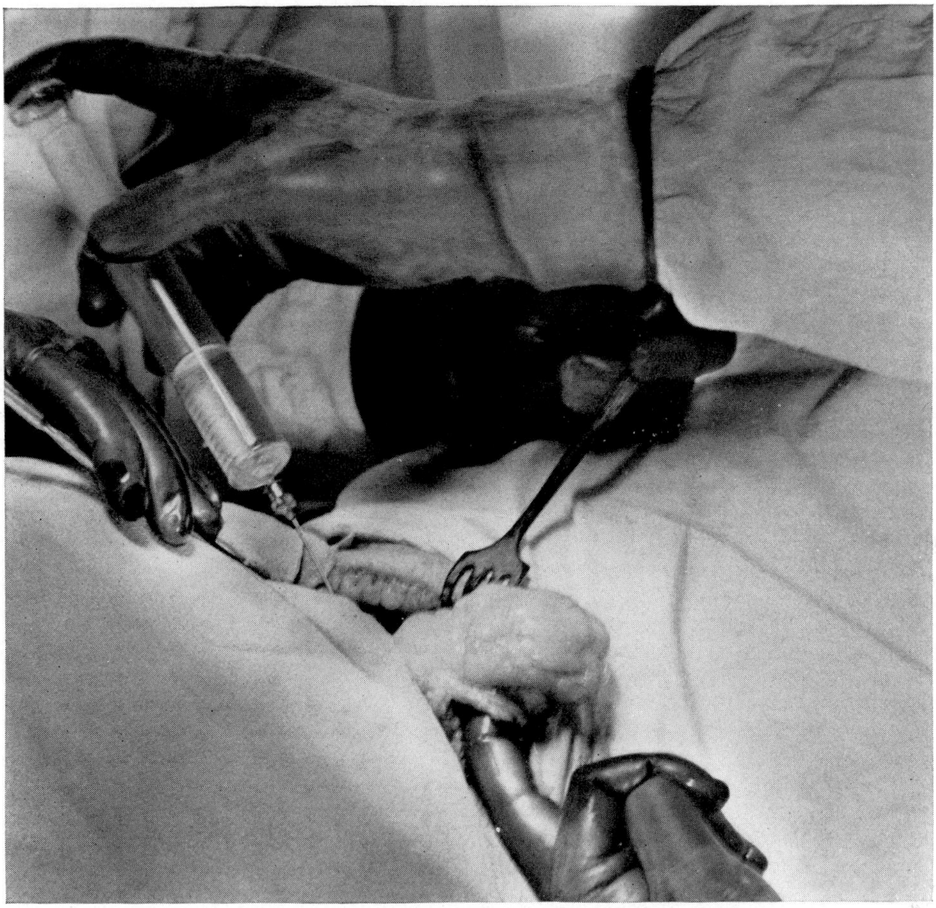

FIG. 84. Infiltration of structures situated in the back of tumor.

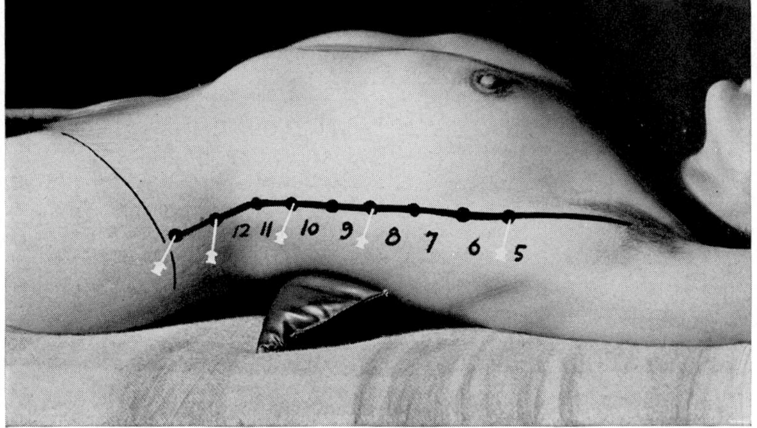

FIG. 85. Block anesthesia of the nerves of the anterior abdominal wall. Where an abdominal incision above the umbilicus is contemplated, it is essential to block the intercostal nerves, from the fifth to the eleventh in this case. If the incision is to be made below the umbilicus the nerves between the eleventh rib and the crest of the ilium are to be blocked.

epinephrine added at the time it is used. Thymol causes a slight stinging sensation when the drug is injected.

The apparatus essential for the administration of local anesthesia consists of a syringe and needles (Fig. 81).

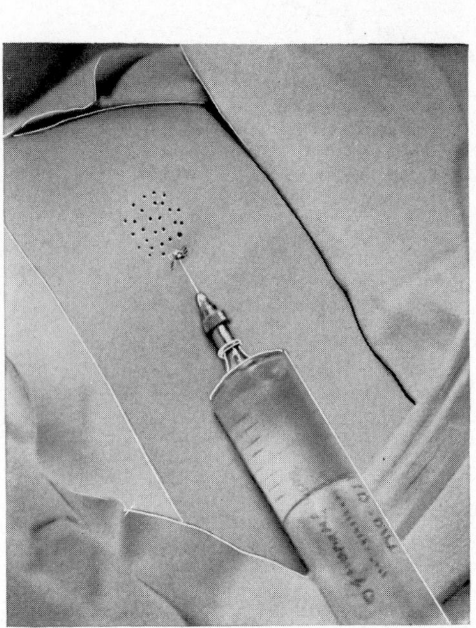

FIG. 86. Local anesthesia. Making endodermal wheal of infiltration.

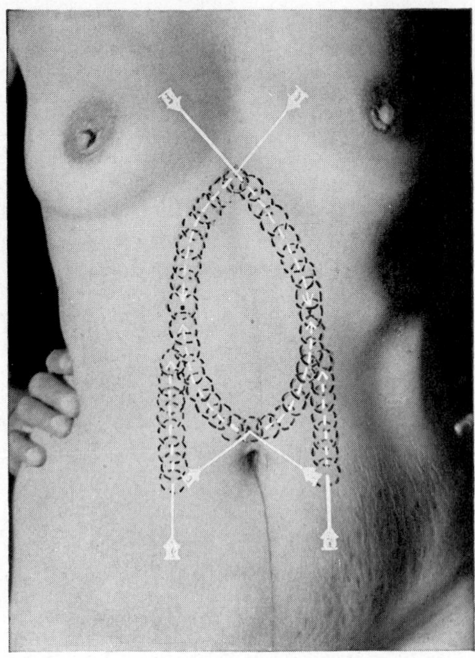

FIG. 87. Block anesthesia in operations on the upper abdomen.

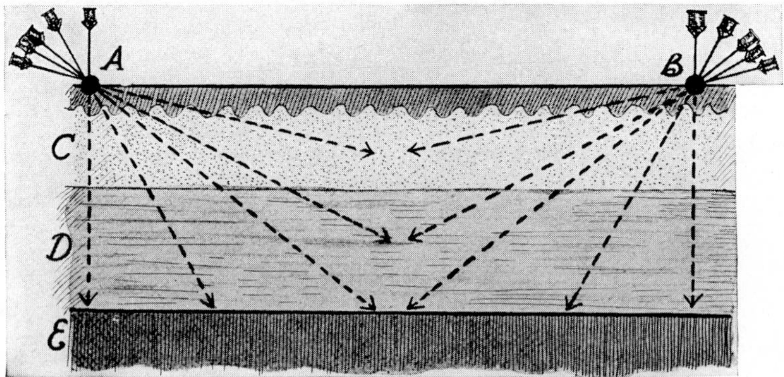

FIG. 88. Diagrammatic representation of bone and overlying tissues infiltrated with anesthetic solution: A.-B. points of entrance of the needle, C. subcutaneous cellular tissue, D. muscle and fascia, E. bone.

If the operation is to be a prolonged one and the patient of the apprehensive, nervous type, a hypodermic injection of ¼ gr. of morphine may be administered an hour or so before the procaine is injected. Hertzler[1] refers to this premedication as "removing the hypertension from the apprehension."

Scopolamine-morphine analgesia may be advantageously combined with local infiltration anesthesia.

[1] Hertzler: Local Anesthesia. C. V. Mosby Co., 1937.

Assurance to the patient and proper suggestion are of inestimable value in local anesthesia. All fears of the patient must be allayed.

TYPES OF LOCAL ANESTHESIA

(Figs. 82, 83, 84, 85)

1. **Endermic Infiltration.** This consists of injecting the papillary layer of the skin where the nerve-endings arborize (Fig. 86).

2. **Subdermic Infiltration.** Here the injection is given under the skin.

3. **Nerve Blocking.** Such nerve trunks as the sciatic, brachial plexus, etc., may be blocked first without exposing the nerves. Smaller nerves (ilioinguinal, radial, ulnar, etc.) one often treated thusly. The anesthetizing fluid is injected into the nerves directly as a rule; however, in some instances the nerve becomes infiltrated by the diffusion of the agent through the tissues. (Fig. 87.)

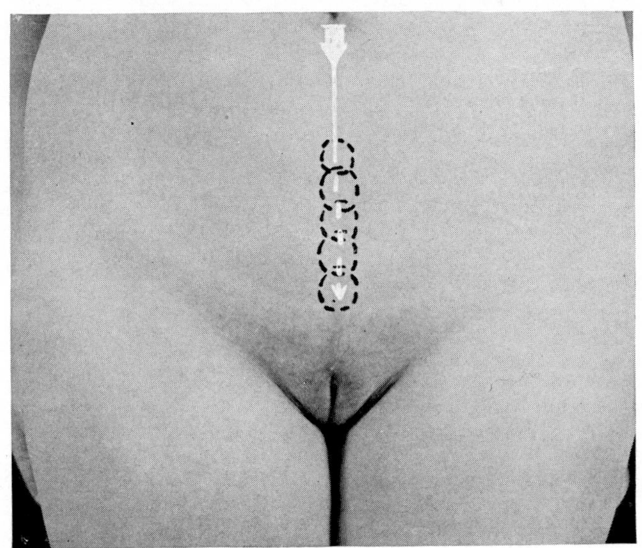

Fig. 89. Infiltration anesthesia for opening the bladder (cystostomy).

4. **Perineural injection** is an infiltration of the tissues around the nerve paths and is resorted to in hernia operations, thyroidectomies, etc.

5. **Edematization (Schleich's Method).** Here also all the tissues surrounding the operative field are injected.

Two or more of the above procedures are usually combined in this type of anesthesia. Endermic infiltration is often used for the skin and some form of nerve-block or edematization for the deeper tissues.

In another method the principal nerve trunk is sought first, necessitating two or more rather deep thrusts of the needle into the tissues, after which the skin is anesthetized.

Descriptions of local anesthesia as pertaining to various operations will be found under the respective operative procedures. (Figs. 88, 89.)

Part II

SURGERY OF THE HEAD AND NECK AND PLASTIC SURGERY

CHAPTER PAGE

7. Surgery of the Scalp and Pericranium 107
8. Surgery of the Skull and Brain 113
9. Surgery of the Ears and Adjacent Structures 178
10. Surgery of the Face 197
11. Surgery of the Sinuses and Tonsils 224
12. Surgery of the Lips, Tongue and Lymph Nodes 243
13. Surgery of the Salivary Glands 267
14. Surgery of the Upper Jaw, Upper Lip and Cheek 281
15. Surgery of the Orbit and Eye 320
16. Surgery of the Nose 352
17. Surgery of the Neck and Cervical Endocrine Glands 375
18. Plastic Surgery 484

ORIENTATION

This part opens with a consideration of the surgery of the scalp and pericranium and is succeeded by a description of surgical operations of the skull and its contents. While neurosurgery is a highly specialized branch of surgical endeavor, the general surgeon, I believe, should be conversant with emergencies that may arise in this connection and he must be prepared to treat these. On the other hand, the student and general surgeon alike should be acquainted with the principles underlying the technic of elective surgical operations of one kind or another which require specialized skill so that they may in consultation with the neurosurgeon intelligently evaluate the problems involved. In this comparatively new field of surgical endeavor the strides made under the leadership of Harvey Cushing (1869-) and his pupils in this country, von Bergmann (1836-1907) and Fedor Krause and others in Germany, Sir Victor Horsley (1857-1916) in England have opened a new horizon for activities and research in this field and the constant improvements as noted in contemporary literature, promises even greater achievements as time goes on.

In Chapter 9 the Surgery of the Ear and Adjacent Structures is discussed. The general surgeon is frequently called upon to do emergency operations on the mastoid process. It is his duty to perform these in an emergency and where no specialized help is at hand and in so doing he must be conversant with the complications of middle ear disease and how to conduct himself in the face of such.

From the apparently simple carbuncle of the upper lip that may, and on occasion does cost the patient's life, if improperly handled, the various forms of fractures, the manifold types of surgical treatment designed for affections of the trigeminal nerve and the Gasserian ganglion are included in the scope of Chapter 10. The operations for the various affections of the accessory sinuses, and diseases of the tonsils are the subject of discussion in Chapter 11. This is followed by a consideration of the surgery of the lips, tongue and lymph nodes, the surgery of which has become standardized in some cases and undergone changes and modifications in others.

The surgery of the salivary glands (injuries, infections, calculi, neoplasms, fistulae) are accorded consideration from the practical point of view and the various surgical methods now in vogue to remedy these are described. Just as the general surgeon is subject to call to perform emergency operations on the ear so must he be prepared to invade the orbit and eye should such occasion arise. He may also choose to practice elective surgical procedures here, provided, of course, his dexterity, knowledge and preparation in this field of endeavor are adequate. Under many circumstances, the scalpel is forced into his hands, particularly when no specialist is available. This holds equally true in surgical affections of the nose (Chapter 16). The Surgery of the Neck (Chapter 17) embraces descriptions of the surgical management of simpler conditions such as burns, and scars of the neck to the more serious affections such as cellulitis, Ludwig's angina, injuries to the neck, emergency tracheotomy, operations on the thyroid gland, the parathyroids and thymus, laryngotomy, laryngectomy, thyrotomy, branchial cysts, thyroglossal sinuses, tumor of the carotid bodies, etc.

CHAPTER 7

SURGERY OF THE SCALP AND PERICRANIUM

INJURIES

WOUNDS OF THE SCALP

Step 1. Shave the affected area. Cleanse it thoroughly by washing with green soap and water followed by bichloride solution (1:1000), ether and, lastly, with tincture of iodine.

Step 2. Remove all foreign materials from the wound. Attend to hemostasis. Temporary hemostasis may be obtained by surrounding the head with a rubber band, bandage, etc. as shown in the illustration (Fig. 90). Crushed edges of the wound should be excised. Individual bleeding vessels in the scalp should be sutured. Do not use ligatures—these will slip off; use sutures of catgut. Approximate the lips of the wound with interrupted sutures (silkworm gut or silk) (Fig. 91). Dress. Inject antitetanus serum.

AVULSION OF THE SCALP

While rare, avulsion of the scalp does occasionally occur in industrial plants.

Step 1. If the avulsed scalp can be located, clip the hair, cleanse both surfaces (bichloride 1:1000, iodine, peroxide, etc.) and replace it onto the defect on the skull after the latter has been thoroughly cleansed and hemostasis has been attended to.

Step 2. Fix the scalp in position by interrupted sutures. Provide for adequate drainage. (Fig. 92.)

TUMORS

MENINGOCELE AND ENCEPHALOCELE

This condition is represented by a congenital globular tumor usually situated in the occipital region (posterior fontanelle). It occurs before the occlusion of the fontanelles and consists of a protrusion of the meninges or the brain and is of variable size. (Figs. 93-94.)

Step 1. Shave the head and render it aseptic. Outline a cutaneous flap leaving sufficient tissues to cover the final wound.

Step 2. Extend the incision through the scalp and fasciae of the neck down to the dura mater. Separate the flaps carefully from the dura. Isolate the sac carefully and make a small opening in it to avoid too rapid an onrush of cerebrospinal fluid.

Where the orifice is very small a ligature is made to encircle the neck of the sac. Superimpose a purse-string suture thus burying the ligature; over this another longitudinal suture is placed.

Step 3. Fashion sufficient fascial skin flaps to allow for proper approximation; excess of skin should be trimmed away. Use silk or Michel clips for the skin closure.

SEBACEOUS CYSTS (WENS)

Step 1. Shave and prepare the skin aseptically: Use local infiltration anesthesia (½ to 1 per cent novocaine) injected around the cystic tumor.

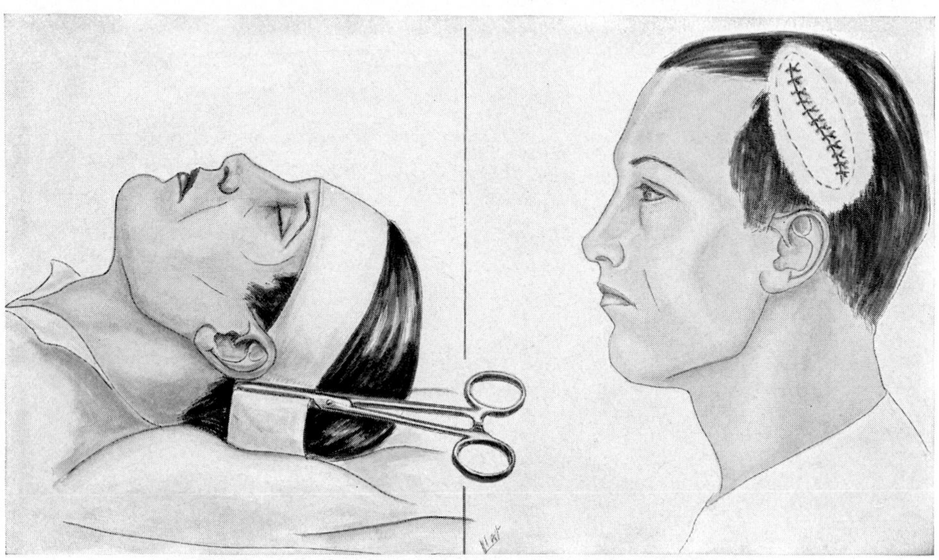

FIG. 90. Temporary hemostasis of the scalp. FIG. 91. Repair of scalp wound.

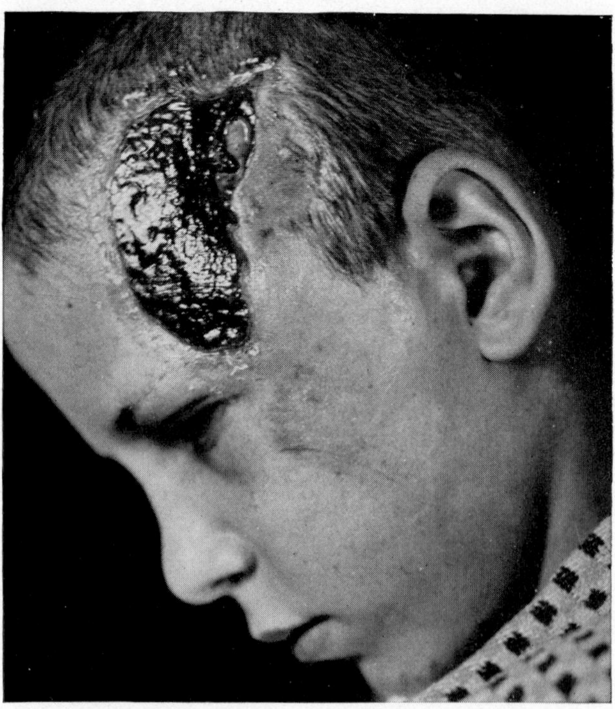

FIG. 92. Partial avulsion of scalp with fracture. Skin grafting. Recovery.

Step 2. Incise the skin overlying the cyst and dissect laterally the tissues overlying it. Attempt to remove the cyst without breaking its capsule.

Step 3. Attend to hemostasis. Close wound with interrupted sutures; dress. (Fig. 95.)

If the cyst is infected and suppurating it should be treated as an abscess (drainage). Wherever possible, it is better to excise it thoroughly together with the infected tegumentary structures surrounding it.

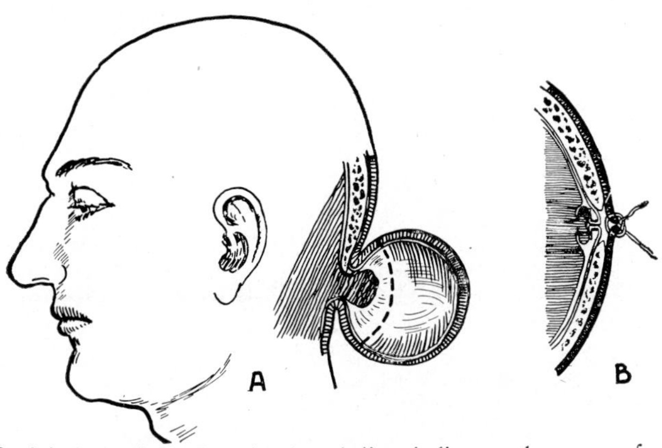

Fig. 93. Occipital meningocele: A, dotted line indicates the area of resection of the internal membrane of the cyst. B, cross section showing reduction of the cerebral hernia and invagination of the collarette, the umbilicus of which is closed with two sutures. Deep and superficial suture of skin with clips (after Doyen).

ANGIOMA OF THE SCALP

When nevi of the scalp require removal by operation, the incision should be made sufficiently far from the nevus so that hemostasis may be easily effected. Rapidly growing angiomas which penetrate the subcutaneous tissues or threaten hemorrhage call for prompt operation. Angiomas over the fontanelles often communicate with the longitudinal sinus. Radical operation should here give way to other measures (radium).

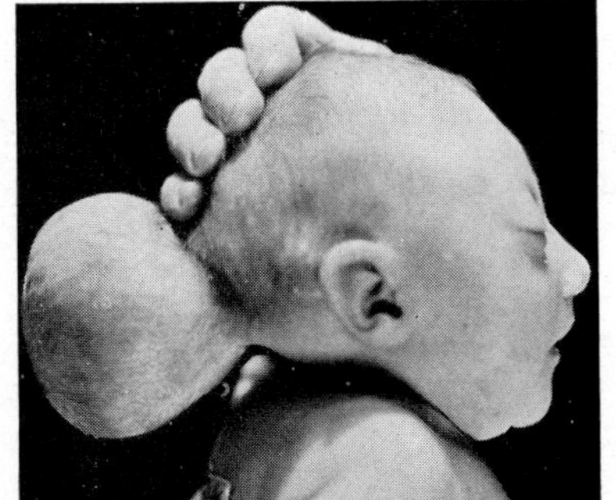

Fig. 94. Meningocele. (Courtesy of Dr. Francis Lederer, University of Illinois.)

Cavernous Angiomas which tend to penetrate the skull should also be treated by radium or electrocoagulation; or by subcutaneous ligation, if surgery is decided upon.

Step 1. Arm a full curved needle with catgut. Pass the needle through the entire thickness of the skin for about 1 to 1½ cm. down to the pericranium.

Step 2. Remove the full curved and substitute a semi-curved needle. With this pass the suture from the point of emergence of the needle back to its point of entry, immediately under the skin. Tie the suture tightly.

Step 3. Repeat this all around the nevus until practically every vessel entering or leaving the tumor is controlled. Each suture should overlap to some extent into the territory controlled by the next stitch.

CIRSOID ANEURYSM OF THE SCALP

Operation for cirsoid aneurysm of the scalp is done in two stages, under general or infiltration anesthesia. Place the patient in an almost sitting position; use a tourniquet wherever possible.

Stage I

Step 1. The incision should extend through the skin and epicranial aponeurosis and embrace the cirsoid mass anteriorly and laterally. Make the incision in steps, using compressions against the bone on each side of the incision until the vessels are secured with artery forceps and ligated. The main vessels should first be isolated and doubly ligated before being divided. When

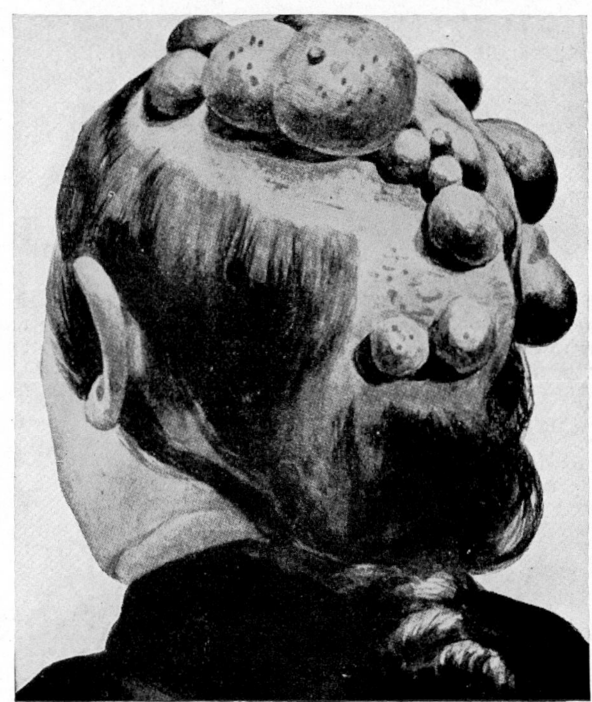

FIG. 95. Multiple sebaceous cysts (fourteen) of the scalp. (Lexer.)

completed, this incision outlines a horse-shoe shaped flap having its base at the occiput. (Fig. 96.)

Step 2. Reflect the flap from the cranium. This step requires the use of numerous ligations because of the free anastomosis with the deep vessels.

Step 3. Place a gauze pack between the flap and the bone. Replace the flap over the gauze. (Bryant). Apply dressings and bandage.

Stage II

Step. 1. After three or four days remove the dressings and excise the tumor. The resulting thrombosis in the blood vessels of the tumor and the loosening of the contiguous connective tissues, the result of edema, now facilitate the excision of the tumor which should not be done at the first sitting.

Step 2. Replace and suture the flap into position. Dress the wound.

MALIGNANT TUMORS OF THE SCALP

Anatomic Considerations. The lymph vessels of the frontal, and the anterior part of the parieto-occipital regions, drain into the parotid lymph nodes which are situated mainly in the parotid region; their removal involves the removal of the parotid gland. Carcinoma of the scalp with metastases into the parotid is usually

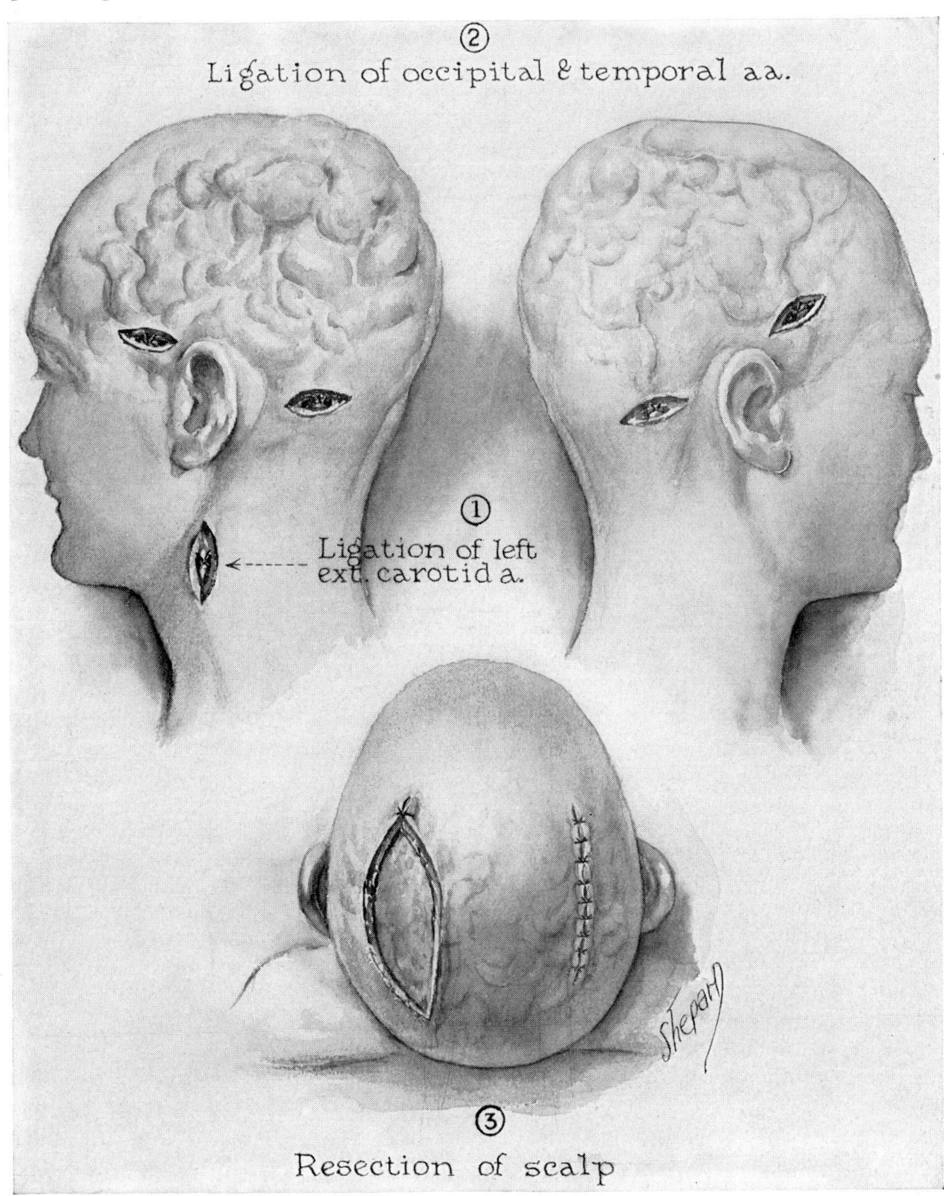

Fig. 96. Cirsoid aneurysm of the scalp. (Courtesy of Dr. R. W. McNealy.)

inoperable. The lymph vessels of the posterior part of the parieto-occipital region drain into the mastoid group of lymph nodes lying on the mastoid portion of the sternomastoid muscle. These may be extirpated with facility. The occipital region is drained by two avenues. From the lateral part, the vessels unite to form a single trunk which courses downwards to a point under the sternocleidomastoid muscle and here enters one of the external nodes of the sternomastoid group. From the mesial surface the lymph vessels course to the occipital nodes.

The surgical principles underlying operative procedures here are the same as obtain elsewhere, viz.,

1. Free excision of the tumor.
2. Removal of the lymph vessels and nodes draining the affected area, whenever possible.
3. Follow up by radiation.

Technic, Carcinoma Being Freely Movable

Step 1. Excise the tumor thoroughly in healthy tissue down to the bone.

Step 2. If possible, cover the resulting defect by undermined or mobilized flaps. If impossible, permit the wound to granulate and later do a skin graft or plastic operation.

Carcinoma Being Adherent

Step 1. As above.

Step 2. Chisel away the external table of bone underlying the involved area.

When the Diplöe Has Been Encroached Upon

Step 1. Remove the entire thickness of the skull, freely.

Step 2. Cover the resulting defect by the Müller-König procedure. In instances where the so-called silent areas of the brain are also involved (frontal, occipital), not only the dura but portions of the cerebral cortex may also have to be removed.

CHAPTER 8

SURGERY OF THE SKULL AND BRAIN

INJURIES OF THE CRANIAL VAULT

SCALP WOUND WITH POSSIBLE FRACTURE

Step 1. Enlarge the wound. If only a **fissure** is seen in the bone and the opposing sides are in good alignment, treat as an ordinary scalp wound.

Step 2. If foreign material (hairs, dirt, etc.) are within the fissure, enlarge the opening with chisel or rongeur. If this offers difficulties, drill a hole on either side of the crack and chisel away a strip of bone along the fissured line, on either side. **Thoroughly remove foreign material!**

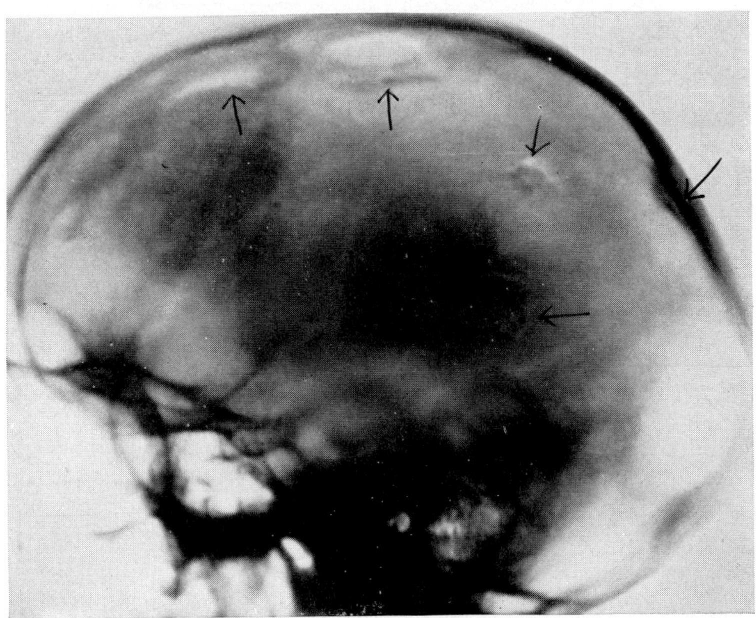

FIG. 97. Multiple fractures of the skull causing no symptoms. The patient was beaten over the head with the butt of a revolver during a holdup. No loss of consciousness but severe bleeding from the scalp. After remaining in the hospital for one day patient insisted on leaving stating he felt perfectly well. (From Author's Service, American Hospital.)

Step 3. Look for injuries of the dura or hemorrhage; deal with these, if present, accordingly. After completing the operation, close the wound; drain. Antitetanus serum.

SIMPLE FRACTURE WITH DEPRESSED BONE

Figure 97 shows deep and multiple fractures of the vault of the cranium which did not produce any symptoms. Occasionally multiple fractures (Fig. 98) may be treated expectantly, provided the patient can be kept under strict observation.

Whether symptoms are present or not the depression, particularly if marked, should be elevated and the subjacent structures relieved from pressure. The inner table is almost always more extensively damaged than clinical signs would indicate. (Fig. 99.)

If **operation** is decided upon, however, the depressed fragment should be delivered into place by introducing a bone elevator (Fig. 100) into a fissure or an opening, made by means of a burr or drill to gain access to the depressed fragment, and liberated; or, an osteoplastic flap designed to have the depressed bone in the center may be made. When the flap and bone are turned downward, digital pressure or light blows from a hammer will bring the depressed bone into normal

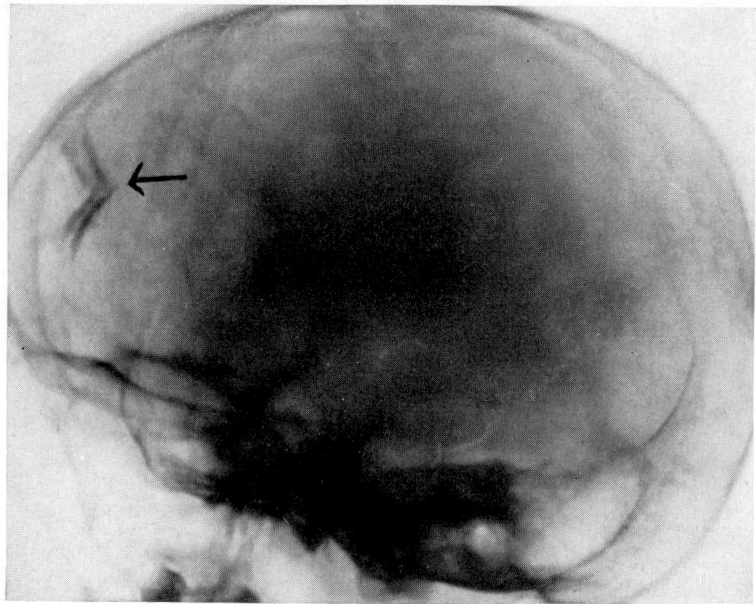

FIG. 98. Depressed fracture of skull.

alignment. The surrounding areas are now inspected for bone spiculae, foreign material or intradural hemorrhage and the flap is replaced. The wound is then sutured in place and a small drain inserted.

COMPOUND COMMINUTED FRACTURE

Step 1. Expose the fractured area.

Step 2. Drill holes on either side of the injured bone.

Step 3. Remove fragmented bone. (Figs. 101 and 102.)

Step 4. Irrigate with hot normal saline solution, washing away debris, blood clots and foreign material (see comment). If the dura is torn, clean it and suture the rent. It is safer to drain than not to drain. Defects in the dura that cannot be repaired should be covered with some aseptic material (foil, cargyle membrane, rubber, etc.) or some duraplastic may be resorted to. Injured sinuses should be packed.

Step 5. Attend to hemostasis. Fragments of bone, if not soiled, may be cleansed and replaced, provided the dura is intact. If not, repair the dura; discard the bone fragments.

Step 6. Close the wound.

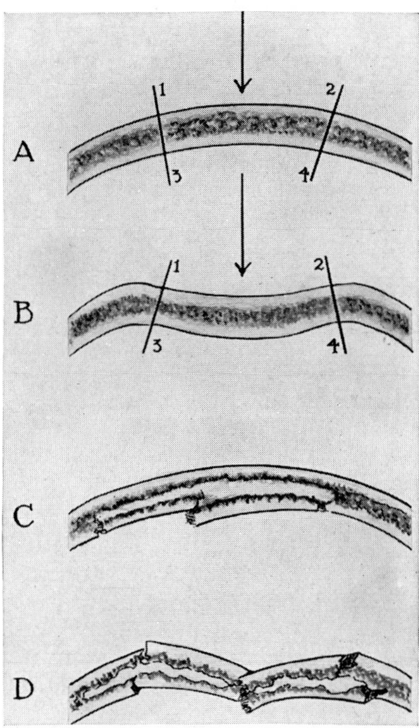

Fig. 99. Local depressed fractures of the vault; the mechanics of their production: A. the normal vault with its outer and inner table, and the interposed diploë. The arrow indicates the force applied at the point of contact, and the lines 1-3 and 2-4 are placed at right angles to both the outer and inner tables, they naturally converge; B. the force applied at the point of contact produces a depression of both the outer and inner tables, and especially of the inner table, as shown by the divergence of the lines 1-3 and 2-4; C. the inner table may fracture and a fragment may be depressed, and yet the outer table may remain intact, either depressed or, as illustrated here, in its original position; D. a complete depressed fracture occurs when the force applied is sufficient to cause a fracture not only at the point of contact but also at the margin of the depressed area, the line of fracture of the inner table is always beyond that of the outer table. (After Sharpe.)

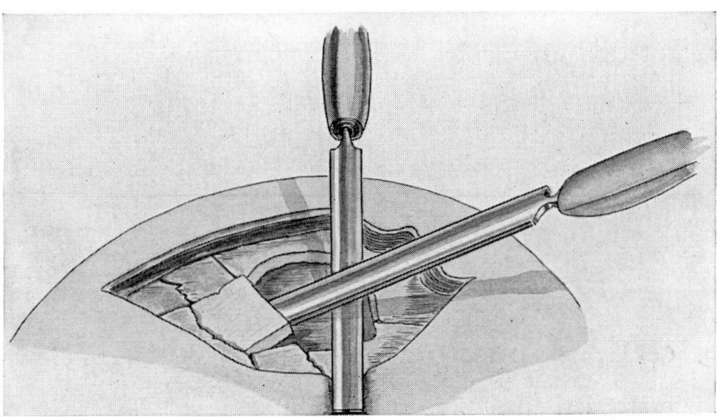

Fig. 100. Method of elevating bone fragments in depressed fracture of the skull.

Comment. At all cost, make sure that nothing is left behind in the wound that may invite disastrous results. If in doubt, make a trephine hole

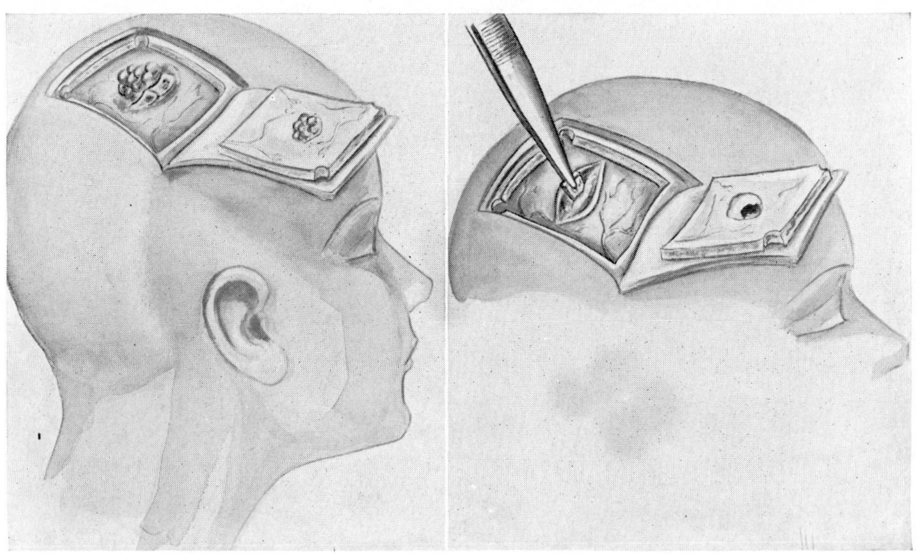

FIG. 101 FIG. 102

FIG. 101. Injury to brain substance, splinters of bone in brain.
FIG. 102. Removal of splinters of bone from brain substance. (Krause-Thorek, Surgery of the Brain and Spinal Cord, F. J. Rebman Publishing Co.)

lateral to the fracture. Explore. Do not exert pressure on the fractured fragments in any operative maneuvers lest injury result to the underlying

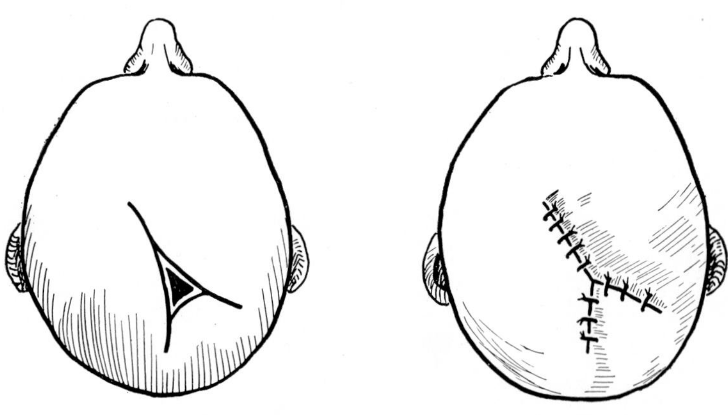

FIG. 103 FIG. 104

FIG. 103. Cushing's tripod incision for wound of the scalp with loss of substance.
FIG. 104. Same incision. Wound sutured.

cerebral structures. A wise rule to adopt in cranial fractures, whether depressed or not, is: When in doubt, explore!

PENETRATING WOUNDS OF THE BRAIN

Step 1. Make a Cushing tripod incision (Figs. 103 and 104).

Step 2. Remove the area of cranial penetration en bloc instead of piecemeal. Bore four holes with a burr or very small trephine outlining a quadrangular area on the outer boundaries of the involved cranial space.

Step 3. With the aid of a Gigli saw remove this square of bone carrying the penetrating osseous wound. Trim away the lacerated edges of the dura.

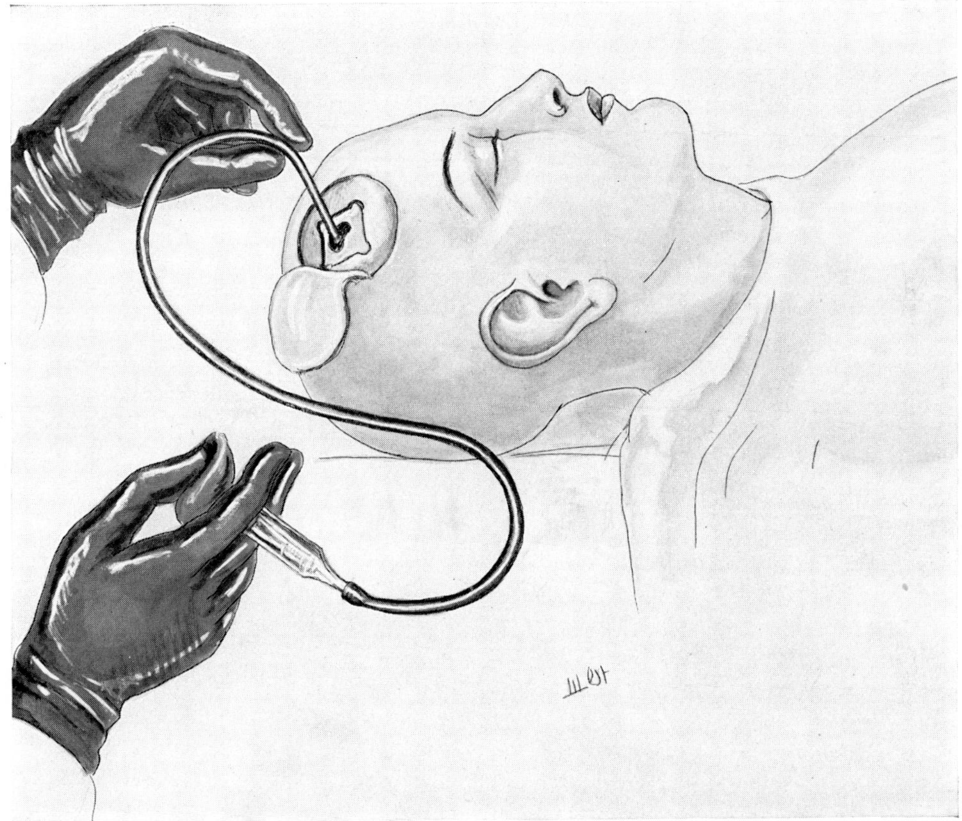

Fig. 105. Removing fragments in penetrating wounds of brain by suction (Cushing).

Step 4. Pass a rubber catheter down to the depths of the wound; do not explore with the finger. The distal end of the catheter is attached to a hand suction bulb or an aspirating syringe through which loose particles of detritus are aspirated or washed away (Fig. 105). Do not attempt to remove bullets unless freely accessible.

Step 5. Close the wound. Drain.

Comment. Bullets entering the cranial cavity may produce death, a great deal of mischief or remain inocuous: all depends on the location of the missile. A flat x-ray plate (Fig. 106) does not give sufficient information as to the exact location of the bullet. Stereoscopic plates and special methods of localization must be employed by the roentgenologist to locate the position of the bullet accurately. If no symptoms are produced by the bullet, leave it alone. If it gives rise to clinical manifestations, remove it.

CONCUSSION OF THE BRAIN

Do not rush the patient to the x-ray room. Get him out of shock first. After shock is combated, get stereo-x-rays to ascertain the presence or absence of fracture and its location.

Masterly inactivity—so aptly expressed by Hamilton Bailey—should be the slogan. Good nursing is here superior to medical meddling.

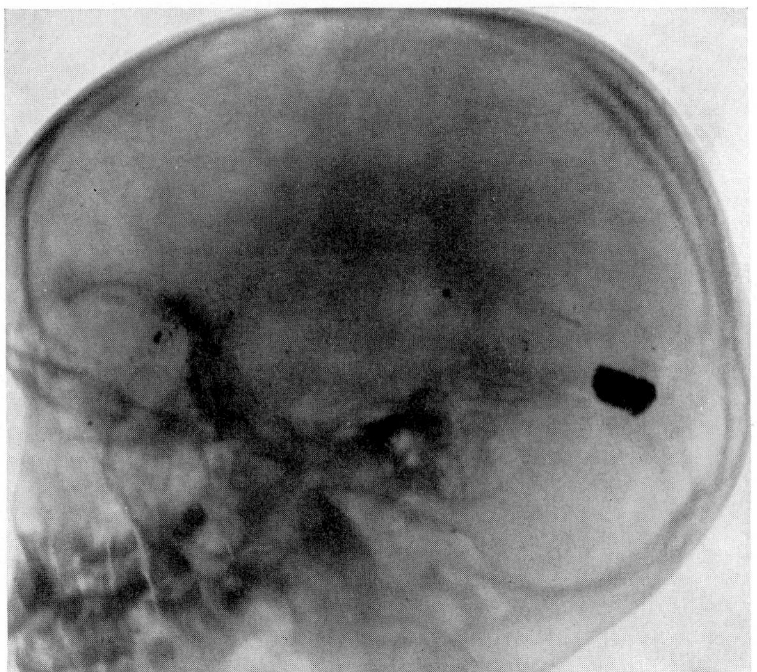

Fig. 106. Bullet in brain causing no symptoms.

METHODS OF REDUCING INTRACRANIAL TENSION

1. **Magnesium Sulphate.** If the patient is conscious, one-half ounce of a saturated solution of magnesium sulphate is given every two hours for twenty-four to forty-eight hours (Hamilton Bailey). Reduce the dose gradually until the seventh or tenth day; then discontinue it. Give no water during this treatment to avoid excessive catharsis. Restricted quantities of barley water, fruit juices and broth are allowed. No catharsis will result when the water intake is restricted.

   If the patient is unconscious give magnesium sulphate per rectum (100 Gm. dissolved in 120 Gm. of water) administered by rectoclysis and repeated every four hours.
2. **Hypertonic Saline Solution by Venoclysis.** This is to be used only in desperate cases (20 cc. of a 30 per cent solution). See that none of the solution finds its way to the contiguous structures lest pain and sloughing result.
3. **Lumbar Punctures.** Abstract slowly about 8-10 cc. of cerebrospinal fluid through a needle reaching the subarachnoid space between the third and

fourth lumbar vertebrae. Repeat the procedure within 24 hours, if necessary. Let the spinal fluid pressure be your guide.

Malone warns against attempting to decompress by any method, if the blood pressure is below normal.

FRACTURES OF THE BASE OF THE SKULL

Treat as concussion.

1. Where cerebrospinal fluid escapes give urotropin intravenously (Tygat) (5 cc. of a 40 per cent solution).
2. Plug the nares or ears to avoid infections.

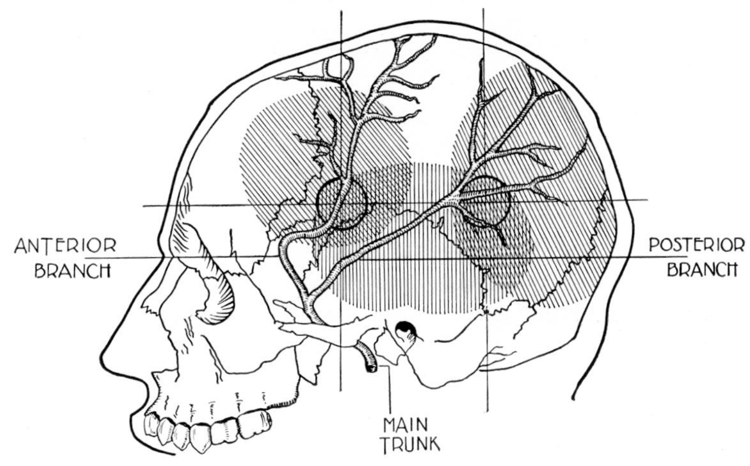

FIG. 107. After injury of the anterior branch of the artery, a hematoma is apt to form in the frontotemporal region; after injury of the posterior branch, in the parieto-occipital region; after injury to the main artery, low down in the temporoparietal region. The two circles intersected by lines designate the regions where the trephine openings should be made.

3. Treat symptoms as they arise.
4. Increased intracranial pressure is combated by one of the methods outlined under concussion.
5. The furor of subtemporal decompression for fractures at the base of the skull (unless definitely indicated) is fortunately passing, except, of course, in definite hemorrhage from the middle meningeal artery (see below).
6. Restlessness is subdued by morphine or paraldehyde (rectally).

INTRACRANIAL BLEEDING

Be familiar with the anatomic position of the middle meningeal artery and its branches. The question to be decided is: Where is the hemorrhage? Is it extra- or intradural? When in doubt and when the condition of the patient is growing worse—explore.

Step 1. Open the skull by any of the methods described on p. 131.

Step 2. If the operation fails to reveal any large collection of blood, do a subtemporal decompression (p. 148).

Step 3. In bleeding from the middle meningeal artery—trephine in the middle of the temporal region, fairly low down, to expose the main branch of the artery.

The common trunk of the middle meningeal artery or the anterior or posterior branch is usually ligated. The locations of hematomas were studied by Krönlein and are shown together with the points for trephining in (Fig. 107). Then continue the operation with A, B or C (see below).

Last Step. After the skull is opened, wash away clots; search and find the bleeding point and ligate it. Be thorough.

(A) Ligation of the Trunk of the Middle Meningeal Artery

There are no fixed relations between any parts of the middle meningeal artery and its branches. The main trunk enters the cranial vault through the foramen spinosum.

Step 1. Select as center for the trephine opening a point that will fall over the artery proximate to its bifurcation, generally about 3.8 cm. behind the external angular process of the frontal bone and 2.5 cm. above the zygoma.

Step 2. Incise and retract the skin and soft parts; ligate the superficial temporal artery and vein, guarding the auriculotemporal nerve and branches of the facial nerve.

Step 3. Carry the incision along the posterior border of the temporal muscle through the periosteum to the bone.

Step 4. Apply the trephine; remove the disc of bone; expose the meningeal artery and ligate it after removing all clots; examine the dura mater and suture the lacerations present, after removing any bone spiculae or other loose tissue. Irrigate the region thoroughly.

Step 5. Close the various layers of the wound in the usual way.

(B) Ligation of Anterior Branch

Step 1. Select as center of the trephine opening a point about 3.8 cm. behind the external angular process of the frontal bone and 3.8 to 4.5 cm. above the zygoma.

Step 2. Make a horseshoe incision, with its center over the above point and its convexity upward, the outer limb being just behind the external angular process; this incision is carried through the skin, temporal fascia, temporal muscle and periosteum to the bone. The soft parts are retracted downward.

Step 3. A ½-inch trephine is applied at the point selected and the further steps in the operation are practically the same as for ligation of the main trunk of the middle meningeal artery.

(C) Ligation of the Posterior Branch Through Trephine Opening Exposed by a Horseshoe Incision

Step 1. As before, a point is selected as trephine center which will fall over the posterior branch of the artery in the groove of the parietal bone, which is taken to be at the intersection of a line drawn horizontally backward on a level with the roof of the orbit and one drawn vertically upward from directly behind the mastoid process; i.e., the point just below the parietal eminence.

Step 2. Make a horseshoe incision, as previously described, with its center over this point, the limbs being from 5 to 5.7 cm. apart.

Step 3. The operation is now performed in general as in the operation on the anterior branch of the artery.

Where an Intradural Clot Is Suspected

Step 1. Incise the dura, or make a dural flap with its base directed upward.

Step 2. Irrigate the clots away with saline solution under **gentle pressure.**

Step 3. If pial vessels are bleeding, ligate them with fine silk carried on curved needles.

Step 4. Gently raise the temporal lobe and explore thoroughly. Wash away clots. If both sides are injured and similar conditions suspected, bilateral exploration should be done.

Where no bleeding is found, do a decompression. It will bring relief (the case may be one of multiple small hemorrhages in and about the brain).

BRAIN ABSCESS

Joseph E. J. King,[1] having observed that the vast majority of abscesses approach the dura to within ½ to 3 cm., has developed the following operation, the technic of which is relatively simple and which has proved very safe in his hands (14 out of 17 recovered). If possible no attempt should ever be made to drain an abscess until it is encapsulated, a process requiring several weeks.

Step 1. Local anesthesia, novocaine 1 or ½ per cent solution with suprarenin alone or combined with avertin. In adults, especially those that are stuporous or in a semicomatose condition, local anesthesia alone will suffice. In children, the combination with avertin is more satisfactory.

Step 2. Incision. In temporosphenoidal abscess a short, straight, slightly oblique incision about 1½ inches long is made through all the soft parts down to the outer table of the skull. An opening with a bone drill is made at a point about 1 inch posterior to and about 1½ inches above the external auditory meatus; this later is enlarged to a mastoid incision if such has not already been made.

In frontal lobe abscess there is usually little brain substance intervening between the abscess and the posterior wall of the frontal sinus or ethmoids; an osteoplastic flap is turned down with incisions along the eyebrow, hairline, and center of the forehead; the flap is turned under and sutured on itself until such later time as it is replaced.

In cerebellar abscess the approach, in the absence of a mastoid incision, is made behind the lateral sinus and should be preceded by ventricular puncture.

In traumatic abscess, incision is through the scar on the skull.

Step 3. A blunt catheter is inserted through a nick in the dura and the abscess wall found (not punctured) and outlined by repeated probes of the catheter. The incisions (in temporosphenoidal abscess) are enlarged to expose the pericranium in an area 3 to 4 cm. in diameter; an opening is made in the outer

[1] Annals of Surgery, 103:647-668. 1936.

table, the dura stripped back to within ¼ inch of the bony defect and the cortex fixed to the dura, and the dural margin, meninges and cortex fused by electrocoagulation.

Step 4. The overlying brain substance is removed by electrocoagulation and the necrotic material by suction.

Step 5. A small amount of abscess material is removed by aspiration to relieve tension, then the outer, presenting portion of the abscess opened with the electrosurgical needle and the pus evacuated by suction. Remaining flakes of pus are removed under direct inspection. There is continuous elevation of the floor of the abscess toward the level of the skull, beginning with the operation.

Step 6. Two layers of iodoform gauze are introduced into the abscess cavity and held snugly against the wall by strips of iodoform gauze. The open end of a small rubber irrigating tube is carried within the overlying gauze and a wet azochloramid gauze dressing applied and held with a bandage.

Step 7. **After-treatment.** Instillation of azochloramid solution is made every two hours. The superficial dressings are removed after 48 hours. The narrow gauze strips are gradually removed, so that by the tenth day the floor of the abscess is level with the skull (too rapid herniation is controlled by lumbar punctures) when the gauze can be entirely removed, care being taken that, if it is adherent, the brain substance is not removed. Epithelialization is rapid. About six months later a scalp plastic may be done to give better protection.

Comment. In frontal lobe abscess in the medial inferior portion, internal to the anterior horn of the lateral ventricle, collapse almost immediately after evacuation will make it difficult to insert anything into the cavity without injuring the wall; a fine meshed silver wire basket covered with a perforated rubber glove finger will serve to lead or guide the floor of the cavity to the surface and prevent collapse and subsequent pocketing.

In cerebellar abscess the abscess wall usually will be widest at the point incised and taper toward the back so that Dakin-tube-size drainage tubes with lateral perforations can be inserted without danger of a secondary pocket after collapse. The wound is loosely packed with iodoform gauze about the tubes. The tubes are irrigated with azochloramid solution and allowed to remain in position about three weeks, then are gradually shortened.

In traumatic abscess, lumbar puncture can be safely done during operation since the cortex is already fixed to the dura. During withdrawal the abscess cavity enlarges so that it can be inspected directly. The cavity is then packed with iodoform gauze or plain gauze dipped in azochloramid oil.

OPERATIONS ON THE SKULL AND BRAIN (GENERAL)

Study of the Patient. The patient who is to undergo an operation on the head should be subjected to an examination by a competent neurologist and oculist whose guidance in the matter of diagnosis and suggested therapy is of equal importance to the surgeon's skill. The patient should be under observation at the hospital as long as is necessary to arrive at definite conclusions and the general condition of the patient brought as nearly as possible to par.

Preparation for Operation. The day before the operation the whole head should be shaved and the cerebral localization outlined with carbol-fuchsin or an alcoholic solution of brilliant green.

After the patient is under the anesthetic and on the operating table, full strength tincture of iodine is applied to the entire scalp; after this has dried, it is removed with a 95% solution of alcohol. (I prefer not to remove the iodine.) Opinions differ as to the manner in which the skin should be prepared. Some prefer to paint the scalp with tincture of iodine; others prepare the field with tincture of green soap and water followed by alcohol and ether or tincture of iodine. As a matter of fact, it does not matter which method is used as long as it is thorough.

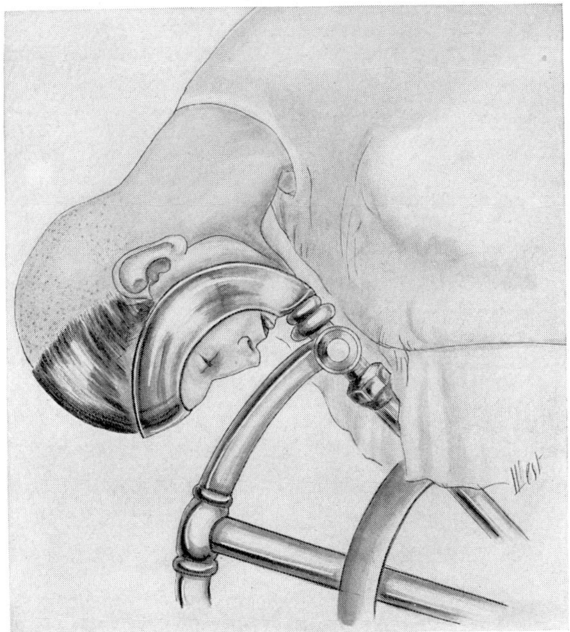

FIG. 108. Position of patient for suboccipital craniotomy.

Position of the Patient on the Operating Table. The patient should be placed securely on the table. The positions are best comprehended by a perusal of the illustrations.

It is of importance that the patient be comfortably placed, that there is no interference with respiration and that the surgeon is afforded free and convenient access to the field of operation.

For anterolateral and frontal operations, the patient should be flat on his back. If lateral or posterolateral exposure is aimed at, the patient is placed on his side and sandbags are used to elevate and steady the head to keep it from rolling from side to side.

For operations on the occipital lobes or cerebellum, the patient is usually placed with his face down. The forehead is placed on a stand near the operating table or on an adjustable headrest and a large sandbag is placed under each shoulder to facilitate respiration. (Figs. 108-109.)

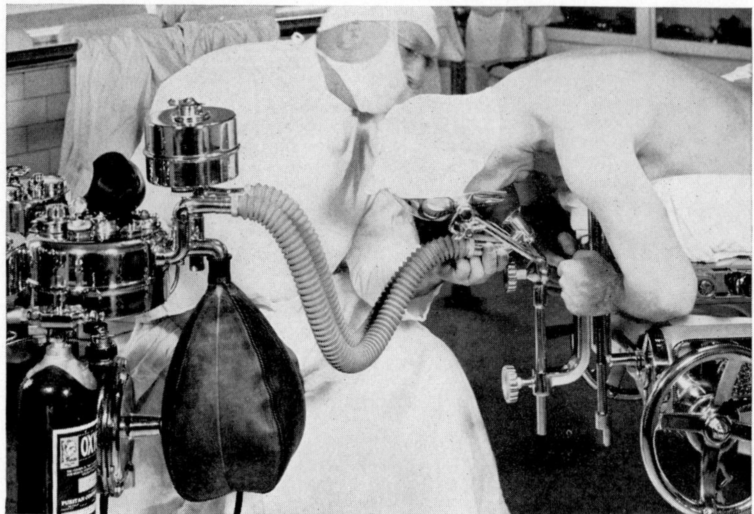

FIG. 109. Anesthesia position of patient for operations on the cerebellum.

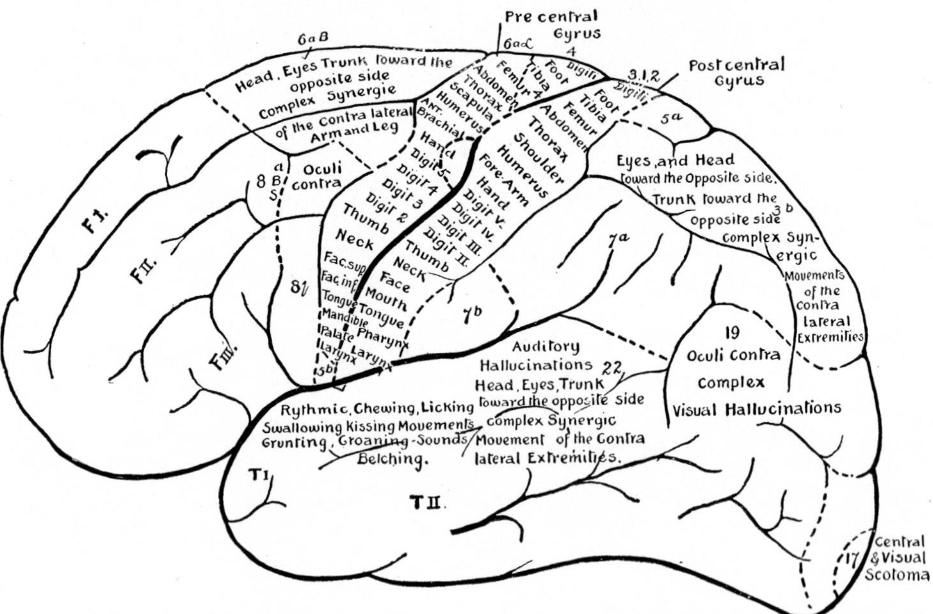

FIG. 110. Diagram of the external surface of the brain to show the localization of movements as mapped out by electrical stimulation (after Foerster).

CRANIOCEREBRAL TOPOGRAPHY

This plays an important role in cerebral surgery. There are many methods of cerebral localization in vogue. (Fig. 110.) Since larger incisions and larger flaps are made nowadays than was the practice formerly, mistakes in determining the exact site of the lesion are offset by adequate exposure. The skilled surgeon readily orients himself on the cerebral cortex. However, if it is desired to locate some certain part of the cerebral hemisphere, the flap may be replaced and the outlines observed in their relation to the surface of the brain.

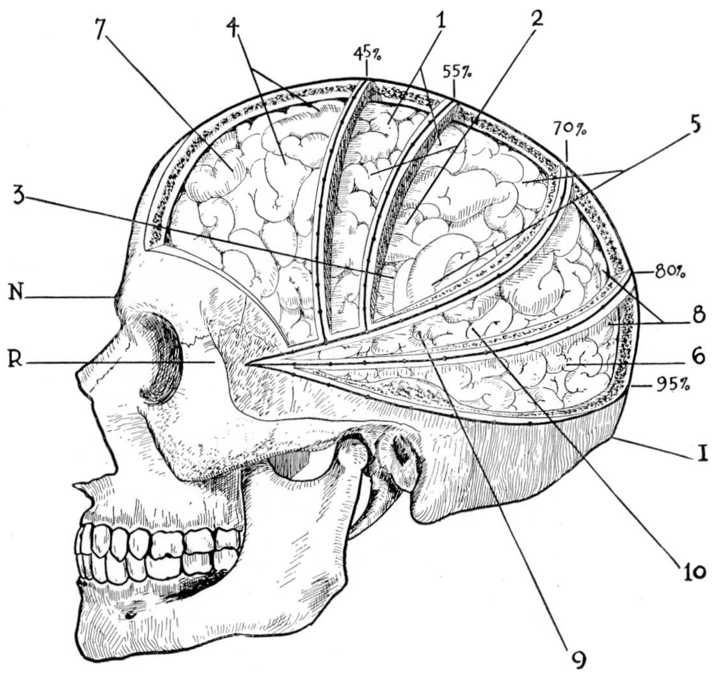

FIG. 111. Chipault craniocerebral topography: N. nasion or nasofrontal suture, I. inion or external occipital protuberance, R. retro-orbital tubercule, 45%, precentral point, 55%, Rolandic point, 70%, Sylvian point, 80%, temporosphenoidal point, 95%, lateral sinus point; 1. motor and sensory disturbance, lower extremities, 2. motor and sensory disturbance, upper extremities, 3. motor and sensory disturbance, face, tongue, jaw, pharynx, and vocal cords, motor aphasia in right-handed people and vice versa, 4. (a) movements of the body (posterior part of the first frontal), (b) movements of the head and neck (posterior part of the second frontal), (e) associated movements of the eyes and head, 5. tactile and muscular sensibility, 6. hemianopsia and word-blindness, agraphia, and paraphasia, 7. intelligence, 8. storage of visual images (cuneus, lingual lobe and calcarine fissure, which lie in the longitudinal fissure between the 70% and 95% points), 9. audition, 10. images for words heard and musical tones (left side). In this same region, on both sides, the sensory motor auditory center exists. The internal frontal convolution lies in the longitudinal fissure opposite the superior frontal convolution. The paracentral convolution lies in the longitudinal fissure between the 45% and 55% points. The quadrate lobe lies in the longitudinal fissure between the 55% and 70% points. The cuneus, lingual and fusiform lobes, first, second and third occipital convolutions, are between the 70% and 95% lines.

I prefer Chipault's Method because it is not difficult to remember, it is easy to execute and is accurate regardless of the type of individual (man, woman, negro, etc.).

THE CHIPAULT METHOD OF CRANIOCEREBRAL LOCALIZATION

The metric system is recommended for making the measurements. The distance is measured from the nasion, over the groove under the glabella, over the sagittal suture, ending at the inion. (Fig. 111.) Measuring from before backward, the following percentages are indicated:

1. 45 per cent—the **precentral** point.
2. 55 " " —the **Rolandic** point.

3. 70 per cent—the **Sylvian** point.
4. 80 " " —the **temporosphenoidal** point.
5. 95 " " —the **lateral sinus** point.

A small prominence opposite the external canthus of the eye, beneath the external angular process of the frontal bone, on the posterior border of the upper part of the frontal process of the malar bone is identified as the **retro-orbital tubercle.**

The position of the **Sylvian fissure** is determined by drawing a line from this tubercle to the 70 per cent point; this line is divided into ten equal parts.

The second and third tenths are joined by a line to the 45 per cent point which denotes the **precentral fissure.**

The **Rolandic fissure** is marked by a line joining the third and fourth tenths to the 55 per cent point.

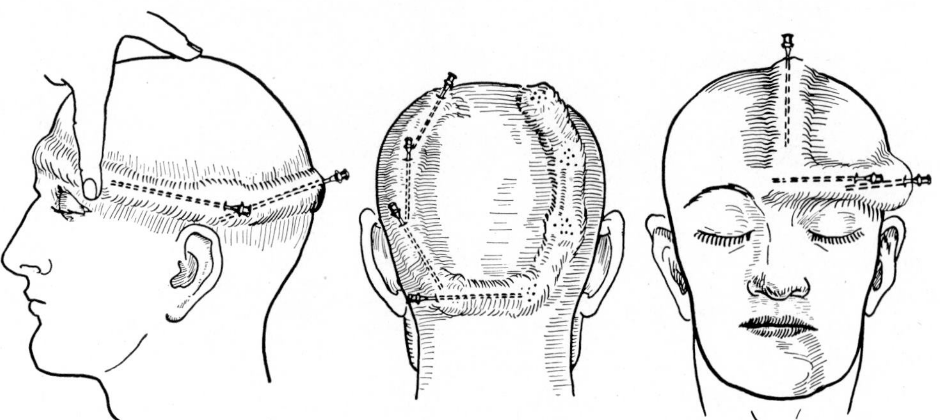

FIG. 112. Block infiltration of the scalp (circumferential).

FIG. 113. Block infiltration of the scalp (circumferential).

FIG. 114. Parieto-frontal block infiltration of the scalp.

The **superior temporosphenoidal fissure** is indicated by the junction of the retro-orbital tubercle to the 80 per cent point.

A line from the retro-orbital tubercle to the 95 per cent point indicates the **lateral sinus,** posteriorly.

For the purpose of minute localization, the above lines are divided into tenths.

The second tenth of the three main lines is transversed by the **anterior branch of the middle meningeal artery.**

By introducing the exploring needle in the superior temporosphenoidal convolution at the junction of the third and fourth tenths on this line at a depth equivalent to one-third of the transverse diameter of the brain here, the posterior portion of the lateral ventricle may be tapped.

If it is desirable to explore the descending horn, the needle is placed in the middle temporo-sphenoidal convolution immediately over the external auditory meatus.

ANESTHESIA IN CRANIOCEREBRAL OPERATIONS

In England and on the Continent, chloroform seems to be the popular anesthetic used in operations on the brain; in America, ether or novocaine-suprarenin analgesia is given preference. I never use chloroform; it lowers the bloodpressure and while it is true that ether raises the bloodpressure and thus favors oozing, it is on the whole, safe. A trained anesthetist is indispensable in these operations. Oxygen and facilities for artificial respiration should be at hand. The bloodpressure should be taken at stated intervals.

Operations of this type which are performed in two stages require anesthesia for the first stage only—it is not essential to anesthetize the patient for manipulating the dura and brain after the osteoplastic flap has been lifted.

Intratracheal or nasopharyngeal insufflation anesthesia works well here, particularly where the patient is placed in the prone decubitus (face downward) with the head projecting over the end of the table. The anesthetist, in such cases, aims to administer the anesthetic from below. In removing tumors of the scalp or in decompression operations, block infiltration may be used as depicted in Figs. 112-113-114.

FORM OF BONE FLAP

Usually the flap is of trapezoid shape and located where the vascularity is ample. In unusual instances, the base of the flap may be anterior, receiving its blood supply from the supra-orbital and frontal arteries or it may be posterior and receive its nourishment from the occipital artery.

The size of the flap varies depending upon the requirements of a given case and it should be sufficiently large so that the various steps of the operative procedure may be accomplished with as little handling of the brain as possible. Certain cases require two flaps; for instance, where the defect is situated near the median line; such flaps should be placed symmetrically and meet about 1 cm. from the midline.

CONTROL OF HEMORRHAGE

Hemorrhage from the Scalp

Tourniquet. Bleeding is controlled by tightly drawing a circular tourniquet which consists of a rubber band or tube around the head over the supra-orbital ridge, anteriorly, extending it far down over the temporal fossa and immediately beneath the occipital protuberance posteriorly. A sterile towel or gauze bandage is placed under the tourniquet to prevent it from slipping.

A **pneumatic tourniquet** may also be used; this consists of a rubber tube equipped with a check valve which is inflated with air after being placed in position.

The drawbacks of the tourniquet method of controlling hemorrhage are: (a) intrusion upon the field of operation; (b) tendency to cause venous oozing, if the tension is not quite right; and (c) interference with the flap when it is being turned down.

Clamp and Suture. Incise boldly all tissues down to the bone, after the assistant has exerted firm pressure with both hands laterally. The bleeding points are caught with artery forceps. Catgut sutures on curved needles are placed in the tissue surrounding the clamp and tied on both sides.

Heidenhain's Continuous Hemostatic Suture (Fig. 115). A curved needle is armed with catgut or silk and is passed through the entire thickness of the scalp surrounding the field of operation down to the bone about 1 or 2 cm. outside the site planned for the incision. The stitches are overlapped in such a manner that the entire blood supply of the scalp is compressed. These stitches are removed after the operation is completed and the flap sutured in place.

Kredel Plates. These plates have notched ends and their upper surface is furrowed. (Fig. 116.) A deep suture extending to the bone about the length of the plate is placed so as to compress the tissues between the suture below and the plate above. The plates are applied to both sides of the intended incision. The object, obviously, is the same as in Heidenhain's deligation method which, in my opinion, is simpler to execute.

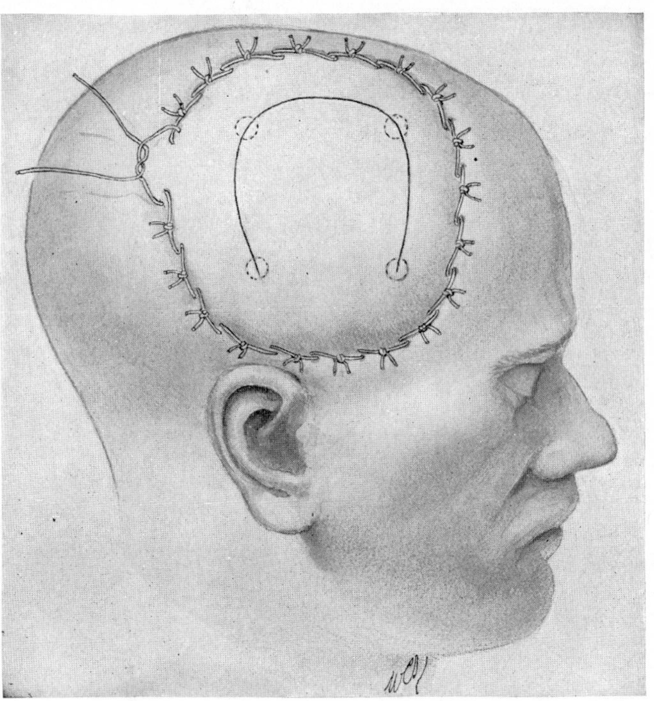

Fig. 115. Heidenhain's deligations to secure hemostasis in operations on the skull and brain.

Hemorrhage from the Bone

Horsley's Bone Wax applied to the bleeding point with the finger or on a piece of gauze or some flat instrument has been found most efficacious for controlling hemorrhage from the bone. A segment of adjacent muscle may be used in the same manner.

Crushing the bone or biting it away with rongeurs often controls bleeding from the bone.

Pieces of sterile wood (such as a toothpick) or Krause's hooks (Fig. 117) may be used to advantage.

Hemorrhage from the Dura

This is controlled by using fine catgut or silk ligatures on each side of the bleeding point, carried on fine curved needles. In passing the needles, care should be exercised not to injure the underlying cortex cerebri.

If a vessel intersects the line of incision while the flap of dura is being fashioned, secure the vessel, ligate it doubly and divide it between the ligatures.

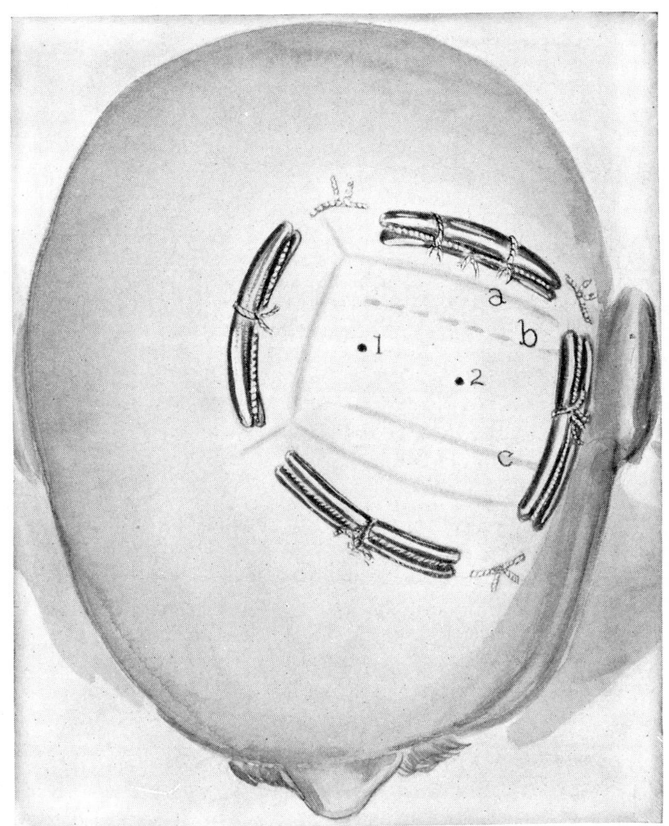

FIG. 116. The use of Kredel plates for hemostasis: 1. incision, 2. central area, 3. precentral area. Neisser's puncture points: 1. leg center, 2. arm center. (Redrawn from Krause-Thoreks, Surgery of the Brain and Spinal Cord, F. J. Rebman Publishing Co.)

In securing the vessel, pass the needle from within outward. This tends to prevent injury to the cortex. Transfixion is essential to prevent the ligature slipping. Silver clips may be used to advantage. Electrosurgical hemostasis has in many cases given me great satisfaction. This consists of grasping the vessel with a fine pointed hemostat and touching the latter with the electrode of a diatherm apparatus. Prompt fusion of the vessel wall causes hemostasis.

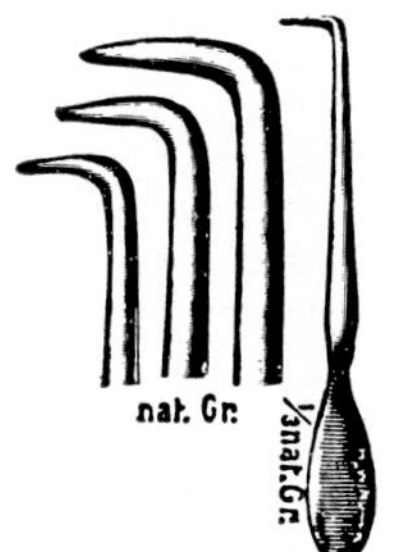

FIG. 117. Krause bone hooks for arrest of bleeding.

Hemorrhage from the Cortical Brain Substance

Bleeding is frequently arrested by placing over the bleeding point a small piece of muscle and leaving it in situ. The use of a small piece of absorbent cotton or gauze impregnated with sterilized vaseline or a piece of Cargile membrane are also frequently useful in effecting hemostasis.

Cyanosis encourages bleeding. Should this supervene, administer oxygen and raise the head of the patient. These measures will tend to check bleeding.

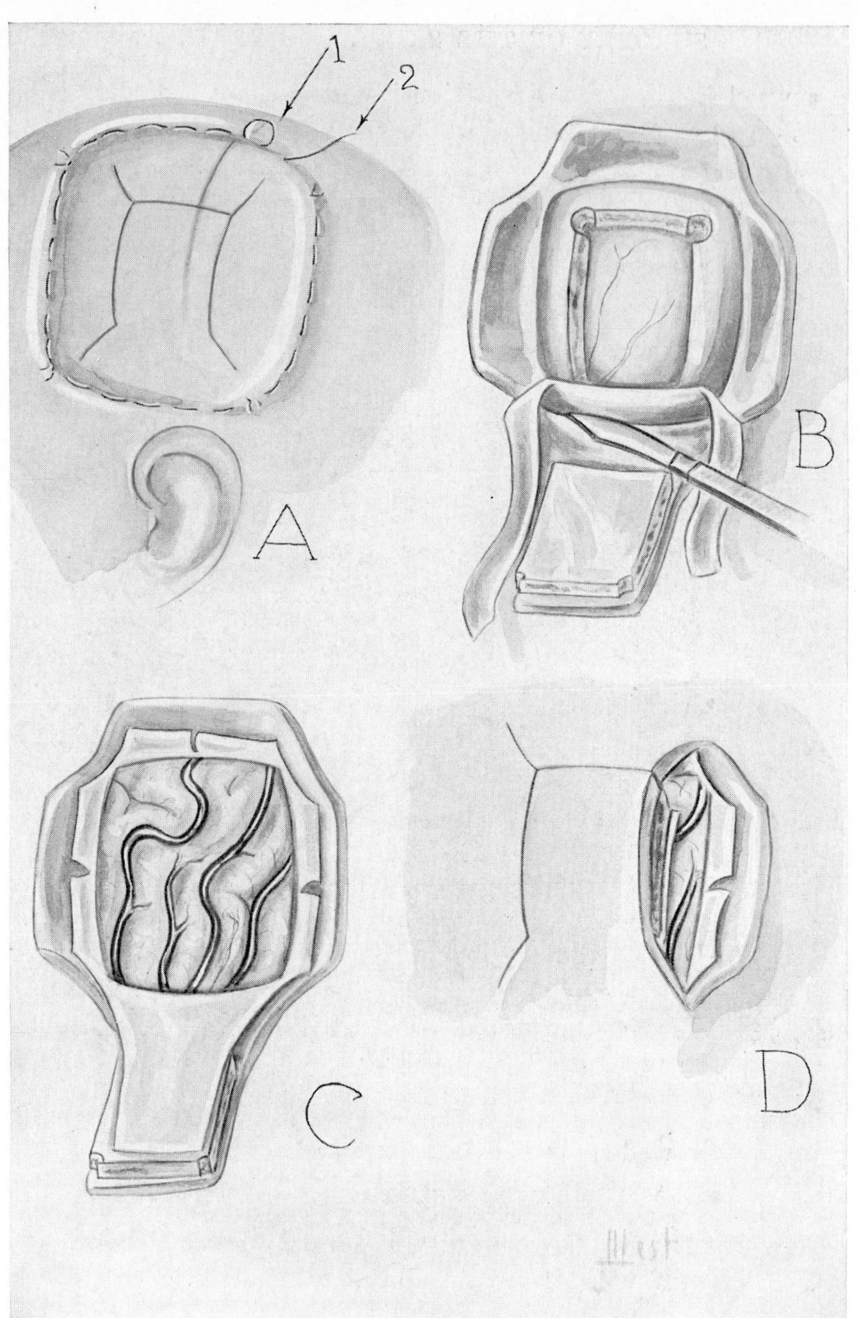

FIG. 118. Technic of valve formation of dura. While Kocher sacrifices bone and dura, the excised portion of bone need not be completely removed. Snipping off 1-2 cm. around the edges of bone is sufficient. A. Line of incision to form cutaneo-aponeurotic flap, avoid injury to periosteum. Note incisions added to each angle of principal flap resulting in three smaller flaps: 1. Rolandic fissure, 2. Heidenhain's deligations. B. After dividing the periosteum at the bases of the flaps and edges of three first incisions, periosteal strips are separated and permitted to remain hanging until removed with the bone flap. C. Bone flaps removed and dura transversely incised and placed over sectioned bone to prevent contact of brain with diploë. Note additional transverse incisions made in dura. D. Large dural flaps replaced and osteoplastic flap sutured exactly in position. The lamina vitrea rests on the principal flap while above, in front and behind, the brain is covered by galea and skin only; a good valve formation results obviating the necessity of wearing plate or shield for protection. (Redrawn from Krause-Thoreks, Surgery of the Brain and Spinal Cord, F. J. Rebman Publishing Co.)

Hemorrhage After the Removal of a Tumor

This usually ceases spontaneously, the contiguous brain substance filling the space occupied by the tumor. Should bleeding continue, packs of vaselinized gauze, a large piece of muscle with fascia attached, or a large piece of fascia may be packed down into the space previously occupied by the tumor. These will arrest the bleeding. Muscle or fascia-muscle strips may be obtained from the outer surface of the thigh and if their need is anticipated, they should be prepared before the operation on the brain is begun. In clean cases omit drainage and packing. Hemorrhage should be controlled before the flap is replaced. External pressure may suffice where a flap is pliable.

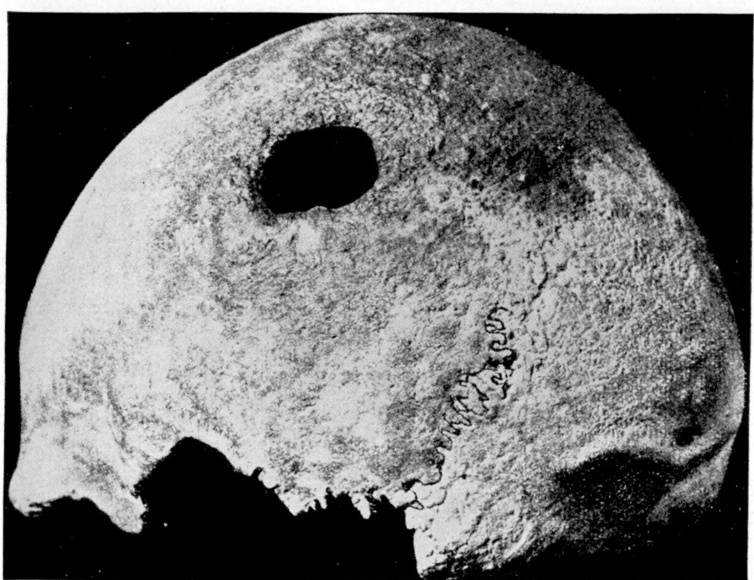

FIG. 119. Prehistoric skull showing healed trephine opening. (Three-quarters natural size, from the collection of Prof. Meyer Steineg.)

METHODS OF OPENING THE SKULL

Trephining

Trephining may be indicated in several conditions, the most common of which are: intracranial tumors, fractures and intracranial suppurations. In many of these cases, patients may be relieved of distressing symptoms such as persistent vomiting, cephalgia and impaired vision due to the presence of the tumor. Decompression operations may be performed in any portion of the cerebral or cerebellar region. However, it is most frequently performed in the temporal region. A valve formation is sometimes resorted to in certain decompression operations. (Fig. 118.)

The use of the surgical instrument known as the trephine to remove a piece of the skull to give access to the cranial cavity or its envelopes is a very old operative procedure; it was known in ancient times, or, at least, certain methods of cutting and removing the bone were in practice. (Fig. 119.)

The modern surgical trephine is merely a hollow steel cylinder, the lower end of which is provided with a saw edge (Fig. 120). To keep this saw edge in

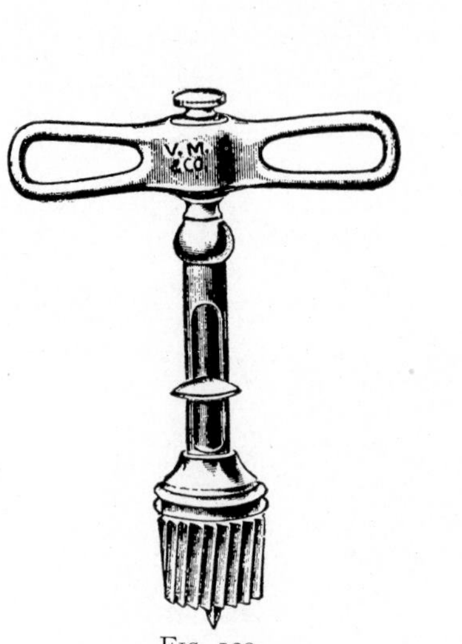

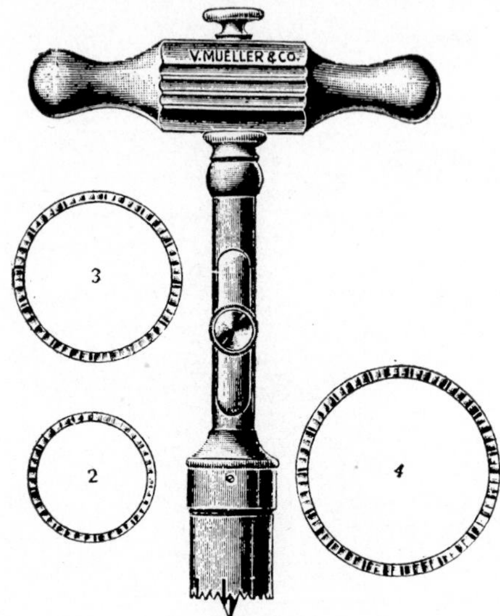

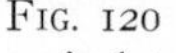

FIG. 120

FIG. 121

FIG. 120. Surgical trephine and bone drill. Stille pattern with one small trephine, four burrs and four drills.
FIG. 121. Galt's trephine.

position on the skull, a pin projects through the center of the cylinder, about one-sixteenth inch beyond the cutting edge; this pin is withdrawn as soon as the trephine has cut a groove in the bone sufficiently deep to keep the trephine from slipping.

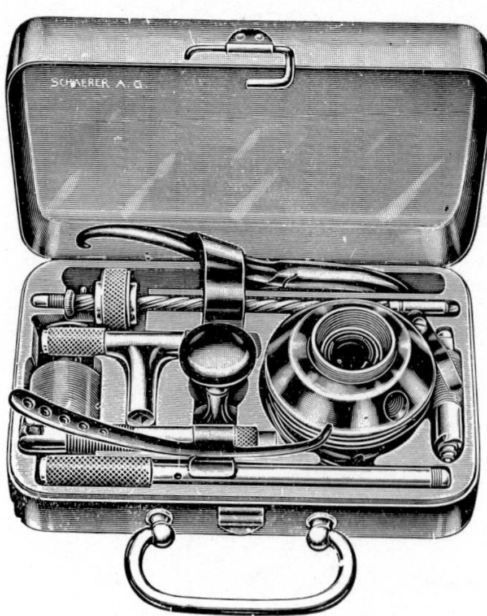

FIG. 122. The Jentzer trephine in carrying case.

In the United States the Galt trephine (Fig. 121) is principally used, the general construction being the same as in that just described except that the cutting part of the instrument is shaped like a truncated cone. There are numerous electrically operated trephines. A most useful instrument is Prof. Jentzer's trephine (Fig. 122). It is distinctly superior and offers many advantages over hand trephines and those operated by electricity. The circular fragment of bone removed by the trephine may be reimplanted and its reunion expected to proceed smoothly. The periosteum is not sacrificed but permitted to remain attached to the cutaneo-muscular flap; its circulation is thus assured. Jentzer prefers local anesthesia for trephining. A small or large opening may be produced with his instrument at will, the latter by contiguous trephining; or, the small trephine may be used to create a small opening and the operation completed with the Gigli saw. Jentzer, as did others, successfully used this trephine in a variety of conditions (simple and subtemporal decompression, removal of tumors of the cerebral hemispheres, hypophysis, etc.).

The component parts of the Jentzer trephine are shown in Fig. 123. The case and instruments may be sterilized in an autoclave, after which the parts are arranged on a small table. To assemble, screw the handbars (13) into the

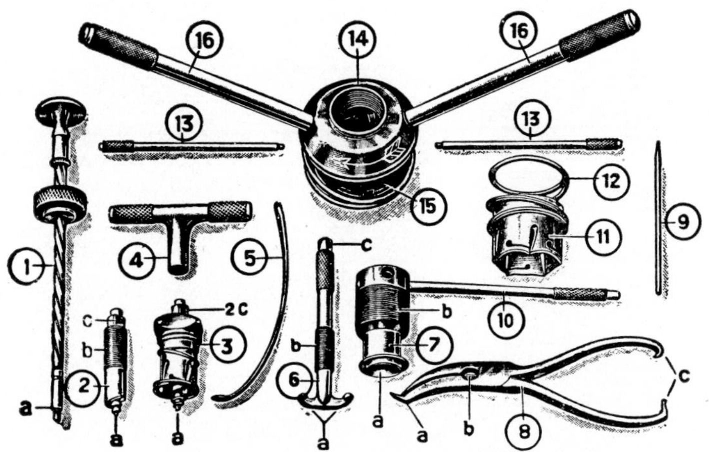

Fig. 123. *The components of the Jentzer trephine.* 1. *Skull perforator* with shoulder (1a). The shoulder prevents too deep penetration. 2. *Short screw device* for trephining thin bone (temporal bone); the long screw is used on thick skulls. The threaded end (2a) is screwed into the orifice created by the perforator until it is thoroughly fixed there; this maneuver is facilitated by using a key (4) which fits the head of the screw device (2c). 3. *Small trephine.* This is placed over the preceding instrument as shown in (3) after which fixation into the opening in the skull is accomplished. *Two handle bars* (13) are used to trephine—always to the right. Use no pressure or force. The trephine cannot penetrate too deeply, because it automatically becomes released and the trephined segment of bone will come away attached to the screw (3a). 4. *Key* for the screw device (2c). 5. *Dura separator.* 6. *Rocker stem* (6a). This is introduced into the cranial orifice created by the small trephine. The threaded axis device (7) is fitted on the channel of the screw (6b) and screwed tight until its lower part (7a) fits perpendicularly into the small trephine. 7. *Threaded axis device.* After being fitted with handle bars or hand on the rocker stem as described above, the trephine with *medium crown* (11) or with the large crown (15) is mounted on threaded axis device (7b). 8. *Special bone forceps.* These are used for the removal of splinters and of bone. The aperture on the forceps (8b) is conveniently used for unscrewing the small trephine (3a). In so doing the short screw device (2c) is tightened with the key 4. For unscrewing the crowns one places properly the hooks (8c) and releases the crowns. 9. *Special probe* for cleaning the instruments. 10. *Handle bar.* 11. *Medium crown.* Observe on the left lower border the protector which, when the resistance of the bone ceases, automatically protects the dura. 12. *Automatic release spring* aiding in the release of the trephine and bone segment. 13. *Handle bars* for small trephine. 14. *Cylindrical segment* the inside thread of which fits the threaded axis device. Arrows indicate the axis of rotation. 15. *Large crown* with spring handle bars.

head of the small trephine and automatic spring. Place the short screw (2) in the threaded axis device (Fig. 124) and cause the threads to engage until the end of the small screw projects beyond the small crown.

Figures 125-126-127 depict and describe the procedure for the large or medium sized trephine.

Force should not be used when the instrument is being assembled. All the screw channels are threaded with such precision that they function perfectly.

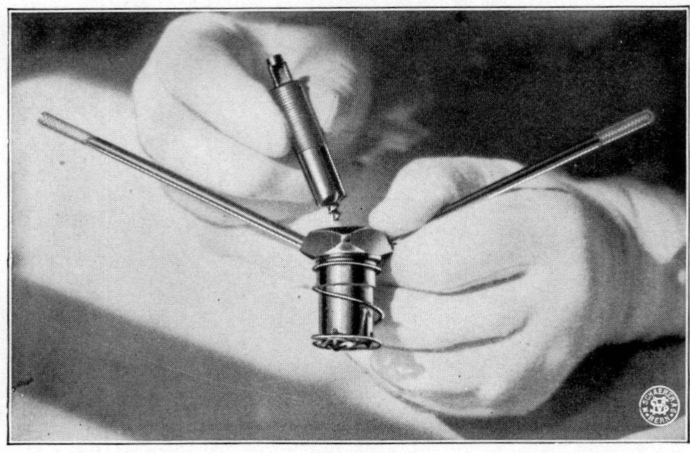

Fig. 124 (*Assembling Jentzer's small trephine*) Fig. 125

Fig. 124. Handle bars screwed into the head of the small trephine.

Fig. 125. Place the short screw device (2) into the threaded axis device; cause the threads to engage until the end of the small screw projects beyond the small crown. Remember that there is a short screw for the temporal and thin bones marked T and a long one for thick skulls.

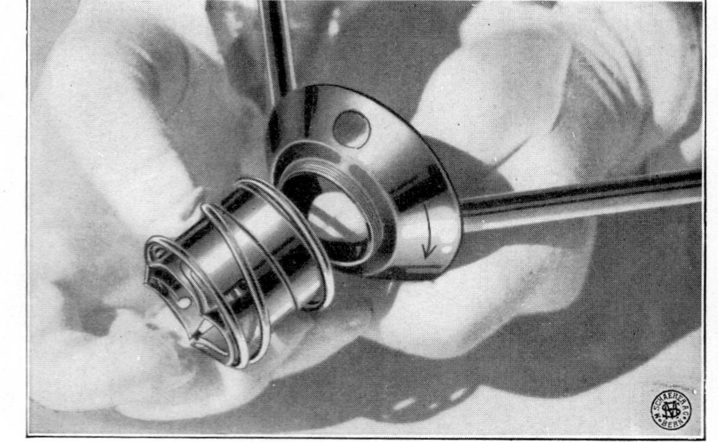

Fig. 126

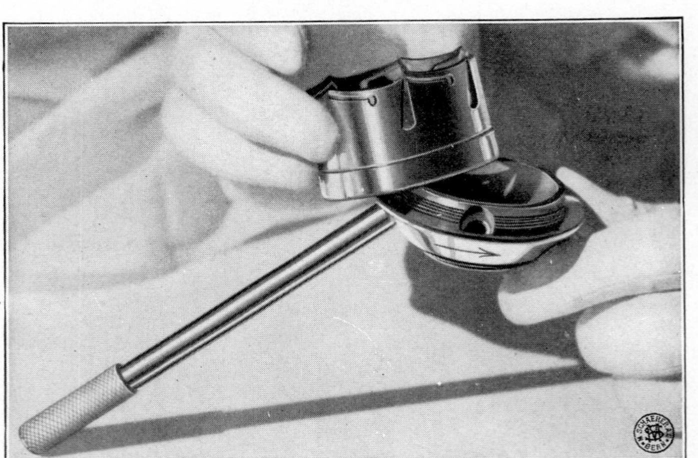

Fig. 127

Fig. 126. *Assembling Jentzer's trephine (medium size).* Observe that this fits on the top portion of the cylindrical part and that the handle

Slight greasing with sterile vaseline will protect the screw channels. The instrument is cleaned with the special instrument shown in Fig. 123(9).

Sterilization is done as usual in an autoclave, in alkaline water (1% sodium carbonate, Na_2CO_3).

TECHNIC OF TREPHINING

Step 1. Mark on the external surface of the cranium the portion the trephine is intended to remove.

Step 2. Form a scalp flap by a semicircular incision comprising the outlined area, the base of the flap being toward the base line of the skull. The soft tissues of the scalp should be, as stated, incised down to the bone.

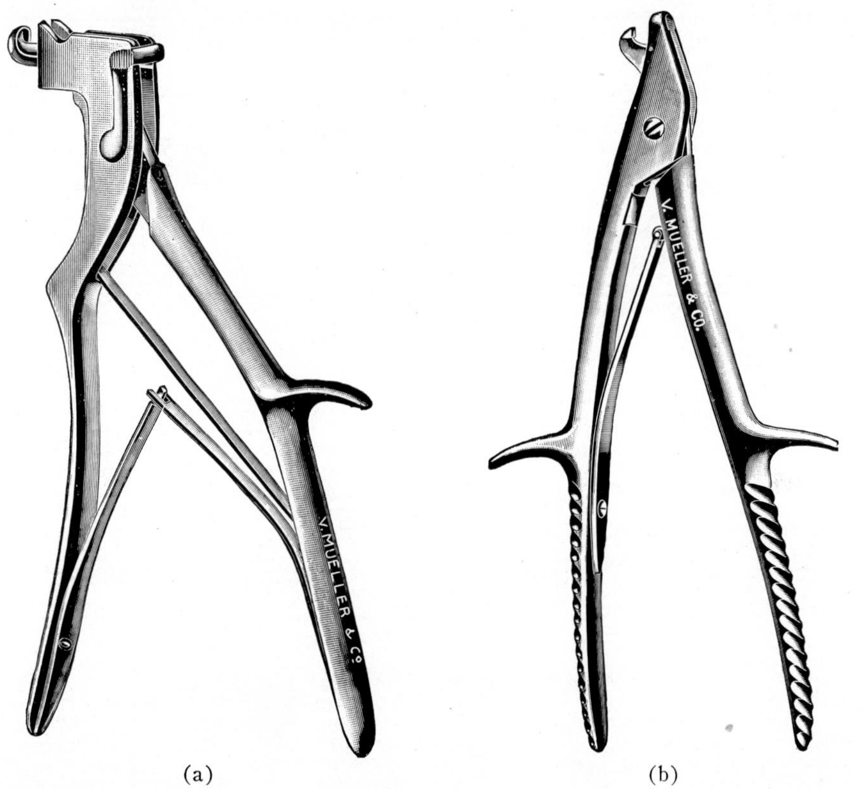

(a) (b)

Fig. 128. (a) De Quervain's skull cutting forceps. (b) Hudson's Rongeur forceps.

Step 3. Detach the periosteum from the bone, the whole of the flap being then turned down and held out of the way. Hemostasis should be attended to.

Step 4. Select a trephine of suitable size. Introduce the center-pin and place it on the center of the piece of bone it is desired to remove. By a series of to-and-fro movements with the hand, the teeth of the trephine are made to cut a circular groove in the bone. When this groove is sufficiently deep, lift the trephine and remove the central pin. Introduce the instrument again without the pin and saw through the circle of bone gradually. Lift the trephine out of the groove occasionally; remove and brush out the accumulated spicules of bone. Do not saw the bone quite through but by side-to-side motion with the trephine when the sawing is nearly complete, joggle the piece of bone up or lift it out with a periosteal elevator, or similar instru-

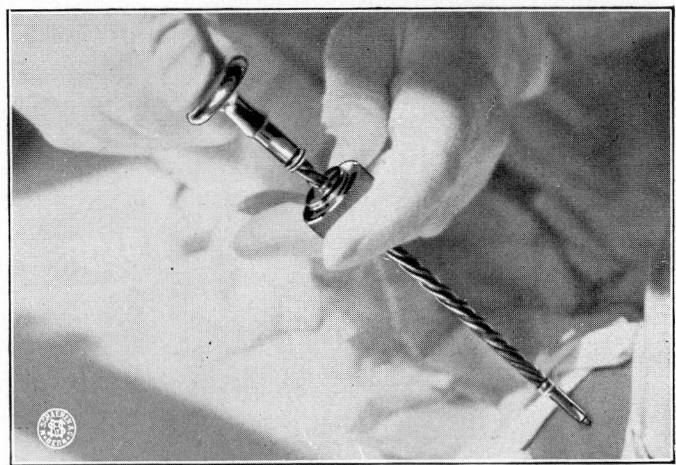

FIG. 129. *Step 1.* Boring a hole in the skull with the perforator.

ment. If the resulting aperture made is insufficient in size, enlarge it with appropriate rongeurs (Fig. 128a and b.)

Steps of Jentzer Trephining

Step 1. (Fig. 129.) Select the place for trephining. Bore a hole in the skull with the perforator (1) using its blunt end.

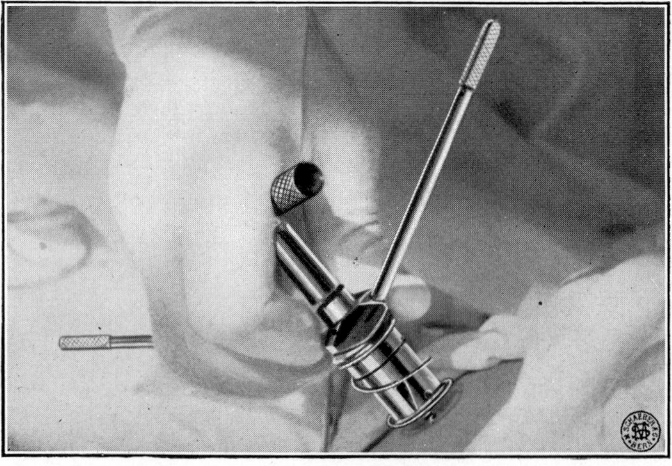

FIG. 130. *Step 2.* Screwing the mounted small trephine into the opening previously made.

Step 2. (Fig. 130.) Screw perpendicularly into the opening thus made, aided by the key (4), the mounted small trephine, until fixation results. Have this fixation firm (an additional quarter or half turn of the screw will accomplish the desired result).

Step 3. (Fig. 131.) Remove the key (4). Grasp the hand-bars, this is usually accomplished without effort, and trephine until the segment of bone is automatically released.

Step 4. (Fig. 132.) **Unscrewing the small round piece.** Replace the key (4) using the special bone forceps (8b) as illustrated. The short screw device

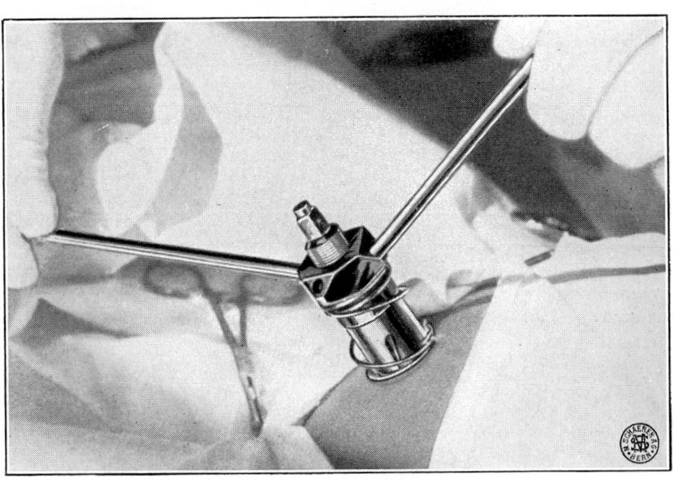

FIG. 131. *Step 3.* The key has been removed. Trephining is done until bone segment is obtained.

(2c) is thus tightened with the key (4). The round section is now unscrewed. Have an assistant hold the instrument while you loosen the round section.

Step 5. (Fig. 133.) With the dura separator, separate the dura mater from the bone, through the opening created in the skull.

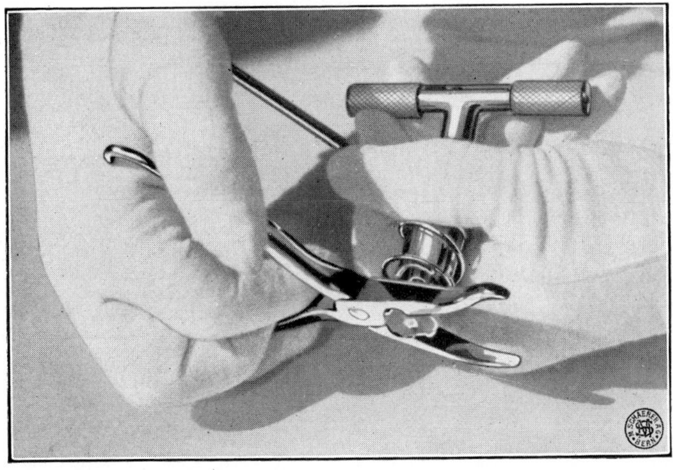

FIG. 132. *Step 4.* Unscrewing the small round piece.

Step 6. (Fig. 134.) Remove any bone splinters with the special bone forceps (8a). This is an important step if one wishes to use the larger, threaded axis device (7).

Step 7. (Fig. 135.) Introduce the rocker stem (6). Hug the lower surface of

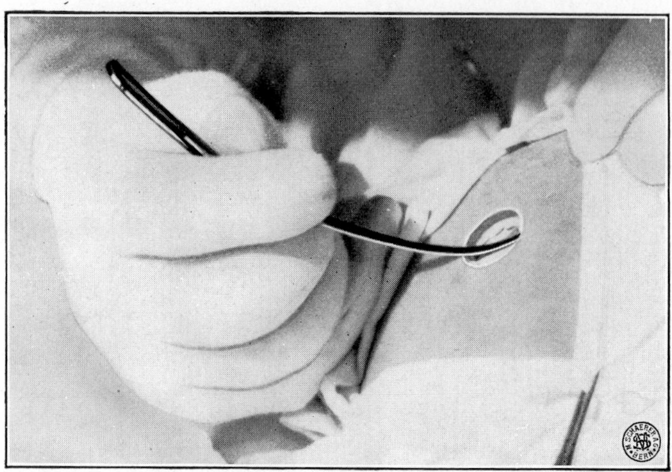

FIG. 133. *Step 5.* Separating the dura with the dura separator.

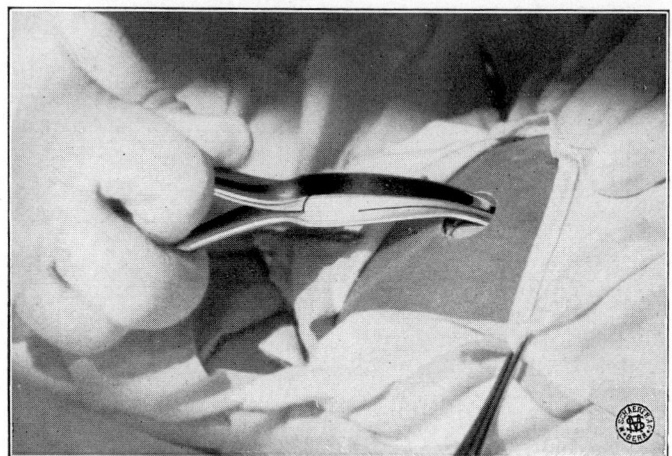

FIG. 134. *Step 6.* Removal of bone spiculae.

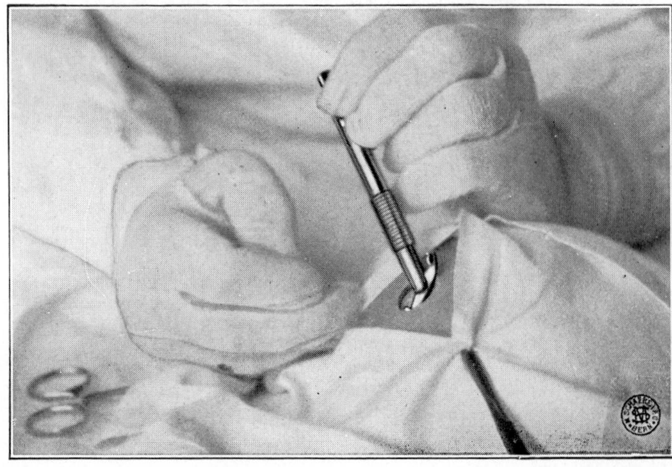

FIG. 135. *Step 7.* Placement of rocker stem (6).

the skull bone. In case of fracture, place the rocker stem perpendicularly, in relation to the line of fracture as seen in the accompanying illustration.

Step 8. (Fig. 136.) Screw the threaded axis device (7) by hand on to the rocker stem until fixation of the axis results.

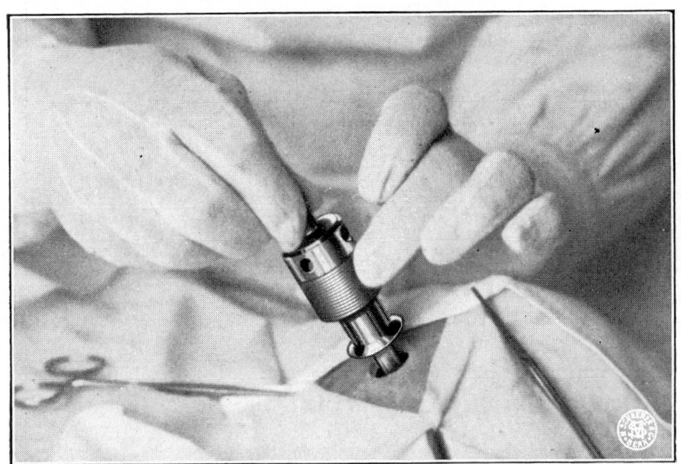

FIG. 136. *Step 8.* Screwing the threaded axis device (7) on the rocker stem (6) until fixation is secured.

Step 9. (Fig. 137). The large crown mounted with hand-bars and spring is now screwed over the external thread of the threaded axis. Never force the adjustment of the thread—you will ruin it. Handle it gently.

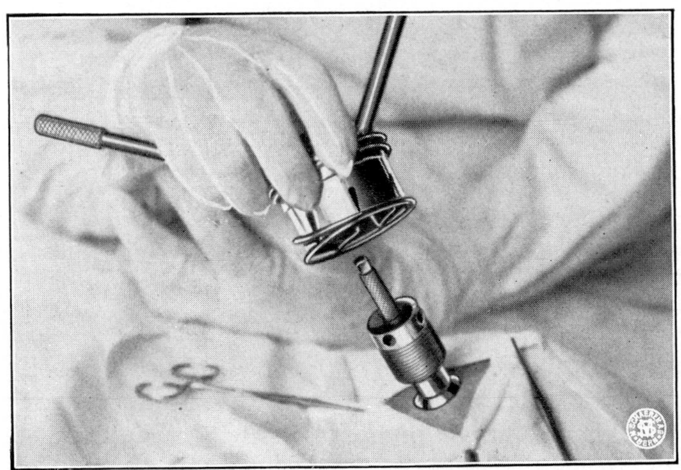

FIG. 137. *Step 9.* Mounting large crown over the external head of the threaded axis. Do not force! Permit threads to engage gently.

Step 10. (Fig. 138.) The trephine is now ready for work. Trephine in the same manner as when using the small trephine. Jentzer urges not to press toward the brain but rather direct the instrument toward one's self. The arrow indicates the direction of the trephine. If this admonition is violated the protecting springs will break.

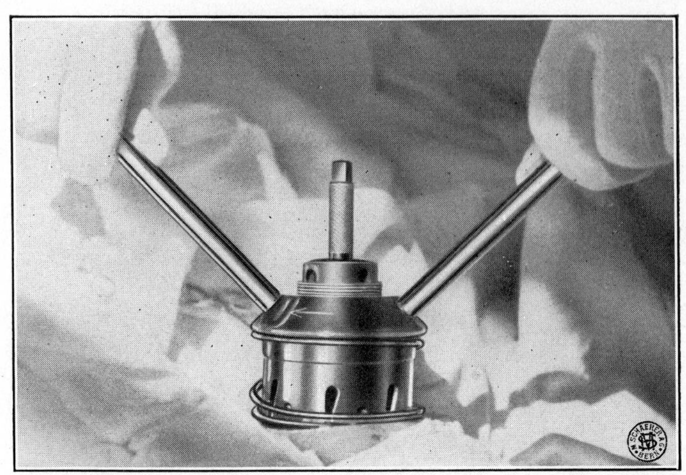

Fig. 138. *Step 10.* Trephine ready for work. Observe proper direction of trephine (arrows) in Fig. 139. Do not push trephine inward (toward the brain)—rather pull it toward you.

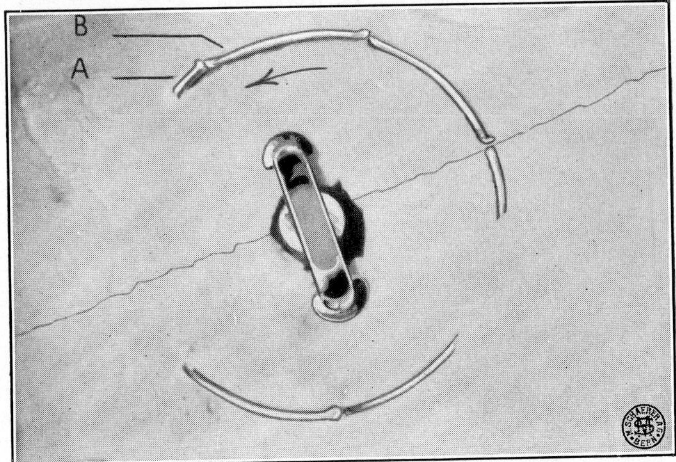

Fig. 139. View of trephined area showing how injury to the dura is avoided.

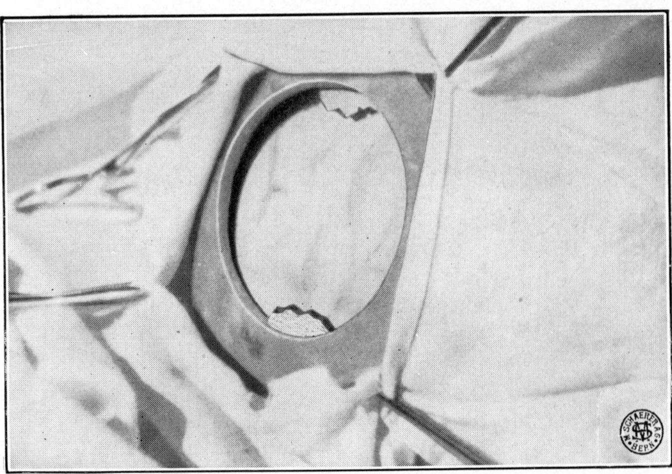

Fig. 140. Bone fragments in trephined area; remove these with the special bone forceps (Figs. 123-8) if deemed advisable.

Figure 139 shows the interior of an area being trephined and how penetration of the dura is avoided.

Figure 140 shows bone fragments in the trephined area; these may easily be removed with the special bone forceps (8).

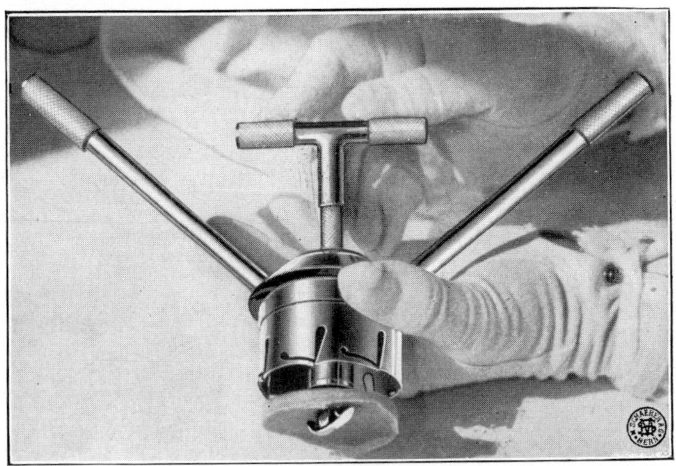

FIG. 141. *Step. 11.* Unsetting of the round section.

Step 11. (Fig. 141.) Unscrew the threaded axis with the key (4) until the trephined segment of bone and threaded axis get out of the crown. Replace the key in the head of the threaded axis. Introduce into one of the lateral orifices of the cylindrical piece a special hand-bar (10).

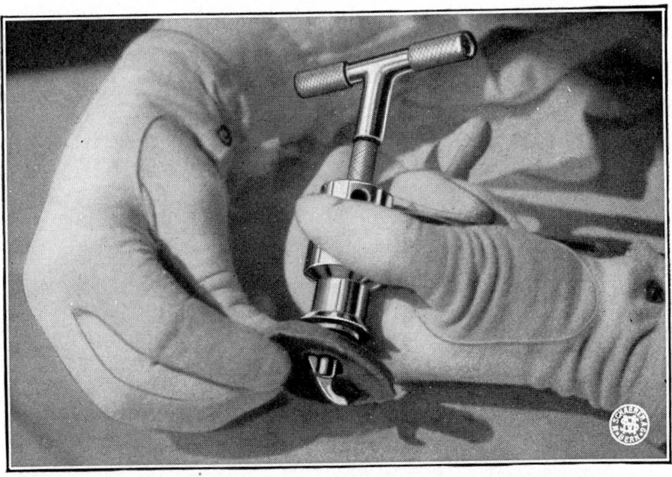

FIG. 142. *Step 12.* Removal of trephined section of skull.

Step 12. (Fig. 142.) This consists of the removal of the trephined section of bone.

Step 13. (Fig. 143.) If desired, replace the trephined portion of bone. Consolidation takes place in about 8 or 10 days; the bones become united with the surrounding structures.

Step 14. (Fig. 144.) Unscrewing of the crown by means of the hooks (8c). Unscrew in the direction opposite to the arrows.

Figures 145-146 depict the technic of combination procedures of Jentzer trephining coupled with the Gigli saw.

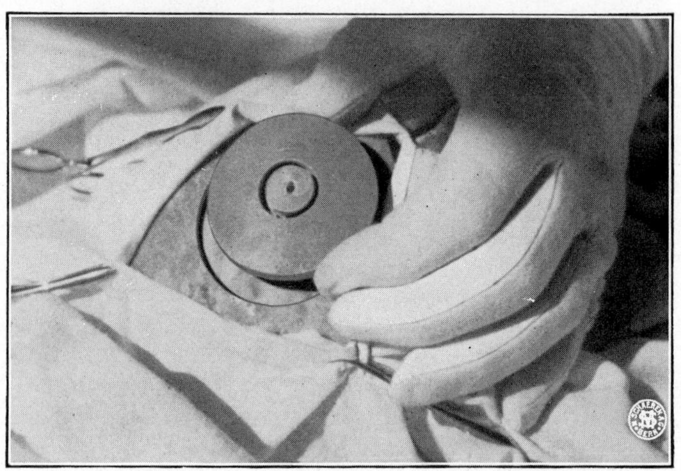

FIG. 143. *Step 13.* Replacement of trephined segment.

As soon as the outer table of the skull is penetrated there will be less resistance felt to the advancing instrument and a greater escape of blood issuing from the diploe will be observed. (Fig. 147.) After traversing the diploe, the hard bone of the inner table is encountered again; here greater caution must be exercised because the inner table is often very thin. For that reason, after

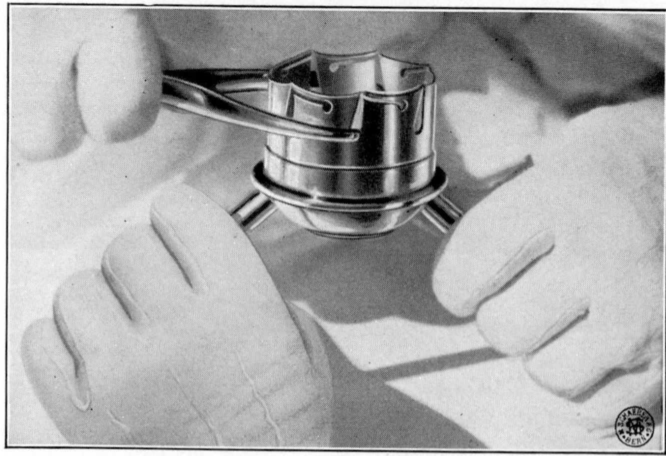

FIG. 144. *Step 14.* Unscrewing the crown.

every few movements of the trephine, the groove in the skull should be probed with a blunt-pointed probe or the blunt point of a straight needle. Furthermore, the convexity and uneven surface of the skull may lend itself to greater penetration in one part of the groove than in another; pressure should, therefore, be lessened at this point, remembering that the tables of the skull are not of

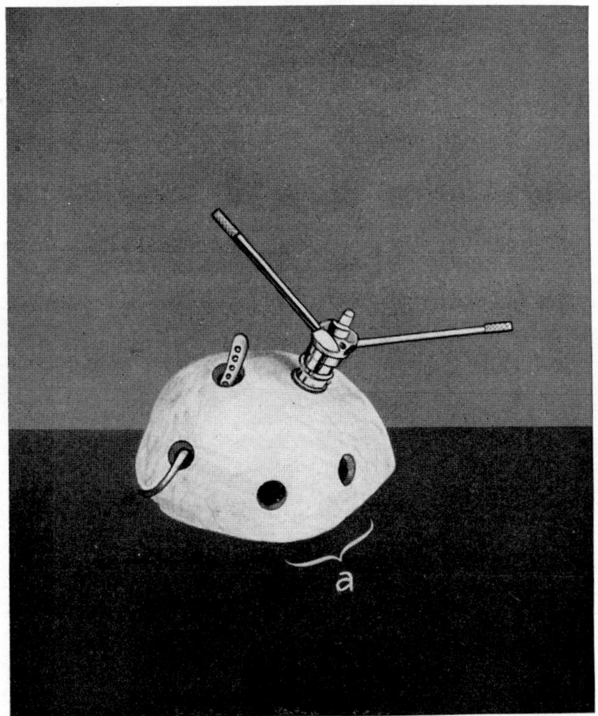

FIG. 145. *Combination technic.* Jentzer trephine coupled with Gigli saw. Introduction of dura separator.

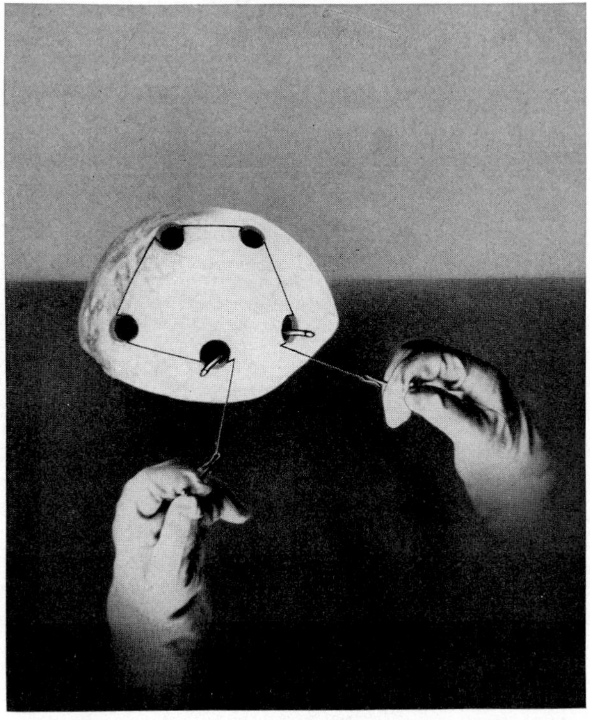

FIG. 146. *Combination technic.* Jantzer trephine coupled with Gigli saw. Sawing through the bone.

uniform thickness and that the inner table may be found cut through at one place before another. As soon as the bone is cut through, the button of bone is removed and the dura mater is exposed. The methods for arresting bleeding from the cut surface of the bone have been discussed above.

The usual size of a trephine is about three-fourths of an inch in diameter; trephines more than one inch in diameter are generally impractical owing to the curving of the cranial vault.

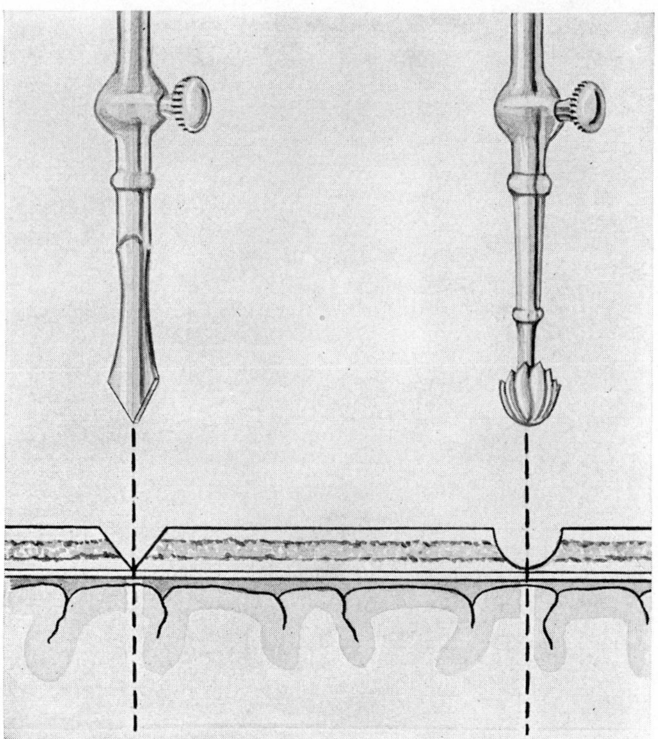

FIG. 147. Diagrammatic cross sections of cranial vault, showing the safe method of opening the skull. A pin-point opening is made with a Doyen perforator; this is enlarged with a Doyen burr, following which rongeurs are used. In this manner the meningeal artery, the dura and cortex are avoided.

When trephining is done for decompression only, unless there are indications to the contrary, it is advantageous to open the skull under the temporal muscle where the bone is thin and nonvascular; besides, the temporal muscle and fascia can be used to form an efficient covering for the brain and prevent undue hernial protrusion ("subtemporal decompression"). In extensive decompressions for tumor, hernia cerebri often results (Fig. 148).

Chisel and Mallet

This is followed by greater shock than when trephining is done as outlined. When, for one reason or another, this method is selected, proceed as follows: Have an assistant steady the head after preparing the skull as described above. After having exposed the skull by fashioning an appropriate flap, place a Doyen's guarded chisel nearly parallel to the plane of the skull and by careful blows of the mallet cause the chisel to cut a narrow groove in the bone. Deepen the groove gradually. Remove the desired segment of bone, thus exposing the dura mater.

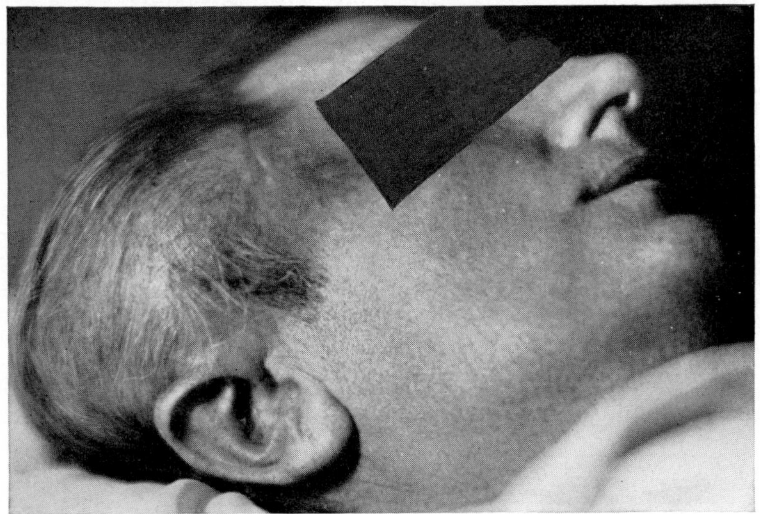

FIG. 148. Hernia following cranial decompression for sarcoma of the brain.

Gigli Wire Saw

This is a splendid instrument for the formation of a trapdoor opening in the skull (Fig. 149.) It enables the surgeon to remove a large area of skull in one piece. A U-shaped flap of appropriate size is fashioned. Reflect the pericranium. At each of the five points of the area to be removed, the skull is perforated with a small trephine or a Doyen's perforator.

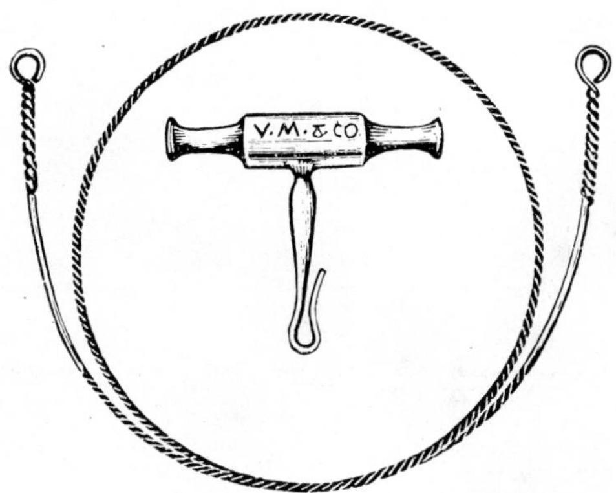

FIG. 149. Gigli wire saw.

The latter is a very efficient and safe instrument conveniently operated by a brace. Before applying the perforator, the outer table of the skull should be drilled so as to permit the rounded perforator to bite. Separate the dura from the skull along the line stretching from one trephine opening to another by means of a dural separator. Introduce now an appropriately shaped grooved di-

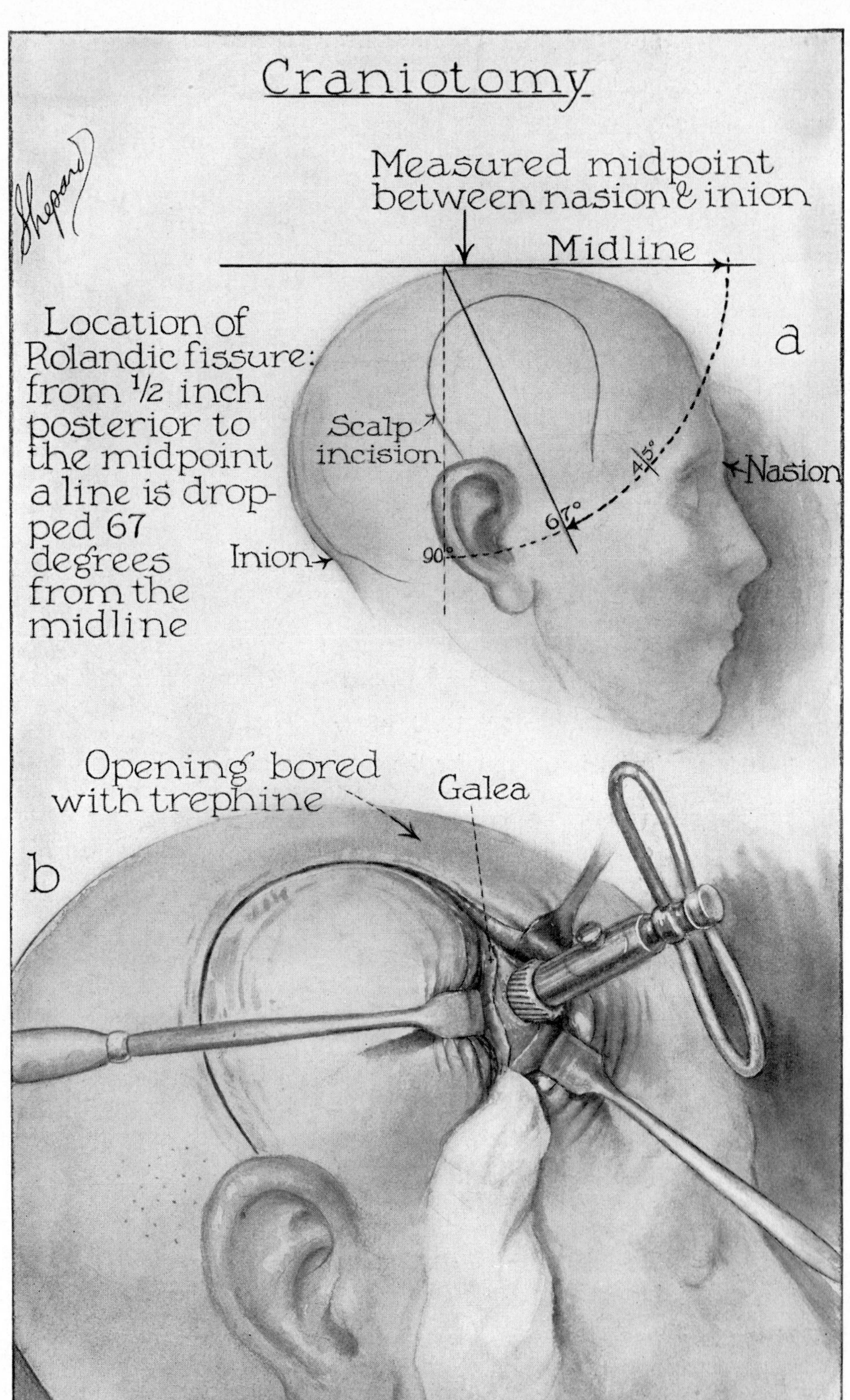

FIG. 150. Cerebral decompression.

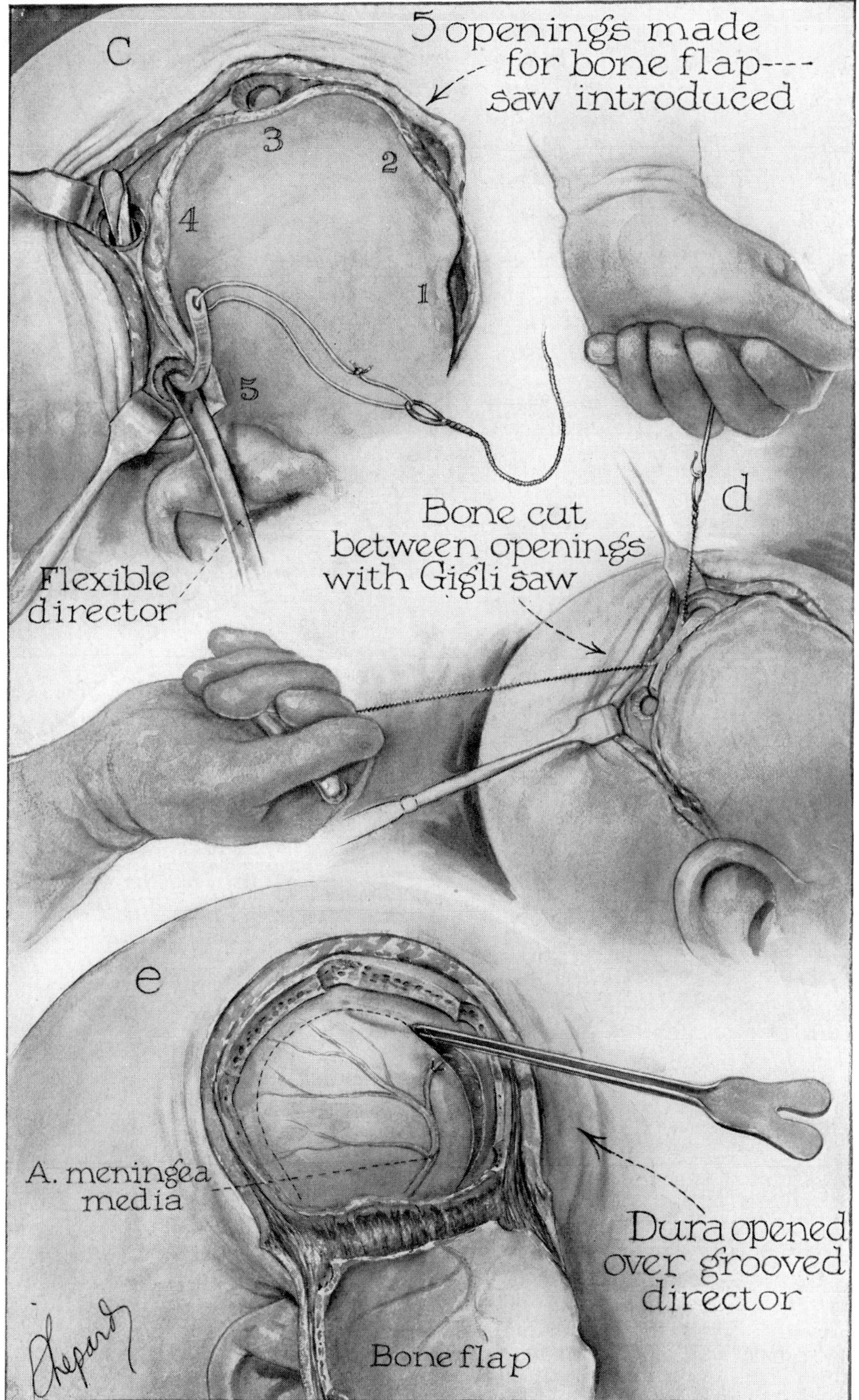

FIG. 150 (continued). Cerebral decompression (for interpretation of illustration see text).

rector to take the place of the dural separator. Pass a Gigli wire saw along the grooved director; leave the director in place to protect the dura. The skull is now divided with the wire saw from within outwards either straight or beveled. Remove the director. This procedure is repeated until the desired area of bone is entirely detached. (Figs. 150 a, and b.)

Forceps

After perforating the skull as described, the bone may be divided between the perforations with bone-cutting forceps, Keen's or DeVilbiss' instruments (Fig. 151) being used instead of the Gigli wire saw. Krause's claw forceps are sometimes used to advantage in turning down an osteoplastic flap (Fig. 152).

Electric Saws, Etc.

Electrically driven circular saws and drills are used by some surgeons as a means of rapidly opening the cranium. A good suction apparatus is of great aid in operative manipulations about the brain.

SUBTEMPORAL DECOMPRESSION

Cushing's Modification

Step 1. Make a semilunar flap consisting of skin and fascia along the temporal crest. Begin the incision in front at a point a little below and behind the lateral angular process of the frontal bone and terminate it posteriorly at the root of the zygoma. Dissect the skin and subcutaneous tissues downwards to the level of the zygomatic arch. Lay the temporal fascia bare.

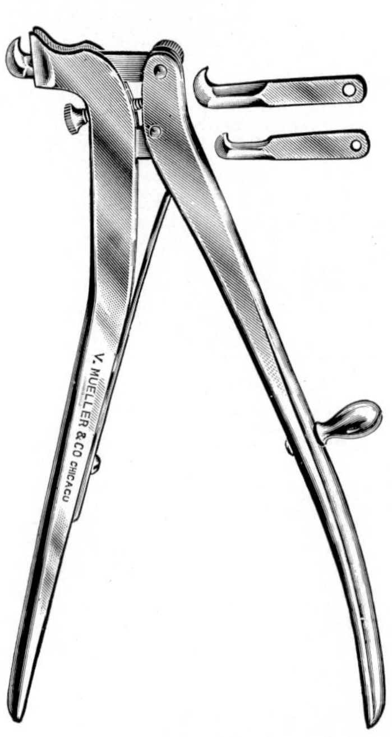

FIG. 151. DeVilbiss cranial forceps.

Step 2. Divide the fascia in the direction of its fibers and continue to just below the temporal crest and to the level of the zygoma.

Step 3. Divide longitudinally and retract strongly the fibers of the temporal muscle in a line extending from the center of the temporal crest to the middle of the zygoma down to the periosteum; this is also divided longitudinally.

Step 4. With a periosteal elevator or rugine, separate the periosteum forwards and backwards until a considerable area of the bone forming the floor of the temporal fossa is exposed.

Step 5. Penetrate the skull with a Doyen burr (Fig. 153) and with a rongeur forceps remove from under the separated soft parts as much of the skull as seems necessary; or, with the aid of a trephine remove a circle of bone from the center of the exposed area as above described. Enlarge the aperture with bone forceps until a sufficiently large opening is created.

Step 6. If deemed necessary, make an incision in the exposed dura mater, taking care to avoid large meningeal blood vessels and to ligate smaller ones which may be divided. (Figs. 154-155-156.)

Step 7. Attend to hemostasis. Unite the fascia with fine chromicized catgut sutures. (Fig. 157.)

Step 8. Replace the skin flap and suture it in position with interrupted sutures.

Step 9. Pass a cigarette drain down to the dura and bring it out through a small opening at the base of the flap. (Fig. 158.)

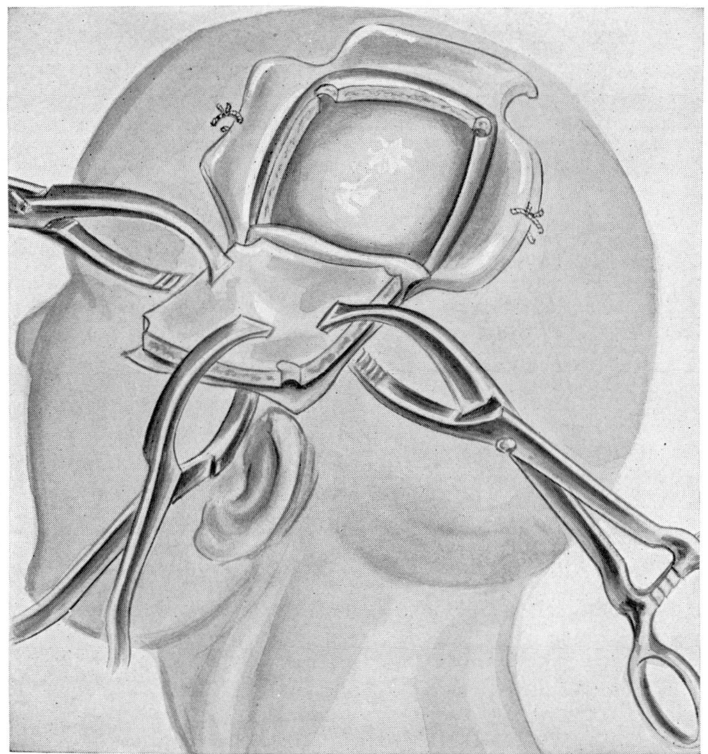

FIG. 152. Use of Krause's claw forceps in turning down osteoplastic flap. (Krause-Thoreks, Surgery of the Brain and Spinal Cord, F. J. Rebman Publishing Co.)

Cushing's Decompression Operation Over the Cerebellum

Step 1. Make a curved incision a little above the superior curved line of the occiput. Add a longitudinal median incision running downwards from the middle of the curved incision. Reflect downwards and outwards the two triangular flaps of skin thus outlined until the upper portion or origin of the flat superficial cervical muscles is exposed. Divide the muscles parallel to and about ¾ inch from their line of origin. Make a median vertical incision between the muscles down to the spines of the upper cervical vertebrae and divide the ligamentum nuchae in the midline. Retract the soft parts. Expose the base of the occiput by separating the periosteum from it and with the periosteum separate the attachments of the deep muscles. (Fig. 159.)

Step 2. Open the skull on each side through the prominent thin bosses of the occiput. Enlarge the openings with rongeur forceps. The ridge of bone in the midline must be attacked with great care because of the occasional presence of the mid-occipital sinus and emissary veins. Cushing finds it helpful "to crowd wisps of sterile cotton ahead of the dural separator when freeing the membranes from this mid-ridge, a procedure which necessarily ruptures and blocks these emissary vessels in case they are present."

Step 3. When the bone defect is large enough, ligate the median occipital sinus and excise the dura corresponding to the opening in the bone.

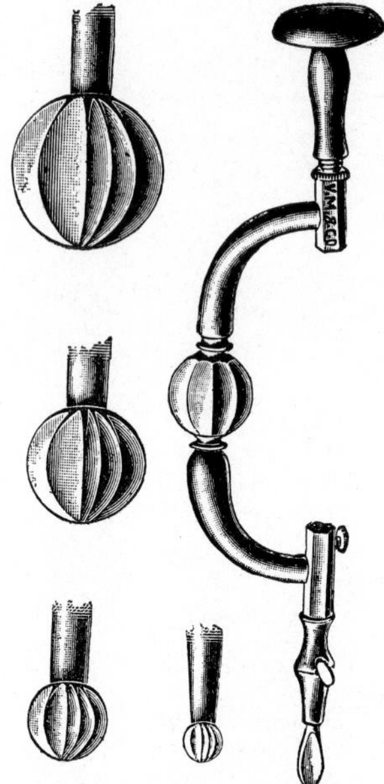

FIG. 153. Doyen's burrs.

Step 4. Close the wound, preferably without drainage. On account of oozing of blood a drain of folded rubber tissue or of oiled silk may be employed. Withdraw the drain within forty-eight hours.

CLOSURE OF CRANIAL DEFECTS

Free, non-pedunculated transplantation of bone in cranial defects is much simpler to perform and is just as efficacious as the Müller-König method which requires dexterity and experience.

1. A portion of the tibia with its periosteum (von Eiselsberg's procedure) is transplanted.

2. Fragments of bone from the outer table of the skull taken at a distance from the defect may be used (Binnie's suggestion).

3. Replacement of the fragment removed by trephining.

4. Replacement of the scalp alone; firm fibrous tissue appears, effectively protecting the brain from external trauma.

MULLER-KONIG METHOD

Step 1. Reflect a skin-periosteal flap exposing the cranial defect (Fig. 160). Clear the defect of all scar tissue. Freshen the edges of the bone with fine chisel or rongeurs.

Step 2. Outline another flap and reflect it as shown in Fig. 161. In shaping this flap include in it a portion of the outer table of the bone of the skull, cut away with the chisel, so that the portion of bone forms an integral part of this flap and corresponds in size and shape to the cranial defect into which it is to be fastened.

Step 3. The graft is now placed into the defect and the edges of the flaps are sutured in place as shown in Fig. 162.

It is difficult during the operative manipulations to avoid detachment of the portion of bone from the pericranium.

Comment. Stieda's Rules. 1. **If the wound can be rendered and kept aseptic, close the defect at once by implantation of the fragments removed (Macewen's method).**

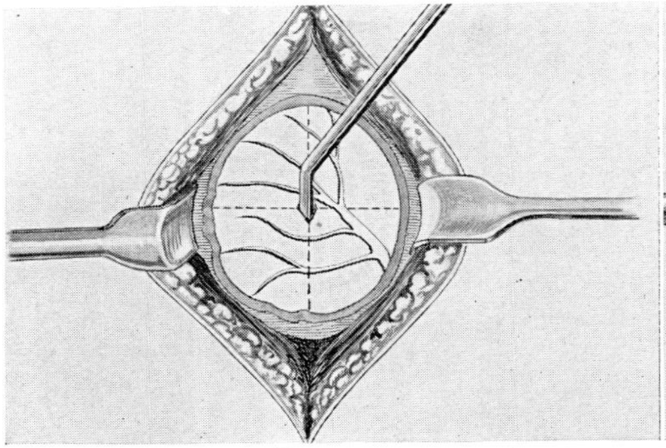

FIG. 154 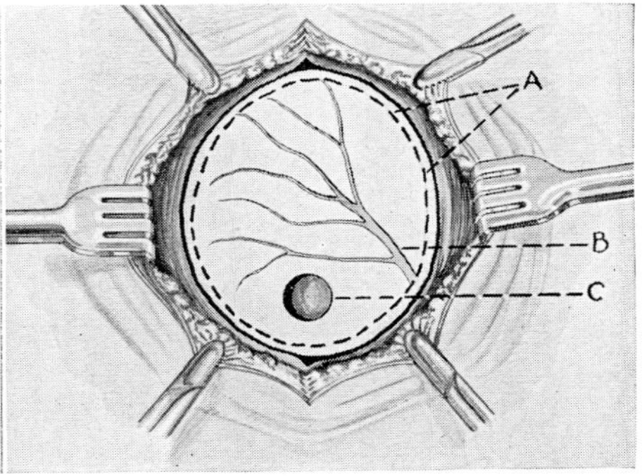 FIG. 155

FIG. 154. Dura incised on a grooved director (subtemporal decompression).

FIG. 155. Subtemporal decompression, area of bone exposed by retracting overlying temporal muscle. The dotted line, A, indicates the extent of bone to be removed; B, shows the course of the underlying middle meningeal artery C. Open the skull in the squamous part of the temporal bone.

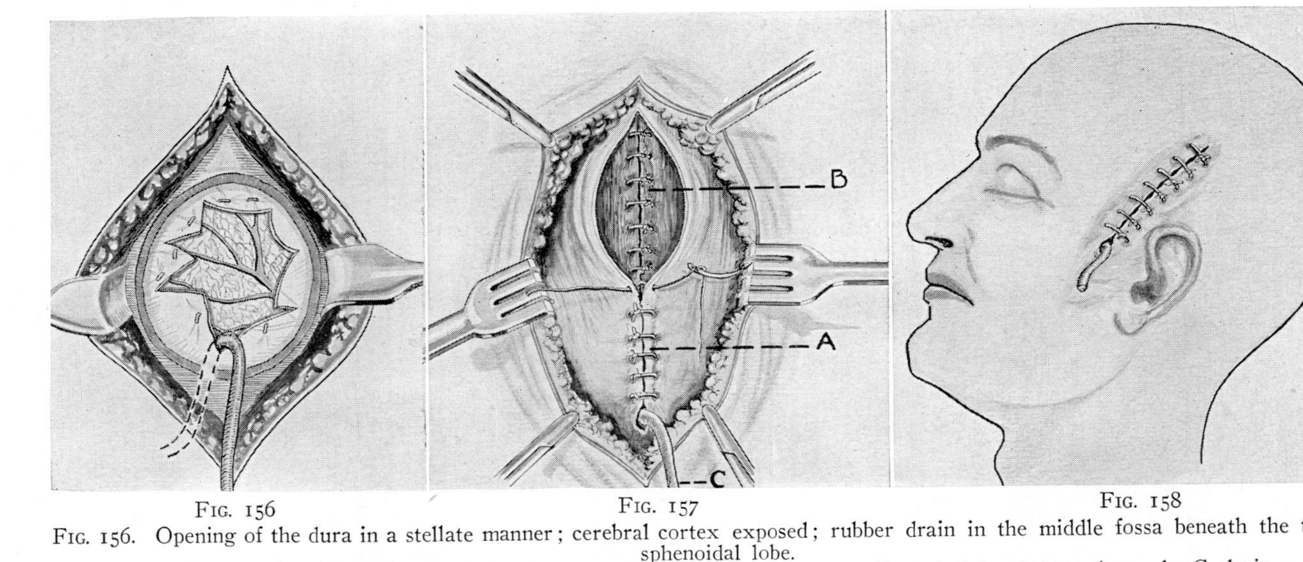

FIG. 156 FIG. 157 FIG. 158

FIG. 156. Opening of the dura in a stellate manner; cerebral cortex exposed; rubber drain in the middle fossa beneath the temporosphenoidal lobe.

FIG. 157. Subtemporal decompression; A, temporal fascia sutured over B, underlying temporal muscle. C, drain.

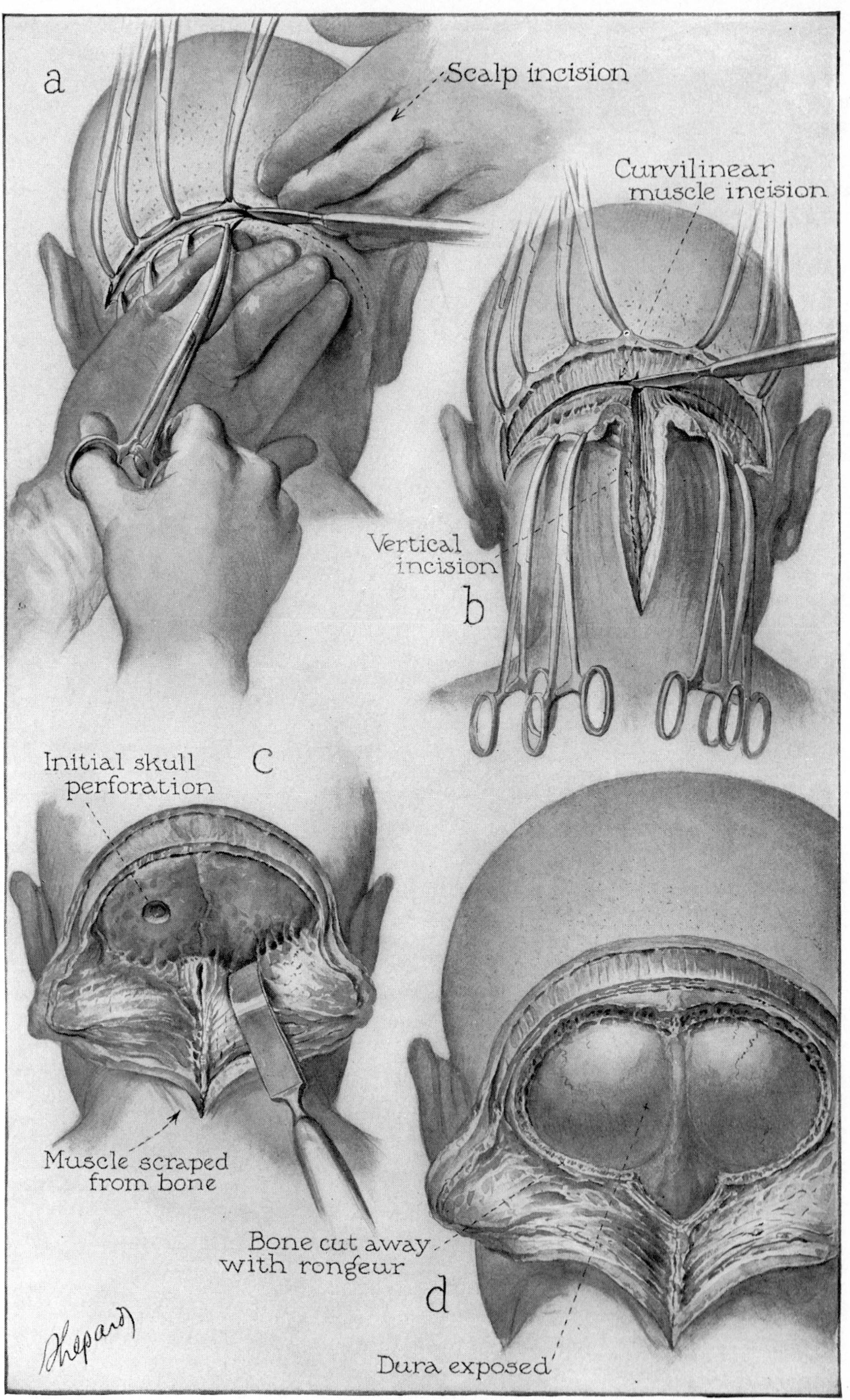

FIG. 159. Cushing's decompression operation over the cerebellum.

2. If the wound is healed—do not wait for epilepsy to develop but excise the scar tissue from the cranial defect and repair it by the Müller-König osteoplastic method.

Macewen's method is applicable only when the bone removed is available for reimplanting.

Autogenous Cranial Transplants

The technic employed is that used by Charles H. Frazier and requires practically the same preparation of the defect as is necessary when the transplant is taken from the tibia or ribs.

Step 1. Make an incision around the boundaries of the old scar and remove the scar tissue (Figs. 163[1, 2]-164).

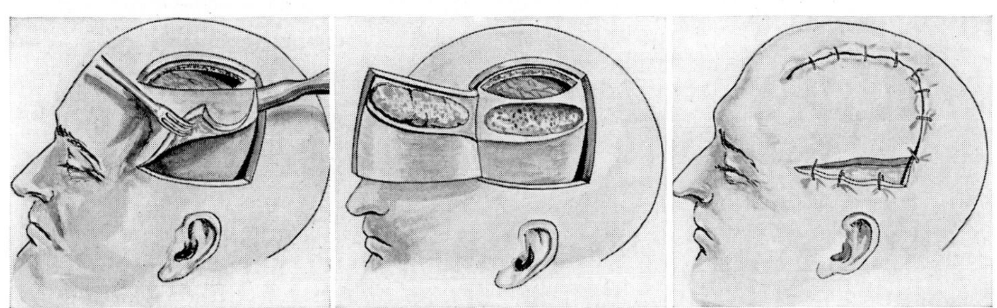

FIG. 160 FIG. 161 FIG. 162

FIG. 160. Müller-König operation for closure of cranial defects. Exposure of cranial defects by reflecting skin-periosteal flap. All scar tissue is cut away from the defect and the edges of the bone freshened.

FIG. 161. Formation of osteoplastic flap.

FIG. 162. Operation completed.

Step 2. Bevel the bony rim with a fine chisel and free the dura. Remove foreign bodies and bone spicules if accessible but do not deliberately open the dura (Fig. 163[3, 4]).

Step 3. Make a pattern of the defect with rubber dam or muslin; place it on the pericranium of the parietal eminence of the same side or of the contralateral side when the defect is large (Fig. 163[5, 6]). Outline the pattern on the bone with a small chisel and remove a thin lamina of bone with overlying pericranium (Fig. 165). The transplant usually curls up during removal and resembles a thick fish-scale mosaic with the fragments held in contact by the pericranial covering. The graft is molded into the desired curve by pressure and placed upon the defect with its bony surface in contact with the dura. Fix the transplant in position by uniting the pericranium around the bony rim with that of the graft using fine interrupted catgut sutures (Figs. 163[7, 8]-166).

Step 4. Close the wound in layers with free rubber tissue drainage over the defect and the area from which the graft is taken. Keep the patient flat in bed about two weeks during which time the protrusion of the intracranial contents which the horizontal position favors will give the thin transplant the proper curve and permit it to set on a plane with the surrounding skull.

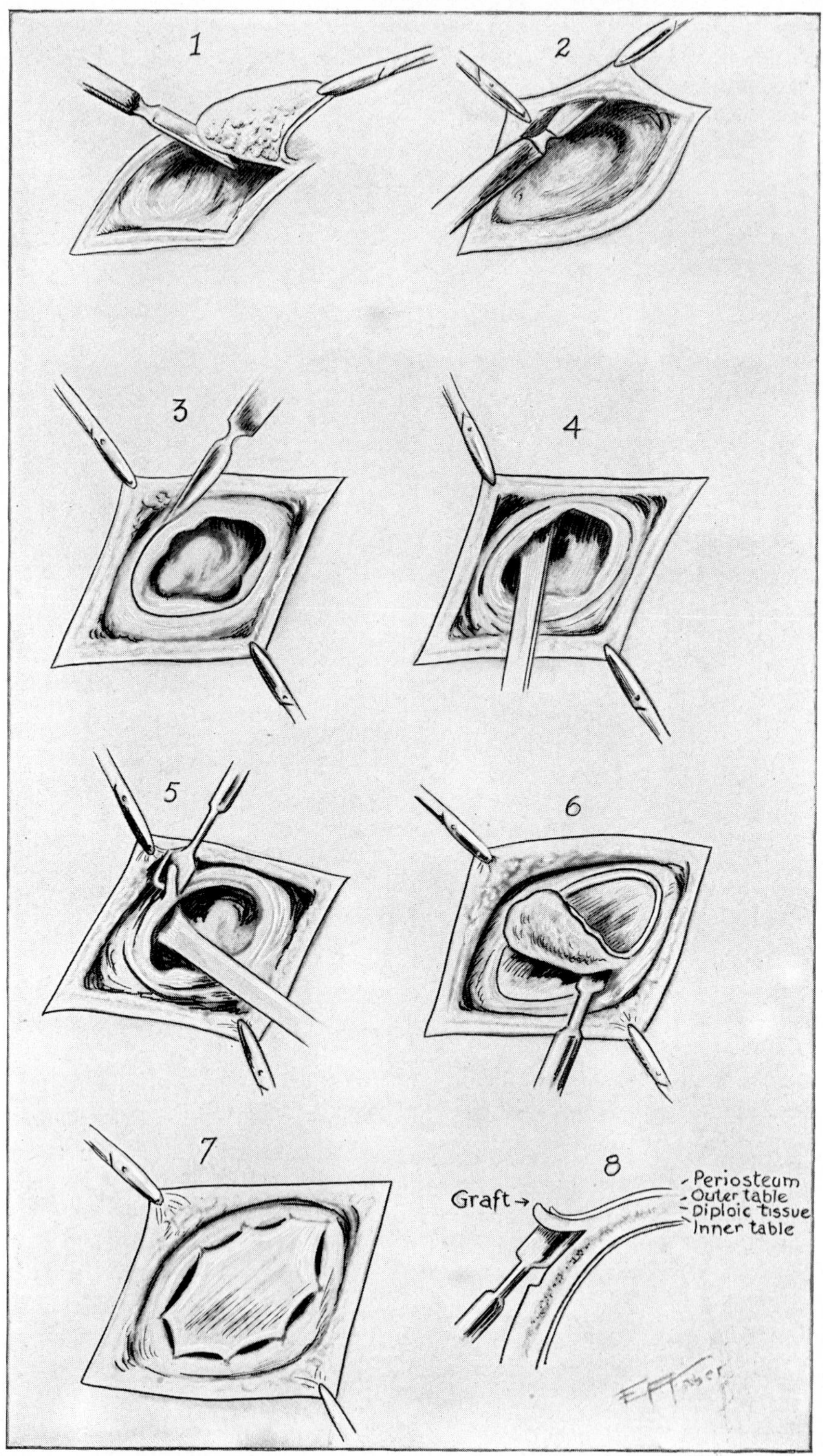

FIG. 163. Repair of cranial defects by autogenous cranial transplants. Consecutive stages of operation: 1. excision of scar from defect; 2. exposure of rim of defect by incision through scar;

GENERAL PRINCIPLES UNDERLYING THE REMOVAL OF TUMORS OF THE BRAIN

The rudiments, at least, of cranio-cerebral localization should be thoroughly understood before a brain tumor is attacked. A competent neurologist should always check on the pre- and postoperative findings. If available, a neurosurgeon should be given preference; the occasional operator should proceed only where the aid of a specially trained colleague cannot be obtained.

The surgeon should acquaint himself with the normal and abnormal appearance of the cortex cerebri.

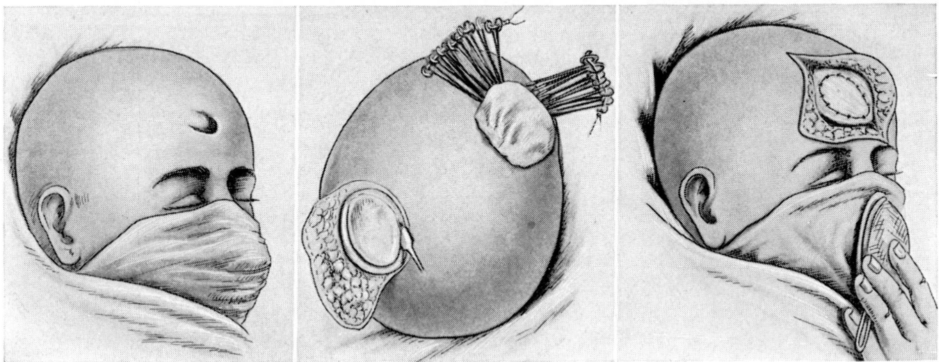

FIG. 164 FIG. 165 FIG. 166

FIG. 164. Repair of cranial defects by autogenous cranial transplants. Sketch of craniofacial defect (courtesy of Dr. C. C. Coleman).

FIG. 165. The defect has been prepared for transplantation. The graft is outlined on the left parietal eminence.

FIG. 166. Complete suture of the graft. The incision in the scalp is usually united with a double row of sutures.

Normally, the dura and pia-arachnoid should not be fused except in the region of the Pacchionian bodies. The vessels of the pia should be easily discernible. Whitish thickenings along the large pial veins are of no moment.

Glioma in the cortex is often difficult to detect; palpation may reveal a difference in consistency.

Infiltrating gliomas or gliosarcomas are of a bluish color, slightly elevated and much more easily discerned.

Small reddish-brown areas resembling tumors are often observed on the cortex in cases of considerable bulging of brain tissue. These hemorrhagic spots often increase in size and, if incised, the brain tissue will be found soft and discolored; these are not to be looked upon as neoplasms.

---

3. incision through pericranium about a quarter of an inch from the edge of the defect, the purpose of the incision being to provide for bone contact with the graft and to free the adherent dura; 4. pericranium within the incision, 3, is forcibly displaced within the defect by an elevator and adhesions of the dura to the edge of the bone are thus freed; 5. beveling the edge of the defect for contact with the graft. The dura is carefully protected from the parietal eminence. The size and shape of the transplant have been modeled by rubber dam and the graft cut to fit accurately; 7. graft partly sutured by uniting the pericranium of the graft with that surrounding the defect, 8. cross section of graft. (Courtesy of Dr. C. C. Coleman.)

EXPOSURE OF THE BRAIN

As a general example of procedure a description of the main steps in the removal of a circumscribed tumor of the central aspect of the brain, by enucleation, through osteoplastic exposure follows:

Step 1. The skull may be opened by chisel and mallet, Gigli wire saw, forceps, electric saws, etc. Focal manifestations are the best guides to the portion of the brain sought.

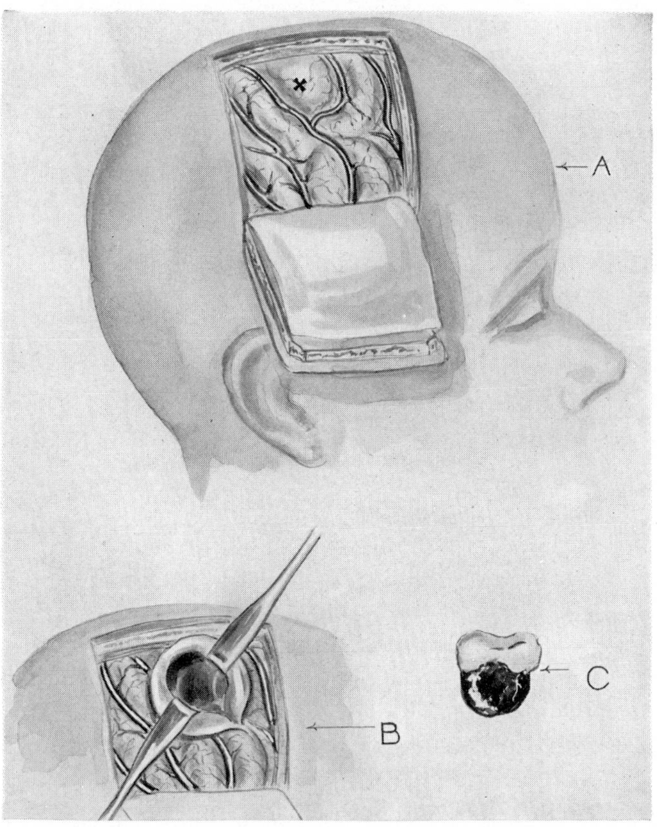

Fig. 167. A. Gliosarcoma, the size of a walnut, of the right motor area, B. field of operation after removal of the tumor, C. tumor. (Redrawn from Thoreks-Krause, Surgery of the Brain and Spinal Cord, F. J. Rebman Publishing Co.)

If there are no guiding localization phenomena, an osteoplastic flap may have to be turned down in the suspected region, as an exploratory procedure, to be extended, if necessary, as subsequently indicated.

Comment. The contour, consistency and the presence or absence of pulsations of the dura will afford valuable information. In tumor or blood-clot there usually is an absence of pulsations and the dura tends to bulge into the trephine opening. Palpation is of great aid in determining the presence of subcortical tumors. The experienced palpating finger has often correctly diagnosed subcortical tumors at a depth of one inch from the surface (Fig. 167).

Step 2. When the location of the tumor has been determined, the dura is incised so as to form a flap with its pedicle situated in the same direction as that of the osteoplastic flap. The flap of dura is seized at each end with Allis forceps and carefully turned downward, slowly elevating it from the brain. Sometimes the tumor will tend to follow tension upon the dura, if a curved scissors or blunt dissector is insinuated between the capsule of the tumor and the brain hugging its contour. Ligation of the blood-vessels facilitates the enucleation of a circumscribed tumor. Double ligatures are placed around the vessels; they are tied; the long ends of the ligature serve as tractors; the vessels are severed between the ligatures (Fig. 168). If the dura is involved in the tumor, the involved portion must also be removed.

Step 3. Binnie recommends an ordinary silver teaspoon aided by gentle dissection for the scooping out of an encapsulated tumor; it is much easier to use than an incision at right angles to the brain surface. Hemorrhage is controlled by ligation, clips, diathermy, compression with gauze or **hot lap sponges.**

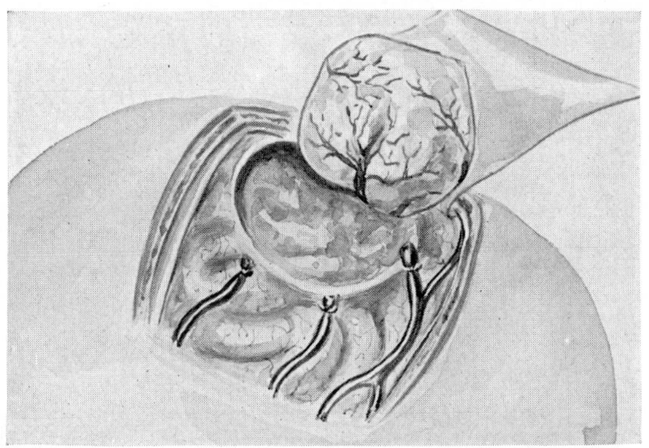

FIG. 168. Ligation of blood vessels around cortical tumor. (Redrawn from Krause-Thoreks, Surgery of the Brain and Spinal Cord, F. J. Rebman Publishing Co.)

Subcortical tumors should be reached by cutting through the summit of a convolution first; expose the tumor mass, gently retract the brain substance and remove the neoplasm with a spoon or scoop.

A small, curved soft metal tube, 3 to 5 mm. in diameter, connected with a continuous suction apparatus, may be used to great advantage to clarify the view of deep-seated, vascular tumors showing slight macroscopic differences between normal and pathological tissues. Trauma to the brain substance is lessened by doing less sponging.

If the condition of the patient is satisfactory, finish the operation in one stage (see Step 5).

Step 4. If the patient shows a drop in blood pressure or an augmented pulse rate after the first part of the operation, suture the flap into place and postpone opening the dura for 5 to 10 days.

In two-stage operations, the dural flap is not sutured; it is simply laid back over the cortex. Part or all of the bone flap is removed.

Step 5. When the tumor is detached from the brain substance but still adherent to its origin from the membranes (meningioma) it is entirely severed from the brain by dividing the base of the dural flap to which it remains attached. The defect in the dura is usually repaired by some form of duraplastic procedure. A fascial flap from the aponeurosis of the fascia lata affords good repair material. The space in the fascia lata, after removing the flap, need not be repaired. While the cavity left in the brain after removal of a tumor sometimes requires drainage, it usually is promptly obliterated by the expansion of the brain.

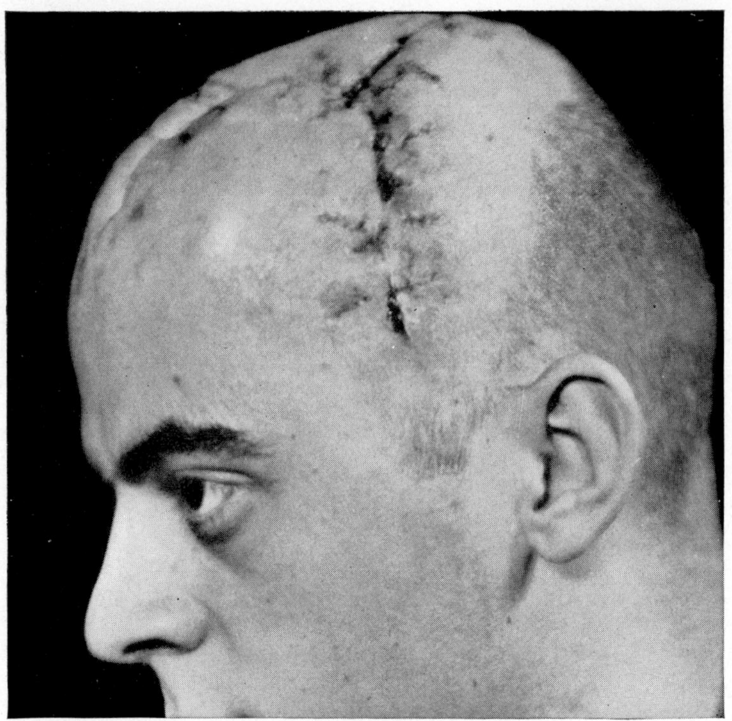

FIG. 169. Malignant meningioma. Patient seven days after operation (electrocoagulation all around tumor mass the size of fist). Normal temperature. No focal manifestations. Dura not opened but coagulated at base of tumor and distance of about 2 cm.

The dura is sutured back into place by either interrupted or continuous sutures. In cases with great tension, the dura cannot be sutured at all; it is simply replaced over the brain.

Disposal of the bone flap is governed by the degree of decompression desired; part or all of it may be removed or it may be replaced in its entirety.

If a trapdoor osteoplastic flap has been made, remove enough bone to permit of adequate drainage.

In tumors occurring on the left side in right-handed persons (and vice versa), and with decided increase in intracranial pressure, there is danger that cortical and subcortical laceration and hemorrhage with paralysis of arm, leg or speech may supervene following a sudden protrusion. Harvey Cushing has recommended that in such cases a preliminary, subtemporal decompression below and behind the Sylvian fissure be performed on the side opposite the tumor.

TUMORS OF THE CONVEXITY OF THE HEMISPHERES

Unless unusually large, neoplasms occurring on the inner surface of the dura mater are usually easily removable. They are completely enveloped and are easily detached from the cortex. The incision should begin to one side of the tumor. Occasionally, a portion of the dura has to be sacrificed. After the attachments of the tumor are severed, it is gently removed from the cortex. Small vessels are ligated with fine silk or catgut; clips or electrosurgical hemostasis may also be employed. Hemostasis is often effected by small cotton pledgets. The depression left by the removal of the tumor usually fills promptly. The edges

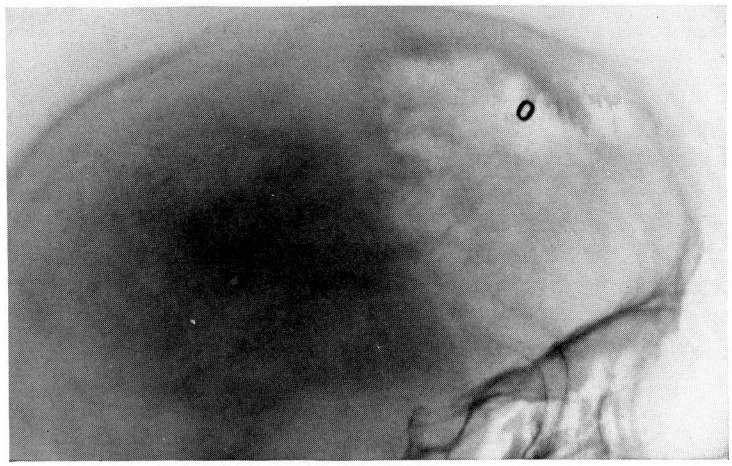

FIG. 170. Malignant meningioma before operation. Same patient as in Fig. 169. (From Author's Service, American Hospital, Chicago.)

of the wound of the dura are held together by interrupted sutures; the bone flap is then replaced and sutured.

In cases where tumors occur on the external surface of the membrane or have perforated the dura, it may become necessary to excise a portion of the dura. If so, the wound is closed by a fascial flap taken from the fascia lata or a flap taken from the outer layer of the dura. Inoperable tumors may often be ameliorated by electrocoagulation. (Figs. 169, 170, 171.)

TUMORS OF THE FRONTAL LOBES

Exercise care to avoid entering the frontal sinus while fashioning the bone flap over the frontal lobes. The flap should be large enough so that all parts of the frontal lobe may be thoroughly examined. Exposure of a subcortical tumor may be accomplished safely by incising the right or left frontal lobe well toward the front avoiding injury to the long motor association tracts. In infiltrating tumors, replace the dura and osteoplastic flap because hernia is apt to follow. In excising a tumor from the inner surface of the frontal lobe, avoid injuring the olfactory bulb.

TUMORS OF THE TEMPORAL, PARIETAL AND OCCIPITAL REGIONS

In operating on the cortex over the Rolandic area proceed cautiously as permanent paralysis of one or more extremities may ensue. If the operation is low down on the left side (right side in left-handed persons) remember that the patient may lose his power of speech.

Tumors occurring in the lower part of the temporal lobe may require extensive sacrifice of bone down to the base of the skull; only by so doing can efficient access to the under surface of the temporal lobe be obtained.

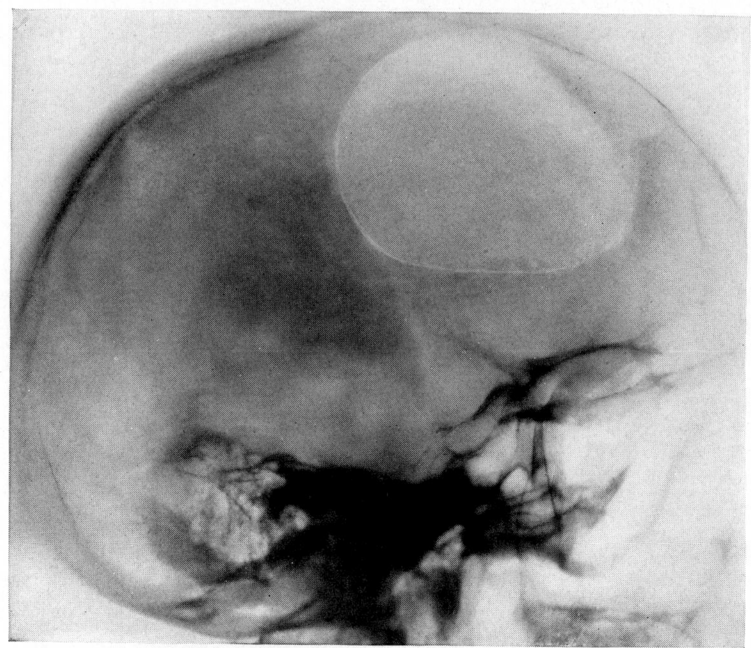

Fig. 171. Malignant meningioma after operation. Trephining. Electrosurgical destruction of tumor mass. (From Author's Service, American Hospital, Chicago.)

If the ventricle has been opened in removing a subcortical tumor, make no effort to close it. A piece of Cargile membrane may be used to cover this opening.

SUBTENTORIAL TUMORS

(Figs. 172, 173-174)

Excision of a tumor from the cerebellar hemisphere or the cerebellopontine angle is more difficult than operating in the cerebral hemispheres. Operations here are usually performed in two stages.

Stage I

Step 1. Incise the dura. Palpate the hemisphere, and if expedient, explore with an aspirating needle.

Step 2. When the tumor is subcortical, ligate the large pial vessels and make a transverse incision. Attend to hemostasis. This is usually not difficult. In infiltrating tumors a large portion of the hemisphere may have to be sacrificed.

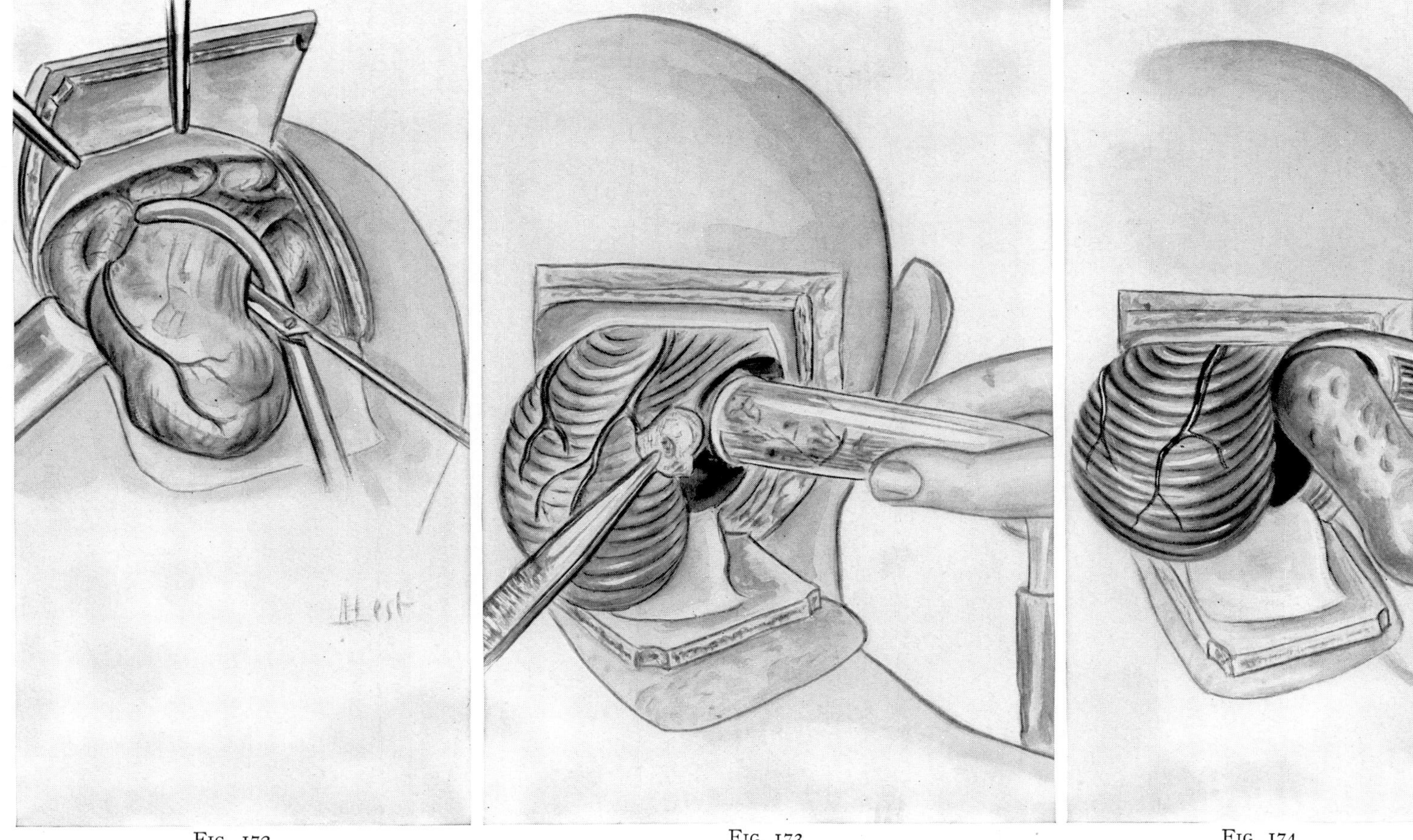

Fig. 172 Fig. 173 Fig. 174

Fig. 172. Removal of tumor of the brain by suction. The tumor has been dislocated and its extensive pedicle, consisting of cerebral medullary substance, was divided with scissors.

Fig. 173. Suction used to deliver a tumor at the cerebellopontine angle.

Fig. 174. Tumor at the cerebellopontine angle. This illustration depicts the possibilities afforded by the use of suction in brain surgery. (The above illustrations were redrawn from Krause-Thoreks, Surgery of the Brain and Spinal Cord, F. J. Rebman Publishing Co.)

Tumors at the cerebellopontine angle tax the skill of the surgeon. Tumors here are usually of long duration and are loosely connected with the nerves and brain. They frequently spring from the **auditory nerve** and resemble a neurofibroma.

Stage II

Step 1. Expose the tumor by retracting the cerebellar hemisphere toward the midline, forcing the whole cerebellum toward the opposite side. Use a medium-sized brain depressor bent to the proper angle.

Step 2. Retract the cerebellum toward the opposite side thus exposing the posterior surface of the petrous portion of the temporal bone. With a suction apparatus or by meticulous sponging, clear the fluid issuing from the lateral subarachnoid cistern which has been punctured.

Step 3. Free the tumor from its mesial attachments, gently working away from the pons and medulla. If the tumor is large it may become necessary to divide the auditory nerve. Avoid injury to the facial nerve.

The manipulation of tumors of considerable size may cause interference with respiration. If the cerebellum is immobile a third operation may be necessary. Protect the cerebellar tissue from injury.

Step 4. After removal of the tumor, attend to hemostasis. Permit the hemisphere to return to its fossa. The wound is closed in the usual manner. The muscles of the suboccipital region sufficiently protect the cerebellum so that suture of the dura is not imperative.

ANGIOMAS (PIAL) OF THE CEREBRAL HEMISPHERES

Obtain good exposure; select a large branch of the principal vessel; doubly ligate it with fine silk and divide it between the ligatures. Hemorrhage is likely here (the vessel walls are easily torn). Work very cautiously. Electrosurgical methods serve here well.

CYSTS AND CYSTIC COLLECTIONS OF FLUID IN THE BRAIN

For an exhaustive description of this condition, the reader is referred to the author's English adaptation of Krause's Surgery of the Brain and Spinal Cord.[1]

Meningitis serosa circumscripta (Oppenheim and Krause) is not frequent and occurs only in the posterior cranial fossa. Brain cysts arise either from an old hemorrhage or from a soft glioma. For method of thorough exposure see Fig. 180, p. 166.

In facing this problem, make sure while aspirating the brain tissue, that a distended lateral ventricle is not inadvertantly aspirated. Fluid from a cyst is usually of a yellowish or greenish color, normal cerebrospinal fluid is quite clear. It is well to remember that an old hemorrhage into the ventricles or tumor near a lateral ventricle may cause the ventricular fluid to present a yellow or greenish hue.

Step 1. Incise the brain tissues and expose the cyst cavity.

Step 2. If the cyst wall is thick, excise it. If this is impossible, endeavor to destroy it by electrosurgical means. (Electrocoagulation.)

The prognosis of simple cysts is favorable although it is at times difficult to differentiate between these and gliomatous cysts.

[1] F. J. Rebman Publishing Co. 1912.

Krause's Transfrontoparietal Intracranial Method for Removal of Tumor of the Hypophysis Cerebri

This operation is performed where x-ray plates reveal a tumor and the diagnosis is based on clinical manifestations produced by the neoplasm. In such cases, the tumor overgrows the sella turcica and involves contiguous areas of the frontal and temporal brain, causing symptoms. The operation is performed in two stages. (Figs. 175-176.)

Stage I

Step 1. Make an osteoplastic flap over the temporoparietal region. This should hinge backward and its dimensions should approximately be 3½ inches anteriorly, 3¼ inches posteriorly, 3¾ inches above and 3½ inches below. Wait about a week.

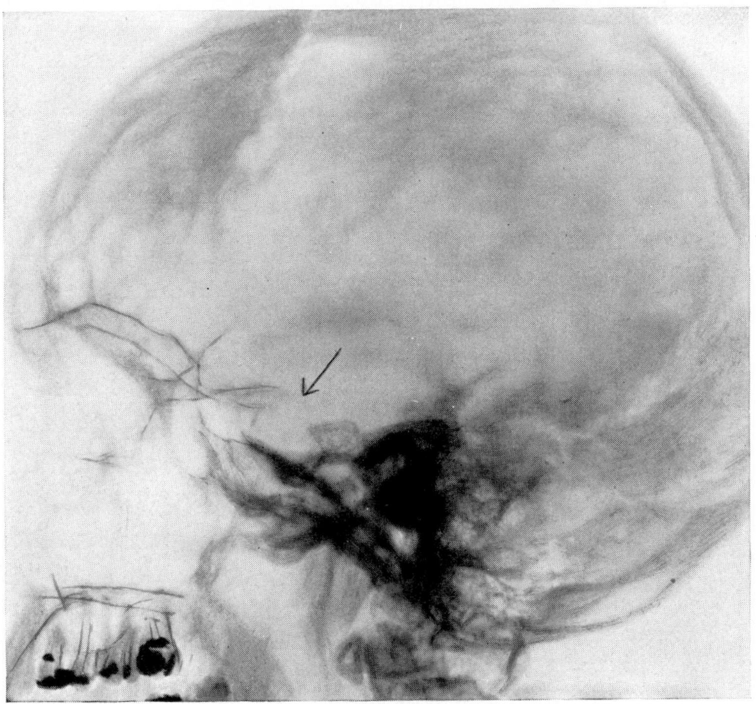

FIG. 175. Tumor of the pituitary gland. Note size of sella turcica and character of clinoid processes.

Stage II

Step 2. About a week later, raise the osteoplastic flap again and turn it back. Fashion a dural flap which hinges downward. Ligate the presenting branches of the middle meningeal artery.

Step 3. With a spatula lift up the frontal brain, from the frontal fossa, exposing the anterior fossa of the skull, the posterior border of the lesser wing of the sphenoid, the sinus running over it, the anterior clinoid process and part of the temporal lobe of the brain posterior to the lesser wing of the sphenoid.

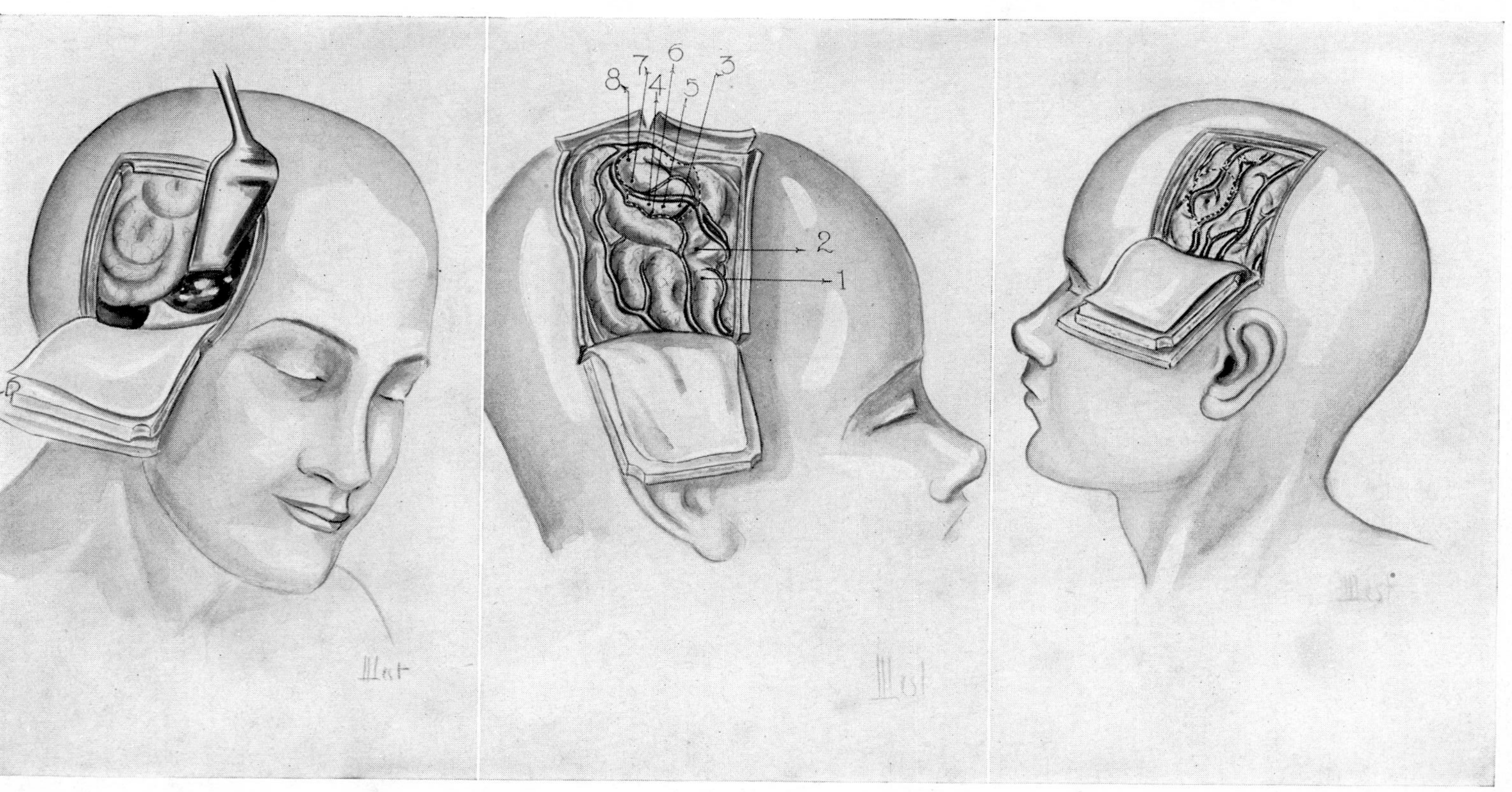

Fig. 176 Fig. 177 Fig. 178

Fig. 176. Large sarcoma of the hypophysis. Removal by the frontotemporal route. Regression of the symptoms of acromegaly.

Fig. 177. Excision of brain substance for Jacksonian epilepsy. The skull has been opened by means of an osteoplastic trap door flap. Points 1-8 inclusive represent areas irritated with specific responses to the Faradic current. The area outlined with dots is to be excised. The blood vessels here are not as yet ligated.

Fig. 178. Excision of brain substance for Jacksonian epilepsy. The excised centrum is outlined by dashes. Unipolar faradic irritation at the point marked in the center of the outlined area, resulted in an epileptic attack, which took its origin in the right facialis and hand. (Redrawn from Krause and Thoreks, Surgery of the Brain and Spinal Cord, F. J. Rebman Publishing Co.)

With a smooth forceps, push the olfactory nerve backward an dthus remove the obstruction on the way to the hypophysis. After the frontal lobe of the brain is moved further away from the fossa, exposure of the hypophyseal tumor and the operative field is accomplished.

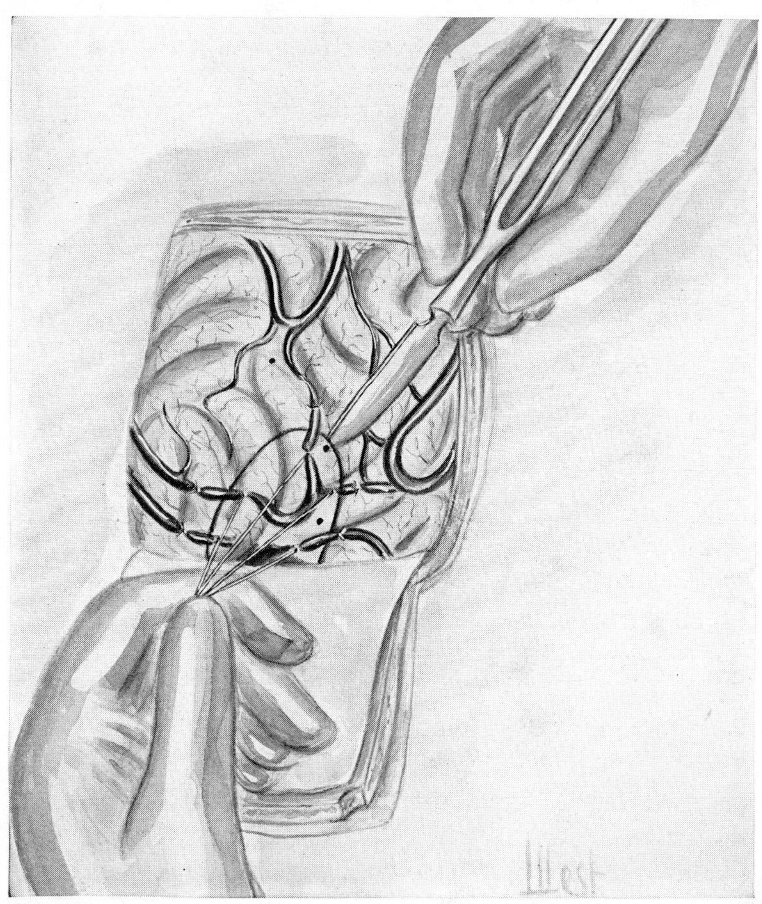

FIG. 179. Excision of the cortex cerebri for Jacksonian epilepsy. After locating the "primary spasm" area by electric stimulation, the center corresponding to the part thus affected is excised together with the contiguous brain substance to the depth of about 8 to 10 mm. To avoid hemorrhage the blood vessels encroaching upon the area to be excised are ligated. Additional ligatures shown in the center of the area are used as tractors to lift the fucus to be removed. The incision is made between the ligatures which are cut short. (Redrawn from Krause-Thoreks, Surgery of the Brain and Spinal Cord, F. J. Rebman Publishing Co.)

Step 4. Further displacement of the brain from the tumor is brought about by means of gauze held in curved forceps. The tumor may be removed by suction, a finger or a spoon.

Effective lifting up of the frontal brain brings to view the sella turcica, dorsum sellae, the anterior clinoid process, the eminentiae capitatae of the roof of the corresponding orbit, the crista galli and both sides of the ethmoid bone. The usual measures are used to check hemorrhage.

Step 5. After the tumor is removed, replace and suture the dural and osteoplastic flaps. Drainage is usually unnecessary.

EPILEPSY

Focal or Jacksonian

In Jacksonian epilepsy the irritation seems to originate in some particular point on the surface of the brain and to radiate to other parts. An endeavor should be made to ascertain the parts affected by cerebral localization (Figs. 177-178-179).

The causes for epileptic seizures are usually (a) depressed fractures; (b) osteophytic growths; (c) tumors; (d) localized meningitis causing adhesions; (e) hemorrhage, abscess, cysts, etc.

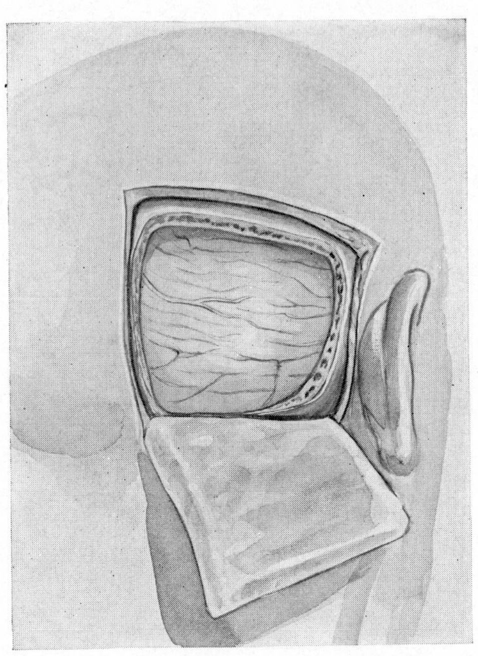

Fig. 180. Exposure of the petrous portion of the temporal bone. (Redrawn from Krause-Thoreks, Surgery of the Brain and Spinal Cord, F. J. Rebman Publishing Co.)

If no macroscopic lesion is found when the skull is opened and the brain exposed, the precise area from which the attacks radiate may be defined by means of stimulation by weak electrical currents. When a definite area is located, excise the gray matter of the affected part together with the pia-mater covering it. Excision of an area of cortex means prompt paralysis of the regions controlled by this area, but such paralysis seldom remains permanent. One may argue that a scar removed from the brain will be supplanted by another scar. True; nevertheless, there is a vast difference between a scar resulting from a violent trauma or inflammation and that occasioned by a clean, aseptic scalpel excision.

Step 1. Form a flap embracing the scar of the original trauma. Dissect the adherent scalp freely from the underlying bone. Inspect the bone thoroughly. Where, in severe injuries, the scalp is adherent to the dura or brain, direct the edge of the knife toward the inner surface of the flap.

Step 2. Examine for fracture. If none is found trephine over the area suspected, because there may be a depressed internal table, subdural hematoma, arachnoid cyst, etc.

Step 3. When a fracture is located, remove the bone directly concerned in the traumatized zone. This applies to both fissured and depressed fractures. (For methods of procedure see under fractured skull.) Avoid injuring the dura which is frequently adherent to the inner aspect of the bone. Use DeVilbiss forceps to bite out the area involved. Where dura, brain, bone-defect and scalp are united in one mass, dissect these out thoroughly and painstakingly. Dissect the dura free from the superimposed structures.

Step 4. **Where the dura pulsates** and has not been injured during the operative manipulations and presents a normal appearance, **stop** and **close** the defect in the skull.

When the dura bulges and there apparently is intracranial pressure, incise the dura crucially. Look for mischief underneath it (hematoma, cysts, etc.). A hematoma should be washed out; a cyst should be shelled out in its entirety; or, if that is not possible, partial excision with drainage may be resorted to.

When the dura is adherent to the brain, dissect it away carefully exposing the loose pia-arachnoid region. Complete the dissection by leaving, as nearly as possible, healthy cerebral tissue.

The cortical scar should be removed (superficial portion)..

Step 5. Attend to hemostasis. Prevention of adhesions between the dura and the brain may be accomplished by interposing silver foil, rubber or a fat-implant.

Step 6. Replace the skull-flap and suture it in place.

Idiopathic Epilepsy

The term "idiopathic epilepsy" is used as a cloak for ignorance and in contradistinction to the focal forms of the disease. The results of a decompression procedure in this domain of surgical endeavor have been good, bad and indifferent.

In many of these cases, scars will commonly be found after careful inspection of the shaved scalp even when no history of trauma has been elicited. Many of these scars are undoubtedly the result of accidents other than that causing the epileptic seizures.

W. W. Keen was so firmly convinced that a scar of the scalp may be the cause of epilepsy that after having excised the scar and having found the bone without evidence of injury, he closed the wound and waited. If after excision the patient failed to recover, Keen then—and not until then—considered the advisability of performing some other operation.

In traumatic epilepsy, Friedrich chose the site of trauma as the site for operation even when the "aura" would indicate some other location as the starting-point of the epileptic explosion.

Theodore Kocher, believing increased intracranial pressure to be the important etiologic factor in so-called "idiopathic epilepsy," trephined the skull, as a general proposition, and excised the dura mater over the right frontoparietal region. This he occasionally supplemented by drainage of the lateral ventricle.

In the absence of evidences of old trauma, Friedrich followed Kocher and operated over the posterior portion of the frontal lobe. He reflected a large flap of scalp, having its pedicle below. The skull was then opened and a segment of bone, from 20 to 48 sq. cm. (8 to 19 sq. in.), excised with forceps or other instruments. An area of dura varying in size from 9 to 33 sq. cm. (3½ to 13 sq. in.) was then carefully removed taking care not to injure the subjacent pia and avoiding as far as possible all hemorrhage.

The flap was then replaced and the scalp sutured.

Causes of Failure After Trephining for Traumatic Epilepsy

(a) Undetected bone fragments.
(b) Extensive thickening of the bone around the site of the injury.

(c) The meninges are too thickened and excessively adherent to the cortex to permit their safe detachment.
(d) Permanent changes in the brain-tissue by reason of the long period that has elapsed from the time of injury.
(e) Systemic conditions.
(f) Trephining without definite justification.
(g) Postoperative complications (meningitis, cerebral abscess, etc.).

DIAGNOSTIC PUNCTURE OF THE BRAIN VENTRICLES AND CISTERNAE

VENTRICULAR PUNCTURE

Usually, no anesthesia is required for ventricular puncture, exceptions to the rule being highly neurotic individuals and patients in delirium.

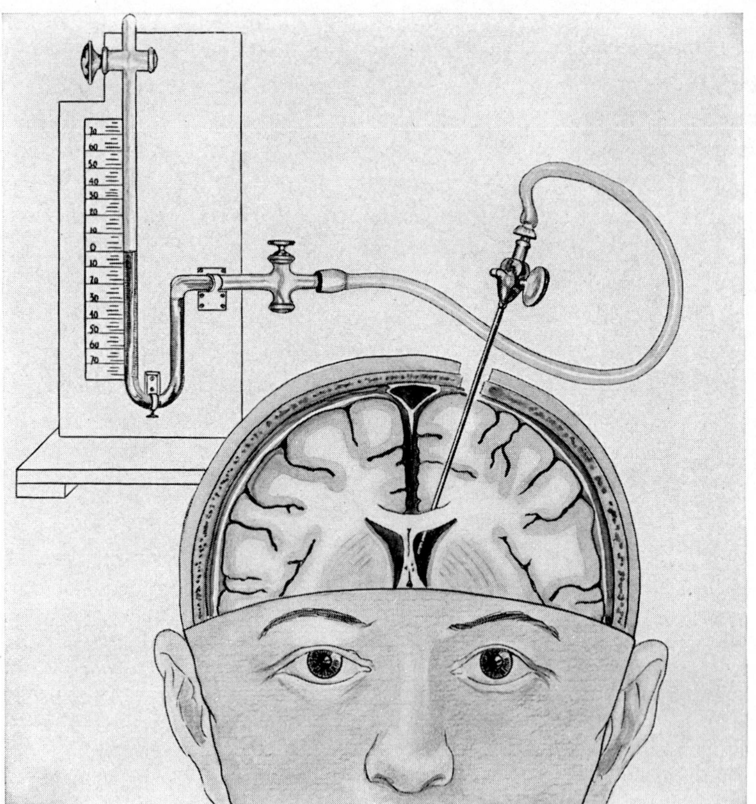

FIG. 181. Ventricular puncture; measuring intraventricular pressure.

Step 1. Place the patient on the operating table in such a manner that the head is elevated; the surgeon stands behind.

Step 2. Prepare the skull as for an operation on the brain in general (see above, except that no iodine should be used). Local infiltration anesthesia is of distinct advantage at the point of puncture.

Step 3. Make a small incision down to the bone which is exposed. Perforate the bone with an electrically driven burr which is placed at an acute angle with the surface of the skull. The work is done more rapidly, with less discomfort to the patient and is not so clumsy as when the hand-driven burr is used.

Step 4. When the dura is reached, the needle with its sheath is introduced at an acute angle. Sometimes difficulties are encountered in finding the opening made by the burr on account of the displacement of the scalp structures. All spiculae of bone and bone-dust resulting from perforating the skull must be meticulously cleared away so that the needle does not, perchance, carry bits of these into the brain substance. The needle should be blunt-pointed. The needle should not be too thin and be of a caliber to permit thick pus to escape should such be encountered. Another advantage of larger size needles

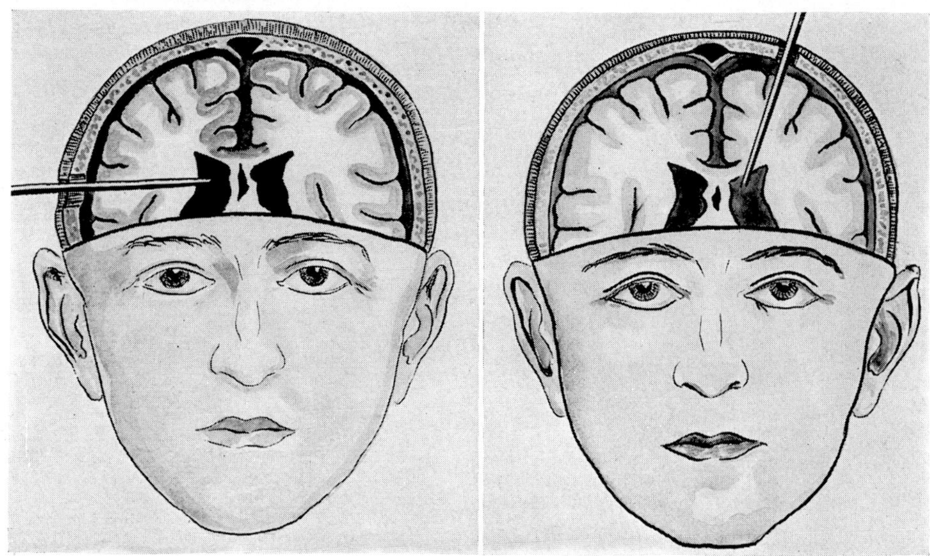

FIG. 182 FIG. 183

FIG. 182. Method of performing ventricular puncture by the lateral route.
FIG. 183. Method of performing ventricular puncture by the superior route.

is that they are not so likely to injure cerebral vessels, in transit, as are finer needles.

Step 5. After the ventricle has been entered ascertain the cerebral pressure with a manometer which is attached to the needle left in situ (Figs. 181-182-183). In order to obtain microscopic particles of tumor from the brain substance, the needle is introduced in the suspected tumor-bearing area and these are removed by suction into an aspirating syringe. These microscopic particles have been used by the German school for diagnostic purposes.

In this country, the majority of neurosurgeons have abandoned this method, preferring in cases where diagnosis of tumor is sought, not to resort to blind puncture but to explore the involved area by exposing the suspected region and investigate it at close range and with less hazard than that incident to brain puncture. To explore a certain area of the brain (ventricles, certain region of the hemispheres) a thorough understanding of craniocerebral topography is essential (see pp. 124-125, Figs. 110-111).

Suction must be carefully avoided in ventricular puncture. The pressure in the ventricle will do all the work that is needed. Suction produces negative pressure in the ventricles and leads to undesirable results.

Step 6. When through, withdraw the needle. Close the puncture wound with collodion. Dress.

Krause also punctured the fourth ventricle. In the two cases in which this was done, the cerebellar hemispheres were exposed, together with the occipital sinus, after which the exploring needle was introduced at a point where the dura marks the junction of the medulla oblongata and the cerebellum. The needle was introduced sagitally and directed forward and upwards at an angle of 45 degrees in relation to the horizontal. The progress of the needle was slow until cerebrospinal fluid issued. As soon as that obtains, one must, of course, stop at once to avoid injury to the important nerves at the floor of the fourth ventricle.

VENTRICULOGRAPHY

Dandy[1] has substituted air for the fluid taken from the ventricles by ventricular puncture. He terms the procedure ventriculography, which by means of x-ray enables one to study the outlines of the ventricles. By ventriculography, one may ascertain the degree of compression of particular ventricles by existing neoplasms. In expert hands the method is free from danger.

Ventriculography via the Anterior Horns[2]

The patient is placed on the operating table in the cerebellar position. The head is extended sufficiently for access to the frontal lobe. Local anesthesia is preferable.

Step 1. The head of the operating table is raised to suit the convenience of the surgeon.

Step 2. The scalp incisions are made in the hair-line, being placed about 1½ inches to either side of the mid-line. Trephine openings are made about ½ inch anterior to the coronal suture line after which the ventricle-needles are introduced at a slight angle to the perpendicular plane of the frontal bone. The points of the needles are directed slightly toward the position of the inferior sagittal sinus.

Step 3. After the needles have entered the cavities of the anterior horns the stylets are withdrawn.

Step 4. Measure the ventricular pressure with a manometer. Accurately measure the collection of the fluid obtained. Lower the head of the operating table so that the patient's head is lower than the body, thus completing ventricular drainage.

Step 5. Inject air through one needle until it escapes from the opposite one.

Step 6. Withdraw the needle into which the air has been injected and inject an extra 5 or 10 cc. of air into the remaining canula until slowly withdrawn.

Step 7. Elevate the head of the operating table. Close the wounds. Turn over the patient to the radiologist for further study.

[1] Annals of Surgery, 68:5,.1918.
[2] The Southern Medical Journal, Vol. 28, No. 12, Dec. 1935.

Comment. Fincher stresses that puncturing the anterior horns through the frontal lobe is anatomically and physiologically well grounded. He points out that some upsetting results using the posterior route have been noted.

Dangers of Cerebral Puncture

1. Injury to vessels. With care, these may be readily avoided. Occasionally by reason of anatomical abnormalities or vascular tumors, death may ensue from injuring a vessel. Pfeiffer reports a death from perforating the artery of the corpus callosum, while Küttner perforated the transverse sinus without ill results and at another time he drilled through the canal of the middle meningeal artery without injuring it. On the other hand, Antone reported two fatalities following injury to the transverse sinus.
2. Entering the needle too deeply; only experience and careful work with the use of proper instruments will tend to avoid such casualties.
3. Infection.
4. Passing the exploring needle through the tumor into healthy territory thus causing implantation metastases.

Tillman reported a case of death of a patient in whom the medulla oblongata was punctured during the exploration. This happened in a case of tumor of the acoustic nerve about the size of a hen's egg which displaced the medulla. Four hours of artificial respiration did not save the patient.

Comment. In doing ventricular puncture (a) be prepared to treat complications that may ensue. (b) In increased intracranial pressure, ventricular puncture is preferred by some to lumbar puncture. (c) In post-traumatic cerebral edema, ventricular puncture is often of inestimable value. Dandy points out that in many instances a bone flap may be saved or a decompression avoided which might otherwise be necessary. Punctures of the ventricles are considered of such value in some cases that one, two or more are often made either in the anterior or posterior horns of the lateral ventricles. They are quite harmless if performed by a skilled surgeon but may be dangerous in the hands of an operator who is not thoroughly versed in the topography of the ventricular system. Dandy's aphorism that a ventricular puncture inexpertly performed is much less safe than a lumbar puncture should be given unreserved heed.

Cisternal Puncture

The same precautions are here observed as in lumbar puncture. While the puncture is made, avoid injury to the tumor or cerebellum; edema and hemorrhage may result if precaution is not taken. In tumors in the posterior fossa of the skull, the cisterna magna is obliterated.

In brain tumor, cisternal puncture is contraindicated; lumbar puncture is much safer and should be preferred. Cisternal puncture is less painful and followed by less severe headache than is lumbar puncture, particularly when performed with the patient sitting instead of lying down.

Technic. Insert the needle just above the foramen magnum to the midline of the occipital bone; do not insert the needle too deeply.

HYDROCEPHALUS

According to Dandy, there are three general types of obstruction producing hydrocephalus: (a) congenital malformation; (b) tumors and other space-occupying lesions; (c) inflammatory sequelae.

Congenital malformations are occasioned by atresia of the aqueduct of Sylvius; failure of the foramina of Luschka and Magendie to develop; failure of the subarachnoid space—either the cisternae or the branches which pass to the surface of the cerebral hemispheres—to become patent.

Tumors of any type and in many locations may occlude part or all of the ventricular system or the subarachnoid space.

Inflammatory obstructions are most frequently located in the cisternae and at the foramina of Luschka and Magendie, but the foramina of Monro and aqueduct of Sylvius may be affected. At times the extension of an infective process surrounding an abscess may occlude the cisterna, the aqueduct of Sylvius, the basal foramina, foramen of Monro, or even the ventricle itself.

"Attempts to drain cerebrospinal fluid into other tissues—the scalp, the subdural space, the cisterna magna, the peritoneal and pleural cavities, the extra-peritoneal tissues—are impractical for one or both of two reasons, i.e., the fistulous tract, whether it be a simple channel in the tissue, a tube of transplanted tissue (veins or fascia) or one of the foreign material (rubber tubes or drains), soon closes; and the fluid soon becomes walled off, owing to the reaction of the tissues.

"The German 'Balkenstich,' or puncture of the roof of the third ventricle is a failure because the connective tissue (neuroglia) repair soon closes the opening and even if the opening could have persisted, absorption of the fluid is impossible because it passes into the non-absorbing subdural space; the fluid cannot, by any conceivable chance, reach the subarachnoid space.

"In children and adults where tumors form the overwhelming percentage of obstructions, the hydrocephalus is automatically cured by removal of the tumor.

"The obstructions prevalent in infancy—strictures of the aqueduct of Sylvius, occlusions at the foramina of Luschka and Magendie, and closures of the cisternae—offer entirely different problems in treatment.

"The fluid can be absorbed only in the subarachnoid space and there is only one part of the subarachnoid space which is large enough to make it mechanically possible for fluid to enter from the ventricular system, namely, the cisternae; elsewhere the subarachnoid spaces are too closely applied to the brain. Moreover, there is only one very restricted part of the ventricular system which is in close apposition with the cisternae—the floor of the third ventricle. And finally, the floor of the third ventricle appears to be the only part of the ventricular walls that is sufficiently thin and devoid of neuroglia to offer a chance of a permanent fistula."

Dandy's Operation for Obstructions at the Aqueduct of Sylvius or the Foramina of Luschka and Magendie—Third Ventriculostomy (Floor of Ventricle)

Commenting on the methods of surgical treatment of hydrocephalus in vogue, Dandy says that repeated ventricular punctures which have been practiced since the time of Hippocrates, and lumbar punctures, are useless because the fluid quickly reforms while a permanent, external fistula quickly ends in meningitis and death.

The original approach proposed by Dandy was under the frontal lobe where it became necessary to divide one optic nerve to gain access to the floor of the third ventricle in the region of the cisterna interpeduncularis. The lateral approach has supplanted the frontal, which has greatly simplified the procedure. The optic nerve is no longer sacrificed, no scar is visible, the floor of the third ventricle is reached much more directly, and at the cisterna interpeduncularis, the stalk of the hypophysis can be seen and avoided, and most important of all, Dandy believes that the formation of an external hydrocephalus will be far less probable because a projecting shelf of dura separates the cisterna from the temporal lobe and acts as a barrier to the flow of fluid into the subdural space. (Fig. 184.)

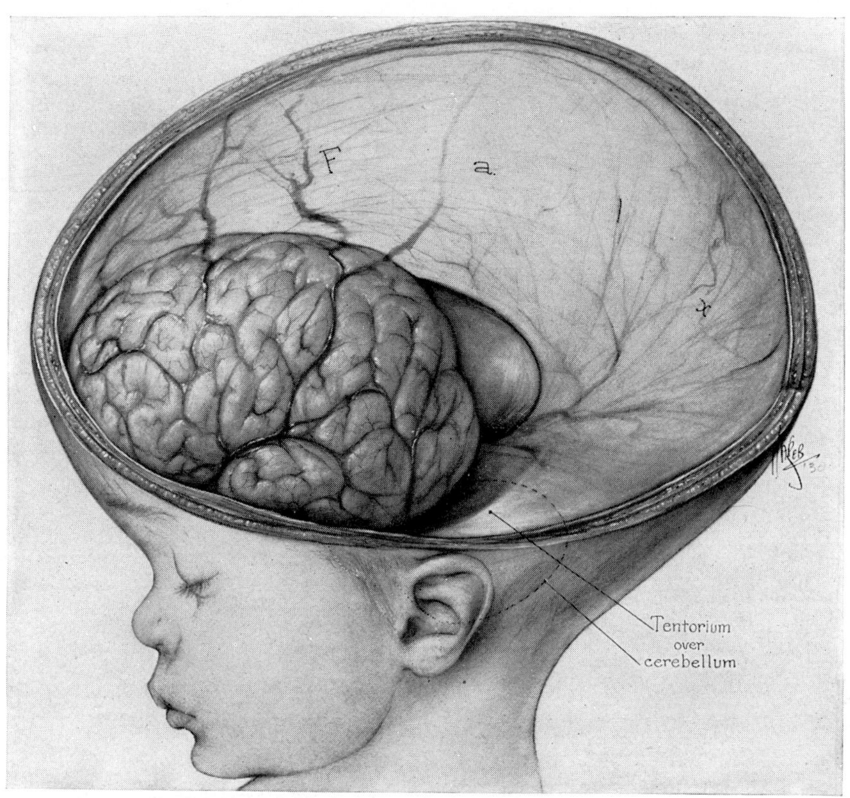

Fig. 184. Drawing of brain showing external hydrocephalus. The fluid is in the subdural space and not in the subarachnoid space. (Dandy in Lewis' Practice of Surgery. W. F. Prior Company, Inc.)

Step 1. A plaster cast is molded to the infant's head. A defect is made in the cast overlying the temporal region of the side to be operated upon. (Fig. 185.)

Step 2. A small curved incision is made in the temporal region (either side), beginning in front of the tragus of the ear and extending upwards and forwards. (Fig. 186.)

Step 3. The temporal muscle is incised.

Step 4. A small area of bone is removed about the base of the skull.

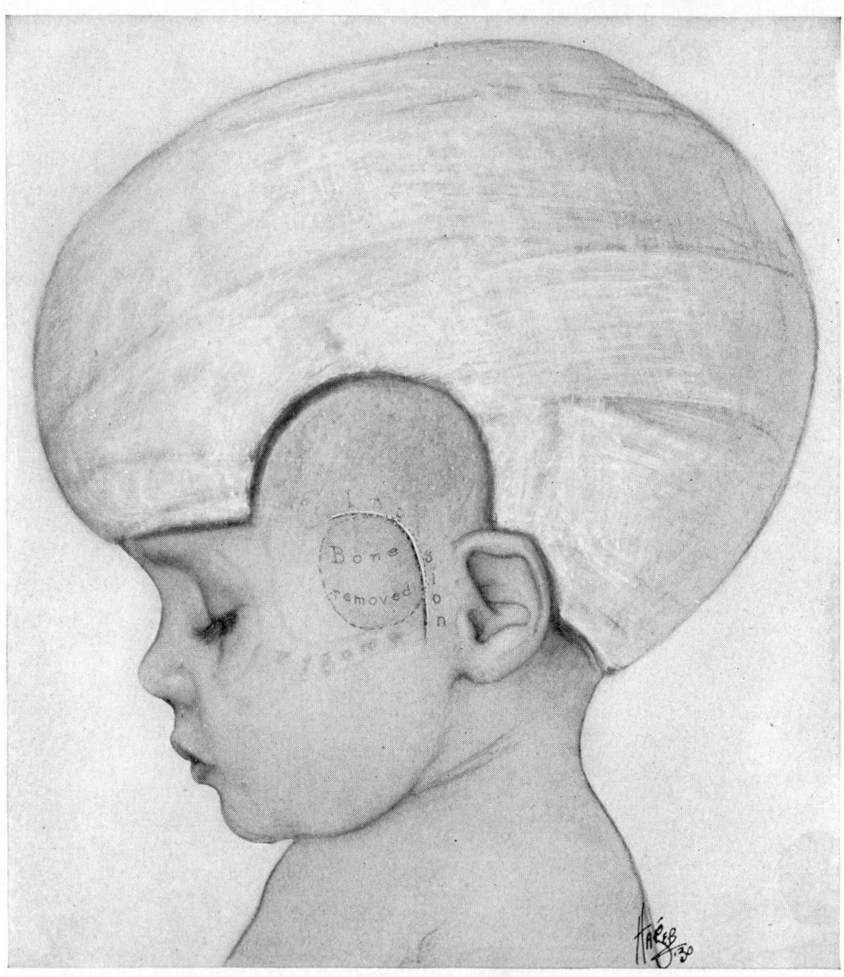

FIG. 185. Plaster cast covering head. This is used to fix the skull so that the head cannot collapse when the ventricular pressure is released. Were it not for the cast, the ununited bones would collapse, and it would not be possible to obtain intracranial room in which to work. Moreover, shrinkage of the head would produce injury to the large intracranial veins and to the brain tissue. (Dandy in Lewis' Practice of Surgery. W. F. Prior Company, Inc.)

Step 5. The flap of dura is reflected toward the base.

Step 6. The head is then lowered about 50°.

Step 7. The descending horn of the lateral ventricle is tapped and 60 to 80 cc. of fluid evacuated. A short flanged ventricular needle is left in place during the operation.

Step 8. The temporal lobe is depressed with a spatula until the lateral wall of the cisterna interpeduncularis comes into view.

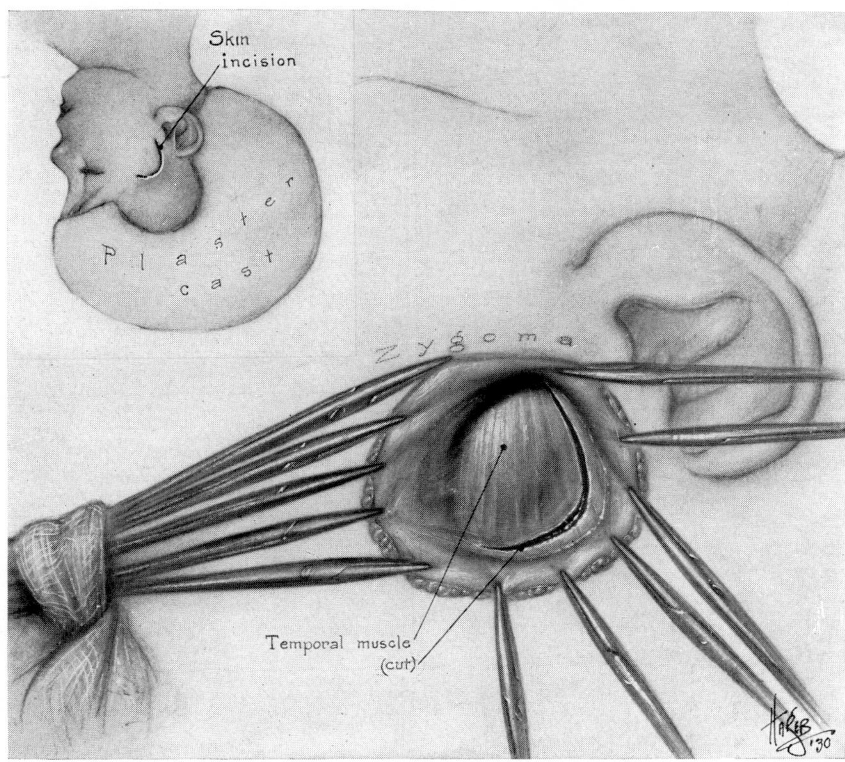

FIG. 186. Operative approach for third ventriculostomy in the treatment of hydrocephalus with ventricular obstruction. (Dandy in Lewis' Practice of Surgery. W. F. Prior Company, Inc.)

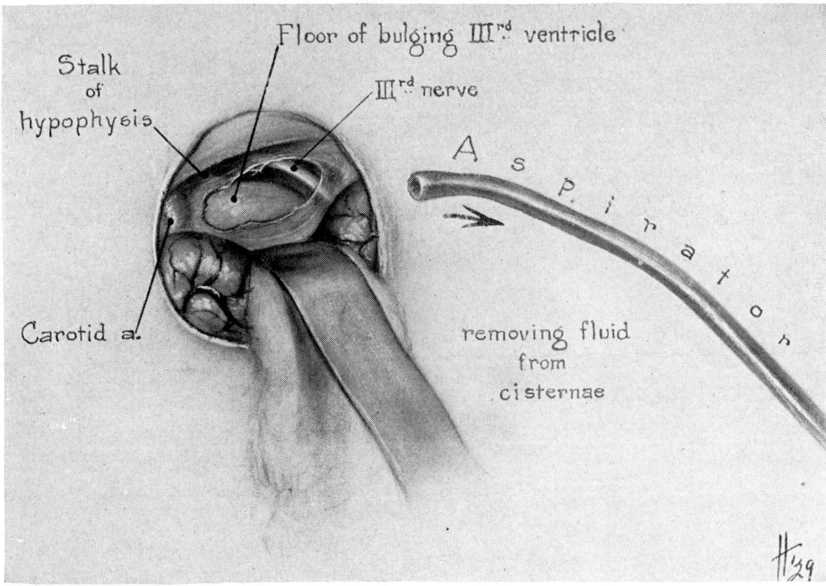

FIG. 187. Bulging third ventricle between the carotid artery and oculomotor nerve exposed through a window in cisterna interpeduncularis. (Dandy in Lewis' Practice of Surgery. W. F. Prior Company, Inc.)

Step 9. The cisternal wall is opened behind the oculomotor nerve, or between the carotid artery and the oculomotor nerve. Both of these structures stand out in the cisternal wall and must be carefully guarded against injury from undue traction (Fig. 187).

Step 10. After the fluid within the cisternae escapes, the bulging floor of the third ventricle is opened as widely as desired (Fig. 188). The opening is preferably made just posterior to the hypophyseal stalk.

Step 11. The space remaining is filled with salt solution. The dura, muscle, galea and skin are closed in layers with interrupted sutures of silk.

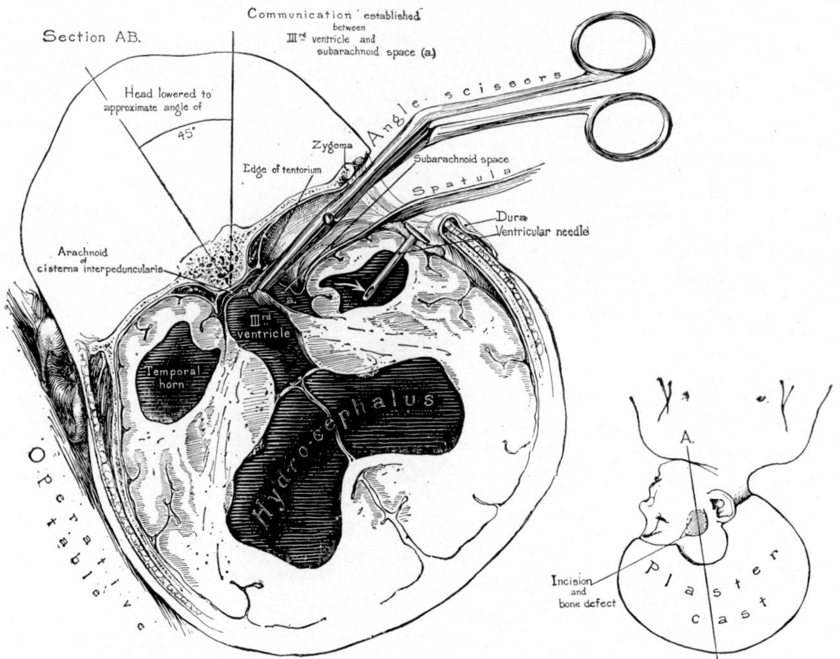

FIG. 188. Method of excising floor of the third ventricle for hydrocephalus due to a ventricular obstruction. (Dandy in Lewis' Practice of Surgery. W. F. Prior Company, Inc.)

Hydrocephalus due to a cisternal block does not appear to offer any prospect of sidetracking the ventricular fluid since the cisternae are obliterated.

Dandy suggested removal of the choroid plexus from both lateral ventricles for this type of hydrocephalus; as yet the survival period has not been long enough to be certain of cures. The reasons upon which the operation is based are:

(a) There is absorption from the spinal subarachnoid space (normally about one-fourth to one-fifth of the amount from the entire subarachnoid space) if we may accept the absorption tests with phenolsulphonphthalein.

(b) The choroid plexus of both lateral ventricles represent perhaps two-thirds or three-fourths of all the fluid-forming organs.

It, therefore, seemed possible that after the removal of the entire choroid plexus from both lateral ventricles, the quantity of fluid formed would be so far reduced that the absorption from the spinal canal would be adequate. In 3 patients from whom the choroid plexus had been removed, a hydrocephalus of this type had changed while under observation to one with ventricular obstruction, doubtless by the slow extension of the old scar in the meninges at the base of the brain. At times the intensity of the color of phthalein in the ventricle is so slight that one suspects a partial ventricular block and subsequently a complete stenosis. Where the ventricular openings are widely patent, the ventricular dye is intense after 20 minutes.[1]

[1] W. E. Dandy. Excision of the choroid plexuses, Ann. Surg., 68:560, 1918.

CHAPTER 9

SURGERY OF THE EARS AND ADJACENT STRUCTURES

OPERATIONS ON THE EXTERNAL EAR

HEMATOMA AURIS

This is usually caused by trauma to the auricle; a dark swelling occurs on the anterior surface of the auricle often associated with severe pain. Treatment consists of aspirating the blood under strict asepsis and applying firm pressure. In extensive cases, an incision must be made and the clot removed with a curet and pressure applied.

CAULIFLOWER EAR

If a hematoma auris is untreated, scar tissue is formed, the contracture of which gives rise to the cauliflower ear.

Don H. Palmer reported the following operation as being satisfactory.

Step 1. Sterilize the outer ear and contiguous region with any good antiseptic except iodine. Introduce cotton in the outer auditory canal.

Step 2. Incise the swelling on the ear at its most projecting portion and remove with a curet or fine gouge all newly formed cartilage or bone as well as blood clots. Continue the cureting until the surface is smooth.

Step 3. Bring the edges of the wound together leaving a small aperture which will allow the insertion of a Eustachian catheter attached to a Pynchon pump which serves to extract the blood which has collected and assists in the approximation of the skin, cartilage and perichondrium.

Step 4. After drying the skin, plug the auditory canal with a fresh dry piece of non-absorbent cotton. Sterile vaseline is applied over the ear and surrounding regions.

Place a cardboard mold around the ear, then

Step 5. Encase the entire ear in plaster of Paris through which the Eustachian catheter is permitted to emerge; this is attached to the pump. The catheter is manipulated as the plaster solidifies so that it may be removed easily when the plaster is completely hardened and the space it occupied is used as a drain. The plaster is held in place with gauze and removed in pieces after ten days.

PROMINENT EARS

Step 1. Remove the skin and fascia between the points 1, 2, 3 and 4 as outlined in the illustration. (Fig. 189.) A semi-ellipse will result on the skull-surface and one on the back of the ear. The skin removed from the auricular surface must be greater than that taken away from the mastoid region.

Step 2. Unite the cutaneous margins with interrupted silk sutures.

Kolle advises the removal of an ellipse of cartilage. This is usually necessary, because if some auricular cartilage is not taken away the resiliency of the cartilage will probably render the operation inefficient and recurrence will result.

Goldstein's operation consists of excising an elliptical portion of the cartilage of a size depending upon the amount of projection present and suturing the margin of the cartilage to the periosteum at that point.

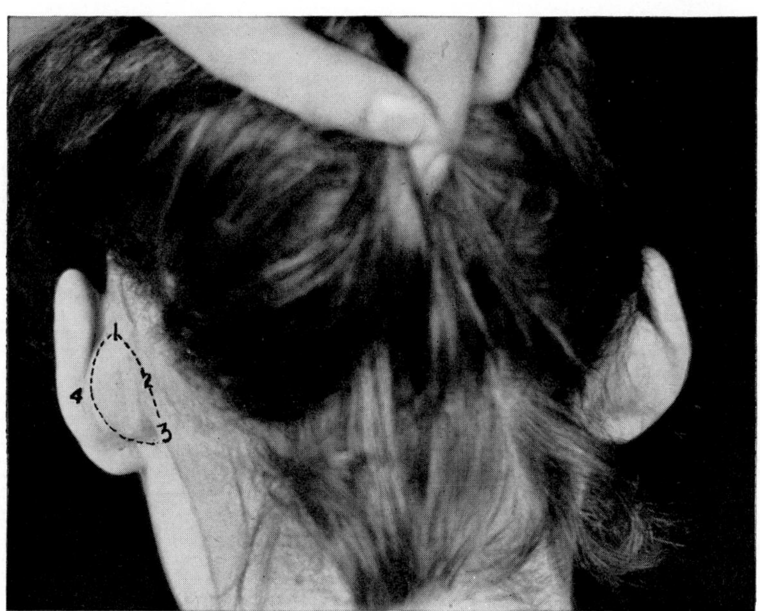

FIG. 189. Protruding ears.

MACROTIA (EXCESSIVELY LARGE EARS)

PARKHILL'S OPERATION

Step 1. Make an incision embracing all the structures of the auricle corresponding to the line and curve of the antihelix.

Step 2. Beginning at each extremity of this incision, make a curvilinear incision towards the outer margins. (Fig. 190.)

Step 3. Excise a small, tongue-shaped flap, extending towards the external border of the ear from the incision last described. This will shorten the long diameter of the ear while the crescentic incision will reduce the width of the incision.

Step 4. Suture the defect.

REMOVAL OF FOREIGN BODIES FROM THE AUDITORY CANAL

The method used for removing a foreign body from the auditory canal is, of course, determined by the size, shape and degree of impaction of the object.

Small objects which are not impacted may be removed by simply irrigating the ear. An article like a button may be removed by hooking a tenaculum in its eye; objects which can be crushed (peas or beans) may be extracted by an angular tenaculum inserted in the compressed substance and withdrawn. Insects should be removed immediately to avoid their injuring the tympanum. Irrigation is often sufficient for their removal; however, they may be killed by pouring melted vaseline in the ear followed by a piece of cotton soaked in chloroform.

Hard, round objects which almost completely fill the canal furnish the greatest difficulties. Care should be taken that they are not pushed in further during manipulations.

Step 1. Illuminate the auditory canal with a strong headlight.

Step 2. Insert delicate forceps; grasp the foreign object and withdraw it.

If this does not seem feasible, an instrument resembling a blunt, curved crochet-needle is inserted in the canal beyond the object while hugging the wall

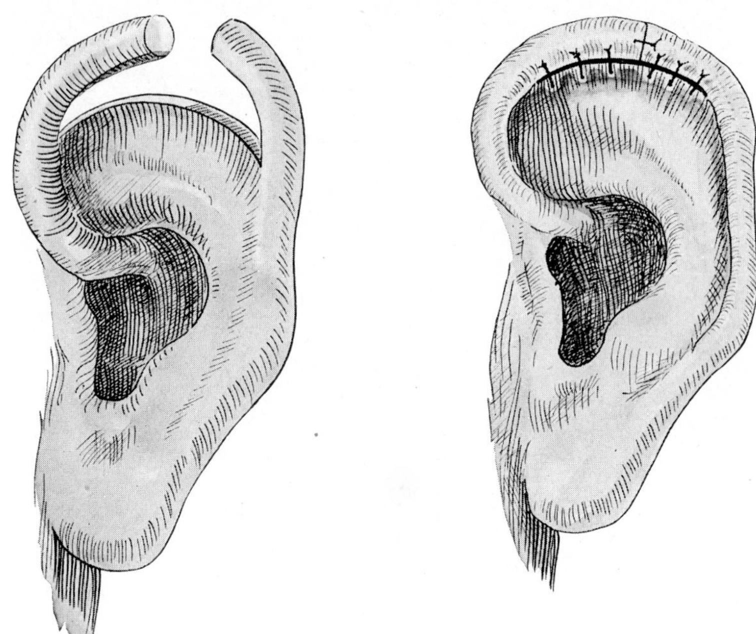

FIG. 190. Parkhill's operation for macrotia.

of the auditory canal, then the hook is applied to the middle of the object and withdrawn.

A straight instrument inserted in the same manner sometimes suffices.

FURUNCLE OF THE AUDITORY CANAL

Furuncles are usually found on the cartilaginous canal walls or on the inside of the tragus. If abortive measures are unsuccessful the furuncle should be opened, followed by sterilization with tincture of iodine which is washed off with alcohol. For analgesic purposes, pure carbolic acid is applied to the point of the furuncle or a mixture of cocaine, carbolic acid, menthol and alcohol. Nitrous oxide is of value in certain cases.

Introduce a fenestrated ear speculum opposite the location of the furuncle. With a proper scalpel thoroughly incise the furuncle. Curet its bed. Swab it with carbolic acid followed by alcohol. Pack with gauze and dress.

REMOVAL OF POLYPI FROM THE AUDITORY CANAL

Polypi are usually found in the tympanic cavity, on the eardrum and the walls of the auditory canal and are always associated with subacute suppurative or chronic otorrhea.

Step 1. Irrigate the ear.

Step 2. Insert a speculum and adjust the snare over the pedicle of the polypus.

Step 3. Draw down the wire steadily and carefully so that the pedicle is detached without any rough manipulations causing damage to the middle ear.

Step 4. Irrigate the canal from which the polypi have been removed and insert a gauze dressing, following which the chronic otitis media must be treated.

Comment. Polypi are often attached to important structures of the middle and internal ear. Even with the greatest care, serious accidents may occur in their removal such as facial paralysis and labyrinthitis. A safer method of removing them is frequent cauterization with strong solutions of silver nitrate.

REMOVAL OF EXOSTOSES OF THE AUDITORY CANAL

The purpose of this operation is to restore the lumen of the auditory canal. Unless exostoses give rise to symptoms (they usually do not) they are best left alone as their removal is often beset with numerous operative difficulties. Smaller growths may be removed through the canal while larger ones may require a post-aural incision. The smaller exostoses made up of compact bone are most satisfactorily removed with a long, slender bone-gouge.

Step 1. If the canal is considered of sufficient size to perform this operation satisfactorily, irrigate the ear with an antiseptic fluid.

Step 2. Insert a speculum into the auditory canal.

Step 3. With a tenotome, or a curved bistoury, make an incision over the tumor in such a way that a small flap is fashioned and placed against the side of the canal.

Step 4. Insert a fine chisel into the canal either while the speculum is in place or after it is withdrawn, until it touches the base of the exostosis. While keeping in mind the danger of injuring the tympanum and other delicate structures close by, the chisel is given a few light taps which are generally sufficient to detach the tumor from the canal wall; if not, the chisel is withdrawn and reinserted to excise a small V-shaped portion of bone, thus forming an acute angle with the first until the base of the bone tumor is detached. Remove the fragments of bone with a forceps.

Step 5. Replace the flap. Pack the canal with gauze.

OPERATIONS FOR INFECTIONS OF THE MIDDLE EAR AND INTRACRANIAL COMPLICATIONS

MYRINGOTOMY

Anatomic Considerations. The tympanic membrane (Figs. 191 and 192) is a delicate, partly transparent membrane which divides the external auditory canal from the middle ear, running downward and upward obliquely with the lower anterior canal walls. In pathologic conditions the marks of identification on the membrane are hidden but they must be kept in mind and not touched. It should also be kept in mind that the drum runs obliquely to the long axis of the canal and that the upper

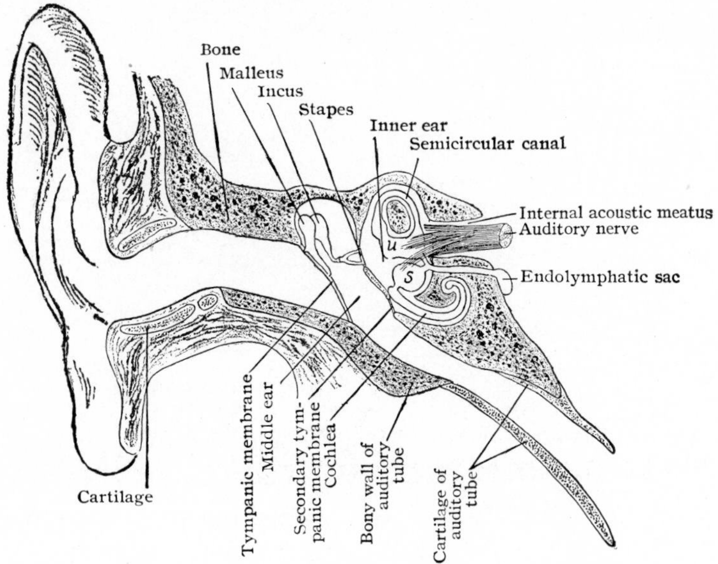

FIG. 191. Diagram showing relations of three subdivisions of ear. (Piersol—modified from Schwalbe.)

portion of the membrane is closer to the surgeon than the lower. The drum membrane is about 2 mm. external to the inner wall of the middle ear and at the back

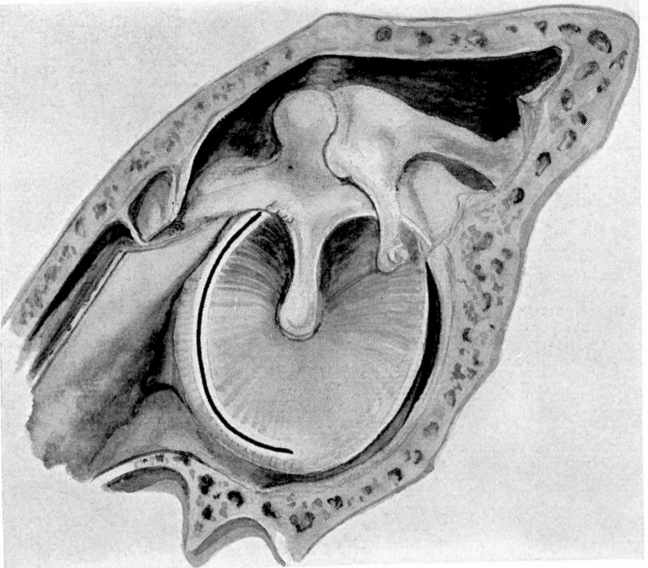

FIG. 193. Drum membrane showing the relation of the landmarks to the usual incision.

portion is found the foramen ovale and stapes above and the foramen rotundum below, which are usually protected by the wall of the posterior canal. The chorda tympani nerve runs through the upper part of the middle ear. Prussak's space is almost completely separated from the atrium so if it is found necessary to drain this space the incision should be extended into the membrana flaccida and over the back fold. Sometimes the jugular bulb is exposed on the floor of the middle ear and on rare occasions in its canal; a fibrous membrane separates the facial nerve from the posterior and inner part of the middle ear. These anomalies occur infrequently so do not warrant any consideration. The lower parts of the drum membrane are best for incision. (Fig. 193.)

Paracentesis tympani is indicated:

1. In acute otitis media, when the membrana tympani is red and bulging.
2. In acute otitis media, when the drum is red and the patient suffers severe pain.
3. In acute otitis media where the membrane is red and when mastoid symptoms are present.
4. In subacute catarrhal otitis media, when fluid (mucus) persists in the middle ear.
5. In cases of otitis media, where resolution is delayed by obstructed drainage.

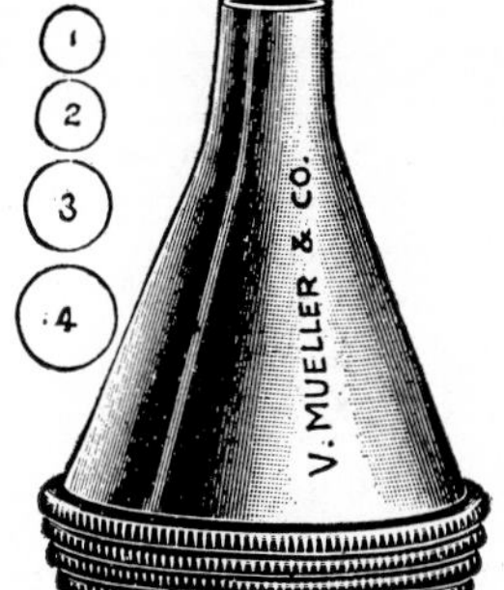

FIG. 192. Boucheron's ear speculum.

Operate under gas-oxygen anesthesia since this is a very painful procedure.

Introduce a large ear speculum (Fig. 192) and obtain a brilliant illumination of the tympanic membrane.

Step 1. Make a long curvilinear incision beginning below at the most dependent part of the ear drum and hugging the posterior border extending upward to the posterior fold. An inexperienced man should make the incision at the point of greatest bulging, from the umbo downward to the floor of the canal. Such an incision will serve for all intents and purposes. (Fig. 193.)

Step 2. Pass the knife through the entire thickness of the drum but not so deep as to injure the mucous membrane of the inner wall.

Comment. The dangers of myringotomy are: dislocation of the stapes; perforation of the foramen ovale owing to inexperience or when the drum is incised from above downward instead of from below upward, and the knife is carried too far inward at the start engaging the stapes and tearing it out of the oval window.

While these phases of surgical intervention require special training, on occasion, the general surgeon is forced to act in an emergency; keeping such contingencies in mind, the author feels the general surgeon should be acquainted with the principles underlying the problems under consideration.

MASTOIDITIS

Operation for Acute Mastoiditis

Opening out from the middle ear is a series of air cells which occupy the mastoid process. This mastoid process frequently becomes the seat of suppurative processes associated with middle ear disease. (Fig. 194 A and B.)

Step 1. Shave the scalp on the affected side for about one and one-half inches about the auricle. Prepare the skin with iodine and alcohol.

Step 2. Make an incision about ¼ inch behind the auricle, parallel to the attachment of the auricle to the skin. This extends from the superior at-

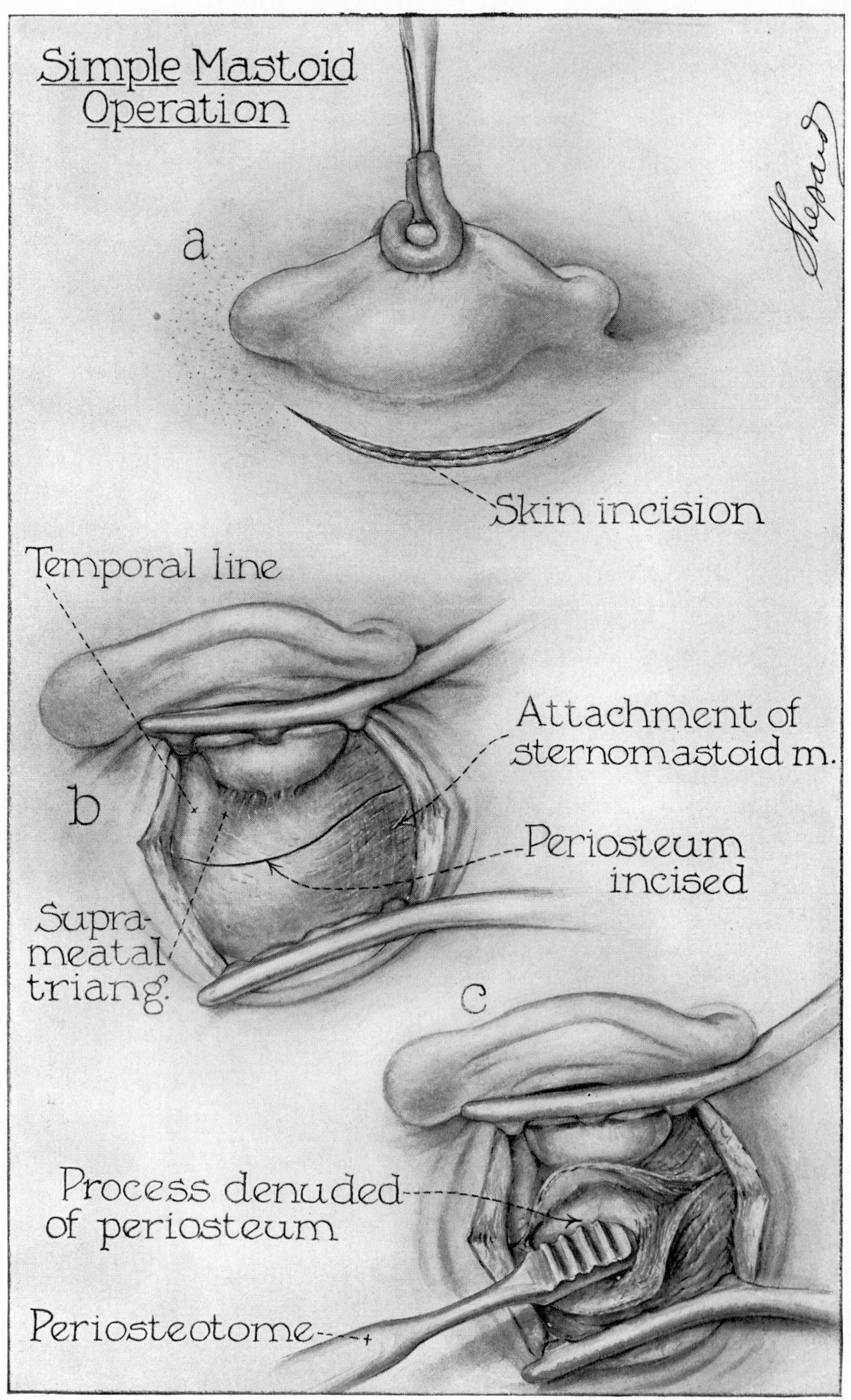

Fig. 194A. Operation for acute mastoiditis. Consult text for steps of operation.

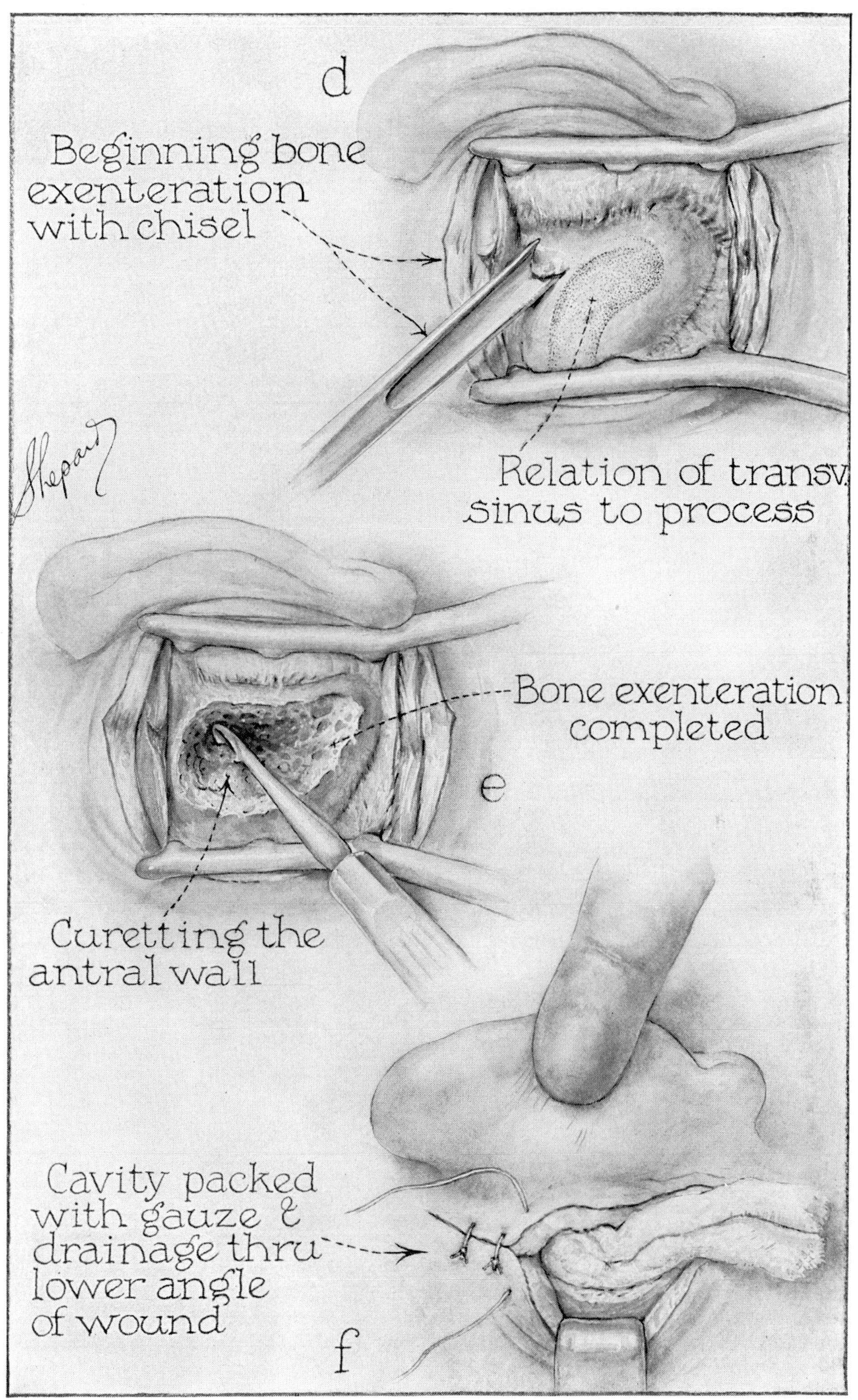

FIG. 194B. Operation for acute mastoiditis. Consult text for steps of operation.

tachment of the auricle to the tip of the mastoid process and is carried through the periosteum to the bone.

Step 3. The periosteum is loosened from the bone with a periosteal elevator, both forward and backward. Care must be taken not to strip the periosteum from the posterior canal wall. Superficial bleeding is controlled with hemostats and ligatures. A self-retaining mastoid retractor is inserted.

Step 4. A search is made for any fistulae caused by the escape of pus through the cortex. If this is found, the mastoid is entered through the fistula. If not, the cortex is removed just posterior to the posterior canal wall from the suprameatal spine of Henle to the mastoid tip. This can be done by chisel and mallet or with an electric burr. The air cells of the mastoid are found beneath the cortex; these are usually infected and contain pus. The necrotic cells are curetted and the overlying cortex gradually taken away in such a manner that one is not working in a depth. One must not go beneath the posterior canal wall anteriorly, as there is a grave danger of injury to the facial nerve. Posteriorly, it is necessary to watch for the hard smooth bone which forms the sinus plate, and superiorly the mastoid cavity is bounded by the hard plate of bone, the tegmen tympani, above which lie the dura and the brain.

Step 5. The operation is not complete until the mastoid antrum leading to the middle ear, is found. This is located by going anteriorly and inward at the superior-anterior portion of the mastoid cavity. When the antrum is located, the entrance is enlarged, care being taken not to enter the middle ear, as there is danger of injuring the ossicles and destroying the hearing.

Step 6. The remaining cells are cleaned out with a curet in such a way that the whole mastoid is converted into one large smooth cavity. This includes the zygomatic cells, the posterior-superior angle cells and the retro sinus cells, if any of these are present.

Step 7. The cavity is carefully cleaned of any bone chips. Iodoform packing is loosely inserted. The end of the packing is brought out to the lower portion of the wound, or a rubber drain is put in the lower part. The upper two-thirds of the wound is closed with silk or dermal suture, the drain emerging from the lowermost portion. Vaseline gauze dressing is placed over the wound and auricle, dry gauze over this and a mastoid bandage applied.

Radical Mastoid Operation

Before proceeding to a radical mastoid operation, rule out suppurative labyrinthitis by appropriate tests. If this precaution is neglected, one is courting danger of meningitis should the labyrinth be involved in the suppurative process.

Anatomic Considerations. (Figs. 195 A and B.) The surgeon should have a very clear picture in his mind concerning the surgical relationship existing between the facial nerve and the temporal bone. The facial nerve passes outward from the internal auditory canal until it reaches the upper, anterior part of the inner wall of the middle ear, just above and posterior to the canal for the tensor tympani muscle. It then passes backward in the inner wall of the middle ear, above the foramen ovale, to the point where it bends beneath the floor of the aditus, descending almost vertically in the posterior canal wall, emerging from the bone at the stylomastoid foramen. The anterior part of the external semicircular canal bears an important relation to the vertical part of its course. The former points outward, over the facial nerve toward the surgeon so that when the posterior canal wall is lowered, the bone can be removed to an imaginary vertical line dropped downward from the convex prominence of the external semicircular canal. The nerve runs through the aqueductus Fallopii, a canal of hard bone which is more delicate and the nerve more likely to be injured in the horizontal part of its course on the inner wall of

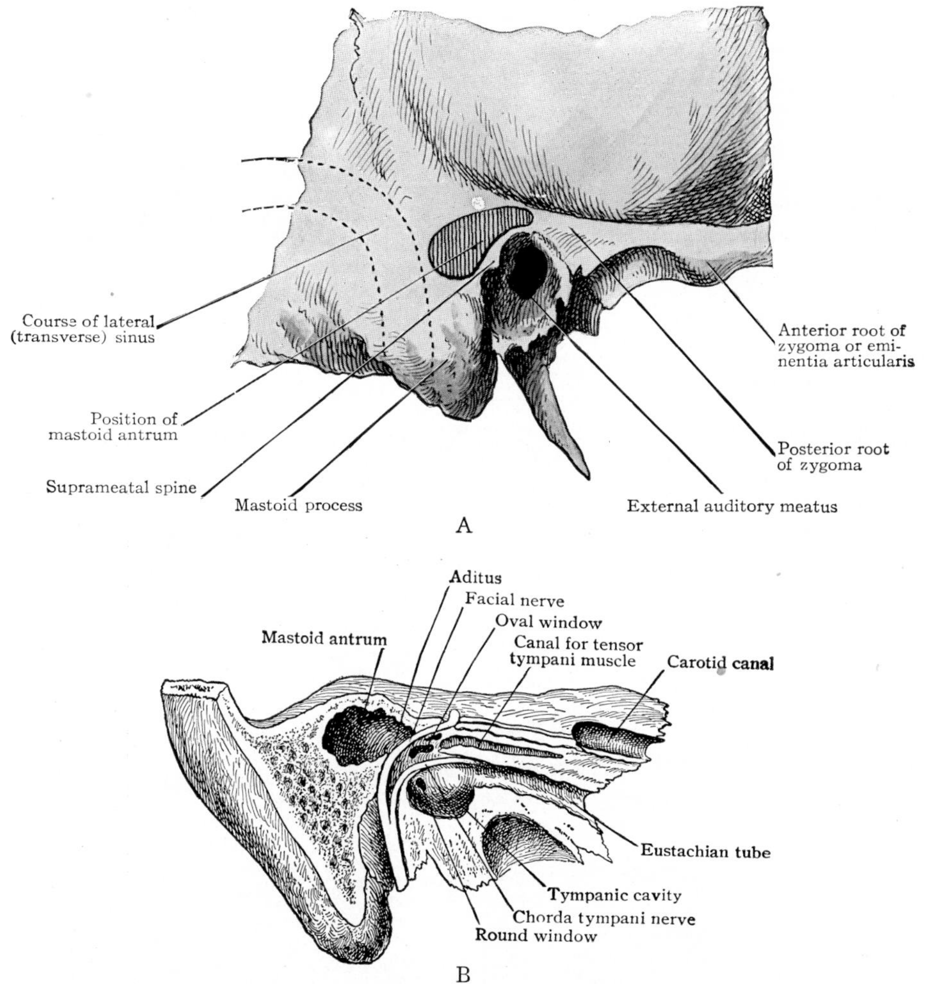

Fig. 195. A. Lateral view of the temporal bone, showing the relations of the lateral or transverse sinus and mastoid antrum, B. right temporal bone showing position of facial nerve and other important structures (Applied Anatomy, Davis).

the middle ear than in its vertical portion in the posterior canal wall. If suppuration has been present, many of the mastoid cells will have been obliterated, the bone will present a dense, ivory-like appearance, and the antrum will be narrowed. In cases of cholesteatoma, the bone beneath the cortex is apt to be soft and the cavities of the ear and antrum made larger. The external semicircular canal should be sought for after opening the antrum. It is covered with white, hard, solid bone and is usually easily discerned. In cases requiring radical operation, the lateral sinus is very apt to be far forward, although its position is extremely variable. The foramina ovale and rotundum lie in the posterior part of the inner wall of the middle ear, anterior to the connecting point of the inner wall and posterior canal wall.

During the radical operation, the foramen ovale, which lies just beneath the turn of the facial nerve, cannot be plainly seen unless the facial ridge has been lowered to its extreme limit. It is usually covered by a mass of granulations that should not be disturbed. The promontory is the bone covering the first and second turns of the cochlea and appears as a rounded prominence on the inner wall of the middle ear anterior to the foramina ovale and rotundum. The Eustachian tube is observed in the hollow space formed by the anterior and inner wall, in the anterior part of the middle ear, and is about 3 or 4 mm. above the floor. The internal carotid artery is found toward the inner side and below the Eustachian tube, separated from it by a thin bony plate which often contains fissures; thus the carotid artery may be injured by careless curettage of the tube. Just above and parallel to the Eustachian tube is the canal for the tensor tympani muscle. The wall of bone between the two canals is often incomplete. The bony wall is extremely thin in the region where the horizontal part of the Fallopian canal is above and behind the canal for the tensor tympani and it is here that care should be taken not to injure the nerve. On the anterior surface of the bony plate forming the anterior osseous canal wall is found the glenoid fossa. This is sometimes entered when the canal is widened, but as a rule no harm results except a slight soreness and stiffness of the jaw. A serious septic arthritis may follow an injury to the synovial cavity.

The technic of a radical mastoid operation consists essentially of the following steps: (Fig. 196).

Step 1. Incision.—This is the same as is used in acute mastoiditis plus elongation of the upper and lower extremity of the incision.

Step 2. Reflect the periosteum. Retract. Drape the margins of the wound. Illuminate thoroughly.

Step 3. Remove the cortex over the outer wall of the attic antrum and posterior wall of the canal for about one-eighth of an inch. In children this step may be omitted.

Step 4. Open the mastoid antrum as described above. In chronic suppurations this step is rendered more difficult because

(a) the osseous structures of the cortex are hardened and thickened,

(b) there is an apparent increase in depth and a

(c) diminution of the size of the antrum.

Work slowly and carefully, beginning at the posterior canal, working inward, forward and somewhat upward. Identify the antrum. Remove its overhanging walls. Orient yourself as to the position of the dural plate and plate of the sinus. In chronic cases there is a tendency for the dura to be low and the sinus situated forward. Remove all suspicious or diseased bone here and in the zygomatic region. Identify the external semicircular canal.

Step 5. Pass a probe from the antrum through the aditus into the middle ear. Remove all the wall of the canal above and extend the probe to the outer portion of the posterior canal (about one-third should be chiselled away). The remaining bridge is now bitten away by a delicate rongeur or by means of a chisel of appropriate size. Avoid injuring the facial nerve.

Step 6. Now lower the facial ridge by means of a chisel or burr. Fine shavings are taken away gradually. At this step an assistant watches the patient's face for twitching which would denote close proximity of the instrument to the facial nerve. External bleeding suddenly appearing may indicate that the artery of the facial nerve, which is here a very small vessel running in

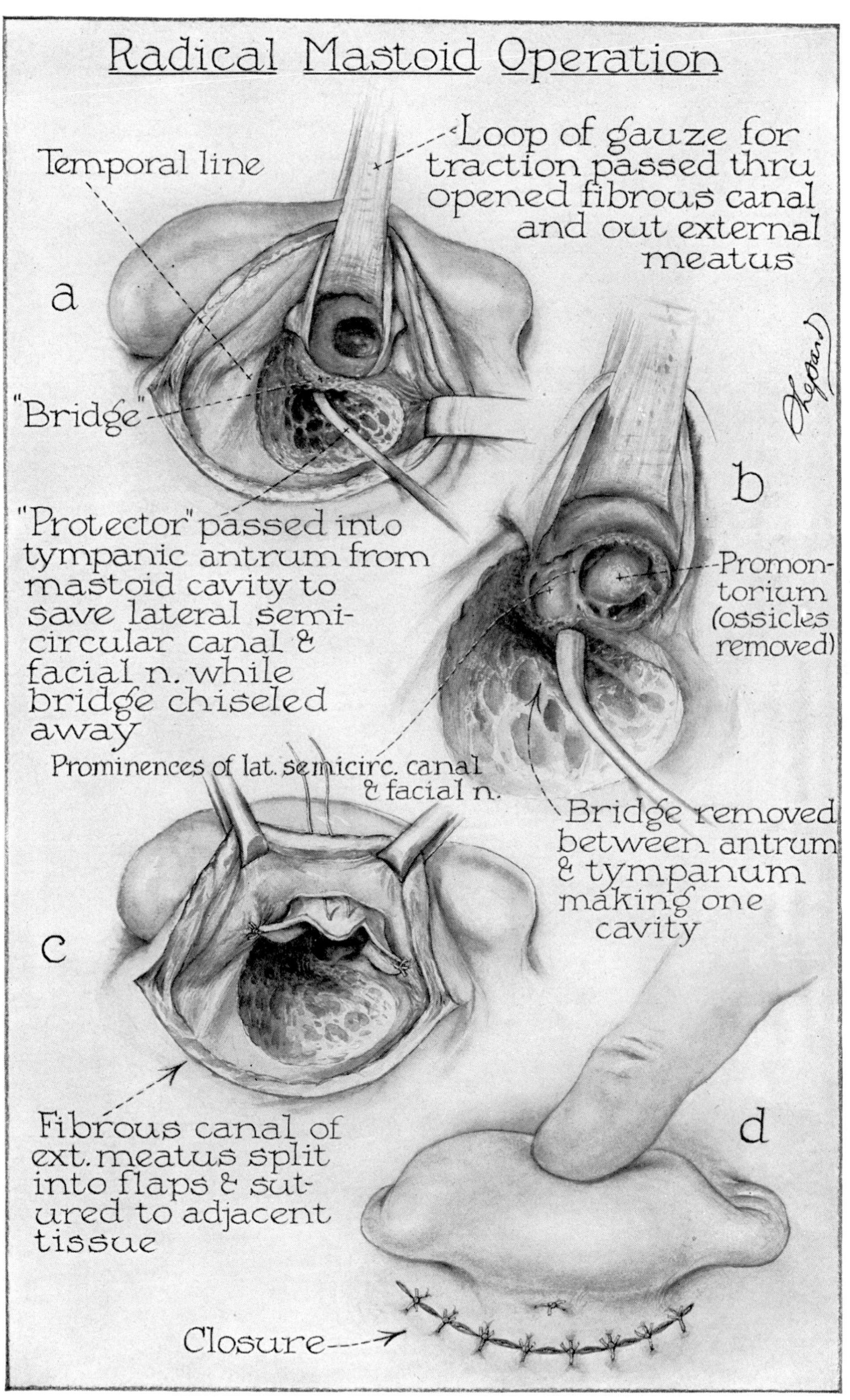

FIG. 196. Radical mastoid operation. Consult text for steps of operation.

the course of the nerve but somewhat external to it, has been divided. Compression easily will stop the bleeding.

Step 7. Remove the outer wall of the attic by means of a sharp bone curet. Remove the malleus and incus but be careful to avoid dislocating the stapes. Dry with appropriate-sized sponges. Oozing is controlled by a pledget of cotton dipped in adrenalin.

Step 8. Obliterate the hypotympanum.—Failure to remove this often results in failure of the operation.

Step 9. Gently curet out the mucous membrane of the Eustachian tube as far down as the isthmus. If this precaution is neglected, a permanent communication with the pharynx will result inviting discharge and infections. Remember the close proximity of the carotid artery to the Eustachian tube. The canal for the tensor tympani muscle should also be obliterated.

Flush the large cavity with normal salt solution. Dry. Steer clear of the promontory and foramen ovale. Unnecessary manipulations here are often followed by labyrinthitis.

Step 10. This step consists of creating a plastic flap in order to enlarge the external auditory canal and to line with skin the cavity created by the operation. A number of methods have been devised to accomplish this object.

Hunter F. Todd describes his method as follows:

A. A long, narrow, curved bistoury is passed down the acoustic meatus so that it projects through the detached end of the fibrous portion, its point being directed backward. The auricle is held well forward and the fibrous portion of the meatus cut through posteriorly, from within outward, for a short distance.

B. The edge of the bistoury is then directed in a slanting direction upward and outward, and the incision continued as far as the cartilaginous portion of the meatus, care being taken not to cut into the concha.

C. The bistoury is then withdrawn and reinserted at the point at which it was first made to turn upward. It is now directed downward and outward and, in a similar manner, the incision is made in a slanting direction toward the inferior margin of the cartilaginous meatus. (In carrying out these manipulations care must be taken that the outer portion of the bistoury does not injure the tragus or other portion of the auricle, a mishap which can easily occur.) The fibrous portion of the meatus is thus divided by a Y-shaped incision into three small flaps; namely, a posterior or external V-shaped flap, and a superior and an inferior flap.

D. The outer flap is fixed to the skin behind the auricle by means of a catgut suture. The auricle is then pulled back into its normal position. By inserting the tip of a finger into the meatus, the upper and lower flaps are pressed upward and downward against the roof and floor of the mastoid cavity, and can be kept in position afterwards by suturing the flaps to the subcutaneous tissue or by packing the cavity through the meatus with a strip of ribbon gauze.

Step 11. Pack the cavity with iodoform gauze. The posterior wound is now closed.

Possible Intracranial Complications: (a) Cellulitis of the flaps; (b)

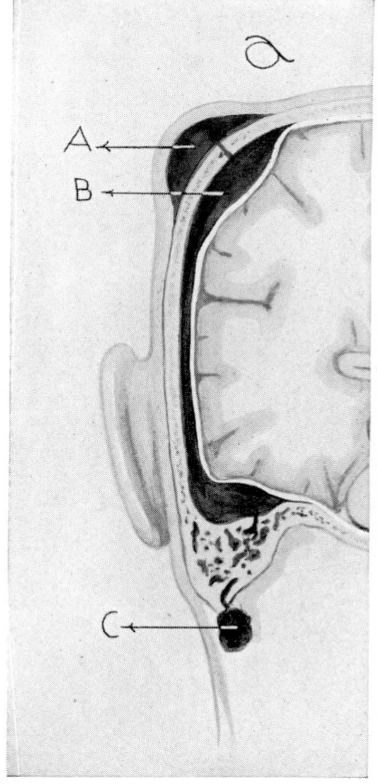

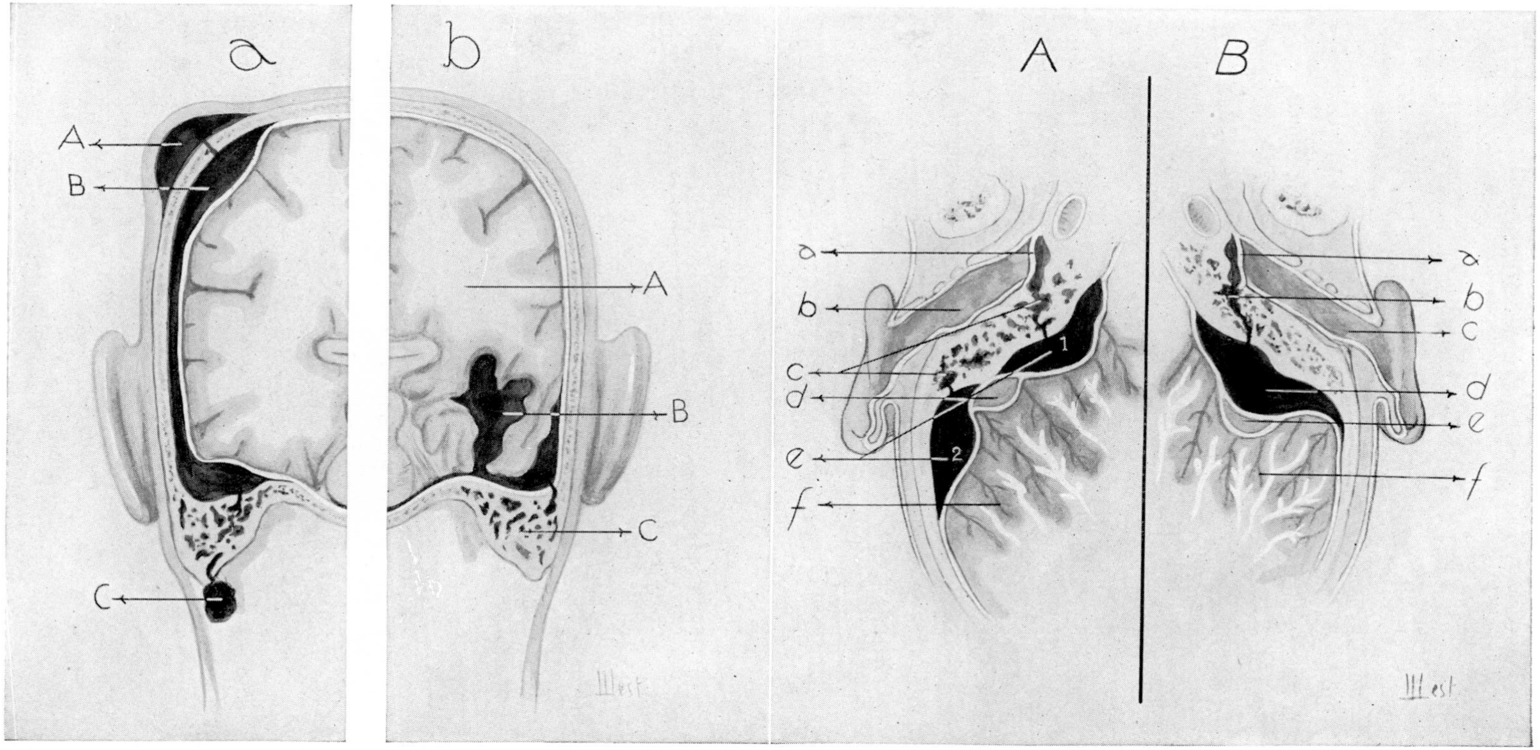

FIG. 197. I. Brain abscess of otitic origin (after Sydney Scott). a: A. Extradural abscess. Coronal section of the head showing abscess originating from mastoid disease and pointing in the parietal region causing subpericranial abscess, B. C. Benzold's abscess. b. Coronal section of the head showing right temporosphenoidal abscess originating from middle ear disease: A. temporosphenoidal lobe, B. abscess cavity, C. mastoid cells.

II. Extradural abscess. Horizontal section of temporal bone through the external auditory meatus and mastoid cells. Subtentorial abscess. A: a. tympanum, b. external auditory meatus, c. mastoid cells, d. sigmoid portion of lateral sinus, e-1. extradural abscess medial to sigmoid sinus, e-2. extradural abscess, f. cerebellum. B: a. tympanum mastoid cells, b. mastoid cells, c. external auditory meatus, d. extradural abscess anterior to sigmoid sinus, e. sigmoid sinus, f. cerebellum.

perichondritis; (c) sinus thrombosis; (d) facial paralysis; (e) brain-abscess; (f) meningitis; (g) acute labyrinthitis; (h) postauricular fistula. Most of these may be avoided by proper technic.

EXTRADURAL ABSCESS

Step 1. Proceed as outlined for simple mastoid operation. Usually a fistula is seen in the middle fossa tegmen, surrounded by granulation tissue. Pus, usually pulsating, may or may not be seen escaping from the fistula.

Step 2. Enlarge the fistula and remove the tegmen very carefully with rongeurs or curet. Extreme care must be taken in this procedure as any injury to the dura may lead to a fatal meningitis. (Fig. 197, I and II.)

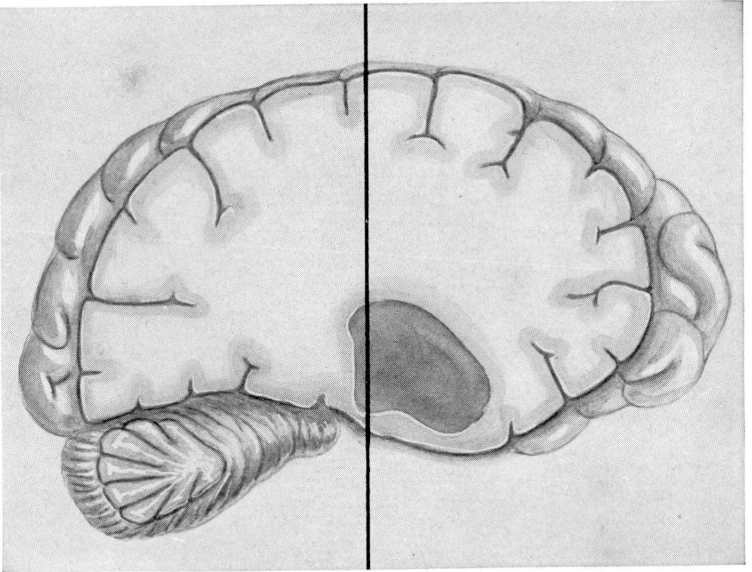

Fig. 198. Temporosphenoidal abscess of otitic origin, vertical section, anteroposterior. Vertical line indicates midcoronal plane. (Modified after Sydney Scott.)

Step 3. Pack the mastoid cavity loosely. Do not close the wound.

Step 4. Bandage the same as in simple mastoid.

OPERATION FOR TEMPORO-SPHENOIDAL ABSCESS

Step 1. Perform the radical mastoid operation as outlined.

Step 2. Expose the dura by removing the middle fossa tegmen quite widely in all directions. (Fig. 198.)

Step 3. With a small electrocoagulation tip, make a circle about ½ inch in diameter in the dura; the cavity is packed loosely and bandage applied. The purpose of the electrocoagulation is to seal off the subarachnoid space in the region where the dura is to be entered.

Step 4. Twenty-four hours later, remove the packing and make a small incision in the dura within the circle.

Step 5. Explore the brain with a Cushing needle; a slight resistance will be felt when the capsule of the abscess is penetrated.

From this point of the operation there are two methods of procedure:

(a) A small catheter may be inserted along the side of the needle into the abscess cavity; the catheter may be used for irrigation or aspiration.

(b) The dural opening may be enlarged with a hemostat and a tract made into the abscess cavity. Insert a Mosher wire basket drain. Pack loosely and as the abscess heals, the basket will be extruded.

OPERATIONS FOR SINUS THROMBOSIS

Anatomic Considerations. (Fig. 199.) The course of the lateral sinus may be outlined by a line drawn from the external occipital protuberance to the center of the external auditory canal. That part of the sinus below the bend or knee which

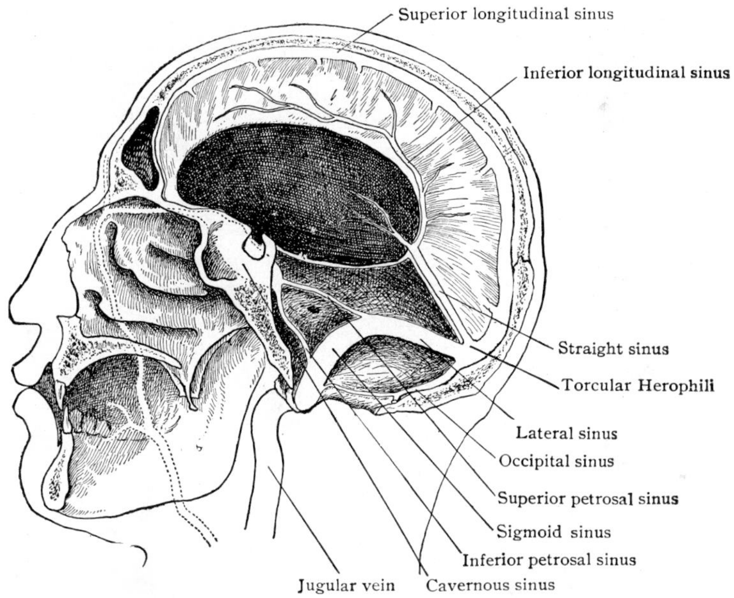

FIG. 199. Cerebral blood sinuses (Applied Anatomy, Davis).

occurs in the posterior part of the mastoid bone, and which extends from the knee to the jugular bulb, is called the sigmoid sinus. This portion of the sinus has no definite surface landmark because it may occupy a variable position on the inner surface of the mastoid bone. Beneath the middle ear the sigmoid sinus makes a sharp turn upward, and expands to form the jugular bulb. The knee of the sinus is joined by a small vein, the superior petrosal sinus. The sigmoid and lateral sinus is simply a large vein which runs on the inner surface of the mastoid process, and is covered by a thin process of dura mater. It is separated from the mastoid cells by a plate of bone of ivory-like whiteness and consistency, the so-called sinus-plate.

No operation is performed on sinuses afflicted by thrombosis without a preliminary exenteration of the mastoid process.

Step 1. This consists of a prolongation of the posterior incision toward the external occipital protuberance. Cut down to the bone; elevate the periosteum; check bleeding.

Step 2. Delineate the sinus plate by removal of the bony structure around its boundary. Use a sharp curet. Do not injure the sinus during this manipulation lest hemorrhage seriously interfere with the operation.

Step 3. Remove the bone over the posterior part of the sinus plate; if hard, use a chisel; if soft, a sharp curet.

Step 4. Remove the sinus plate with powerful rongeur forceps. A grooved director is inserted between the plate and the sinus to avoid injuring it; this is an important step and must be carried out with care and gentleness. The sinus is thus bared of plate on top and on its sides to the extent desired.

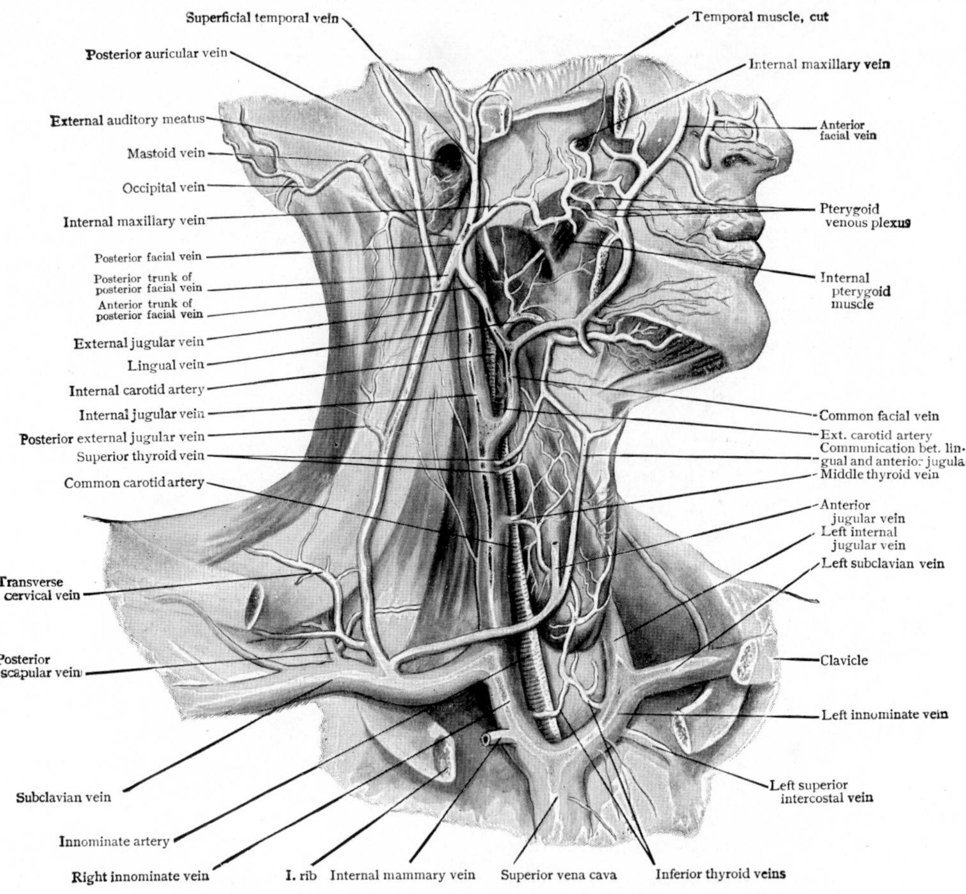

FIG. 200. Dissection showing deep veins of neck and head.

Step 5. An assistant compresses the upper and lower segments of the sinus with iodoform plugs of appropriate size held in forceps, while the surgeon opens it in its long axis with a scalpel to the length desired. When the sinus is opened and

(a) there is no bleeding, there is a clot in its interior. When (b) there is free bleeding, determine its source. Make pressure on the jugular end. If bleeding ceases there is a clot at the torcular end. If bleeding continues slightly, it issues either from the mastoid emissary vein (superior petrosal sinus) or a partially obstructed torcular end. Exert pressure on the torcular end, release the pressure from the jugular end. No hemorrhage indicates a clot in the jugular end of the sinus. Slight bleeding indicates partial clotting. Free bleeding does not as a rule clot, for the blood may issue from the inferior petrosal sinus. If there is a clot at the torcular end, endeavor to dislodge it gently with a dull curet; if unsuccessful open the sinus further until you find the clot and free bleeding takes place.

A firm clot at the jugular end is an indication to stop operative manipulations and to proceed to ligate, or excise the internal jugular vein. If that can be removed and free bleeding takes place some surgeons wait 24 hours; if no septic symptoms are present, the clot is removed with a dull curet and the sinus packed with iodoform gauze.

Step 6. Trim the edges of the open sinus; pack it with iodoform gauze. Pack the mastoid wound as usual. In packing the sinus, do it gently, remember too much pressure may cause injury to the contiguous brain. Leave the packs in situ for 5 days. If on removing the packs bleeding recurs, pack again.

LIGATION AND RESECTION OF THE INTERNAL JUGULAR VEIN

Anatomic Considerations. (Fig. 200.) The internal jugular vein is the continuation of the lateral (transverse) sinus, and begins in the postero-external compartment of the jugular foramen. It descends vertically, at first on the outer side of the internal carotid, and subsequently on the outer side of the common carotid, and ends behind the inner end of the clavicle by joining the subclavian vein to form the innominate vein. In the upper part of its course, the vein rests upon the rectus capitis lateralis and the transverse processes of the upper cervical vertebrae; it is crossed by the spinal-accessory nerve, the posterior belly of the digastric and the stylohyoid muscles, and also by the occipital and posterior auricular arteries. It is overlapped lower down by the anterior border of the sternomastoid, and is crossed opposite the cricoid cartilage by the anterior belly of the omohyoid. The terminal part of the vein, which lies deeply between the sternal and clavicular heads of the sternocleidomastoid, under cover of the infrahyoid muscles, passes in front of the first part of the subclavian artery. During its course, the vein receives the inferior petrosal sinus, the common facial, the lingual, the pharyngeal and the superior and inferior thyroid veins.

Place a sandbag under the patient's shoulders. Turn his head to the opposite direction.

Step 1. Make an incision along the course of the sternocleidomastoid muscle beginning about half an inch from the mastoid process and extending to the clavicle. The scalpel divides the skin, subcutaneous tissue and platysma muscle. (Fig. 201.)

During this manipulation the external jugular vein is encountered; ligate it and divide it.

Step 2. Locate the anterior border of the sternomastoid muscle. Retract it. Separate the delicate layer of the deep cervical fascia. The common carotid sheath embracing the common carotid artery, the internal jugular vein and the pneumogastric nerve will be exposed. The vein is external, the artery internal and the nerve posterior in position. The vein is bluish in color and expands with the respiratory movements.

Step 3. Open the carotid sheath in the region of the omohyoid muscle. In so doing avoid injury to the vein. Open the sheath of the vein by gentle dissection from the omohyoid below to above the entrance of the facial veins. Dissect the vein bluntly from its posterior attachments. Avoid injury to the pneumogastric nerve. Ligate and divide the large venous branches entering the vein (middle and superior thyroid, lingual, facial and occasionally a branch from the external jugular vein).

Step 4. After sufficient exposure of the vein has been obtained, ligate it doubly below and divide it between the ligatures.

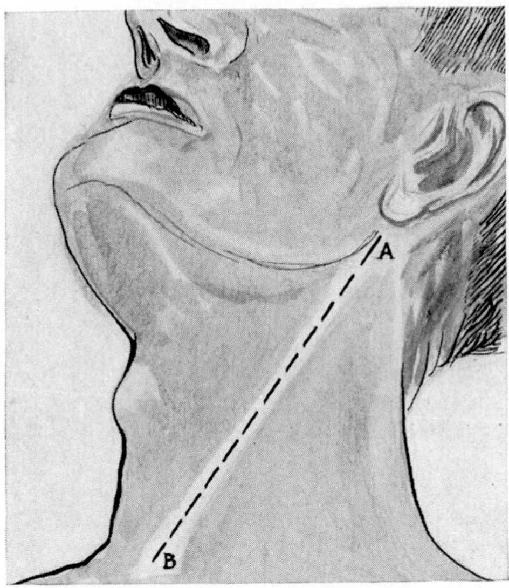

FIG. 201. Incision for ligation and excision of internal jugular vein. Line of incision.

Step 5. Deliver the main trunk of the vein into the wound as high as possible; ligate it doubly with plain catgut above and divide it below the ligature; ligate branches as encountered.

Step 6. Irrigate the cavity with normal salt solution. Insert a cigarette drain to the stump above and another drain into the lower angle of the wound. Suture the platysma and deep fascia with interrupted plain catgut sutures.

Step 7. Close the wound and dress securely.

CHAPTER 10

SURGERY OF THE FACE

INFECTIONS

CARBUNCLE OF THE FACE

The favorite location for this lesion is the upper lip. Death ensues in many cases; the fatality is preceded by the formation of a blood-clot in the cavernous sinus.

One or both angular veins are ligated under local anesthesia as a means of preventing the spread of the infection. (Fig. 202.)

The resistance of the patient is sufficient in some cases to control the spread of the infection.

Caution: If the temperature rises and edema appears and extends from the lip to the inner canthus of the eye accompanied by suffusion of the eyelids, do not hesitate—act.

Half an hour before the operation, administer a hypnotic.

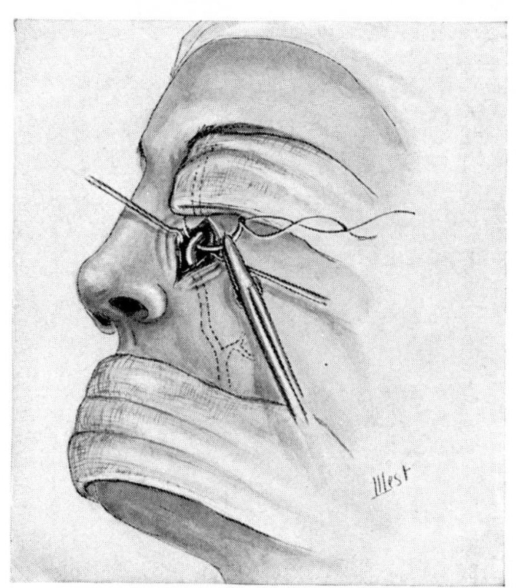

Fig. 202. Ligation of angular vein in infections of the face. (After Hamilton Bailey.)

Step 1. Drop castor oil into the eye and cover the eyelids with damp gauze so that no iodine can reach the conjunctiva.

Step 2. Cover the lip with gauze dampened with perchloride solution. The junction of the nose and cheek forms the external marking for the angular vein.

Step 3. After the area has been analgesized, make an incision about an inch long, beginning a little below the inner canthus of the eye and extending downward slightly obliquely. Gauze saturated with adrenalin will control oozing.

Step 4. Inject more novocaine about the tissues and expose the levator labii superioris alaeque nasi muscle through the wound. Carefully separate the fibers of the muscle in or between which is found the angular vein.

Step 5. Ligate the vein and divide it between ligatures; suture the skin and apply dressing.

X-ray Treatment of Furuncles and Carbuncles

Considerable has been written lately in the current medical journals of x-ray therapy in certain types of inflammatory lesions. Especially good results have been obtained in furuncles and carbuncles. All authors agree that such lesions should be treated early and the dose of x-ray must be small.

Furuncles: In acute furunculosis a dose of 100 to 150 "r" units (in air) using a voltage of 74 to 100 kvp, is administered over the inflammatory area, blocking out the normal surrounding tissues. By such treatment early undeveloped lesions may be completely aborted in 12 to 24 hours. Relief from pain often occurs in a few hours. In chronic furunculosis better results are had with a filtered ray. 125 "r" units, 125 kvp, 5-6 mm. of aluminum may be given once a week for several treatments, if necessary.

Carbuncles do not respond quite so well as furuncles to x-ray therapy. A somewhat heavier dose is suggested, rarely exceeding 150 "r" units. Filtered rays are better because the lesion is more deeply situated. With this form of

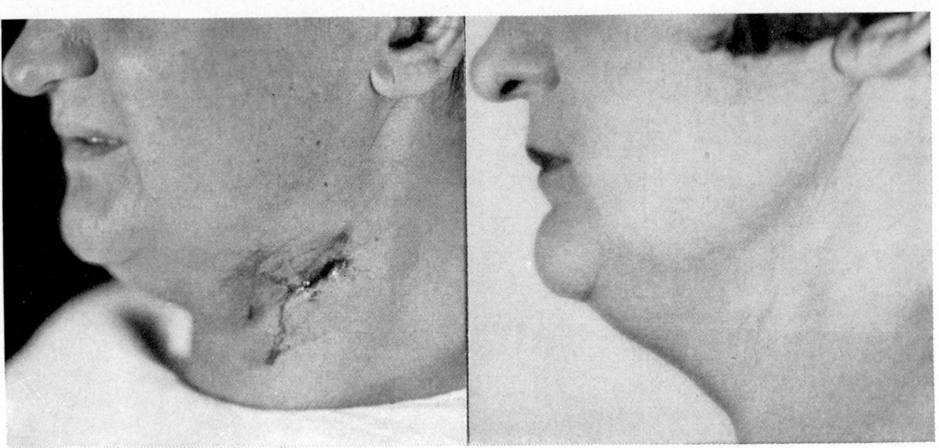

FIG. 203 FIG. 204

FIG. 203. Patient 39 years of age; swelling in neck; diagnosis, abscess in neck, tuberculous glands, possible malignancy. Examination of pus revealed characteristic findings of actinomycosis.

FIG. 204. Same patient after treatment with potassium iodide and radium.

therapy the course is definitely shortened, drainage is increased and pain often relieved.

X-rays have no bactericidal effects. The modus operandi resulting in the changes as a result of irradiation is not definitely known. We do know, however, that leukocytes and lymphocytes are very sensitive to x-rays and as a result of their premature destruction some type of antibody may be liberated, or a metabolic change occurs which is antagonistic to the invading microorganism.

ACTINOMYCOSIS OF THE FACE

As a prophylactic and cure, serotherapy proved unsuccessful in treating actinomycosis of the face. The iodides administered internally seem to possess some merit and the internal use of iodides combined with surgery seem to meet the situation best. So-called "lumpy jaw" seems to have the best chance for recovery. The microscope confirms the diagnosis. If all mycotic infiltration is obliterated, a cure may be effected. If the condition does not yield to conservative measures (curetment), complete excision should be done regardless of the disfigurement it may cause. (Figs. 203-204.)

Dark and irregular portions of skin and subcutaneous fascia often harbor cavities and pus pockets. The infected areas should be incised to the deepest points and recesses of infiltration. Soft tissues and sloughs should be cureted thoroughly and the cavities painted with tincture of iodine. Such operations may require repetition.

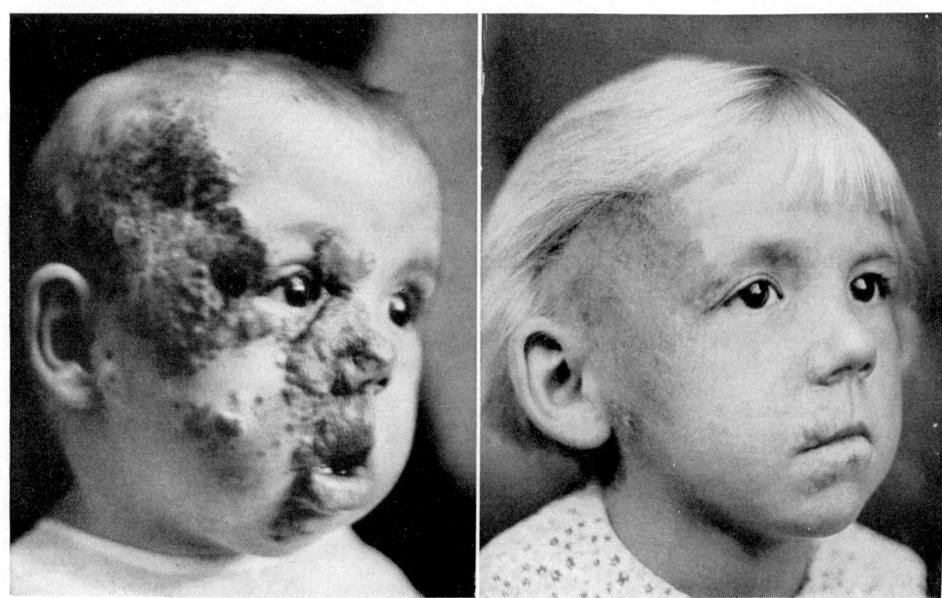

FIG. 205 FIG. 206

FIG. 205. Hemangioma of the face, girl, 18 months of age.
FIG. 206. Same patient four years after radium treatment. (Courtesy of Dr. Frank E. Simpson.)

TUMORS OF THE FACE

Hemangiomas are best treated by radium (Figs. 205-206). Occasionally, epithelioma of the face lends itself much better to the same treatment than to removal with the scalpel (Figs. 207-208).

PLASTIC REPAIR OF DEFECTS OF THE CHEEK (MELOPLASTY)

A multitude of operations are advised for the repair of loss of substance of the cheek from one cause or another. (Figs. 209, 210, 211.) Of these may be mentioned simple suture, and the use of pedunculated flaps from the frontal, temporal, maxillary or mandibular region. Such operations are often beset with many difficulties. (Figs. 212, 213, 214.) Failures often result from insufficient blood supply and infection. No given method will suit all cases. Careful selection is essential. As a type of procedure aiming at supplying nutrition, the following will serve the purpose:

DEFECTS WITHOUT CICATRICIAL MAXILLARY OCCLUSION

CHEYNE AND BURGHARD'S PROCEDURE

Step 1. Dissect up the cheek freely on each side of the defect. The detachment should be more liberal below than above in order to avoid undue displacement of the eyelids.

Step 2. Accurately unite the edges by interrupted sutures.

If this fails, recourse should be had to the following procedure:

Step 1. Outline a single flap having a broad pedicle. Turn the flap forward on its pedicle in such a manner that the skin surface faces toward the interior of the mouth. It is well to have the pedicle attached a little distance behind the posterior margin of the defect.

Step 2. At the end of about two weeks, sever the flap. Use any remaining portion of tissue to cover part of the area from which the flap was taken.

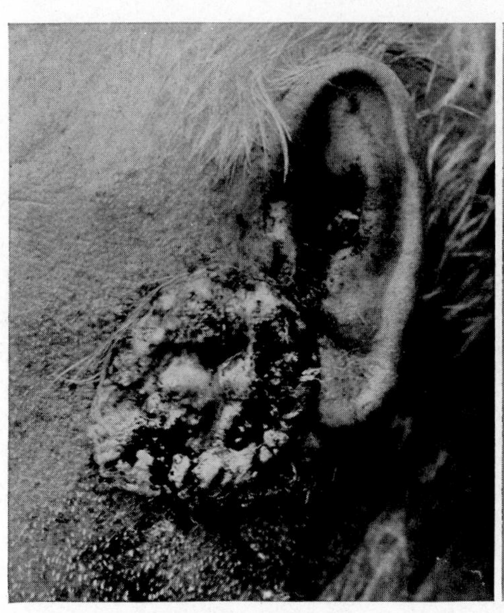

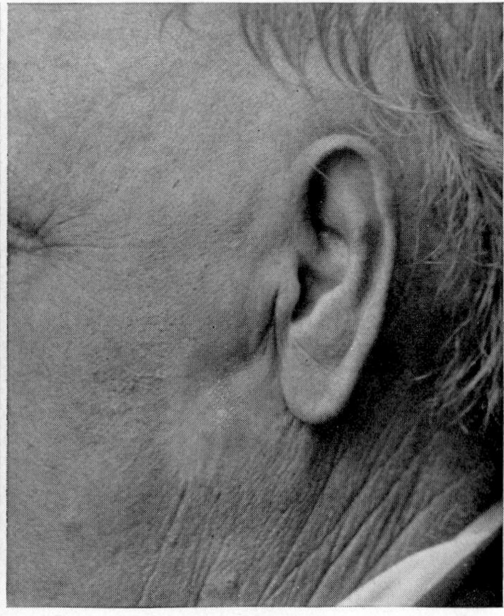

Fig. 207 Fig. 208

Fig. 207. Epithelioma of the face before treatment with radium.

Fig. 208. Epithelioma of the face after radium treatment. Clinically well 10 years (courtesy of Dr. Frank E. Simpson).

Step 3. Cover the external surface of the flap with skin grafts or a superimposed flap from the tissues lower down (jaw, neck).

Step 4. Later reshape the angle of the mouth.

In case of large defects resort to

ISRAEL'S OPERATION

Step 1. Make a very long pedunculated flap, taken from the neck and reaching from the front of the ear in the maxillary angle as far down as the clavicle, if deemed advisable. This flap is to replace the mucosa (Fig. 215).

Step 2. Attach the flap to the margins of the defect with its skin surface facing toward the interior of the cheek.

Step 3. Close the wound in the neck (Figs. 216-217).

Step 4. Between the second and third week following the previous step, divide the pedicle and turn it on itself over the raw surface of the healed flap, the skin side now facing outward. Suture it into place.

Step 5. Reshape the angle of the mouth.

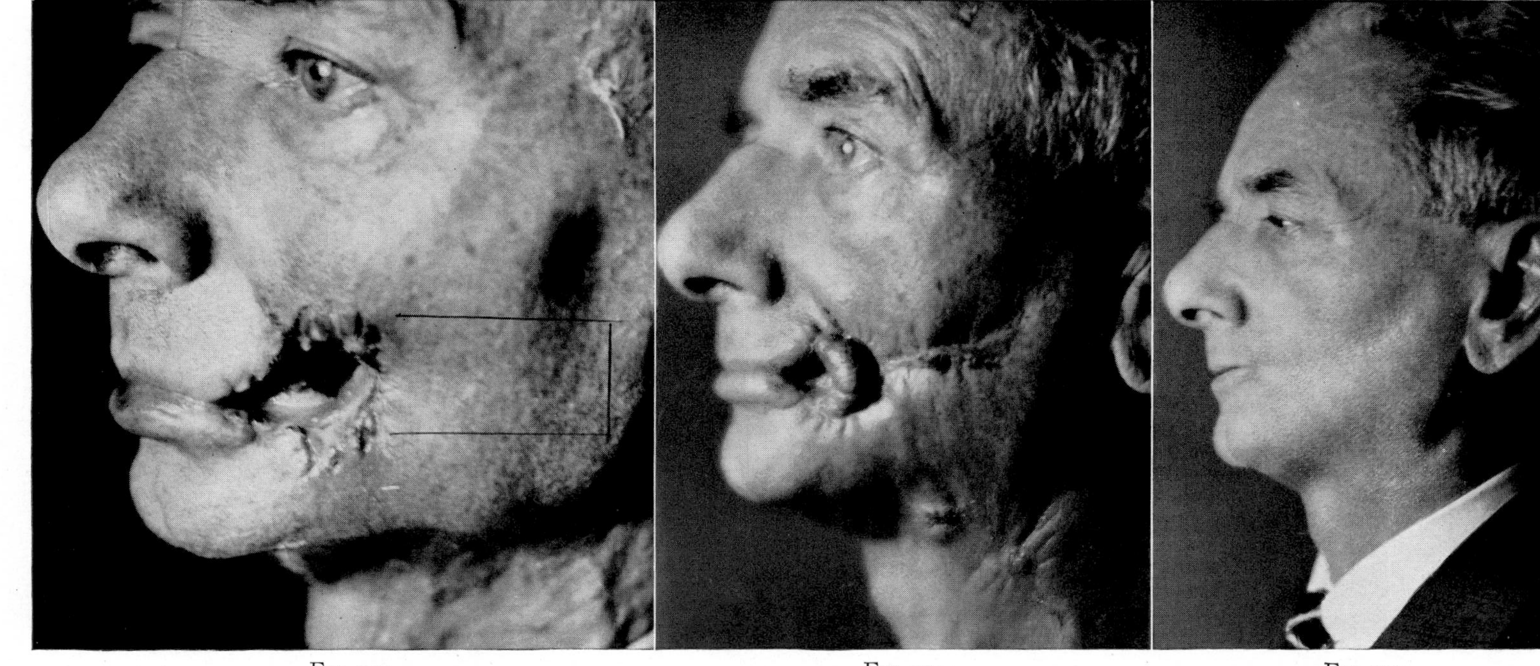

Fig. 209 Fig. 210 Fig. 211

Fig. 209. Defect in chin the result of carcinoma. Note outline of contemplated flap for meloplasty. Implanted flap as outlined proved failure. A migrating flap from the neck was then resorted to.

Fig. 210. Same patient as in preceding illustration showing migrating flap taken from neck in place.

Fig. 211. Same patient after plastic operation. (From Author's Service, American Hospital, Chicago.)

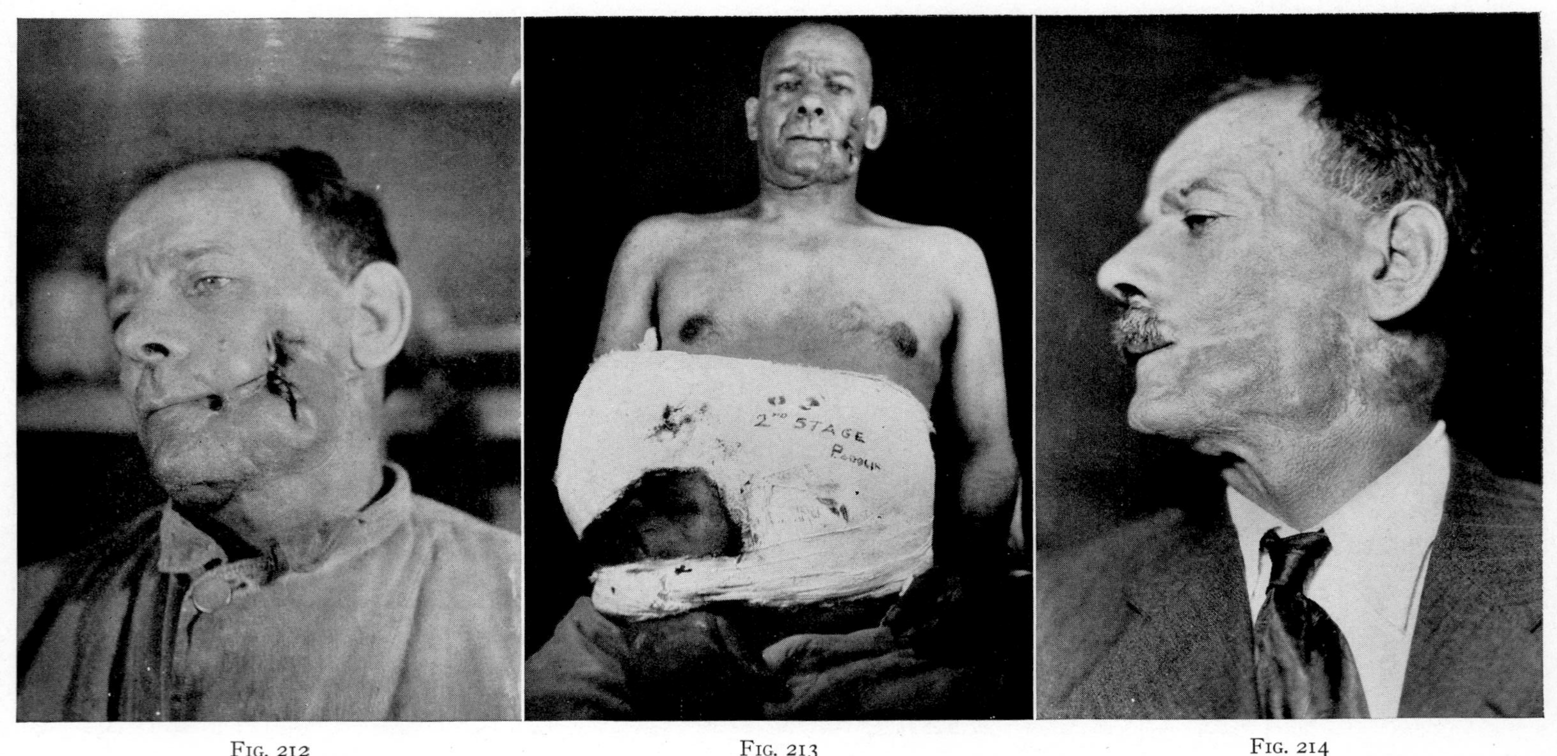

Fig. 212 Fig. 213 Fig. 214

Fig. 212. Arrested epithelioma on alveolar ridge.

Fig. 213. A pedicle flap was raised on the abdomen and attached to the forearm. After it had picked up a secondary blood supply from the forearm, it was cut from the abdomen and transferred to the mouth.

Fig. 214. The skin of the cheek was cut from the ear to the angle of the mouth. The pedicle flap was then carried into the mouth with the skin surface toward the tongue and palate. The end of the pedicle flap was sutured into the masseter region, also into the upper and lower buccal sulci. The skin incision was sutured together over the raw surface of the flap. After the flap had again picked up a blood supply in this position, it was severed from the forearm; a double transfer of the pedicle flap. (Courtesy Dr. A. E. Schaeffer's Service, Cook County Hospital.)

OTHER PROCEDURES

1. **Pedunculated flaps from the forehead** enclosing the temporal artery.

2. **Flaps from the arm (Lexer).**

3. **Flaps from the chest (Hahn).**

4. **Immediate closure of a defect** following excision of a tumor of the mucous membrane by using the mucous membrane at the base of the tongue (Weissl—1906) and (Willard Bartlett—1907).

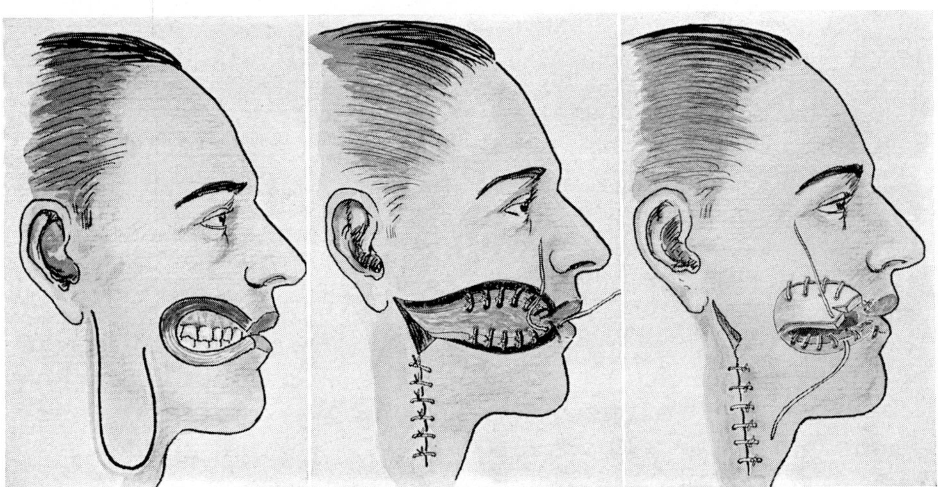

FIG. 215 FIG. 216 FIG. 217

FIG. 215. Israel's method of meloplasty. Flap of neck is outlined with pedicle near the mandible; the flap should extend to the clavicle.

FIG. 216. Freshen margins of gap in the cheek. Turn the flap in such a manner that its cutaneous surface faces interior of mouth. Suture the flap in position. Close defect in the neck.

FIG. 217. Cut pedicle after satisfactory union of previously united tissues. Fold flap on itself so that the raw surfaces face one another; suture folded flap as outlined in drawing.

DEFECTS WITH CICATRICIAL MAXILLARY OCCLUSION

GUSSENBAUER'S OPERATION

This operation consists in dividing the cheek and implanting double flaps into the defect. This operation can only be successfully used when sufficient healthy skin is available. The operation is performed in two stages.

Stage I

Step 1. A portion of skin and subcutaneous tissue, which is slightly wider at its dorsal end than at its anterior end, is separated upward and its pedicle placed at the anterior border of the masseter muscle. The cicatricial tissue is dissected from before backward and the mouth widely opened.

Step 2. The skin flap is turned into the imperfection in such a manner that its free anterior margin is inside the mouth; its edges are stitched to the edges of the defect and the deep surface of the flap is sutured to the inner aspect of the internal pterygoid muscle.

Stage II

Step 3. After about four weeks the pedicle is separated and the posterior part of the flap is carried into the anterior part of the defect and sutured to its refreshed margins. In this way the skin surface of the flap is directed toward the mouth, and the exposed raw surface is covered by a superimposed flap taken from the lower jaw.

INJURIES TO THE BONES OF THE FACE

FRACTURE OF THE UPPER JAW

Direct injury may result in a partially or completely fractured process of the superior maxilla; the malar bone may be forced into the antrum, or the jaw may be separated along the midline. The prognosis in most cases is favorable, about five weeks being required for complete recovery. Callus formation is slight. Occasionally it becomes imperative to remove the tear duct. Displacement of the fragments often tax the surgeon's skill to insure alignment so that a deformity will not result. Remove no fragments unless imperative (infection, necrosis). Have a skillful dentist apply an interdental splint.

LOTHROP'S OPERATION

Step 1. General anesthesia (preferably rectal). Have the patient in a sitting position.

Step 2. Draw the cheek back from the teeth. Incise the mucous membrane at the upper margin of the alveolar process to the extent of about an inch, directing the incision from the canine ridge backward.

Step 3. Separate the bone from the soft tissues of the cheek with a periosteal elevator.

Step 4. After the fracture-fissure has been located by the surgeon's finger, introduce a probe into it and with it raise the fractured portion of bone into its normal position.

Step 5. Where the fissure cannot be located, force the probe into the antrum immediately over the second bicuspid tooth and raise the broken wall of the antrum. If the probe does not seem strong enough to accomplish the desired result try a No. 22 or 24 French male urethral sound, inserting it on top of the probe which is used as a guide.

Step 6. Introduce one or two small gauze drains into the deepest portion of the wound; remove the drains in one or two days. Irrigate the mouth frequently with diluted iodine solution or some other mild antiseptic. If the face is swollen, apply hot, wet boric acid dressings.

Instruct the patient not to touch the affected side or lie on it, in order to avoid displacing the fragments.

FRACTURE OF THE MALAR BONE

Steps 1 to 3. These are the same as those in the foregoing procedure.

Step 4. Introduce a urethral sound (No. 21 to 24 French) into the apex of the antrum where it joins the malar bone. Have an assistant steady the patient's head while the surgeon holds the sound in both hands, his left hand serving as a fulcrum holding the sound near the curve and his right hand grasping the handle.

Step 5. Exert firm pressure upon the fragment; push it back into its normal position. Detached portions of bone are removed with forceps.

Drain into the mouth. Order liquid diet for a week and general treatment as in Lothrop's operation.

FRACTURE OF THE ZYGOMA

The main objective is usually to correct deformity.

Step 1. General anesthesia. Make an incision with its center over the depressed fragment.

Step 2. Retract the soft tissues from the bone with proper retractors.

Step 3. Replace the fractured fragments of bone by manipulation. It generally will remain in position; if not, suture it to the sound part of the bone.

Step 4. Close the wound. Apply dressings in such a manner that no pressure is exerted upon the incision (opening in the center of the dressing). In uncomplicated cases, healing takes place in about two weeks. Do not permit the patient to lie on or manipulate the affected side of the face.

OPERATIONS ON THE DIVISIONS OF THE TRIGEMINAL NERVE AND THE GASSERIAN GANGLION

TRIGEMINAL NEURALGIA (TIC DOULOUREUX)

Anatomic Considerations. (Fig. 218.) The trigeminus (fifth) nerve comprises two roots (motor and sensory). These are connected to the anterior surface of the pons Varolii. From here they pass forward on the apex of the petrous portion of the temporal bone, where the sensory root becomes flattened and joins the Gasserian (semilunar) ganglion lying on the apex of the petrous portion of the temporal bone where it is enclosed by a thin-walled recess of the dura mater (Meckel's cave) to which it is partly adherent. From the anterior border of the ganglion arise the three divisions of the nerve: (1) The ophthalmic; (2) superior maxillary and (3) the mandibular.

The number of injections necessary for relief depends on the accuracy with which the alcohol is placed; one injection within the nerve sheath will suffice to stop the pain at once. An injection near, but not in the nerve is not without value because the alcohol undoubtedly diffuses sufficiently to reach it; relief comes after some minutes or hours but does not last long. Hence it is wise to continue the injections even though the patient is having no pain, until the characteristic sensory phenomena (pain and feeling of swelling and stiffness in the area supplied by the nerve; analgesia in area) announce marked action on the nerve. If pain returns there is no objection to secondary injection.

Treatment by Injection

Usually 80 per cent alcohol is used for injecting the affected nerve and from 2-4 cc. are deposited directly into the nerve trunk. The object is to destroy the nerve by producing degeneration and absorption in the nerve structure except its neurilemma. (Figs. 219, 220, 221, 222, 223.)

The site of point of entry of the needle is anesthetized with some local anesthetic (novocaine 1 or 2 per cent). A special needle of considerable length and strength is required; it should be graduated indicating centimeters and supplied with a stylet capable of extending to the point of the needle. The attachable syringe should be of from 2-4 cc. capacity. (Figs. 224, 225, 226, 227.)

Step 1. Locate the position of the affected nerve trunk. Do not incise the skin.

Step 2. Introduce the needle slowly; steadily push it onward toward the nerve until its sheath is entered; this is usually manifested by a sensation of pain felt by the patient, which radiates over the entire course of the peripheral distribution of the particular nerve.

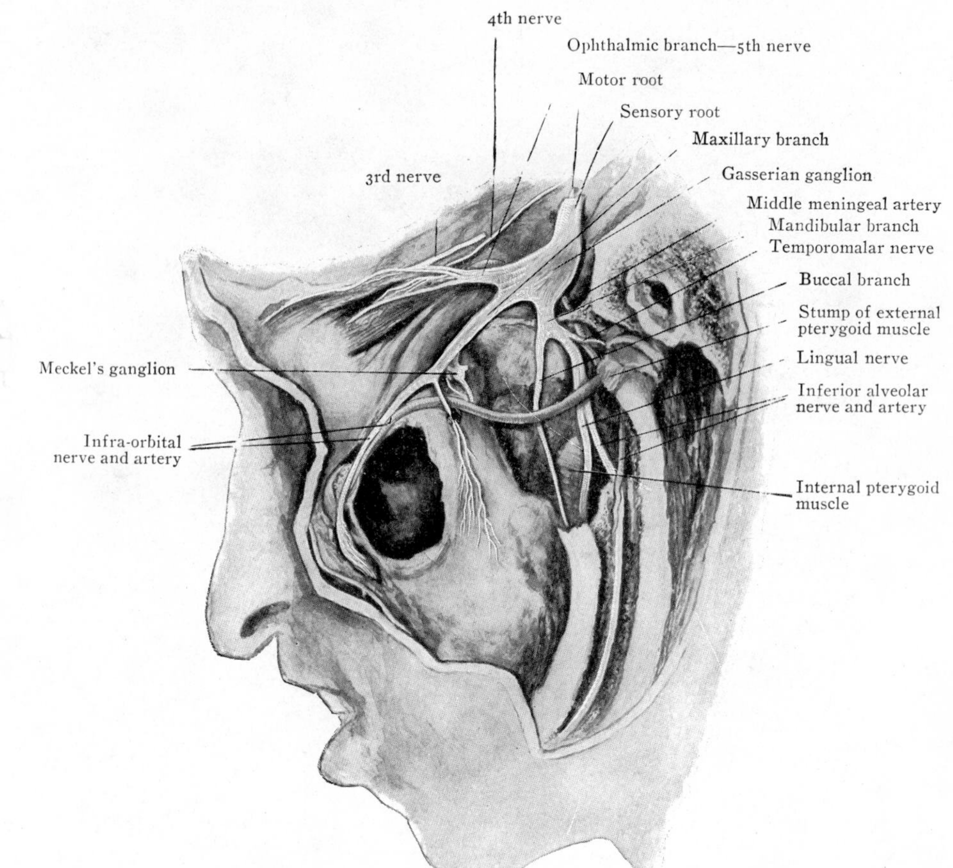

FIG. 218. The fifth or trifacial nerve with its various branches. (Davis, Applied Anatomy.)

Step 3. Withdraw the stylet; adjust the syringe to the needle and inject the alcohol into the nerve slowly and steadily. Detach the syringe and leave the needle in position for a minute or two and then withdraw it slowly. Seal the puncture point with collodion or sterile zinc oxide plaster.

OPHTHALMIC NERVE (LEVY-BAUDOIN METHOD)

The first branch of the fifth nerve divides inside the cranium, hence it is difficult to attack its trunk. The nasal route is scarcely accessible in the midst of the important motor nerves which surround it. The orbital route is indicated to reach the frontal and lachrymal nerves. Insert the needle at the external wall of the orbit at the level of the inferior extremity of the external angular process of the frontal bone, pass it below the lachrymal gland and follow the periosteum without injury to the eye or to any important organ. The injection is made at a depth of 35 or 40 mm., after withdrawing the mandrin. The patient should have his eyes closed. The needle has some difficulty in penetrating the outer portion of Tenon's capsule which is very thick.

SUPERIOR MAXILLARY NERVE (MURPHY'S METHOD)

Step 1. Draw an imaginary line vertically downward beginning at the external angular process of the frontal bone; introduce the needle directly under the zygoma where this line crosses its inferior margin. The needle is inserted somewhat upward and inward until it comes in contact with the back of the superior maxilla.

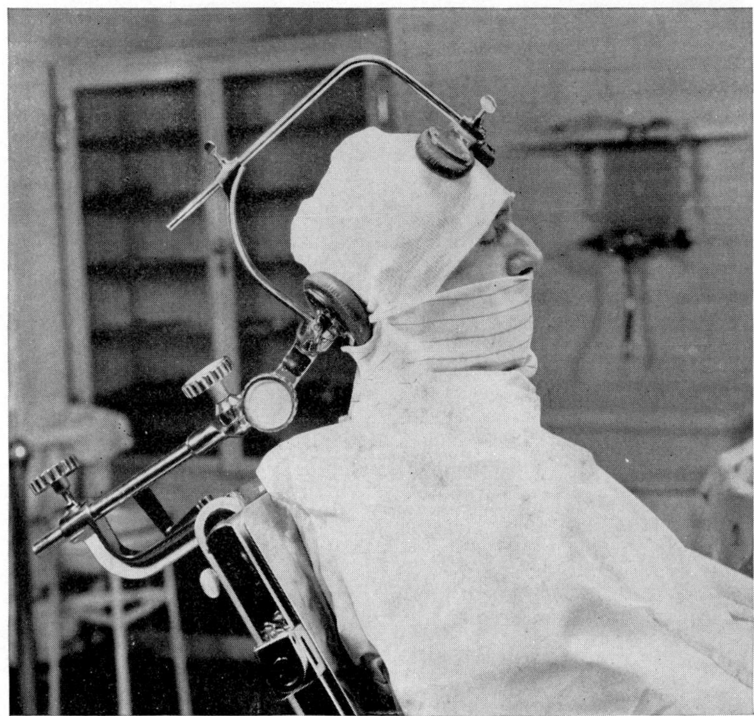

FIG. 219. Position of the patient in approach to the branches of the Gasserian ganglion for injection treatment.

Step 2. Using the maxillary bone as a guide, push the needle on until its point has penetrated about 1¾ inches (4½ cm.) or slightly more, from the surface of the malar bone and has reached the foramen rotundum. Intraoral approach of the superior dental nerve is shown in Fig. 230, p. 211.

INFERIOR MAXILLARY NERVE (MURPHY'S METHOD)

The needle is introduced at a chosen point in the middle of the upper edge of the zygoma and passed directly inward until the squamous portion of the temporal bone or the great wing of the sphenoid is struck and directed by these passes over the foramen ovale at a depth of 1½ inches (4 cm.) from the outer surface of the zygoma.

INFERIOR DENTAL OR MANDIBULAR NERVE

This nerve may be blocked as it leaves the skull in the foramen ovale, but the most desirable point of entry for the needle seems to be inside the lower

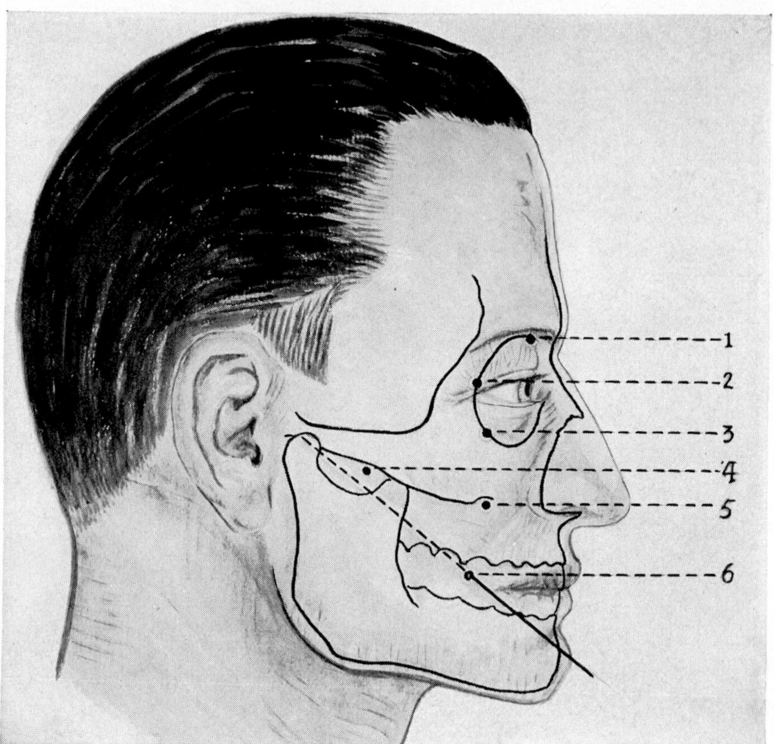

FIG. 220. Points of injection for blocking the various branches of the trigeminal (fifth) nerve (lateral view): 1. supra-orbital nerve, 2. lateralorbital nerve, 3. pterygopalatine fossa through the orbit, 4. otic ganglion, 5. pterygopalatine fossa from the side, 6. Gasserian (semilunar) ganglion.

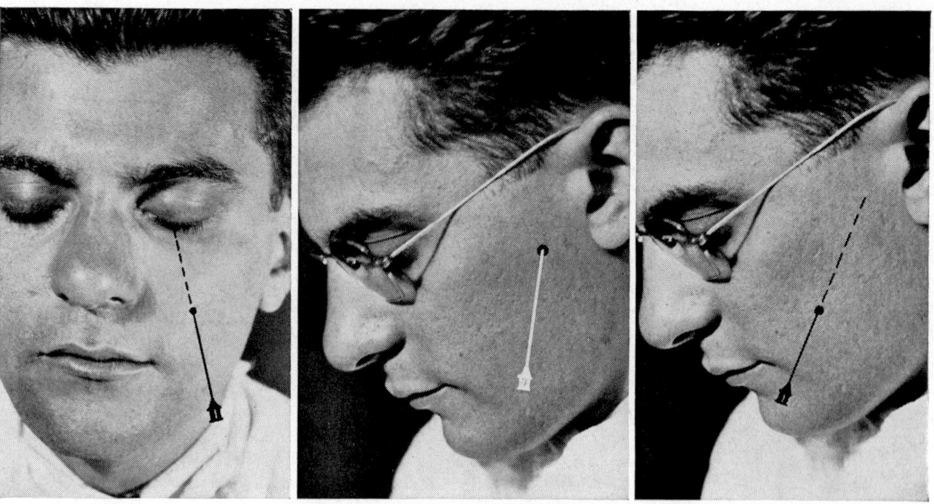

FIG. 221 FIG. 222 FIG. 223

FIG. 221. Tic douloureux. Direction of passing needle through the cheek to reach the Gasserian ganglion. According to Hartel, the needle is entered at a point about 3 cm. from the angle of the mouth and passed upward in a plane that bisects the pupil of the eye.

FIG. 222. Tic douloureux. Block anesthesia of the second and third branches of the trigeminal nerve by an external approach. The needle is introduced at the point about the middle of the zygomatic arch.

FIG. 223. Tic douloureux. Direction of passing needle through the cheek to reach the Gasserian ganglion. Same as preceding lateral view showing the direction of the needle in a plane that bisects the auricular tubercle (after Hartel).

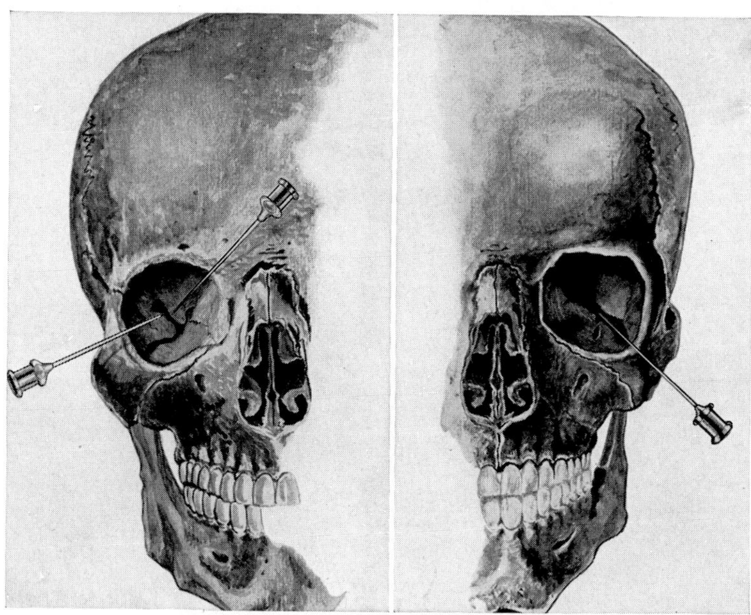

FIG. 224 FIG. 225

FIG. 224. Medial and lateral position of the needle for blocking the branches of the first division of the trigeminal nerve.

FIG. 225. Position of the needle for blocking the second division of the trigeminal in the pterygopalatine fossa through the orbit. The needle is inserted in the inferior orbital fissure.

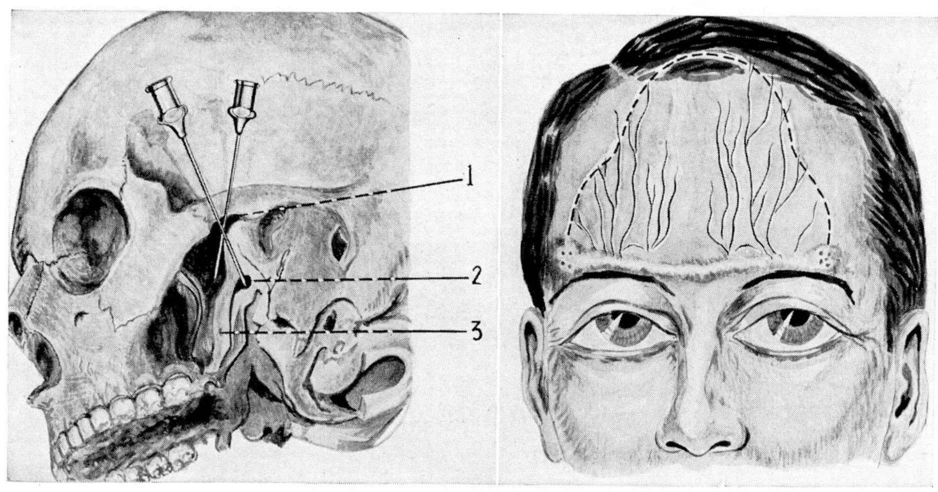

FIG. 226 FIG. 227

FIG. 226. Blocking the third division of the trigeminal at the foramen ovale. The needle is directed slightly forward and is inserted at the center of and under the zygomatic arch. It strikes at first the outer lamella of the pterygoid process, and is then slightly withdrawn and directed backward, where it enters the foramen ovale. 1. Insertion point at the middle of the lower border of the zygomatic process, 2. foramen ovale, 3. exterior lamina of the pterygoid process.

FIG. 227. Bilateral blocking by subcutaneous infiltration across the forehead and the eyebrows.

jaw near the lingula. A long needle is used for this injection. (Figs. 228, 229, 230, 231.)

Step 1. The needle should be entered near the canine tooth, directed parallel to the biting surface of the teeth across the mouth until the bone is reached after forming a wheal in the mucous membrane over the nerve. The bone is then followed posteriorly until the needle reaches a point immediately in front of the trigonum retromolare.

Step 2. Five to ten cc. of a 1 per cent solution of novocaine-adrenalin solution is sufficient to anesthetize the corresponding half of the lower jaw and about half of the tongue. Insertion of the needle in the mental foramen under the first and second bicuspid teeth, will produce anesthesia in the anterior branches of the nerves.

According to Braun, the most direct way of reaching the foramen ovale is from the outside. By inserting the needle immediately under the border of the zygoma and carefully observing the suggestions of Offerhaus, the anesthetic solution is almost certain to be injected into the trunk of the mandibular nerve as it leaves the skull. After carefully measuring fifty skulls, Offerhaus discovered that the connecting line of the articular tubercle is anterior to the maxillary joint and divides the two points a short distance below and usually the same distance anteriorly from both foramina ovale. Since the mandibular nerve is directed forward and downward after leaving the skull, the intertubercular line intercepts these nerve trunks exactly at the foramen ovale. (Fig. 226, p. 209.)

OFFERHAUS' METHOD

Step 1. A wheal marks the articular tubercle on the side to be injected and a blue pencil marks the point on the opposite side. With an ordinary compass, measure, externally, the length of the alveolar process of the maxilla back of the last molar teeth and measure the length of the intertubercular line with an Offerhaus compass. For instance, if the measurements are 5 and 14 cm., the points will be 4.5 cm. from the point at which the needle should be inserted.

Step 2. By placing a small cork on the needle about 1 cm. beyond the desired length the surgeon is able to determine how far the needle should be inserted—it should be inserted no further.

Step 3. The needle is inserted in the direction indicated by the points of the Offerhaus compasses which have been placed on the head; the patient will experience pains in the lower jaw at this point. The thick nerve trunk offers resistance to the needle here although at times it can be penetrated.

Step 4. If the needle has entered the nerve trunk a 2 per cent novocaine-suprarenin solution suffices; if the needle enters near the nerve trunk 5 cc. are necessary. Blocking of the nerve often takes place in an instant although never more than 5 or 10 minutes are required.

FARR'S METHOD

This method of injection of the foramen ovale is supposed to be simpler than the above.

Step 1. Insert the needle transversely; a skull which is marked by a sound is held beside the patient to determine the direction.

Step 2. After being inserted 4 or 5 cm. the needle reaches the pterygoid process and is then about 1 cm. from the foramen ovale, the movable piece of cork marking the distance on the needle.

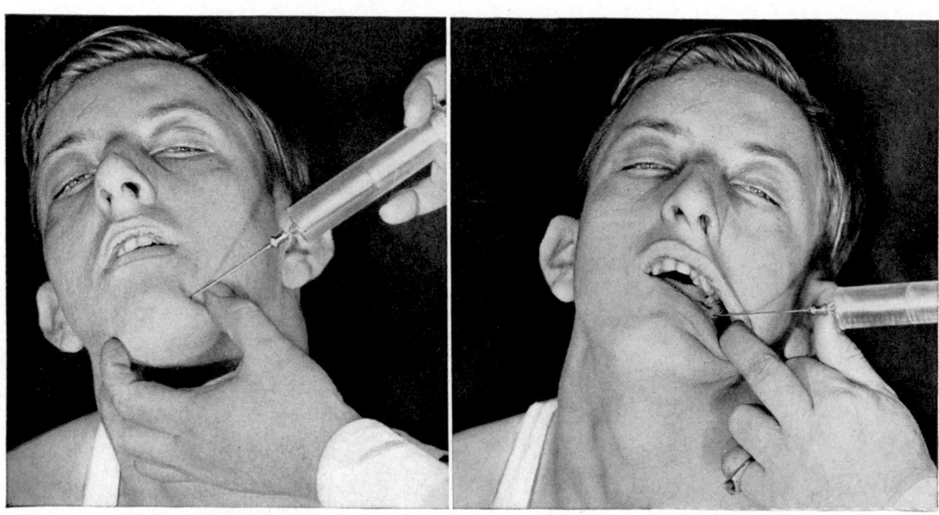

FIG. 228 FIG. 229

FIG. 228. Infiltration blocking of the inferior dental nerve. External approach.
FIG. 229. Infiltration anesthesia of the inferior dental (maxillary) nerve. Intra-oral approach.

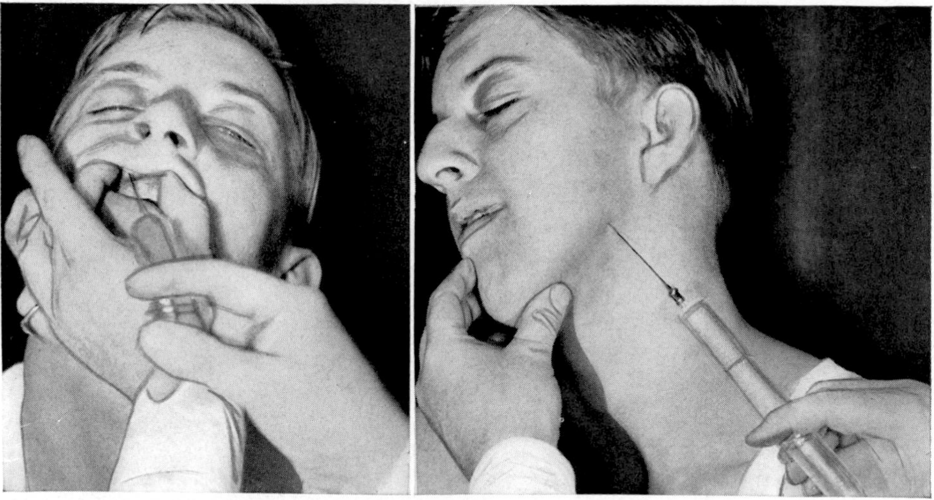

FIG. 230 FIG. 231

FIG. 230. Infiltration anesthesia of the superior dental nerve. Intra-oral approach through the mental foramen.
FIG. 231. Infiltration anesthesia of the inferior dental nerve. Extra-oral approach (at the mental foramen).

Step 3. After retracting the needle as far as the subcutaneous tissue it is again inserted at a slight angle to the same depth or deeper. The patient now complains of the usual radiating pains.

Comment. The complexity of this method may be further decreased by determining the exact depth of the foramen ovale. Farr utilizes both methods while inserting the needle but directs it back farther than Offerhaus in his search for the base of the pterygoid process. The needle is then directed a little posteriorly and .5 to 1 cm. deeper than the distance first figured. Undesirable secondary effects such as hematoma, etc., need not be feared if the foramen ovale is injected from without.

In case the injection of alcohol or other substance (osmic acid) fails to relieve the symptoms, neurectomy is resorted to.

Neurectomy

NEURECTOMY OF THE SUPRAORBITAL NERVE

Step 1. Locate the supraorbital notch or foramen. Make a horizontal incision parallel to and a little below the eyebrow. (Fig. 232.)

Step 2. Separate the fibers of the orbicularis palpebrarum muscle. Retract the divided tissues and expose the nerve as it passes through the supraorbital notch.

Step 3. Isolate the nerve for a short distance. Seize the undivided nerve trunk with a pair of narrow bladed hemostats and twist the hemostat in such a manner that the nerve is wound round it. Reverse the direction of rotation. Work slowly. Repeat the procedure as often as is necessary until all of the peripheral portion of the nerve and a section of its central part are avulsed. Close the wound. Dress. (Fig. 232a.)

NEURECTOMY OF THE INFRAORBITAL NERVE

Anatomic Considerations. The superior maxillary nerve originates at the middle of the Gasserian ganglion. It passes horizontally forward and leaves the skull through the foramen rotundum of the sphenoid bone. It crosses the spheno-maxillary fossa. Here it becomes the infraorbital nerve and enters the infraorbital canal of the superior maxilla through which it reaches the face to break up into terminal branches. To locate the infraorbital foramen, draw a line from the supraorbital notch to the interval between the two lower bicuspid teeth. About half an inch below the lower margin of the orbit and along the line described, the infraorbital foramen is located. The nerve may be resected (a) at the infraorbital foramen or (b) at the foramen rotundum (more difficult to perform but more satisfactory in results).

RESECTION OF THE INFRAORBITAL NERVE AT THE INFRAORBITAL FORAMEN

Step 1. Raise the head of the patient on a sandbag or pillow. Turn the head slightly toward the affected side. Locate the infraorbital foramen as suggested above.

Step 2. A slightly curved incision about half an inch in length is now made running parallel and close to the lower margin of the orbit. The incision is slightly concave; it is dissected upward and is so planned that its center will cross the infraorbital foramen. (Fig. 232b.)

Step 3. Divide the orbicularis palpebrarum muscle in a direction parallel to its fibers. The levator labii superioris (caput infraorbitale) is now exposed and it also is split in the direction of its fibers.

Step 4. Elevate the periosteum from the floor of the orbit exposing the infraorbital nerve in its canal. As it leaves the infraorbital foramen the infraorbital nerve divides into a number of branches. Seize the nerve in a nar-

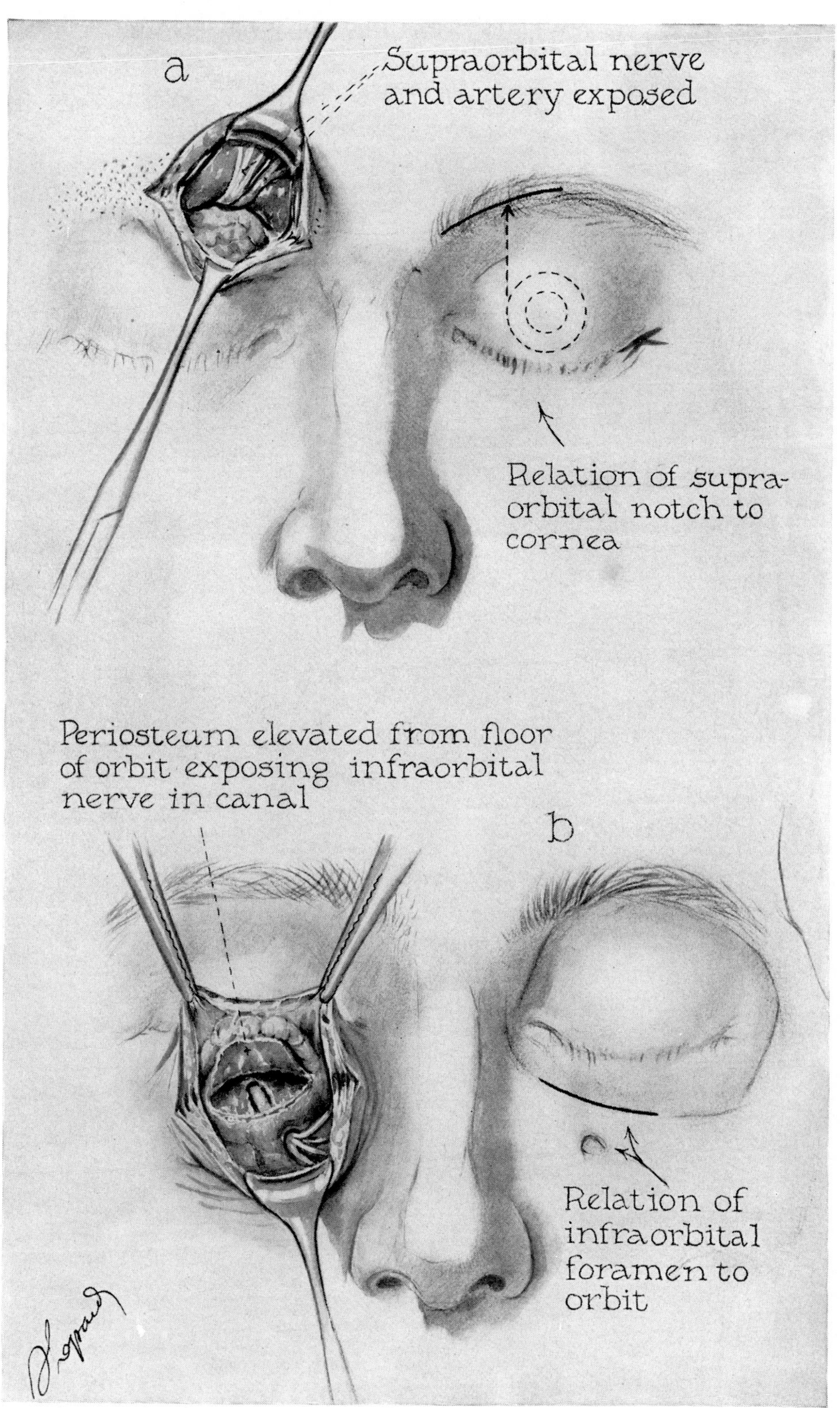

FIG. 232. a. Neurectomy of the supraorbital nerve; b. neurectomy of the infraorbital nerve.

row bladed artery forceps and by traction and torsion extract as much of its trunk from its bony canal as is possible. With the patient at ease a great portion of the nerve may thus be avulsed.

There is often considerable hemorrhage due to injury to the infraorbital artery and vein. An adrenalin tampon will control the bleeding.

Step 5. In order to prevent a recurrence of the neuralgia, plug the bony canal, with a bone peg, silver screw, etc. This operation is not so successful as the removal of the nerve. This may be accomplished at the foramen rotundum. With the nerve, Meckel's (sphenopalatine) ganglion is also removed.

RESECTION OF THE INFRAORBITAL NERVE AT THE FORAMEN ROTUNDUM

(See Fig. 218, p. 206.)

Step 1. In this procedure the nerve must be followed up through the superior maxillary bone to the foramen rotundum. Make a Kocher incision; this commences just below the inner edge of the infraorbital margin and runs obliquely downward and outward to the lower angle of the malar bone. The incision should be ample enough to give good exposure of the anterior surface of the superior maxilla from the canine fossa to the lower margin of the orbit.

Step 2. Separate the fibers of the levator labii suspensoris (caput infraorbitale). Expose the nerve at the infraorbital foramen as in the previous operation.

Step 3. Surround the nerve with a ligature for identification and traction. Clear the anterior surface of the superior maxilla of muscles and periosteum.

Step 4. Chisel away a square opening, the sides of which should be about an inch in length. This opening is so planned that the infraorbital opening is slightly below the center of the square and the upper edge is to be just below the margin of the orbit. During the chiseling watch the nerve constantly and avoid injuring it. It is left hanging through the opening.

There usually is considerable oozing after the antrum of Highmore is opened. Pack the wound with small cotton tampons dipped in 1:1000 adrenalin solution. Do not proceed with the operation while oozing continues.

Step 5. When the field is clear, illuminate the area with a head-mirror and remove the lower wall of the antrum with a fine chisel. Guard the nerve. If it be torn, the guide for further steps will be lost.

Step 6. After the entire floor of the infraorbital canal has been chiseled away as far back as the posterior wall of the antrum, a slightly smaller opening is created on the posterior wall of the antrum. The nerve now protrudes through the openings made.

Step 7. Dry the field. Pull the nerve taut; trace it to the foramen rotundum. Identify Meckel's (sphenopalatine) ganglion. Grasp the nerve with a pair of forceps near the foramen rotundum, pull it out forcibly or divide it flush at the foramen with a pair of scissors. In either procedure the ganglion will come away with the trunk of the nerve. Pull the nerve out of the foramen as much as possible. Attend to hemostasis. Unite the structures. Drain. Close the skin wound. Dress.

NEURECTOMY OF THE THIRD DIVISION OF THE TRIGEMINAL (FIFTH) NERVE

Anatomic Considerations. (Fig. 233.) The third or inferior maxillary (mandibular) division of the fifth nerve leaves the skull through the foramen ovale and divides into two main branches, the anterior (smaller) giving off the following branches, the masseteric, buccal and external pterygoid. From the posterior (larger) the following branches are derived, the auriculo-temporal, lingual and inferior dental

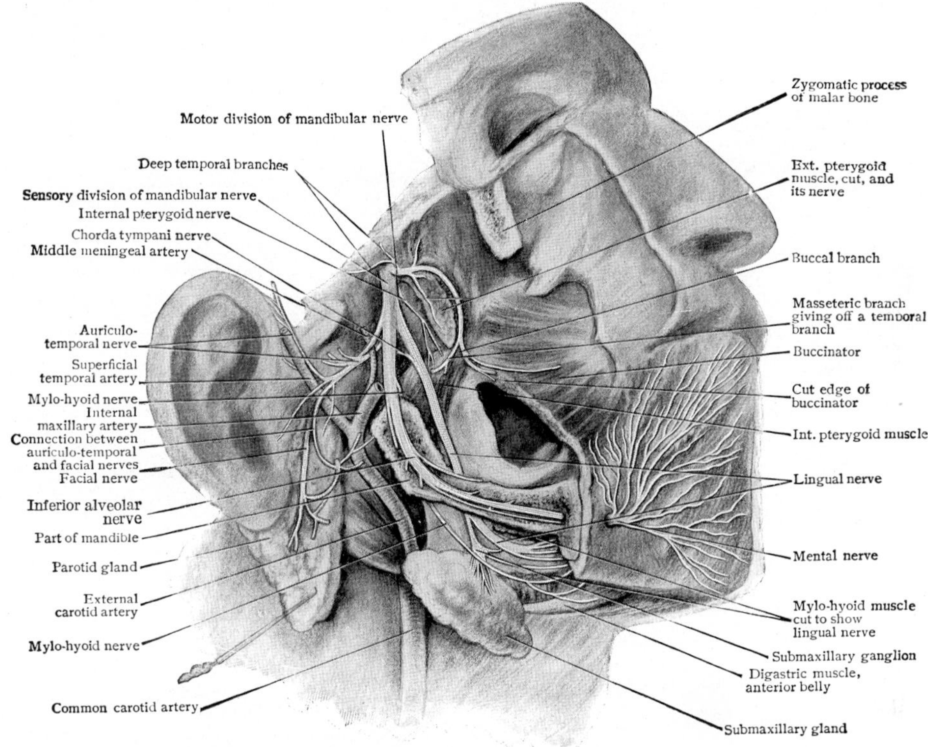

Fig. 233. Dissection showing mandibular nerve and its branches; mandible has been partially removed, exposing inferior dental nerve in its canal.

(alveolar). Oftentimes, in neuralgia of the third division of the trigeminal, neurectomy fails and removal of the Gasserian ganglion has to be resorted to. The lingual and inferior dental nerves have a close surgical relationship. They are generally conjointly involved if either of them is affected by neuralgia. Their excision may be considered as part of one operation.

Step 1. Make a curved incision around the angle of the jaw. Displace the supramaxillary branch of the facial nerve downward. Respect the facial artery.

Step 2. Separate the masseter muscle with a periosteal elevator and slight touches of the knife. Trephine an opening in the center of the ascending ramus of the inferior maxilla (Velpeau's rule). If necessary, the trephine opening should be enlarged with appropriate rongeur forceps. Pull out the nerve by twisting it about a clamp.

The nerve may also be reached by exposing the mental foramen (Fig. 234)

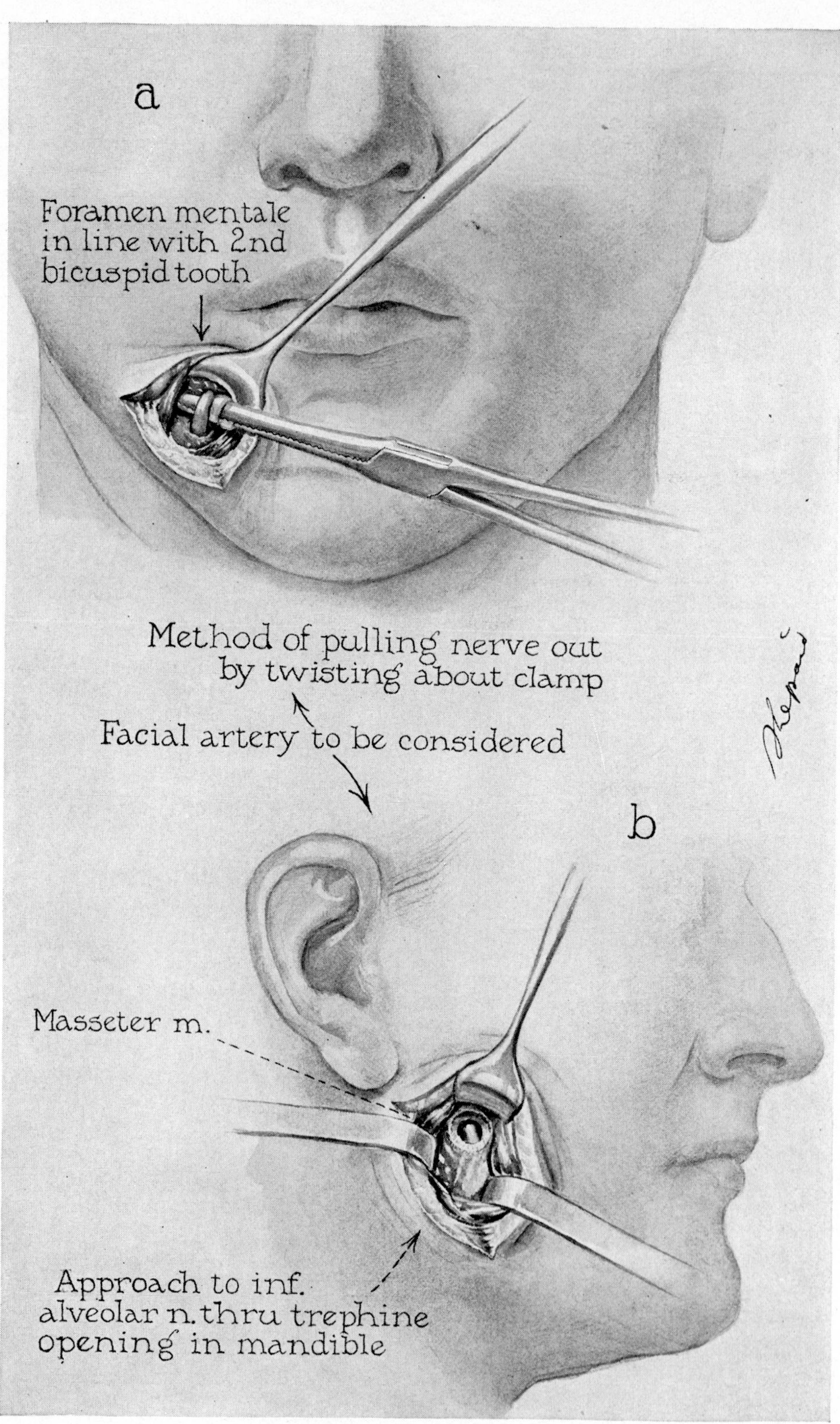

FIG. 234. Neurectomy of the inferior maxillary (mandibular) nerve.

in line with the second bicuspid tooth. This approach, as will be seen, produces more or less scarring. The nerve may be reached through an intraoral approach. This is technically more difficult, of course, but in many respects preferable.

INTRAORAL APPROACH

Step 1. Open the mouth of the patient widely with suitable mouth gag. Good illumination is essential. Transfix the tip of the tongue with a stout linen suture. This is to act as retractor. Keep the tongue out of the field of operation.

Step 2. Make an incision one inch long running parallel with the anterior border of the ascending ramus of the mandible. Separate the mucoperiosteum from the bone.

Step 3. Expose the inferior maxillary (mandibular) spine, situated above the commencement of the inferior dental (mandibular) canal.

Step 4. With a fine, blunt-pointed scissors detach the long internal lateral (sphenomandibular) ligament which is attached to the mandibular spine.

Step 5. Behind this, identify the inferior dental (alveolar) nerve. Bring it into the wound with a hook. Keep the field dry. (Plug with adrenalin tampon until oozing stops.) Remember that the nerve lies in front of the inferior dental vessels. Avoid injuring these.

Step 6. Avulse or excise the nerve. The wound is permitted to heal by granulation.

Tic douloureux frequently recurs after even the most extensive excision of the nerve-trunks involved. Keen and Spiller have shown that marked degeneration is present in the Gasserian ganglion. When injections or even neurectomy fails to be followed by relief, the Gasserian ganglion should be removed.

REMOVAL OF THE GASSERIAN GANGLION

Anatomic Considerations. The Gasserian ganglion (ganglion semilunare) nerve-fibers and cells lie in a slight depression on the apex of the petrous portion of the temporal bone. In shape it is a flattened crescent with its convexity forward, measuring from 1.5-2 cm. in width and about 1 cm. in length. The surface of the ganglion presents an irregular longitudinal or reticular striation. From the anterior expanded convex border of the ganglion arise the ophthalmic and maxillary nerves and the sensory portion of the mandibular nerve while its narrow concave posterior margin is continued into the sensory root of the fifth nerve. The ganglion lies in Meckel's space (cavum Mecklii), a cleft produced by a delamination of the dura mater, and comes in relation internally with the cavernous sinus and the internal carotid artery. Beneath, but unconnected with it, are the motor root of the trifacial and the great superficial petrosal nerve. In structure it resembles a spinal ganglion, being composed of the characteristically modified neurones, from whose single processes proceed the peripherally directed dendrites and the centrally coursing axones. In addition to the three large trunks given off from the anterior margin, the branches of the Gasserian ganglion include some fine meningeal filaments which arise from the posterior end of the ganglion and are distributed to the adjacent dura mater.

HARTLEY-KRAUSE OPERATION

Shave the patient's head and prepare it as outlined under operations on the brain. The face and external auditory meatus are also cleaned and asepticized thoroughly. Pack the external auditory meatus with iodoform gauze. (Fig. 219, p. 207.)

Step 1. Make a curved incision beginning on the zygoma immediately in front of the tragus. The convexity of the incision is directed upward; it ends on the zygoma at a point about one and one-half inches in front of its starting point (Fig. 235). The flap thus outlined is about 2½ inches in height, 2 inches wide at its broadest part, and presents a pedicle about 1½ inches wide. Attend to hemostasis. With chisel and mallet, a gouge with V-shaped cutting edge or an electric saw or, preferably, with a Jentzer trephine, divide the skull along lines corresponding to the wound. Turn down the flap consisting of the skin, temporal muscle, periosteum adherent to the bone and the bone. Break the bridge of bone opposite the pedicle. The soft parts act as a hinge. The line of fracture at which the bone-flap is reflected is opposite the zygoma, therefore at a higher level than the base of the skull. With rongeur forceps bite away the bone immediately below the opening in the skull, until the true floor of the middle fossa of the skull is reached. This removal of bone after the bone-flap has been reflected is an extremely important step in the operation.

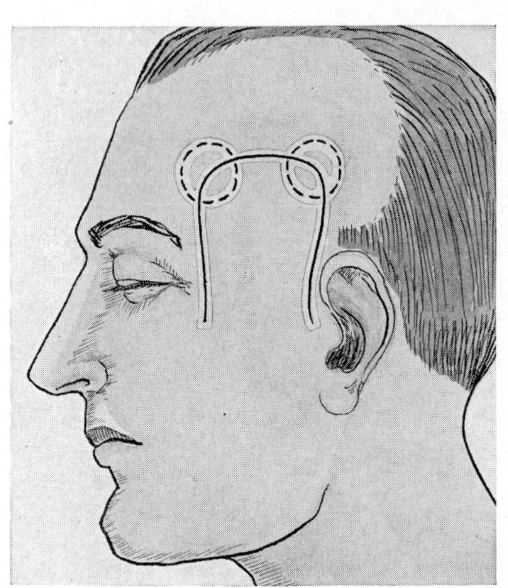

Fig. 235. Hartley-Krause operation. Incision for the removal of the Gasserian ganglion.

With the finger, quickly separate the dura from the base of the skull until the foramen spinosum and middle meningeal artery are reached. (Fig. 236.) Fedor Krause recommends quick work with the finger, this being without danger and producing less venous bleeding than slow separation with a blunt raspatory. However, this step is followed by brisk venous bleeding; control it by gauze pressure. When the foramen spinosum is reached, gently lift up the brain, covered by the dura mater, with a spatula bent at a right angle.

Pussep made the important observation that when the patient's head is hanging downwards and somewhat to the side, the brain recedes, the wound cavity thus becomes wider and it is no longer necessary to retract the brain with a spatula. On the other hand, with the head in this position, the venous bleeding is more profuse. Retract the brain sufficiently to afford good exposure of the deep structures.

Step 3. The middle meningeal artery is ligated doubly and divided. The artery often runs in a deep groove or even in a canal in the skull and may be, and often is, torn while the bone is being removed. In such event, control the bleeding by packing the foramen with a thin strip of gauze or with Horsley's wax. Separate the dura mater further from the bone with a blunt instrument in the direction of the ganglion. Bleeding at this step is usually brisk but packing with gauze against the bone for a few seconds will usually control it.

Step 4. When the ganglion is reached, recall that its upper surface is often firmly adherent to the dura; separate it by blunt dissection. Should the dura be opened while separating the ganglion, cerebrospinal fluid will issue, but this is of no importance. Seize the posterior portion of the ganglion transversely with the jaws of a hemostat. Identify and outline the second and third divisions of the fifth nerve; divide them with a tenotome at the foramen rotundum and ovale, respectively. Do not attempt to isolate the first division of the nerve because it is closely united with the cavernous

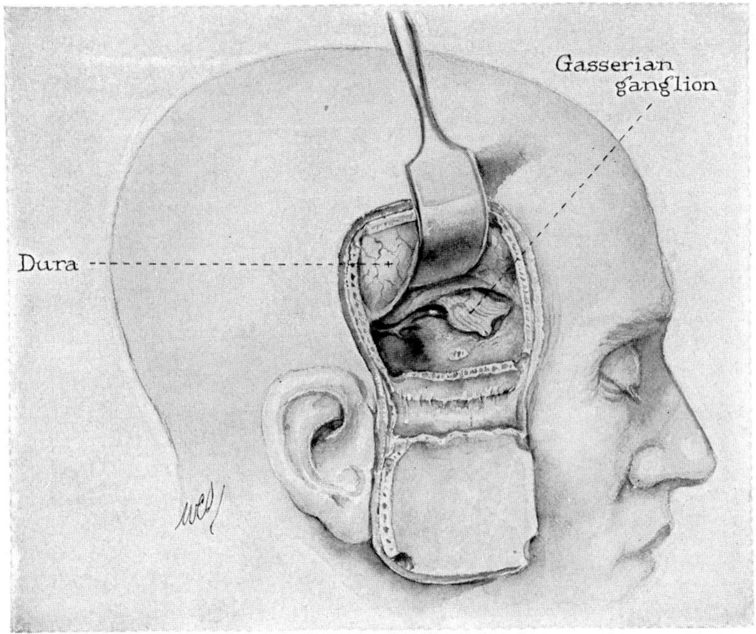

FIG. 236. Extradural exposure of the Gasserian ganglion.

sinus which may be injured. Bleeding accompanying the division of the second and third divisions of the nerve is easily stopped by pressure or by boring a blunt instrument into their foramina. With the forceps previously applied to the ganglion, make traction along the axis of the nerve. This pulls the ganglion out and with it a longer or shorter portion of its root is delivered.

Step 5. Replace the brain. Suture the temporal osteoplastic flap into place. Provide drainage, if deemed advisable. Dress.

Step 6. For several weeks after the operation, danger threatens the eye of the side involved. Being rendered anesthetic it is subject to injury (dust, contacts, etc.); it should therefore be kept protected and clean by means of boracic acid lotion. The eyelid is closed by one or two sutures so placed that while the eye is closed the boracic solution may still be applied. Remove the sutures from the eyelids after two or three days. Protect the eye by a watchglass-shield held in place by adhesive plaster.

Comments. Should threatening hemorrhage ensue during the operation, suspend the operation. Pack the wound with gauze, dress and keep the patient in bed for a few days. Resume the operation when the condition of the patient warrants it. Should the cavernous sinus be injured during removal of the ganglion, the gush of blood can always be easily checked by gauze pressure because the blood-pressure in the sinus is very low.

ABBÉ'S OPERATION

In order to avoid the dangers of hemorrhage, shock and prolonged operation, Abbé has given up attempts formally to resect the Gasserian ganglion. He performs an intracranial neurotomy or, preferably, neurectomy, and then prevents reunion of the divided nerves by interposing a layer of thin rubber tissue. To lessen hemorrhage from the middle meningeal artery, Abbé ligates the external carotid artery just above the thyroid, although Cushing and others see no benefit from ligating the external carotid artery, because most bleeding is venous.

Step 1. Ligate the external carotid (optional).

Step 2. Make a straight incision in the temporal fossa above the zygoma; split the temporal muscle, scraping it widely from the bone, and enter the skull by a small trephine opening, rapidly enlarged by rongeurs to 1½ inches in diameter.

Step 3. Expose the second and third branches from the Gasserian ganglion to the foramina. Seize each at the foramen by a narrow clamp, cut it, and resect a half-inch, or tear it from the ganglion; push the dura well back beyond the foramina.

Step 4. Arrest bleeding by pressure, and spread over the bone a piece of sterile rubber tissue (sterilized in bichloride solution and washed in saline), more than enough to cover both foramina, one inch wide by an inch and a half in length. This must be pressed upon the bone by a strip of gauze packed over it for a couple of minutes.

Step 5. When the gauze is removed, the rubber tissue lies in close contact with the skull and the dura is allowed to settle down to its place upon it. The wound is then closed by a few fine catgut sutures and drained for a day at its lower angle.

G. R. Fowler recommends Crile's plan of temporary occlusion of both common carotids as a useful procedure. Abbé's operation gives excellent results and seems preferable in every way to the more formidable excision of the ganglion.

Exposure of the Gasserian Ganglion and the Three Divisions of Fifth Nerve by the Direct Infra-Arterial Route (Cushing's Method)

Step 1. The head is shaved and the patient laid on one side and supported by a pillow. The surgeon stands at the side of the head either in front of or behind the patient and his assistant opposite. The zygomatic arch is outlined. A horseshoe-shaped incision is made, the ends of the two limbs extending to the outer and inner ends of the zygomatic arch about 4 cm. apart and the upper part of the convexity reaching about 5 cm. above the zygoma. The temporal vessels are secured.

Step 2. A second horseshoe incision, somewhat smaller than the first, is made through the temporal fascia; its base passes through the periosteum along the outer aspect of the zygoma, mesially. With the exception of the periosteum along the attachment of the masseter muscle, the zygoma is freed of its periosteum through this incision. With a Gigli saw, divide the zygomatic arch at its inner and outer ends after first drilling on each side of the saw-cut as a preparation for future ligatures.

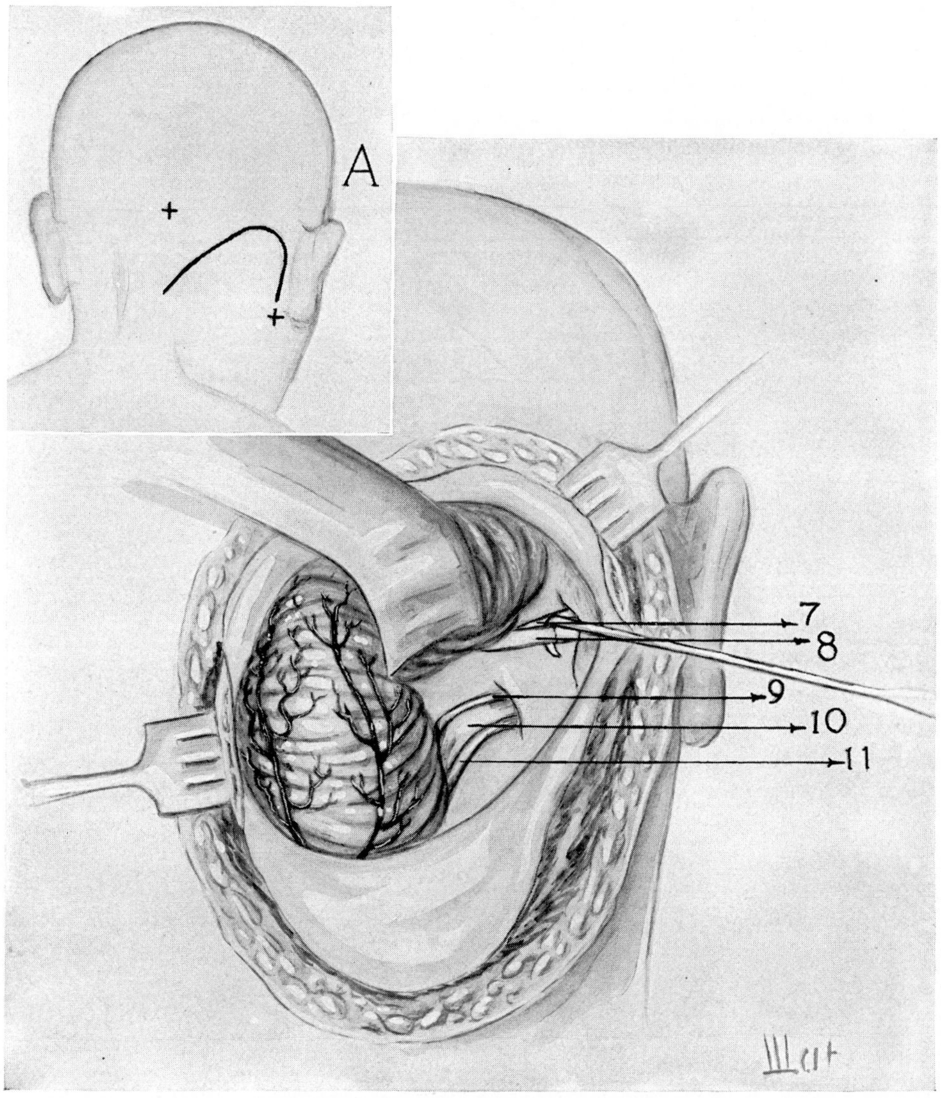

FIG. 237. Intracranial section of auditory nerve for Ménière's disease. Complete division of the eighth nerve, avoiding injury to the underlying facial nerve. A. Scalp incision for intracranial exposure of the fifth, eighth and ninth nerves. (Dandy.)

Step 3. Divide the temporal muscle down to the bone along the line of the legs and convexity of the preceding horseshoe incision and turn the flap of soft parts, with zygoma attached, downward, retracting it in order to expose the zygomatic crest (infra-temporal ridge), the lower part of the temporal fossa and the starting point of the pterygomaxillary fossa.

Step 4. Make an incision with a 3 cm. trephine in the prominent portion of the sphenoid wing exposing the dura in the middle fossa of the base of the skull at a point to the outer side of and about midway between the foramina ovale and rotundum—near these foramina and below and to the outer side, the middle meningeal artery emerges from the foramen spinosum.

Step 5. After carefully detaching the dura from the bony wall of the middle fossa, the Gasserian ganglion and its three branches are exposed. Meckel's cavity, which should be recognized and opened before contacting the Gasserian ganglion and its branches, is incised along its outer aspect between the second and third nerves where they enter their foramina. The upper part of the roof of Meckel's space is gently opened by blunt dissection exposing the ganglion and its second and third branches upon the floor of this space. The floor is now detached from these tissues by blunt dissection until the ganglion is lifted from it. The dura is dissected on the inner side toward the first division where it contacts the cavernous sinus and sixth nerve. With blunt hooks, the second and third divisions are stretched and divided close to their foramina. With forceps, the body of the ganglion with the origins of the first, second and third divisions is torn out.

Step 6. Avoid wounding the middle meningeal artery. Temporary packing controls hemorrhage from the cavernous sinus, small arteries and veins. The wound is closed entirely if continuous packing is unnecessary; the structures, including the zygoma, are sutured back into normal position. The eye is relieved from all pressure by a rubber protective.

Comment. Serious hemorrhage is avoided by approaching the ganglion from below the middle meningeal artery. The necessity of a bone-covering is less here than in operations which reach the ganglion through the temporal fossa because of the small size and protected locality of the opening through the skull. The ganglion should not be removed until it has been freed from the envelope of reflected dura which should be done first, from above thus lessening the danger from hemorrhage. Oftentimes the sixth nerve is injured when the ophthalmic division of the nerve is freed; on account of its intimate relation, the sympathetic nerve is always hurt, but these accidents are rarely serious. Sometimes the zygoma is not sutured into position but is permitted to settle into a less prominent position as the muscles of mastication atrophy. Ligation of the middle meningeal artery is sometimes necessary.

NEURECTOMY

Acoustic Nerve

This is on occasion resorted to in intractable Ménière's disease. It consists of sectioning the eighth (auditory) nerve. Local or general anesthesia may be resorted to.

Step 1. Make a curved incision (Fig. 237-A) having its convexity upward and situated low over the occiput on the affected side. (Dandy.) Begin the incision laterally at the level of the tip of the mastoid process, curving upward and then medially and downward to the midline to a point on a level with its beginning. The muculocutaneous flap thus obtained is freed from the bone and retracted downward.

Step 2. Make an opening in the occipital bone of about 1½ inches in diameter over the posterior fossa of the skull and just medial to the mastoid bone. This affords the most direct approach to the cerebellopontine angle.

Step 3. Make a dura flap by an incision corresponding to that in the skin. Multiple radiating incision may, on occasion, be resorted to.

Step 4. Expose the cisterna magna and the lateral cistern; puncture these with an appropriate needle and evacuate the contents by suction. This affords a greater operative field and greatly facilitates retraction of the cerebellum.

Step 5. Retract the cerebellum, gently, medially; expose the seventh, eighth, ninth, tenth and eleventh basal nerves. The seventh (facial) nerve is practically covered by the eighth (acoustic) and cannot be seen until the latter is lifted from it by a small hook. The acoustic nerve is lifted gently upward and backward well away from the underlying facial nerve and then the acousticus is divided using a fine-pointed knife (Fig. 237-B). Sometimes, when deafness is not complete, an attempt is made to cut only the vestibular part of the nerve leaving the auditory portion intact.

Step 6. The dura may be closed or left open. It is never closed if radial incisions have been made. The muscle, fascia and skin are closed in layers. No drains are used.

Comment: Anomalies of the bloodvessels may add difficulties to the operation. Exposure of the eighth nerve may be hindered by an artery from the cerebellum which may cross it and even supply it with a twig. Occasionally a branch of the auditory artery may lie within the nerve and severing it will result in annoying hemorrhage. Temporary, and even permanent, facial paralysis may ensue. This may result from trauma to the seventh nerve during manipulations or from pressure by the swollen stump of the eighth nerve. Vertigo is, as a rule, abolished by this operation. Temporary unsteadiness or dizziness on suddenly moving the head, however, may be present following surgery but this gradually disappears. Tinnitus is not always completely relieved but it is usually favorably modified.

Neurectomy of the Glossopharyngeal Nerve

Division of this nerve is performed for glossopharyngeal neuralgia. Intracranial section of the nerve is the procedure of choice because here regeneration of the nerve is impossible and because possible injury to the vagus nerve is obviated. For these reasons the extradural route is not used.

Step 1. The nerve is exposed by the same steps as for exposure of the eighth nerve.

Step 2. As the cerebellum is gently retracted medially, the ninth, tenth and eleventh nerves can be seen converging toward the jugular foramen. The most anterior of the three is the ninth nerve. It is about 1 mm. in diameter and leaves the skull through a separate canal. It is caught up by means of a small hook and divided, using a fine pointed knife or scissors.

Step 3. The wound is closed in layers with the exception of the dura which is usually replaced and left alone.

CHAPTER 11

SURGERY OF THE SINUSES AND TONSILS

OPERATIONS ON THE SINUSES

FRONTAL SINUS

Extranasal Approach

There are enormous individual variations in the size and shape of the frontal sinuses, hence no operation should be undertaken here without a stereoscopic x-ray study. There are two methods of approach to the frontal sinuses: intranasal; extranasal. The intranasal approach is more dangerous than the extranasal route (limited space; distance of operation field). As a matter of fact the only advantage of operating intranasally is that the disfigurement resulting from

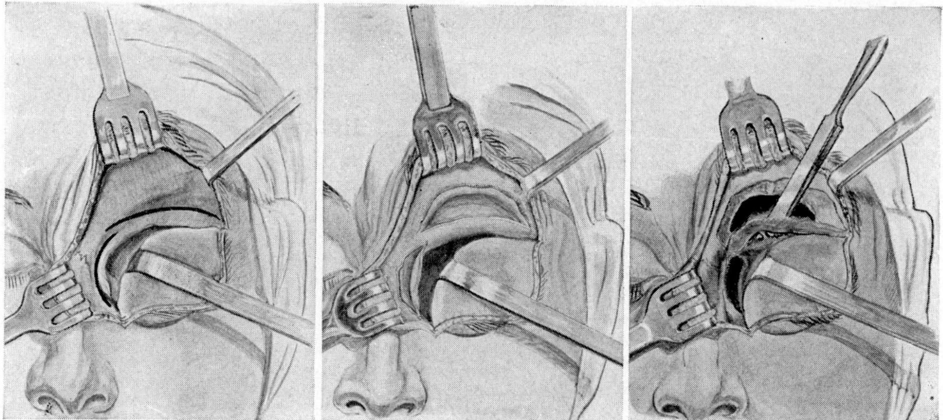

FIG. 238 FIG. 239 FIG. 240

FIG. 238. Killian's operation on the frontal sinus. Direction of incisions in the periosteum overlying the frontal sinus.
FIG. 239. Periosteum reflected, bone exposed ready to be chiseled open.
FIG. 240. Sinus opened.

the surface approach is avoided. Most modern surgeons abandoned the blind intranasal approach to the frontal sinus in favor of the external approach.

THE KILLIAN OPERATION

This is indicated in frontal sinus suppurations especially if complicated by disease of the ethmoid. It exposes and drains the frontal sinus by the external route. Local anesthesia. (Fig. 242.)

Step 1. Make an incision down to the bone extending along the whole length of the eyebrow just above the orbital margin. Continue the incision at its inner end down the middle of the nasal process of the superior maxilla (Fig. 238).

Step 2. Make two incisions in the periosteum (Fig. 239). The upper one is to be about 6 mm. above and parallel with the supraorbital margin and ends over the glabella; the lower one corresponds with the skin incision running along the supraorbital margin. Enter the sinus with a chisel and mallet.

Step 3. Make a furrow with the chisel and mallet through the bone immediately above and parallel to the margin of the orbit; with forceps remove the whole anterior wall of the frontal sinus above the furrow (Fig. 240).

Step 4. Clear out the sinus and remove its mucous membrane thoroughly.

Step 5. Standing behind the patient and having good illumination of the field of operation, make an opening with the chisel in the floor of the sinus avoiding injury to the supraorbital arch. After the opening is made remove the rest of the floor with a bone forceps.

Step 6. Resect the frontal process of the superior maxilla and the rest of the floor of the sinus.

Step 7. Resect the anterior and middle ethmoidal cells and the respective parts of the middle turbinates because these structures are usually also affected.

Step 8. Irrigate the wound with salt solution. Close the wound. Provide drainage with a rubber tube passing from the temporal end of the incision down through the external orifice of the nose.

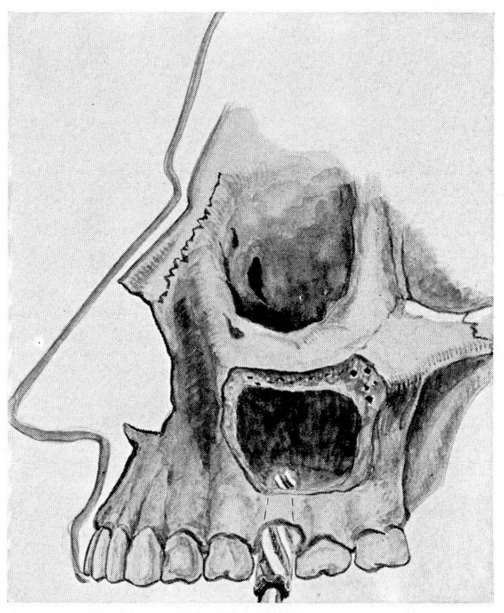

FIG. 241

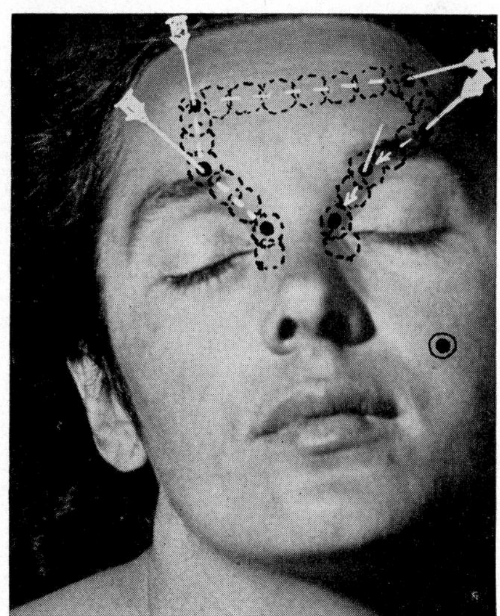

FIG. 242

FIG. 241. Oral operation on the maxillary sinus. Küster's operation through the alveolus.
FIG. 242. Method of block anesthesia of the frontal sinus. The isolated point on the cheek indicates infiltration blocks for operations on the maxillary sinus.

MAXILLARY SINUS

Empyema of the Antrum of Highmore (Maxillary Sinus)

Maxillary antrum suppurations usually result from propagated infection from the stump of a decayed tooth in the upper jaw or from an intranasal infection (Fig. 241). If dental, such an abscess may be temporarily drained by the extraction of one of the premolar teeth or, if nasal in source, by a drainage tube introduced from the nose into the sinus.

NASAL APPROACH TO THE MAXILLARY SINUS

Step 1. Local anesthesia suffices (Fig. 242). Puncture the nasomaxillary wall through the interior of the nose with a trocar. The point of the trocar (Fig.

243) should be turned outward, touching the nasal wall of the antrum under the inferior turbinate bone.

Step 2. Exert steady pressure until the instrument enters the antrum. Permit the pus to escape and wash out (irrigate) the antrum. If the opening is insufficient to allow free drainage, a window may be created with biting

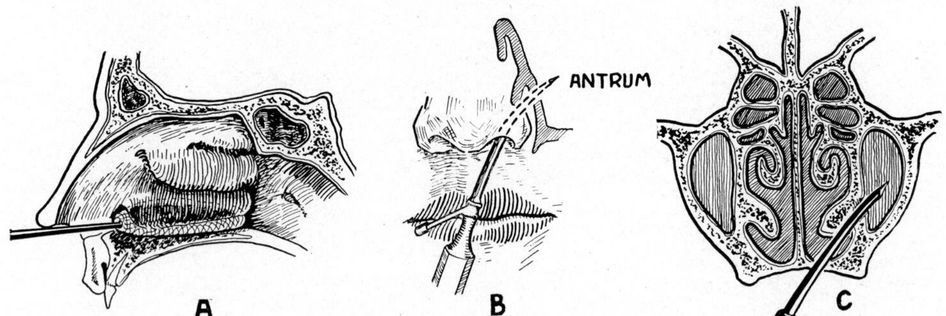

FIG. 243. A. Anesthetizing inferior meatus; applicator under inferior turbinate. B. Plunging trocar into maxillary sinus. C. Diagrammatic section showing trocar in maxillary sinus.

forceps. Sometimes a part of the inferior turbinate may have to be removed to facilitate free drainage.

Vail's intranasal operation consists of making a rather large circular opening in the naso-antral wall by means of the Vail saw. The steps of the Vail operation are as follows:

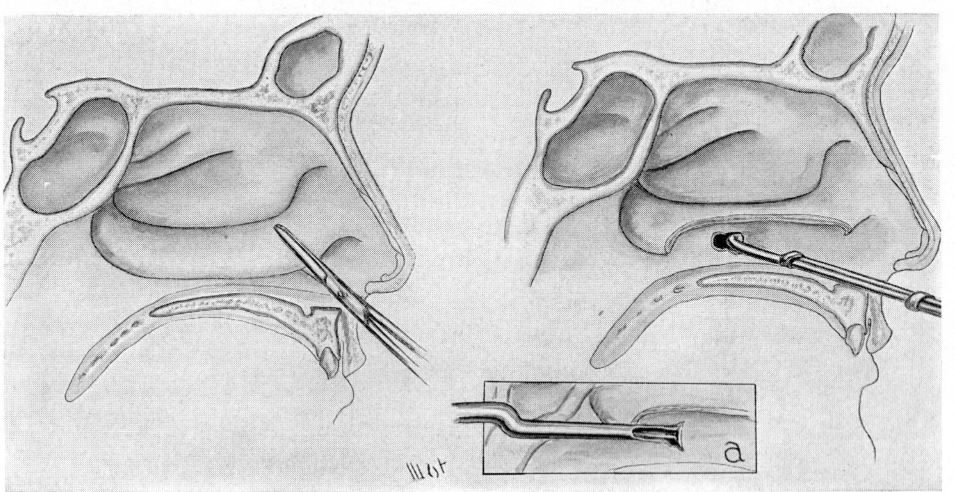

FIG. 244 FIG. 245

FIG. 244. Resection of the middle turbinate.

FIG. 245. Removal of nasal wall of maxillary sinus with Wagner's punch forceps. Insert: Opening of a sinus with chisel.

Step 1. The mucous membrane covering the naso-antral wall and the inferior turbinate bone is completely anesthetized by local application of cocaine.

Step 2. The anterior part of the inferior turbinate is now removed with a curved scissors. (Figs. 244-245.)

Step 3. The naso-antral wall is punctured at a low point with a perforator.

Step 4. The point of the instrument is introduced into the puncture, and an oval opening is made. The size of the aperture can be regulated by the surgeon and should be large enough to allow the removal of granulations which have a tendency to close the aperture.

In chronic cases more radical procedures are called for.

EXTRANASAL ROUTE (CALDWELL-LUC OPERATION)

Step 1. Use general anesthesia. Pack the cheek and mouth with gauze. Raise the upper lip and make an incision through the mucous membrane about ½ cm. below the gingivo-labial fold (Fig. 246). Cut down to the bone. Reflect the mucoperiosteum upward. Expose the canine fossa.

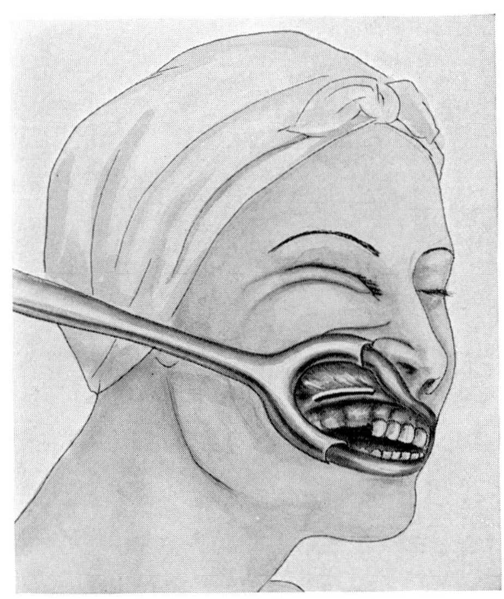

Fig. 246

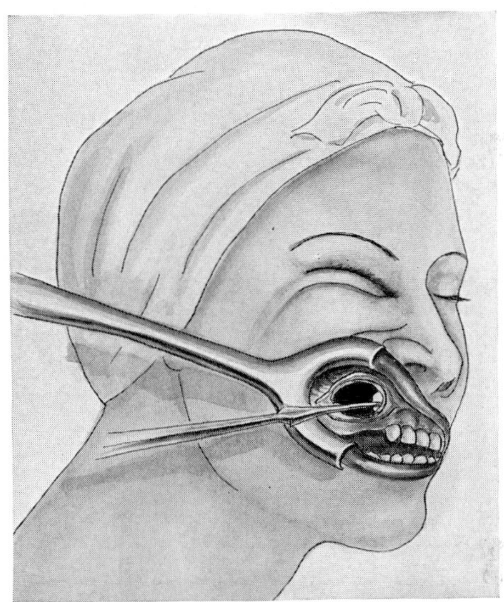

Fig. 247

Fig. 246. The Caldwell-Luc incision for operation upon the maxillary sinus.
Fig. 247. Caldwell-Luc operation on the maxillary sinus. The nasal wall of the maxillary sinus is broken through below the level of the attachment of the inferior turbinated bone.

Step 2. The bone forming the front wall of the upper jaw is then opened up by means of hammer and chisel, gouge or small trephine and freely removed by enlarging the opening with rongeurs to the extent of about half an inch. A counter opening is made from the inner wall of the antrum into the nose, making a hole into the latter cavity large enough to allow the passage of the tip of the finger (Fig. 247.) Free bleeding usually ensues immediately after opening the sinus; it is promptly controlled by adrenalin packing.

Step 3. The cavity is cleaned of pathologic products (curetted) and is tightly packed with gauze; the end of the gauze pack is brought out through the nostril and the cheek is allowed to fall into position without any sutures. The gauze is allowed to remain in place for one or two days and is then loosened gradually by irrigation with peroxide of hydrogen until the discharge ceases.

Generally, three operations are made use of for suppurations in the antrum of Highmore; these vary according to the degree of suppuration:

1. Tapping the antrum through the alveolar process.

2. The radical operation, as outlined above, in which the antrum is exposed through the canine fossa.

3. Drainage through the nose, here a portion of the naso-antral wall and inferior turbinate are taken away.

Intranasal Operations on the Frontal, Ethmoid and Sphenoid Sinuses

Anatomic Considerations. (Fig. 248.) The ethmoid cells consist of numerous thin-walled cellular cavities, duplicated within the ethmoid bone on either side, placed between part of the orbit which forms its outer wall and part of the nasal fossa which forms its inner wall. These cells are developed when the indi-

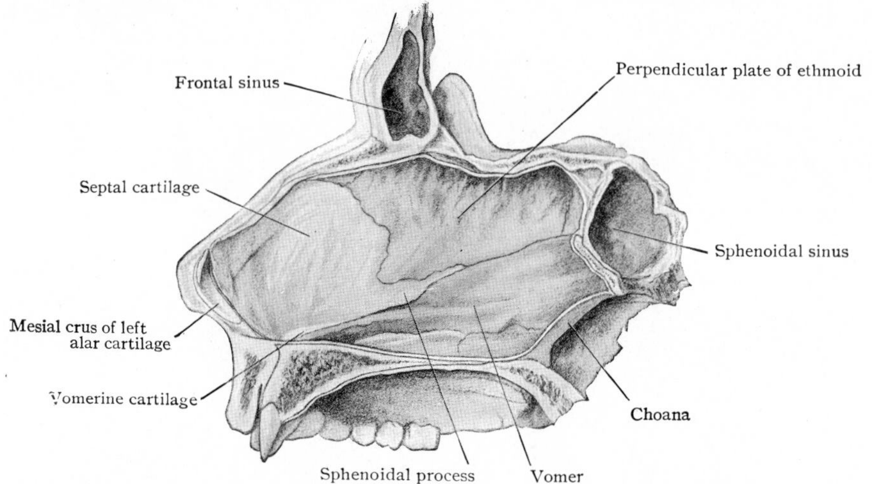

FIG. 248. Nasal septum viewed from left side; mucous membrane has been partially removed. (Piersol.)

vidual is five years of age. They are surrounded, superiorly, by joining with similar cellular cavities which bound the ethmoidal notch of the frontal; posteriorly, by joining with similar cellular cavities which consist of the sphenoidal turbinated bones and the orbital processes of the palate bones; anteriorly, by joining with the lacrimal bones and the nasal processes of the superior maxillae; below, by joining with the superior maxillae.

Descriptions of the ethmoidal cells vary; they are sometimes said to consist of three groups, walled off from each other, viz., anterior, middle and posterior; at other times they are said to consist of an anterior and posterior group. Independent openings or a common opening connect the anterior and middle cells with the fore-part of the middle meatus of the nose. The frontal sinus communicates through the anterior ethmoidal cells by way of the common infundibulum ethmoidale; when the communication is by a single opening, with the middle meatus. The posterior part of the superior meatus communicates with the posterior ethmoidal cells or sometimes with the sphenoidal sinus. On a few occasions the ethmoidal sinuses communicate with the maxillary sinuses.

Remove the anterior end of the middle turbinate.

Step 1. With a long-handled curet, enter the agar nasi cell which is situated just anterior to the anterior attachment of the middle turbinate. With a backward-downward motion, remove all of the ethmoid cells as far back as the sphenoid, care being taken to remain lateral to the middle turbinate, to avoid entering the cribriform plate. (Figs. 249-250.)

Step 2. The middle turbinate will then be hanging loosely in the nose and can be removed with a snare. The remnants of the ethmoid cells and mucosa are gently curetted until the orbital plate is felt to be perfectly smooth.

Step 3. The curet is now directed against the ascending process and the anterior cells removed. This gives an opening to the naso-frontal duct and a probe can be passed into the frontal sinus. With a Goode rasp, the naso-frontal duct can be enlarged. Care is taken to rasp forward only so as to prevent a stenosis of the duct and intracranial complications.

Step 4. When the ethmoid is completely exenterated, the front wall of the sphenoid can be easily seen. (Fig. 251.) The ostium is now enlarged with a curet and the entire anterior wall taken down with a sphenoid punch. (Figs. 252-253.) Some operators prefer a burr for this procedure. Care must be taken to avoid injury of the sphenopalatine artery which runs along the lower border of the anterior wall. Anomalous internal carotid arteries are occasionally found traversing the sphenoid cavity.

Step 5. When this operation is completed, it is best left unpacked, but in the presence of moderate bleeding, a light vaseline gauze pack is inserted; this should be removed in 24 hours.

External Operation on the Ethmoid and Sphenoid Sinuses

Step 1. This operation can be done under general or local anesthesia. If general anesthesia is used, a tampon is inserted into the nasopharynx to prevent the blood and debris from entering the trachea and bronchi.

If local anesthesia is desired, sufficient premedication is given. The eyelids are closed by a marginal suture of horsehair. One per cent novocaine solution in a syringe carrying a long needle is used. This is inserted through the upper lid and follows the superior medial bony border of the orbit for about 1½ inches. Injection is slowly made on the removal of the needle; the purpose is to infiltrate the anterior and posterior ethmoid nerves. Subcutaneous injection is made along the site of the incision described below.

Step 2. Make a curved incision from the supra-orbital notch about ⅜ of an inch medial to the inner canthus of the eye, and down to the lower edge of the nasal bone. This is carried down to the periosteum.

Step 3. The periosteum is divided and reflected laterally and medially by means of a periosteal elevator. The lacrimal sac is reflected with the periosteum, being turned laterally out of its bed in the lacrimal groove. The periosteum is elevated from the orbital plate of the ethmoid for about 1 inch. Here the posterior ethmoidal artery can be seen. This is ligated by means of the Yankauer instruments.

Step 4. Ferris-Smith self-retaining retractor is inserted to give adequate exposure.

Step 5. The ethmoidal cavity is entered through the lacrimal groove; the bone is thin here and can be entered with a curet. This opening is enlarged anteriorly and superiorly, the ascending process of the superior maxilla

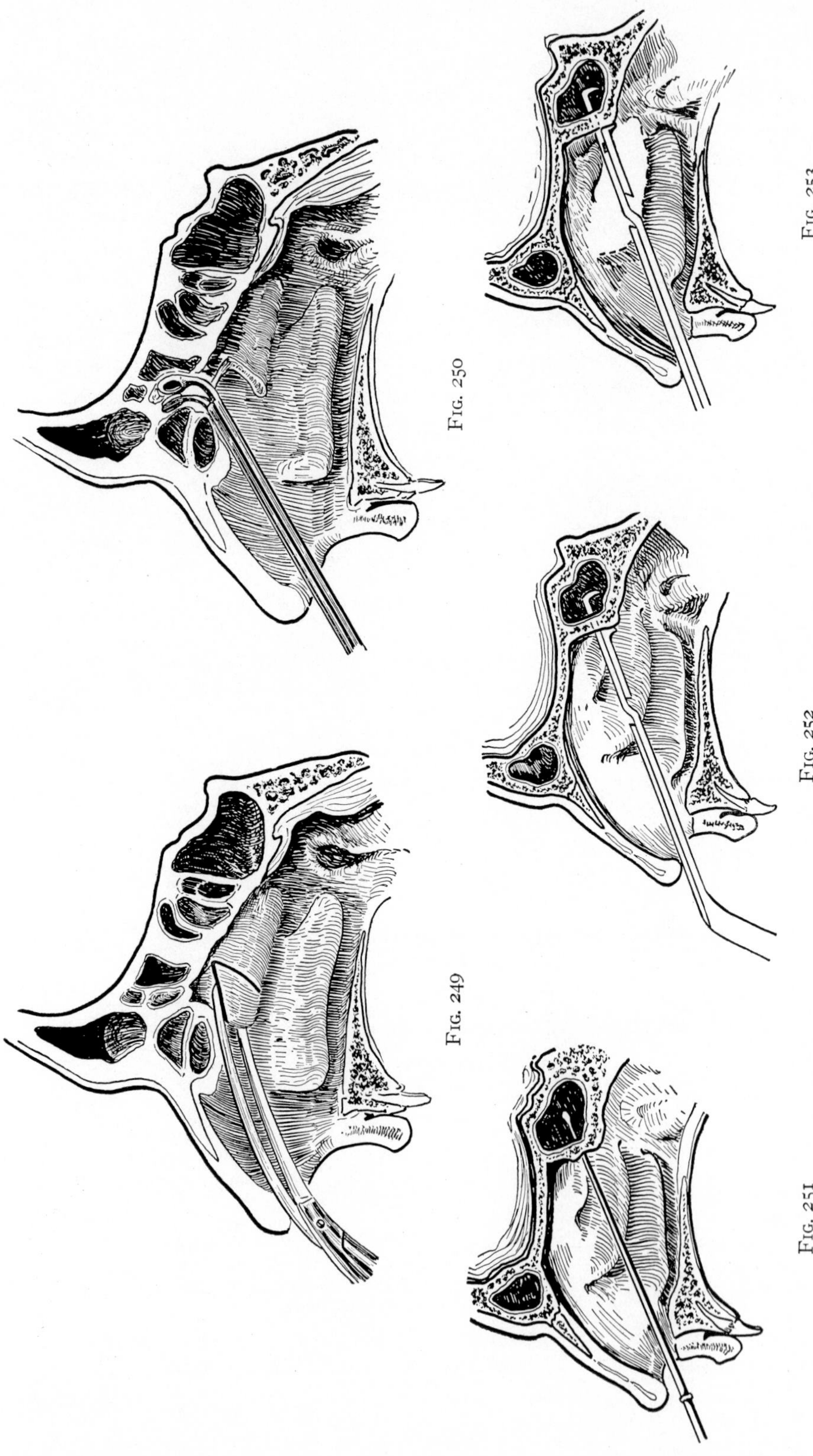

Fig. 249 Fig. 250

Fig. 251 Fig. 252 Fig. 253

Fig. 249. Removal of the ethmoid cells. Resection of the anterior end of the middle turbinate bone.

Fig. 250. Removal of the ethmoid cells. The anterior end of the middle turbinate has been removed. A double curette removed the ethmoid cells.

Fig. 251. Probing the sphenoidal sinus.

Fig. 252. Enlarging the sphenoid ostium with backbiting forceps. Turbinates intact.

Fig. 253. Opening of sphenoidal sinus. Enlarging the sphenoid ostium with backbiting forceps. Middle turbinate removed.

being removed with a Kerrison rongeur. This will give a good external approach to the ethmoid labyrinth.

Step 6. The anterior third of the middle turbinate is removed with a scissors and snare, through the nares. A Grünwald punch is introduced through the nose, and, by direct vision through the external opening, the ethmoid cells are removed. Care must be taken to remain between the attachment of the middle turbinate and the orbital plate, so as not to enter the cranial cavity in the region of the cribriform plate. The cells are removed until the orbital plate of the ethmoid and the roof of the ethmoid are perfectly clean. Anteriorly, the removal of the ethmoid cells exposes the opening of the naso-frontal duct and the frontal sinus can be entered with a probe.

Step 7. When the ethmoid is exenterated, the remaining portion of the middle turbinate is removed. This exposes the front wall of the sphenoid. The ostium is located and enlarged and the front wall is taken down.

Step 8. A small rubber tube is now passed from the sinus out through the nose, smeared with vaseline and covered with a Thiersch graft (skin side out) to points above and below the opening in the bone. This forms a drainage duct and at the same time the graft adheres to the underlying muscle and periorbita and prevents these structures becoming adherent to the bone. The skin is closed with silk and an eye-pad and a firm bandage applied to the eye. Beginning with the fifth day, secretion is removed by gentle suction. No intranasal dressing is used.

OPERATIONS ON THE TONSILS

TONSILLECTOMY

Anatomic Considerations. In theory the faucial tonsils are two oval-shaped collections of adenoid tissue located between the faucial pillars on either side of the oropharynx. They are from 20-25 mm. long, 15 mm. wide and 10 mm. thick. In children the tonsils generally appear as projecting, globular masses; if they project to any degree beyond the faucial pillars, they are enlarged. After middle life, the protrusion is usually negligible. The size of the deep surface is not indicated by the shape of the free surface. They are enveloped in a capsule which is intersected by a delicate layer of muscle fibers on both the deep and free surfaces. The layer from the free surface originates from the palatoglossus; the deep layer begins at the superior constrictor and extends to the tongue. The free surface contains numerous crypts varying in depth. The supratonsillar fossa is a small opening above the tonsil in front of which frequently appear numerous pits surrounded by adenoid tissue, buried under the anterior pillar behind and forming a pocket under a fold referred to as the plica triangularis.

Blood Supply. (Fig. 254.) The tonsils obtain their blood supply from different sources; tributaries from the ascending pharyngeal and facial arteries enter its base while branches from the descending palatine and lingual arteries enter it under the mucous membrane. The veins form a venous plexus connecting with those of the pharynx. The lymphatics connect with those of the dorsum of the tongue and the nodes found close to the angle of the jaw.

Nerves. The fifth and glosso-pharyngeal nerves furnish the nerve supply for the tonsils.

The pharyngeal tonsil is frequently referred to as the third tonsil. It is located in the posterosuperior wall of the pharynx and reaches its greatest size about the age of twelve, gradually diminishing in size after that. It is about 1 cm. thick mesially. Since the pharyngeal tonsil consists of many lobes, the swellings frequently occur around a central depression resulting in numerous pockets. The central one is often erroneously referred to as the bursa pharyngea. However, it has no relation with the canal from the mouth to the sella turcica. (Fig. 255.)

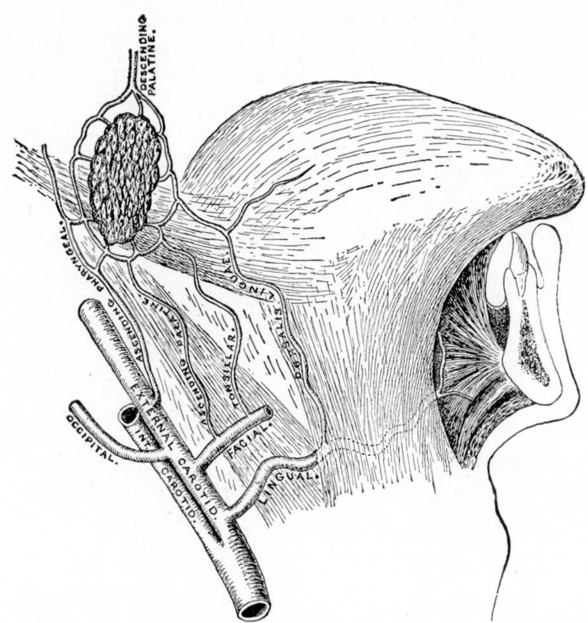

Fig. 254. Diagram illustrating blood supply of faucial tonsil (Davis, Applied Anatomy).

Anatomical anomalies in the tonsillar region while not common, do occur. The internal carotid may be in close relation to the outer surface of the tonsil, and

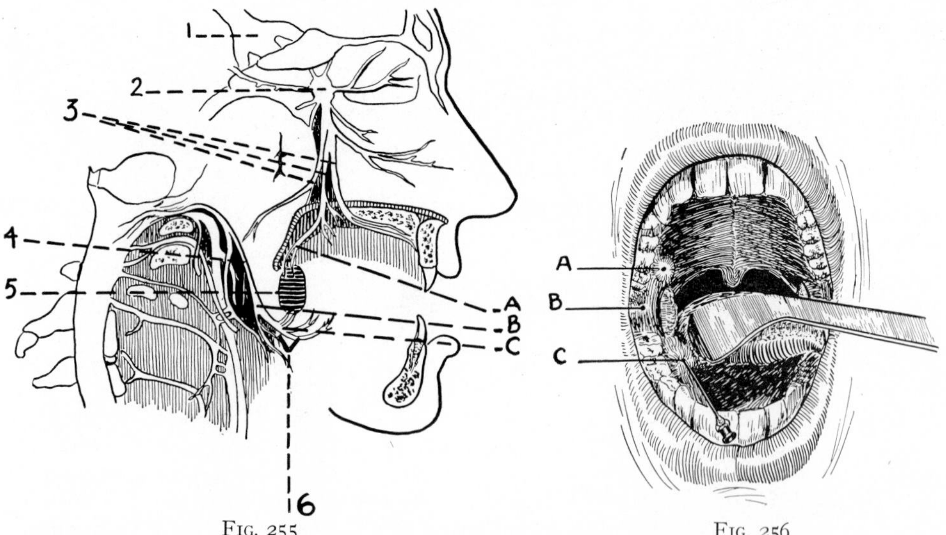

Fig. 255 Fig. 256

Fig. 255. Nerve supply of the tonsil (after Farr): A. palatine, B. glossopharyngeal, C. rami tonsillares; 1. semilunar ganglion (Gasserii), 2. sphenopalatine ganglion (Meckel), 3. anterior, posterior, and middle palatine, 4. glossopharyngeal, 5. tonsil, 6. rami tonsillares.

Fig. 256. Points of injection in tonsillectomy under local anesthesia.

occasionally a rather large artery is seen passing over its oral surface. Pathological changes (due to syphilis, tumors or disease of adjacent structures as well as aneurysm of the internal carotid artery, etc.) are quite frequent.

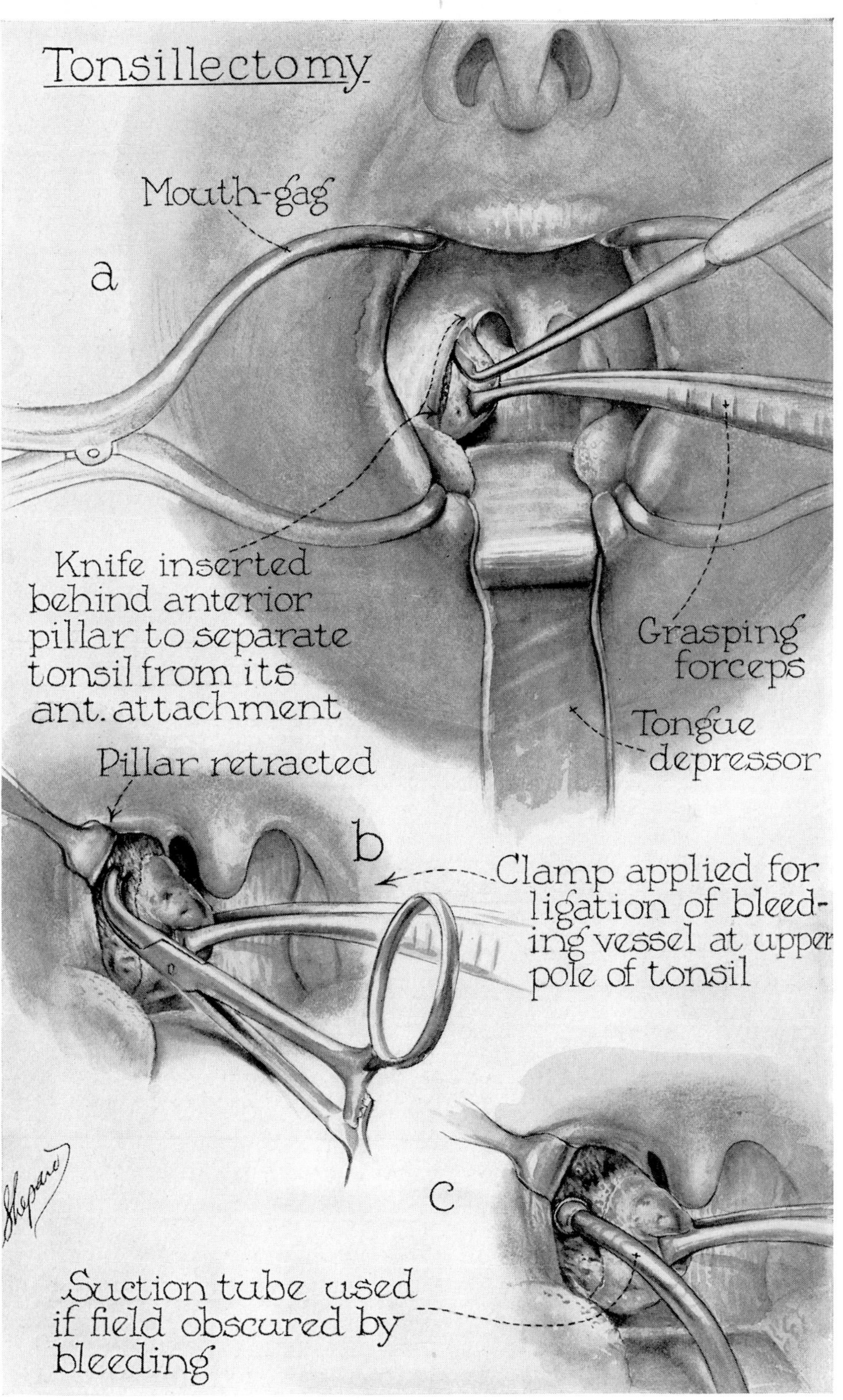

FIG. 257. Steps in tonsillectomy operation. (See next illustration.)

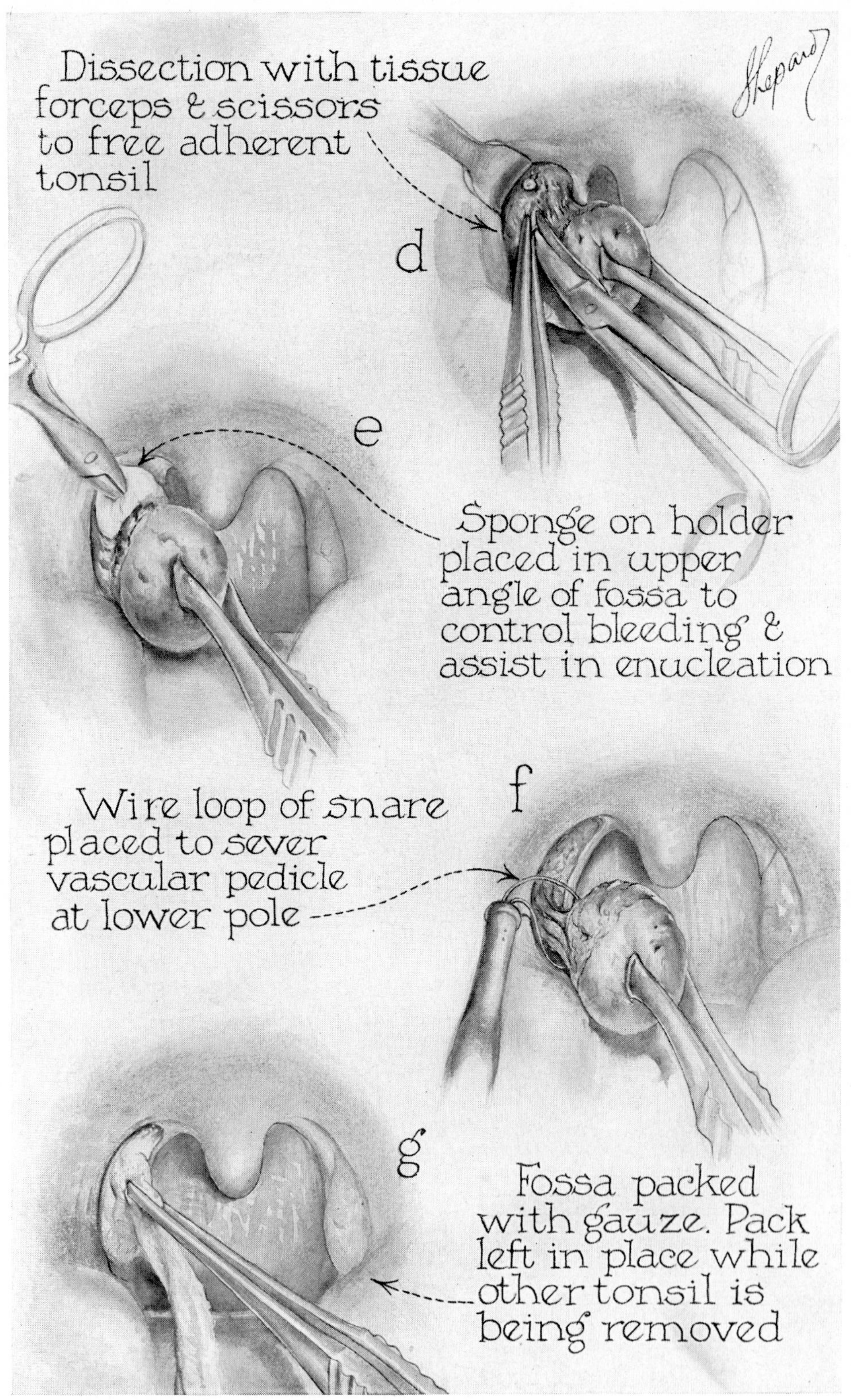

FIG. 257 (continued). Steps in tonsillectomy operation.

Anesthesia. For children under 15 years, use ether. Never use chloroform. Nitrous oxid and oxygen often give rise to uncomfortable cyanosis. Infiltration anesthesia with novocaine is frequently used in those more than 15 years of age. Neither the patient nor the surgeon should be of a nervous disposition when in-

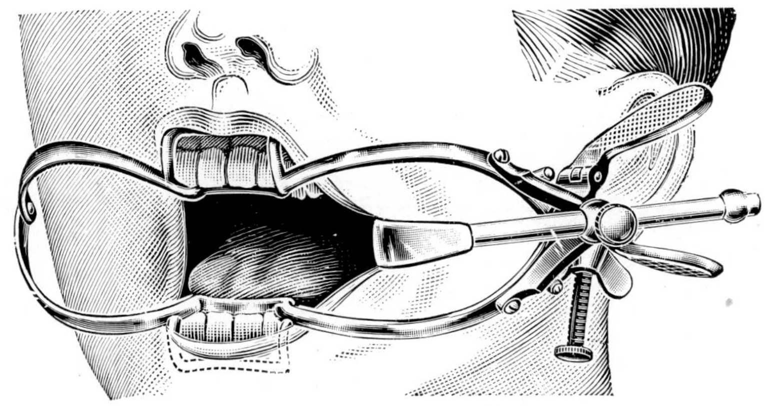

Fig. 258. Boettcher's modification of Jenning's mouth gag with Alter's lip retractor, Boettcher anesthesia tube and cheek retractor combined. Anesthesia tube, and cheek retractor are attached by means of a swivel socket and easily removable when not wanted.

filtration anesthesia is used. One-half of one per cent novocaine in a weak adrenalin solution should be used after first swabbing the fauces, pillars, soft palate, and the posterior pharyngeal wall with a 5 per cent cocaine solution. Quinine urea hydrochloride (2 per cent) may also be used. The solution used for infiltration should be freely injected into the pillars, the capsule of the tonsil and the extratonsillar space. (Fig. 256.)

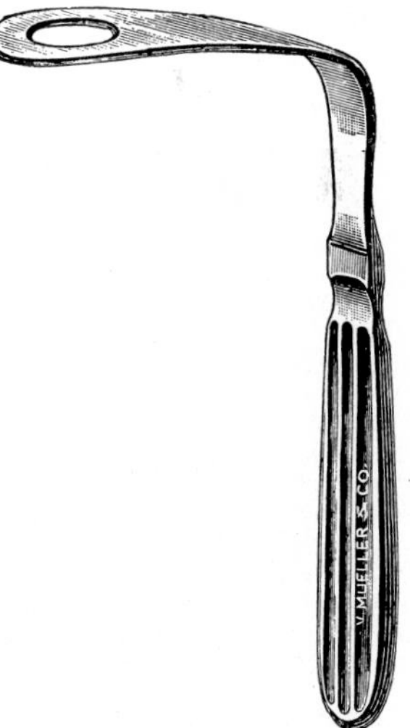

Fig. 259. Bosworth's tongue depressor.

Position of the Patient. When local anesthesia is used, have the patient in the sitting position. Under general anesthesia the reclining position with the head turned to one side is the only safe one. An anesthetized patient should never be put in the upright position.

Instrumental Dissection of the Tonsils. (Fig. 257A and B.) Three things besides the skill of the surgeon are necessary for the successful performance of this operation (a) a good anesthetist; (b) a skilled assistant; and (c) faultless illumination.

Step 1. Introduce a proper mouth-gag (Fig. 258) and depress the tongue (Fig. 259). Seize the tonsil with proper forceps or volsella and draw it toward the opposite side (Fig. 260).

Step 2. Incise the plica triangularis at its anterior border with a proper tonsil knife or proper scissors allowing the tonsil to be partly drawn from its bed. Pass a curved blunt instrument or the tip of the gloved forefinger into the exposed space and pass these rapidly above and external to the tonsil, stripping it from its bed and from the posterior pillar until it lies free, attached only by its vascular pedicle.

Step 3. Complete the removal of the tonsil by the snare (Fig. 261). Make sure that the loop of the snare is well placed. Clamp and tie bleeding points, if necessary. The opposite tonsil is then removed in a similar manner.

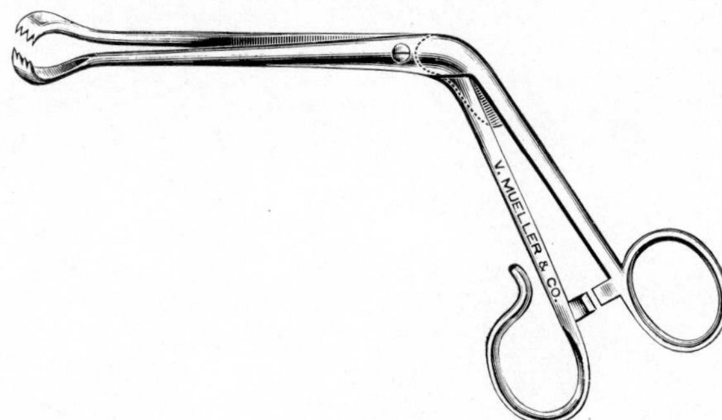

FIG. 260. MacManus' tonsil forceps. The jaws of this forceps are shaped so they will firmly take hold of the gland with the minimum amount of damage to the surrounding tissue.

There are many methods of dissecting the tonsils but the principles underlying the procedure are the same in all, viz., incision of the plica triangularis and blunt or sharp dissection of the tonsil.

The Sluder Guillotine Technic

Step 1. Place the patient in the upright position. Local anesthesia. Introduce the Sluder guillotine (Fig. 262) through the left angle of the mouth until the

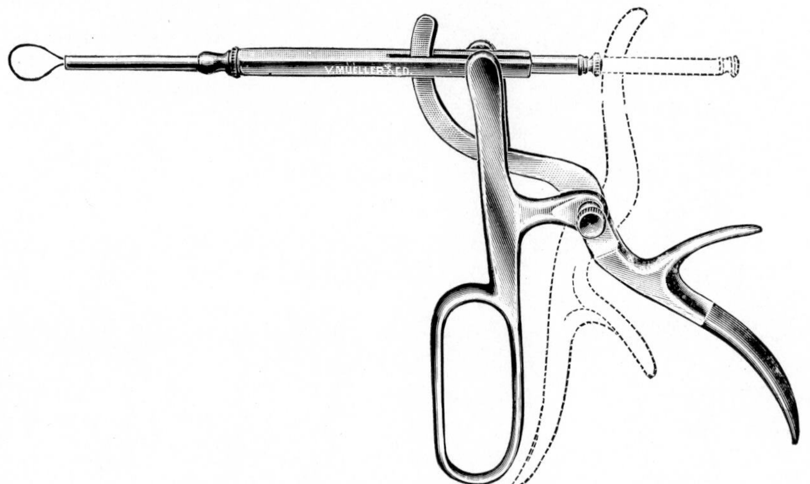

FIG. 261. Tydings' tonsil snare, original model.

far part touches the lower and back part of the tonsil. The instrument is held firmly against the structures which are displaced anteriorly and superiorly for about 2.5 cm. from the tonsil.

Step 2. The tonsil is pulled forward until the far border of the fenestrum of the instrument lies nearly upon the summit of the eminentia. The handle of the guillotine is then lowered sufficiently to bring the upper part of the border of the fenestrum into close contact with the lower part of the tonsil.

Step 3. The tonsil is pushed through the window of the guillotine by pressure with the finger from the surface overlying the tonsillar area, the blade of the instrument being slightly pressed against the anterior part of the tonsil to steady it while the rest of the tonsil is pushed through the ring. Advance the blade of the guillotine by thumb pressure until the tonsil passes through the fenestrum; the blade is further advanced until only the thin, soft mucous membrane of the anterior pillar and posterior pillar intervenes between the finger tip and the far border of the ring of the instrument.

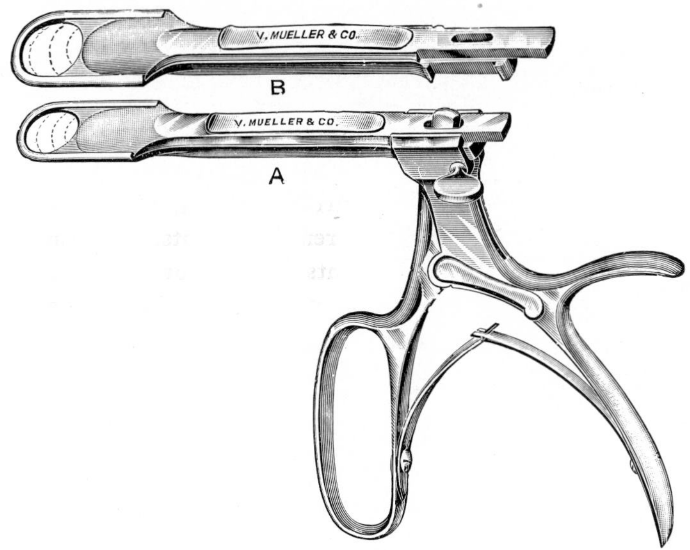

FIG. 262. Sluder's tonsil guillotine.

Step 4. Push the blade of the instrument firmly home, thus completely severing the tonsillar connections and bringing away the tonsil in its intact capsule.

Judging from the literature, complete success with the Sluder operation is attained in only about 60 per cent of the cases. The rounded, protruding tonsils, even although well buried, are easily removed by this method, but the flat, soft or very fibrous ones are difficult to dislodge, especially if the pillars of the fauces are infiltrated.

Dangers and Complications. Because many thousand pairs of tonsils are successfully removed daily in the civilized world, the operation, nevertheless, carries with it a certain degree of risk. It is not a minor operation. No operation is a minor operation if major catastrophes, though remote, may result. The removal of tonsils in physician's offices and out-patient clinics is to be condemned. Tonsillectomies, like other operations, require skill and experience. On more than one occasion have I turned my head when a general surgeon after completing (?) the operation removed much around the tonsil and left most of the tonsil behind. I have heard much of tonsils that "grew again" and I often wondered if so-called recurrences are really not tonsils incompletely enucleated.

Besides hemorrhage, shock and aspiration pneumonia, there remains the possibility of injury to the uvula, the pillars and the tongue. If, at the beginning, the right cleavage plane is found and is followed with care, there usually should be no difficulty except in "submerged tonsils" and in cases with much inflammatory infiltration.

The most dangerous complication of tonsillectomy is infection. The cavity resulting after the operation heals by granulation. Oral sepsis is responsible for infection to a greater or lesser extent. Fortunately the drainage here is free and, as a rule, the reaction following the operation is slight. The subparotid nodes swell occasionally but suppuration is rare. Nevertheless, general sepsis, while rare, is a possibility.

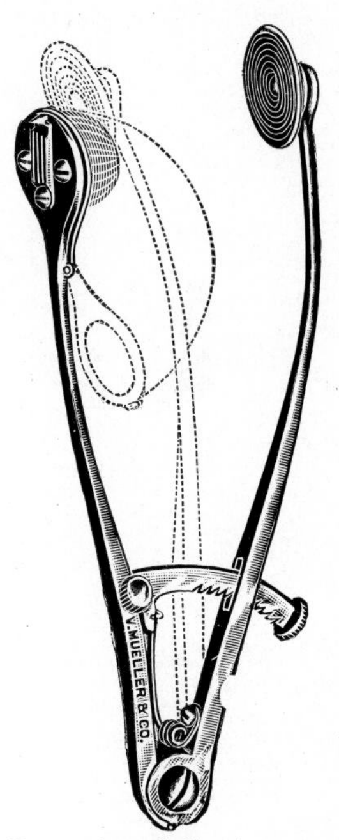

FIG. 263. Cullom's tonsil hemostat.

Hemorrhage immediate or delayed, is the most common complication. It is usually venous in type but may be arterial. Prompt recognition of the source of bleeding is essential. Treatment consists of removal of clots, compression by special instruments (Fig. 263), or clamping and ligating the bleeding vessel or suturing together of the anterior and posterior pillars or uniting them over a plug of gauze. It cannot be too strongly emphasized that a child will bleed at times even to death, without visible signs of hemorrhage (Bryant). Constant watchfulness is the only safeguard. Shock must be treated on general principles after the bleeding has been checked.

The immediate results of tonsillectomy are sore throat, pain behind the ears and dysphagia. A pseudomembrane forms in the tonsil-bed and healing takes place in about a fortnight. If the pillars have been injured, healing is considerably delayed. Not much harm follows partial removal of the anterior pillar—the patient usually complains that his tongue is tied to the roof of his mouth. Injury or removal of the posterior pillar results in more or less serious impairment of the singing voice. Mediastinal complications and aspiration pneumonias are more frequent following tonsillectomies than is reported.

REMOVAL OF PHARYNGEAL ADENOIDS

Anatomic Considerations. (Fig. 264.) The pharyngeal tonsil is a mass of adenoid tissue lying back of the soft palate, between the eustachian tubes, and extending from the base of the occiput to the lower edge of the axis, being separated from the bone by the pharyngeal aponeurosis and the superior constrictor of the pharynx. It varies greatly in shape, from the flat and fibrous to the rounded and soft protruding mass. Similar but smaller patches of lymphoid tissue are to be found scattered all over the pharynx and even the posterior surface of the posterior pillars of the fauces, from which it may readily be seen that the complete removal of adenoid tissue from the throat is an impossibility. The points of surgical interest are the posterior edge of the vomer above, the internal openings of the Eustachian tubes on either side, and the uvula in front. (Fig. 265.)

Step 1. Put the patient in the Rose position (Fig. 266). Extend the head moderately. Insert a mouth gag separating the jaws widely. Introduce the left forefinger into the nasopharynx; hook the uvula out of the way.

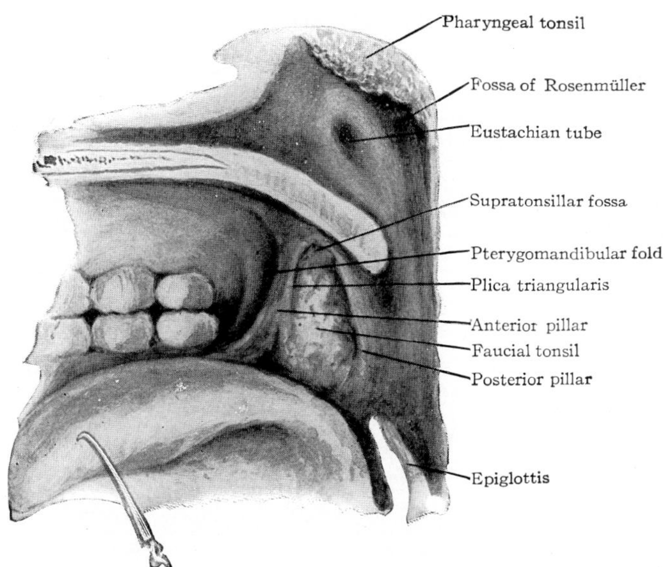

Fig. 264. Lateral view of the faucial tonsil and pharyngeal region. (Davis, Applied Anatomy.)

Step 2. Insert the adenoid curet carefully until you feel the vomer; depress the handle of the instrument as far as possible. With one sweep of the instrument, curet downward, thus removing briskly the main mass of adenoids. A dull curet or too light pressure will not accomplish the object. Experience and judgment must be the guides. Too great pressure will cause injury to the pharyngeal aponeurosis or even to the vertebrae.

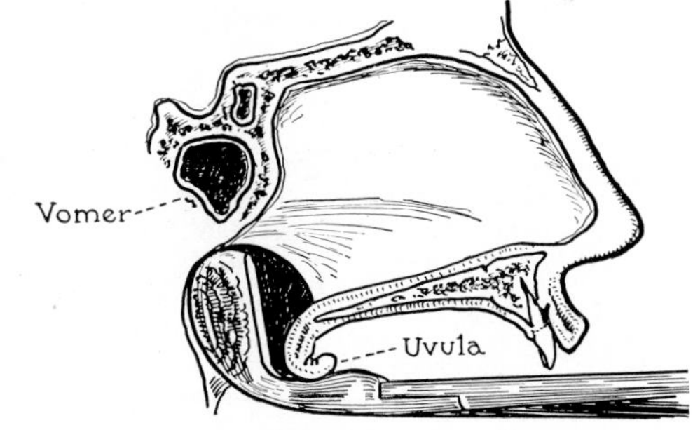

Fig. 265. Anatomic points of interest in removal of adenoids. Position of adenoid curet in removing adenoids.

Step 3. Repeat the same maneuver on either side of the median line, pressing the curet well over into the lateral sulci. The forefinger is then passed well up into the posterior nares on either side and remnants of adenoid tissue searched for which should also be removed with the curet. Clear the space with dry sponges.

Comment. The principal danger of the operation is aspiration pneumonia. To avoid this, operate quickly and turn the child promptly on its face. Clumsy work jeopardizes the uvula and may injure the vomer, the vertebrae or the Eustachian tubes. Use judgment in wielding the curet.

Injury to the Eustachian orifices should be avoided for it may eventuate in otitis media. Acute septic meningitis and death have been known to follow. An adenotome may be used instead of a curet. (Fig. 267.)

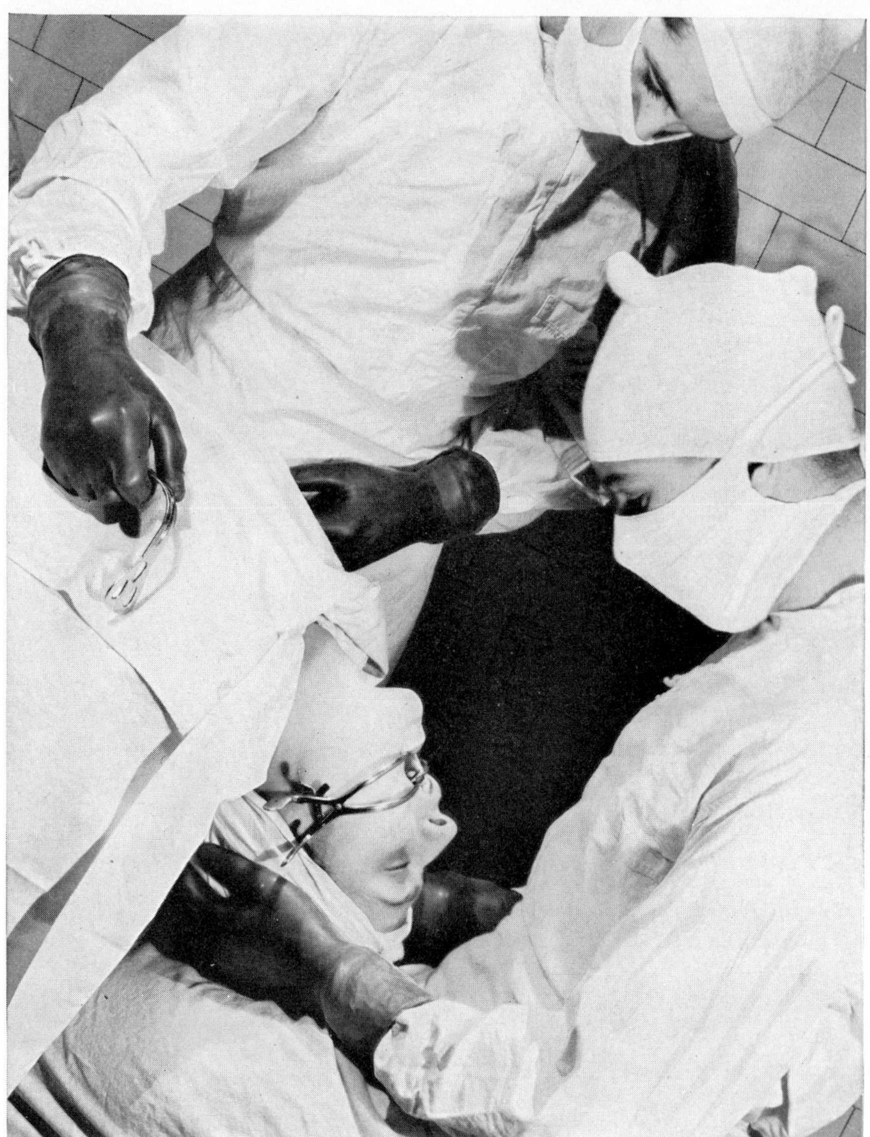

FIG. 266. Rose's position of the head for operations on the palate or oropharynx.

REMOVAL OF THE LINGUAL TONSIL

The lingual tonsil rarely requires operative treatment. It may be removed by suitably curved punch-forceps, or by a curet.

INFECTIONS

PERITONSILLAR ABSCESS

Chance punctures in the region where the pus "ought to be," more or less probing before pointing, are methods to be condemned. Where the abscess is definitely "pointing," a slight incision and dilatation of the opening are sufficient. In "blind cases" it is much better to insert a curved blunt instrument behind the anterior pillar and separate it from the tonsil. A whiff of nitrous oxide should be used in the latter case. Operate in the stage of analgesia after

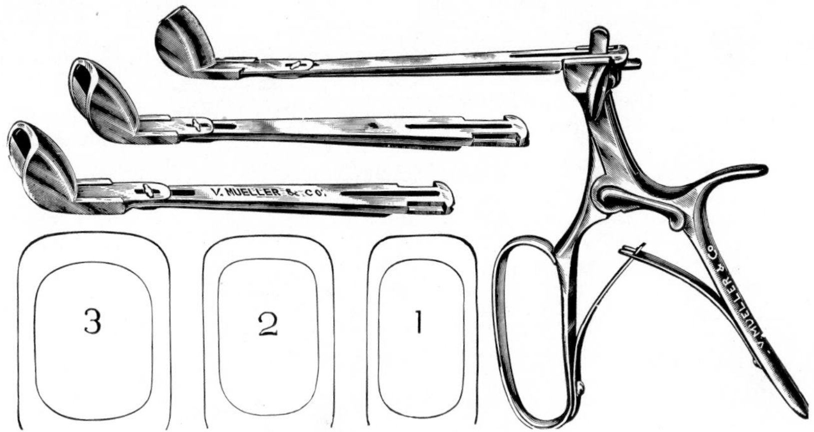

Fig. 267. LaForce's adenotome.

consciousness has returned. Aspiration of pus may be followed by serious consequences. Drainage by this method is efficient.

OPERATIONS FOR RETROPHARYNGEAL ABSCESS

The opening and draining of retropharyngeal abscesses may be accomplished by the intra-oral route or the suppurative focus may be approached through the exterior of the neck. When the abscess is of ordinary size and the patient can still open the mouth, the intraoral approach is generally employed.

Step 1. Locate the fluctuating point with the index finger in the posterior pharyngeal wall, through the opened mouth. Make a controlled stab-incision alongside the guiding finger, preferably in the median line (Fig. 268). Wrap the blade of the cutting knife with zinc oxide adhesive plaster to within a short distance of its point, thus controlling the depth of the incision. When pus issues, the incision is enlarged as the knife is withdrawn.

Step 2. Irrigate and drain the abscess cavity.

Cervical Approach for Retropharyngeal Abscess

A. POSTERIOR ROUTE

Step 1. Prepare the skin surface and locate the posterior border of the sternomastoid muscle.

Step 2. Make an incision along the posterior border of the sternomastoid, beginning at the mastoid process and descending as far downard as deemed necessary. Incise the fascia and ligate the superficial vessels. Avoid the transverse and descending superficial cervical nerves. With a blunt dissector, follow the anterior surface of the scalenus anticus muscle, thence through the connective tissues until the outer border of the longus colli muscle is reached. Pass beneath the longus colli, reaching the prevertebral areolar tissue of the retropharyngeal space; evacuate the pus. This route is comparatively free of important structures.

Step 3. Establish free drainage from the bottom of the wound.

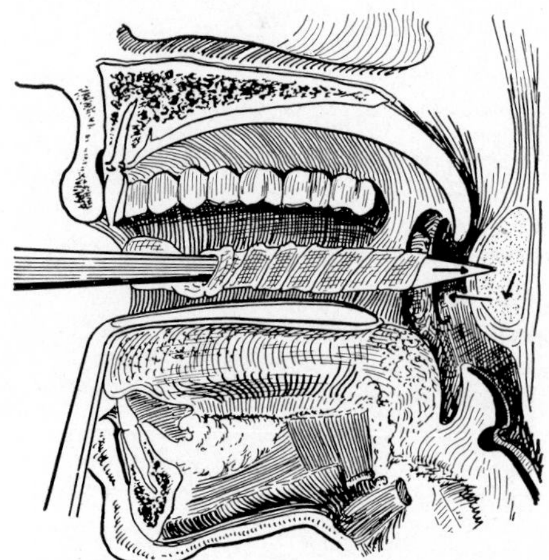

FIG. 268. Opening retropharyngeal abscess.

B. ANTERIOR ROUTE (BUCKHARDT'S OPERATION)

Step 1. Approach the retropharyngeal space by an incision made along the anterior border of the sternomastoid muscle on the level of the larynx. This incision passes in front of the great vessels of the neck. Retract the vessels and the sternomastoid muscle backward and the thyroid, larynx, trachea and anterior cervical muscles forward, thus exposing the fascia covering the longus colli muscle passing anteriorly to it, transversely across to its inner side, into the retropharyngeal space.

Step 2. Evacuate the pus.

CHAPTER 12

SURGERY OF THE LIPS, TONGUE AND LYMPH NODES

SURGERY OF THE LIPS

PLASTIC SURGERY OF THE LOWER LIP—CHEILOPLASTY

Triangle or V-Resection

Anatomic Considerations. The lips are formed chiefly by the interlacing fibers of the buccinator and orbicularis oris muscles and connective tissue. The lips are covered on the outside by skin and on the inner aspect by mucous membrane. Blood Supply: The coronary branches of the facial (external maxillary) artery which freely anastomoses with its opposite fellow. The blood vessels lie superficially beneath the mucous membrane.

Step 1. General or infiltration anesthesia with 1 or 2 per cent novocaine with adrenalin. The shoulders and head of the patient are elevated and the head, slightly flexed, rests on a firm pillow or sandbag.

Step 2. Murphy's intestinal clamps are applied as near the angle of the lower lip as possible. Complete incision through the lip should be made. Each of the two incisions forming the "V" should be made with one cut of a sharp scalpel and the excision should result in a very acute angle. (Fig. 269 A, B, C and D.) In making the incisions, the scalpel is introduced into the lip not quite at right angles with the skin, sloping inward, so as to remove a larger portion of skin than mucous membrane. The coronary artery is ligated, in order to control hemorrhage. Slight venous oozing is of no moment. If the portion removed is not more than a third of the lip, it is possible to secure satisfactory approximation without much pull on the united tissues.

Step 3. Three or four fine silkworm-gut or silk sutures are generally inserted at right angles to the skin down to but not through the mucous membrane and are sufficient to give perfect apposition and stop all oozing. Perfect alignment of the vermilion border and of the skin is necessary. Doyen believed that a stronger and firmer lip results when the mucous membrane is sutured first, then the skin, with all the sutures placed superficial.

CARCINOMA OF THE LOWER LIP

The general principles underlying the treatment of carcinoma of the lip are those observed elsewhere—free excision of the primary growth and the lymph nodes draining the area involved. In early cases good results are often obtained from electrocoagulation of the primary lesion followed by thorough irradiation of the areas draining the affected field. When should the lymph nodes be removed? Some surgeons complete the entire operation (removal of the growth, removal of lymph nodes and the plastic reconstruction of the lip) in one sitting. I prefer graded operations, because they are safer for the patient and because one can work in an aseptic field without fear of infection from the mouth.

Each step of the operation being of necessity a prolonged one (particularly in advanced cases), the best interests of the patient are served by painstaking graded operations.

Inoperable cases are best left alone. The degree of involvement should be gauged before operation is undertaken. If after beginning the operation the surgeon finds that fixation is considerable, it is wiser to abandon the operation

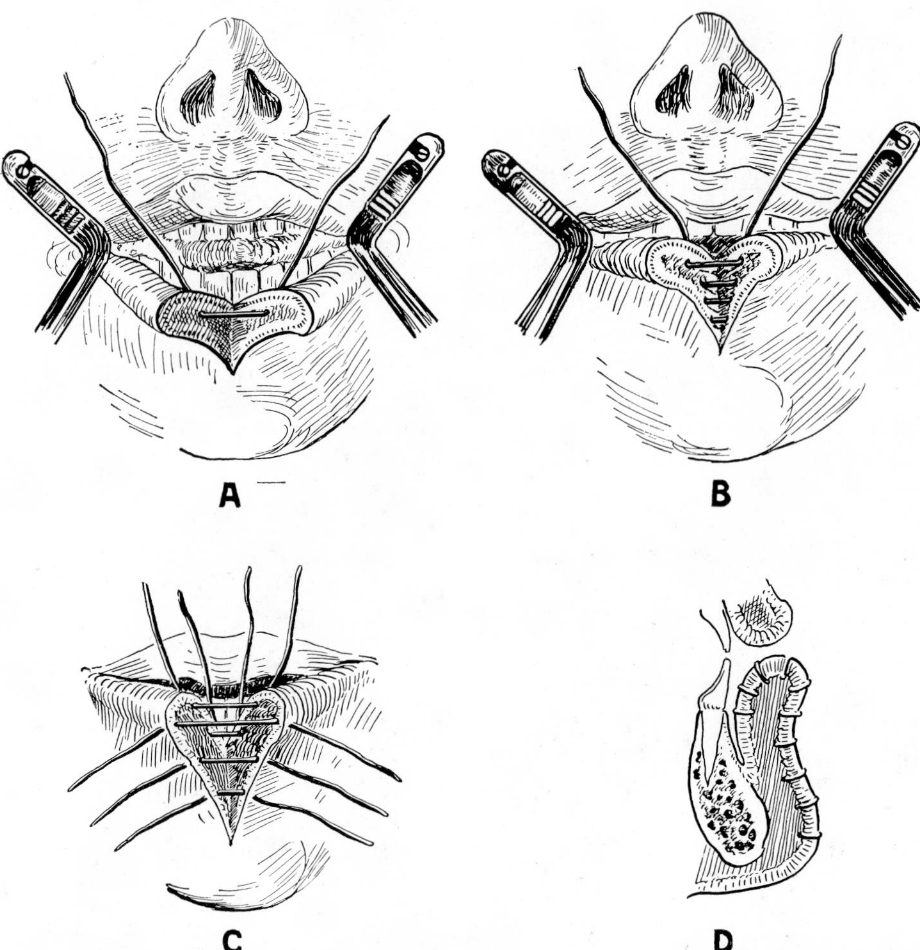

Fig. 269. A. V-shaped resection of lip. Placing of first muco-mucous suture. B. Suture of vertical portion of mucous membrane is almost completed. C. Diagram showing the position of the mucous and cutaneous sutures. D. Cross section of completed operation.

and close the wound. A precipitate catastrophe may thus be averted. In such cases the benefits of radiation (deep x-ray, radium) should be accorded the patient.

Comments. The sooner a correct diagnosis is made and the malignancy removed the better the prognosis. A thorough knowledge of the anatomy of the parts is essential. Opinions as to results of forms of treatment differ. According to Waring, radium is of no value. He considers diathermy more effective. Stevens is partial to electrocoagulation. Kennedy believes radium to be the sovereign remedy for carcinoma of the lip. Perthes prefers x-rays; he favors radium for inoperable cases. I am inclined to disagree with Waring. The appended photographs tell their own story (Figs. 270-271-272).

Dogmatization is obviously dangerous. Careful selection of cases and the use of a combination of properly indicated and selected methods will give the best results.

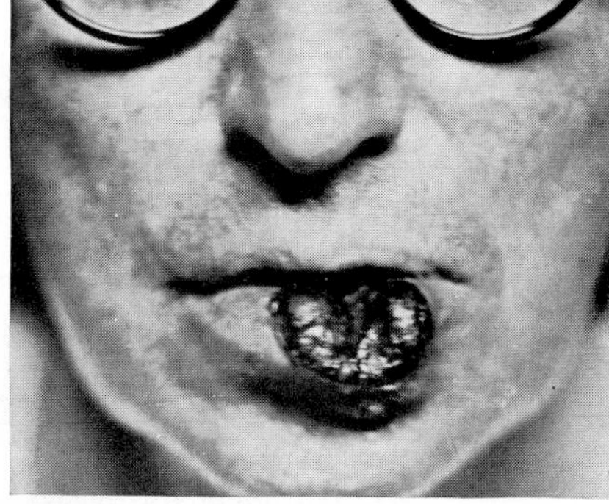

FIG. 270. Squamous-celled carcinoma of lip.

Olan R. Hyndman in discussing carcinoma of the lip concludes as follows:[1]

"1. About 80 per cent of epidermoid carcinomas involving not more than one-half of the lower lip will not be associated with regional metastases. The indiscriminate use of radical surgical intervention and irradiation is neither necessary nor to the best interest of these patients.

"2. A small percentage of carcinomas of the lip are nonkeratinizing and metastasize early. In these cases there are not more than 50 per cent of cures. It is the impression that these lesions arise from the buccal mucous membrane and bear the characteristics of buccal carcinomas elsewhere, while the relative benign, keratinizing cancer of the lip bears the characteristics of epidermoid carcinomas of the skin in general.

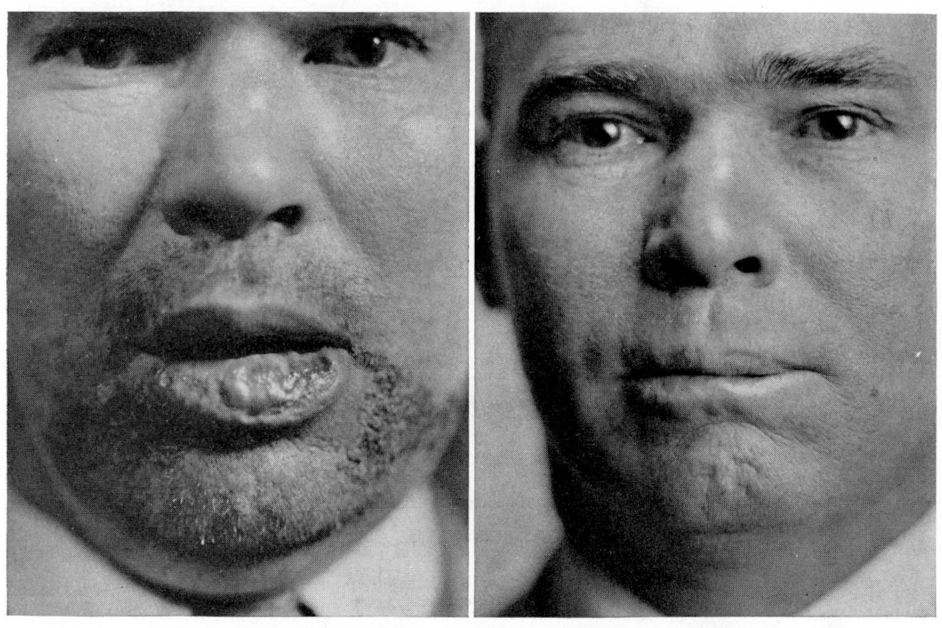

FIG. 271 FIG. 272

FIG. 271. Carcinoma of the lip, January 29, 1935; submaxillary lymph nodes palpably enlarged.

FIG. 272. Same patient as in previous illustration, April 16, 1935; after radium treatments.

[1] Arch. of Surg., August, 1933, Vol. 27.

The operation consists of three phases, viz., removal of the lymph nodes, removal of the tumor, and restoration of the contour of the lip. It is best to remove the lymph nodes first, then the tumor. The primary removal of the lip and restoration of its contour often lulls the patient to a sense of false security. He feels that no second procedure is needed and refuses further intervention. This often leads to disastrous consequences.

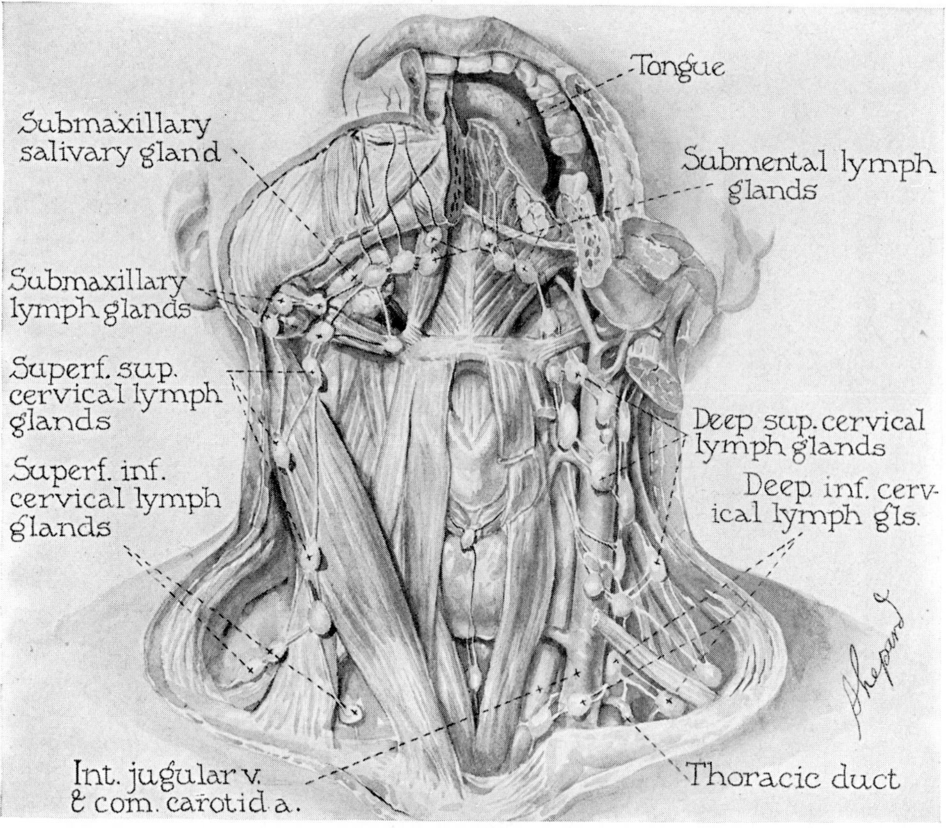

FIG. 273. Lymph vessels and nodes of the tongue, submental, superficial and deep cervical regions.

In advanced cases, all lymph nodes as well as the submaxillary salivary glands should be removed.

Removal of Lymph Nodes of the Neck

A thorough knowledge of the position of the lymph nodes and their topographic relationship is of utmost importance (Fig. 273). For convenience the lymph structures are divided into three main groups:

1. The superficial cervical nodes.
2. The deep superior groups.
3. The deep inferior groups.

Anatomic Considerations. The superficial cervical lymph nodes are rather small and inconstant and may be divided into three sub-groups: A. The external jugular nodes, situated along the external jugular vein, receive afferents from the pinna of the ear and the parotid region; they open into the superior deep cervical nodes. The anterior superficial cervical nodes, inconstant and variable in situation (anterior surface of larynx, anterior and lateral surfaces of trachea), receive afferents from the larynx and trachea. Their efferents drain into the lower deep cervical nodes. B. The superior deep cervical nodes are ten to sixteen in number and are situated along the internal jugular veins beneath the sternocleidomastoid muscle; they are united by stems and extend from the mastoid process to the posterior belly of the omohyoid muscle. The principal lymph node of the tongue belongs to this group. It is constant in position (opposite the bifurcation of the common carotid artery). They receive afferents from the posterior auricular, occipital, retropharyngeal, parotid, submaxillary and submental nodes, also from the tongue, nasal mucosa, palate, pharynx and larynx. C. The inferior deep cervical nodes also called supra-clavicular nodes. They lie below the omohyoid and rest upon the scaleni muscles and the tracheal plexus. They receive afferents directly from the superior deep group, the integument of the lower part of the neck, the upper part of the pectoral region, the occipital region and the tip of the tongue. Their afferents form the jugular lymphatic trunk which opens on the right side into the right lymphatic duct and on the left side into the thoracic duct. Both the right and the left trunk, however, frequently open directly into the subclavian vein.

Note. In applying to clinical practice the anatomical connections of these and other lymph nodes, it should be remembered that in disease the lymphatic vessels may become obstructed and the lymphatic flow thereby reversed. Widely separated groups are thus liable to be involved and an enlargement of the nodes on the side opposite to that of the lesion are rather frequent.

Step 1. The incision must be so planned as to afford a thorough exposure (Fig. 274). It follows the line of the sternomastoid muscle and has another incision joining it at right angles and extending forward to the chin. (Butlin's incision.) Free the skin from its underlying surfaces up to and slightly above the border of the mandible. The whole outer surface of the parts to be removed is now exposed to view.

Step 2. Remove the contents of the submaxillary triangle (submaxillary and submental nodes, areolar tissue, fat and nodes). Begin the dissection from below, at a considerable distance from the enlarged nodes. Clear the muscular floor of the space of all connective tissues. Dissect carefully, step by step, in an upward direction. The mass dissected en bloc is now turned outward.

Step 3. Ligate the facial and lingual arteries when encountered. The common facial vein is also ligated. The submaxillary duct is delivered and ligated as near the mouth as possible. Carcinomatous lymph nodes may lie between the salivary gland and the jaw, being firmly attached to the periosteum. These should be removed, of course, together with the platysma, and if need be, with the periosteum of the mandible.

Step 4. In deep dissections of the neck care must be taken to preserve the hypoglossal, spinal accessory, descendens hypoglossi, recurrent laryngeal and, in very deep maneuvers, the vagus nerves. The carotid, the superior and inferior thyroid arteries, and the jugular veins and their branches must be respected. If the surgeon is working in the left supraclavicular fossa he should avoid the thoracic duct.

Step 5. In more extensive dissections for recurrences appearing in the upper part of the neck, the result of carcinoma of the mouth or originating from branchial cysts, the whole lymph-node bearing area from clavicle to mandible should be removed. In such cases the sternomastoid muscle is divided at its clavicular attachment. Both the external and internal jugular veins are ligated and divided. Avoid injury to the phrenic nerve. The dissection is carried backward and the whole fascia is lifted away from the deep muscles of the neck. The entire dissection is best accomplished from below upward.

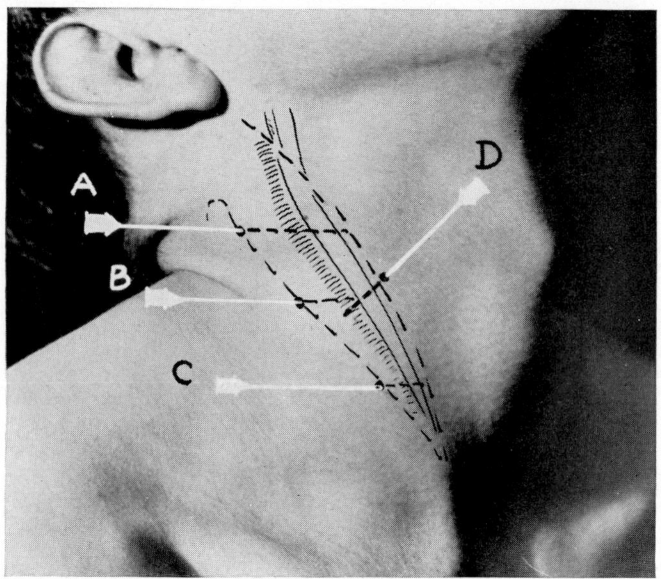

FIG. 274. Block dissection of the lymph nodes of the neck. Needles A, B & C indicate deep infiltration of the novocaine solution in front of the carotid sheath. Needle D deposits the solution between the carotid sheath and the trachea. (After Hertzler.)

Removal of Carcinoma of the Lip

Step 1. The shoulders and head of the patient are elevated, the head is slightly flexed and is made to rest on a firm pillow or on a sandbag.

Local or general anesthesia is given. The coronary arteries may be controlled by an assistant by pressure with the fingers and thumb. Aspiration of blood should be avoided. The incisions should be made at least ¼ inch from the tumor. Bleeding vessels are picked up with delicate, pointed hemostats.

By referring to Fig. 275 a good idea is gained of the principles of the operation. Figure 275 (a) depicts the triangular resections necessary to accomplish the desired result. Observe particularly that the distance 1-1 plus 2-2 equals the distance 3-3. The incisions should be traced as shown in the illustration. The size of the triangles depends upon the size of the tumor to be removed.

Step 2. Resection of the tumor-bearing area is now done and other triangles are fashioned. The mucous membrane of each triangle is preserved (Fig. 275c).

Step 3. The sutures are placed in such a manner as to approximate 1-1 and 2-2. The entire thickness of the lip, excluding the mucous membrane, is

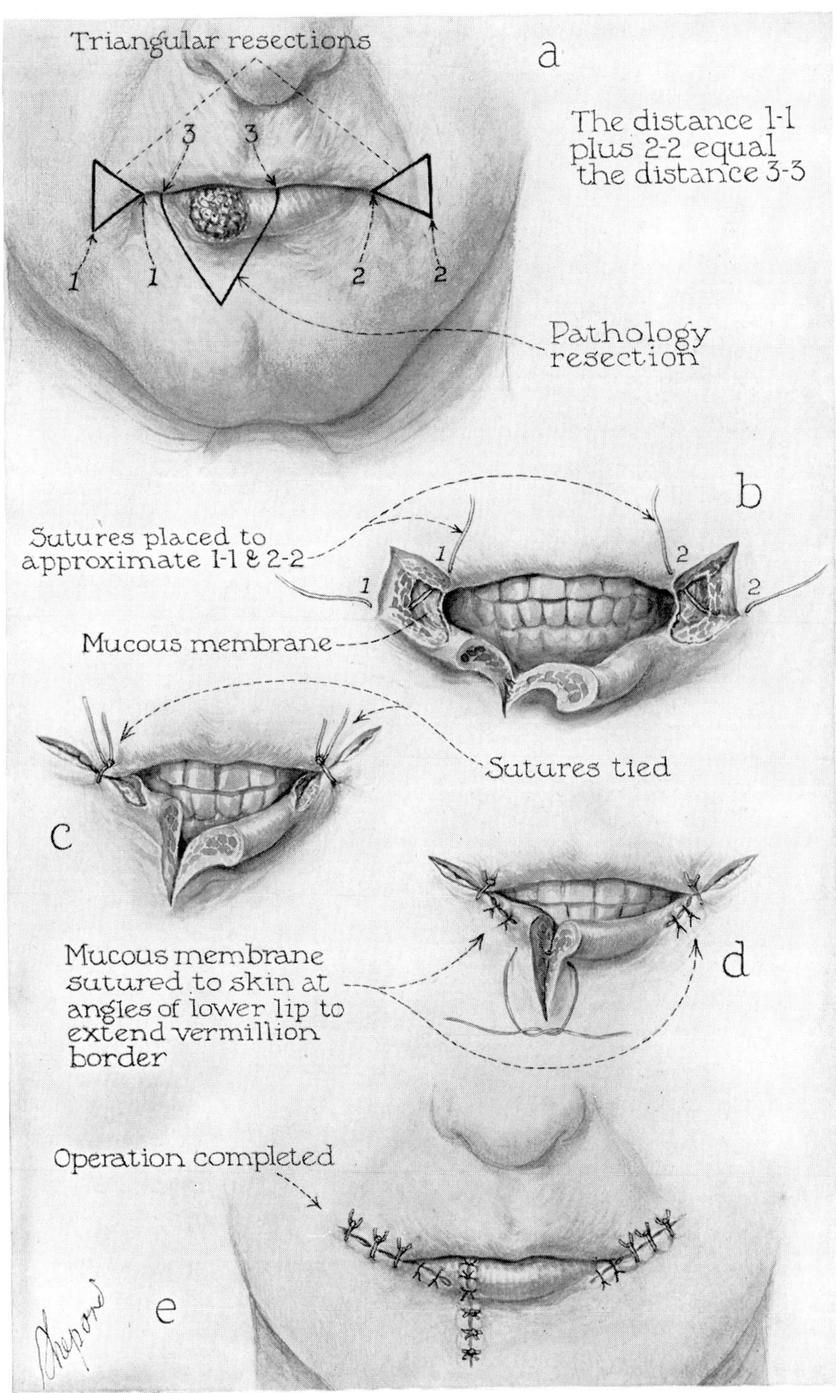

FIG. 275. Excision cancer of the lip.

embraced by the sutures, using delicate silkworm gut or Pagenstecher linen. The mucous membrane (Fig. 275c) is united to the skin by interrupted linen sutures in such fashion as to form the vermilion border (d) after being trimmed into proper shape.

Step 4. Vertical resuturing of the lower lip is now begun. Interrupted sutures unite the mucous membrane. Three or four such sutures usually suffice, depending on the extent of the resection. The skin is next approximated, the first suture being placed at the junction of the skin with the mucous membrane. Care should be taken that the labial commissures be properly reconstructed. Strangulation of the tissues should be avoided. Approximation only is necessary. Attend to hemostasis. Aim at a good plastic result. (Fig. 275e.)

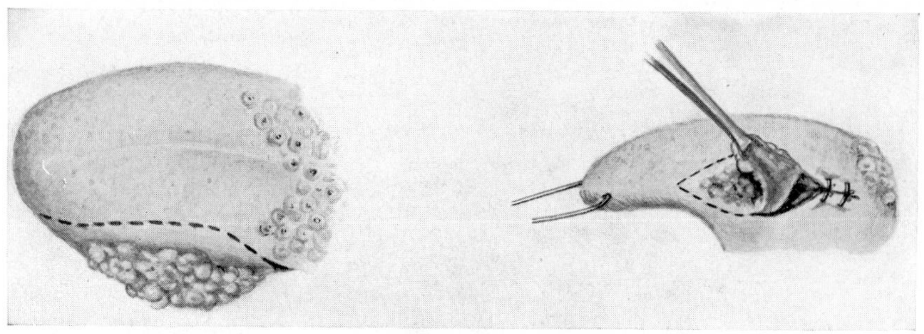

FIG. 276 FIG. 277

FIG. 276. Removal of tumor from the lateral margin of the tongue. Outline of portion to be resected.

FIG. 277. Same operation. The dissection proceeds from the back forward. Sutures placed.

OPERATIONS ON THE TONGUE

REMOVAL OF ANGIOMA OF THE TONGUE

If the size of the tumor is not excessive it may be excised after injecting a sterile 3 per cent novocaine solution all around it. Bleeding is slight unless the ranine arteries are severed. Suture the edges with silk—this also helps to control hemorrhage.

Electrosurgical methods or radium often yield gratifying results. In large-sized tumors, use general anesthesia (intratracheal).

Step 1. Open the mouth with a gag.

Step 2. Pass a silk loop through the tip of the tongue and pull it forward. An assistant should exert pressure on the tissues immediately outside of the anticipated wound.

Step 3. Quickly dissect out the growth with scissors followed by

Step 4. Suturing with catgut bringing the raw surfaces together and checking hemorrhage. If better approximation of the surface epithelium is desired, additional sutures may be inserted. Use a mouth wash frequently until healing takes place. (Figs. 276-277.)

ACUTE ABSCESS OF THE TONGUE

Step 1. Use general anesthesia through nasal tubes. Make free incisions into the affected substance of the tongue and prevent the inflammatory process from extending to the cervical planes. The incisions should be made in the long axis of the tongue on each side of the median raphé and, if necessary, should extend to the foramen cecum. Make the incisions deep enough to separate the submucous fibers, thus lessening tension.

Step 2. Open deep abscesses with blunt artery forceps. Keep the abscess cavity open for a short time by means of an appropriate drain.

RANULA

Ranula (Fig. 278) is a cyst of salivary origin situated in the tissues of the floor of the mouth. They may be either sublingual or submaxillary depending

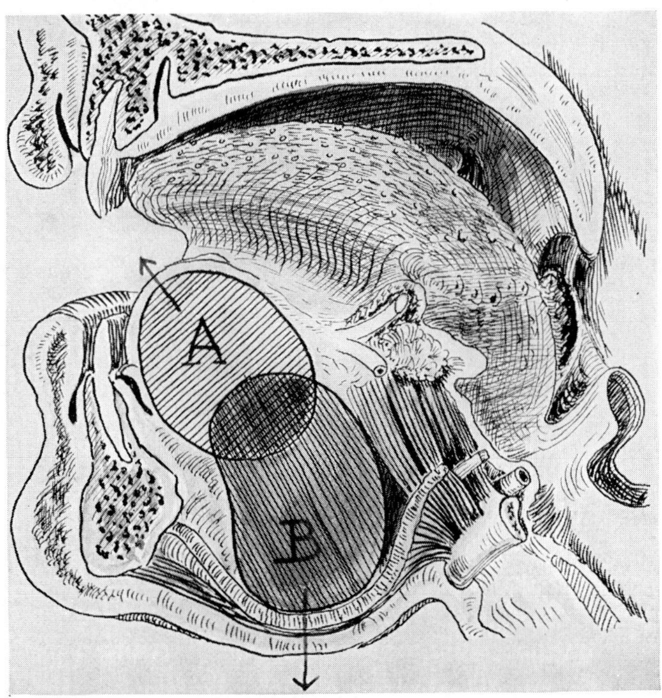

Fig. 278. Diagrammatic drawing of the evolution of a ranula. A. Upward toward the frenum linguae. B. Downward toward the submaxillary region.

upon the respective position they occupy. The cysts have a thin wall and are of bluish color and are generally derived from the mucous glands of the mouth or from the incisive glands. Occasionally, they are derived from either the duct of Wharton or one of the ducts of Rivini. Dermoid cysts in this region are occasionally met with. They are generally derived from the upper part of the thyroglossal duct.

Step 1. Separate the jaws with an appropriate mouth gag. Engage the tongue in a proper tongue forceps. Pull it out of the way.

Step 2. When the cyst is small, excise as much of its wall as possible. These cysts can only rarely be dissected out entirely although this should be attempted. The content of the cyst is usually a thick, glary mucoid fluid. The portions of the cyst wall which cannot be removed should be treated with the application of a strong solution of silver nitrate or thermocauterization.

Step 3. Where complete dissection of the cyst is possible the wound in the floor of the mouth should be united with interrupted linen sutures which are removed after about three days.

DERMOID CYSTS

Dermoid cysts in this region are removed by making an incision in the median line from the chin to the hyoid bone. Separate the mylohyoid muscles; divide the other deeper structures until the capsule of the cyst is exposed. Dissect it out bluntly. Close the wound, avoiding dead spaces. Drain, if deemed advisable.

REMOVAL OF FOREIGN BODIES FROM THE TONGUE

When x-ray or palpation confirms the suspicion that a foreign body such as a sharp piece of metal, wood or bone is lodged in the front part of the tongue, the mouth is rendered aseptic and a piece of sterile gauze is used to hold the tongue forward.

Step 1. Inject a few drops of 2 per cent novocaine solution over the most sensitive part and make an incision with a scalpel down to the foreign body. Hemorrhage may be controlled by pressing with the fingers on either side of the incision.

Step 2. If possible, the foreign body should be removed in the opposite direction from which it entered the tongue. The incision should be sutured with silk and drainage, provided if the wound is a large one; otherwise, the incision is permitted to heal without suturing. If the foreign body is lodged in the back part of the tongue, general anesthesia may be necessary. Have a tracheotomy set ready in case of unexpected emergencies.

TONGUE-TIE

Where the frenum is so short that the tip of the tongue cannot be protruded beyond the lower gum-line (interference with nursing), divide the frenum, remembering while doing so the ranine arteries located beneath the mucous membrane on the under surface of the tongue on each side of the frenum. Immediately under the ranine vessels on the floor of the mouth are the sublingual vessels.

Step 1. In order to avoid these vessels, inject a few drops of 1 per cent novocaine solution into the frenal region, elevate the tip of the tongue and sever the frenal band with a scalpel.

Step 2. If this is not sufficient to bring up the tip of the tongue, enlarge the incision posteriorly exactly in the middle. Control hemorrhage with a ligature of fine catgut carried on a small curved needle and passed immediately under the wound. Leave the incision open.

An antiseptic mouth wash should be used several times daily.

Comment. Look out for hemophilia; several fatalities have been reported from this cause. If the infant is able to nurse satisfactorily, postpone the operation until the baby is about 6 months old.

Acquired Tongue-Tie. This usually results from scar tissue formation following infections. The tongue becomes attached to the mucous membrane of the gums or cheeks. Sever these attachments under novocaine anesthesia. Incise carefully. Interpose sterile rubber strips between the freshened surfaces until tissue granulation ensues, thus avoiding reunion of the raw surfaces. Maintain oral asepsis.

EXCISION OF THE TONGUE

Removal of the tongue, either in whole or in part, is indicated whenever malignant conditions within the limits of operability are present; these include primary carcinoma or sarcoma of the tongue in the early stage; lymphangioma, nevus and macroglossia of the tongue; although non-malignant tumors, may, according to their severity, size and stage of progression, be indications for removal of a greater or lesser segment of the organ.

In all cases of malignant disease of the tongue an attempt should be made to remove the cervical lymph nodes which receive the lymph vessels from that portion of the tongue which is involved in the disease as well as the fascial tissues surrounding them. The submaxillary gland should also be removed because, if it is left behind, the nodes associated with it usually escape notice. When the lingual artery is ligated to control hemorrhage, the lymph nodes associated should be removed at the same time.

Except in cases in which less than half of the tongue is removed, it will be found, as a general rule, better technic to carry out resection of the tongue as the primary operation and then a fortnight or so later, to remove the lymph nodes and tissues in the neck. Some surgeons prefer the opposite.

No matter whether the operation is a partial resection or a complete excision of the tongue, the greatest attention must be given to place the oral cavity in a surgically clean condition, as a preliminary to operation. All defective teeth should be removed. These precautions are necessary in order to frustrate, as far as possible, any provocation to septic pneumonia. For the same reasons special precautions must be taken during the operation to prevent the swallowing of blood. Some surgeons prefer to do a preliminary laryngotomy. In most cases it will suffice to plug the lower part of the pharynx with a sterile marine packing material and to use a suction apparatus during the operation for the removal of blood and fluids.

Both before and following the operation the mouth should be washed out several times daily with a suitable antiseptic solution. This may be done easily by suspending an irrigator filled with the antiseptic solution above the head of the patient's bed and attaching to the irrigator a long rubber tube controlled by a clip and ending in a glass nozzle. The patient can thus irrigate his mouth at frequent intervals by holding his head over a receptacle for the reception of the ejected solution. Not less than a week should be spent in this preparation, if the mouth is unclean, unless contraindicated by more important considerations.

The operations usually carried out on the tongue are:

1. Resection of a wedge-shaped piece.
2. Resection of half of the tongue.
3. Excision of the whole tongue.

The first is only permissible for a benign tumor or for a malignant condition of quite recent date and entirely limited to the lateral margin of the tongue. Most other early cases, if limited in extent, i.e., where the disease has not extended to the fibrous tissue which forms the median septum, and is still operable, can be sufficiently dealt with by resection of half of the tongue. In extensive cases of malignant disease still within limits of operability, excision of the whole tongue is called for. Nitrous oxide and oxygen anesthesia, administered intratracheally through a tube, is usually the best for these types of operation. If contraindicated use massive infiltration anesthesia at the base of the tongue (Fig. 279).

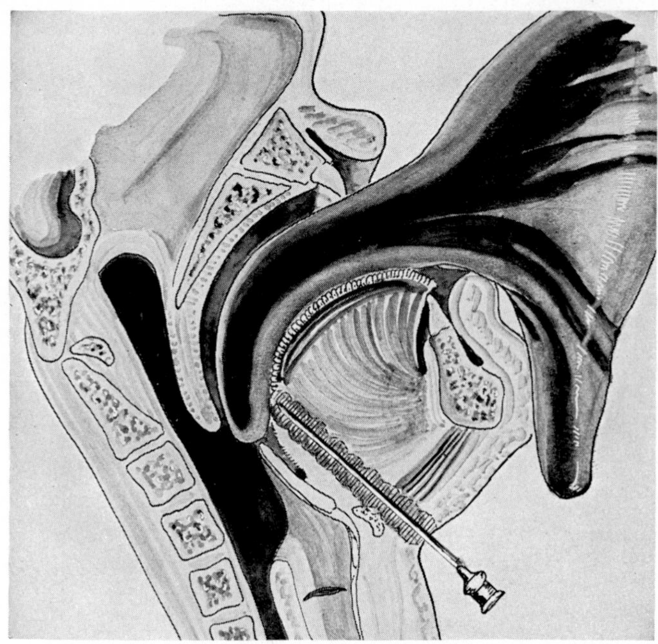

Fig. 279. Massive infiltration at the base of the tongue for operations on the tongue.

Macroglossia

REMOVAL OF A WEDGE-SHAPED PIECE OF TONGUE

This is a pathologic increase in the size of the tongue and demands operative correction; the same operation is used for delimited, benign growths. (Figs. 280-281.)

Step 1. Circumscribe the section of tongue to be removed by two semi-elliptical incisions.

Step 2. Perform a cuneiform resection of the segment thus outlined with a scalpel or scissors. Spurting blood vessels are seized with Kelly artery forceps and secured by ligatures carried on curved needles of appropriate size.

Step 3. Approximate the raw surfaces of the tongue with interrupted silk or Pagenstecher linen sutures. Aim at exact coaptation. The bite of the needle must be deep to avoid dead spaces at the bottom of the resected segment.

Chronic Glossitis

BUTLIN'S MARGINAL RESECTION

This operation is indicated where the tongue is too large for the mouth and where it shows signs of being irritated to a dangerous degree by the teeth.

Handley's modification of Butlin's operation does not require laryngotomy. The anesthetic is given in the same manner as for cleft palate operation.

Step 1. For purposes of traction and control, the tongue is drawn well back by a strong silk suture. (Fig. 282.)

Step 2. Make a transverse incision about 1½ inches long in the dorsal aspect parallel to the end of the tongue. Make a corresponding incision on the under surface. Excise a wedge-shaped piece through these incisions but leave the piece fastened by its two ends to the tongue.

Step 3. Hemostasis is effected by drawing the mobile portion away from the tongue and closing the wedge-shaped incision with sutures.

Step 4. Continue the wedge-shaped excision along the margin of the tongue inserting sutures to prevent hemorrhage. Dissection is completed when

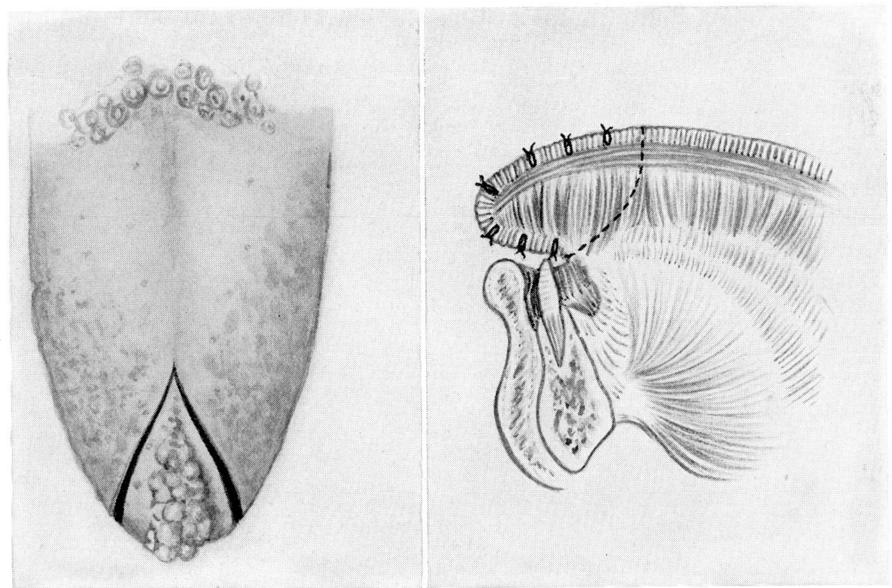

FIG. 280 FIG. 281

FIG. 280. Removal of papilloma from tip of the tongue by V-shaped resection.
FIG. 281. Same as preceding in anteroposterior section.

the level of the last molar tooth is reached (Fig. 283.) Resect the opposite side in like manner. The lower incision is made where the smooth mucosa of the under surface of the tongue joins the papillary mucosa of the dorsum. Make the dorsal incision internal to the tissue to be excised. The infralingual mucosa forms a flap for reconstructing the tongue margins (Fig. 284).

Excision of Half of the Tongue

This may be carried out either (a) through the mouth; (b) through a submaxillary incision or (c) after section of the cheek and division or removal of a part of the lower jaw. (Fig. 285.)

Choice of Operation. Removal through the mouth is indicated when the malignant disease is limited and there is no apparent infiltration to adjacent tissues. When the disease principally involves the lower aspect and outer margin of the tongue, and has extended thence to the adjacent portion of the floor of the mouth and lower jaw, it is better to split the cheek and remove the portion of the lower jaw involved as well as the involved half of the tongue. When the jaw is uninvolved and the floor of the mouth is the chief seat of infiltration, median division of the lower jaw should be the operation of choice. If the lateral and dorsal portions of the tongue are mainly involved, the diseased half of the

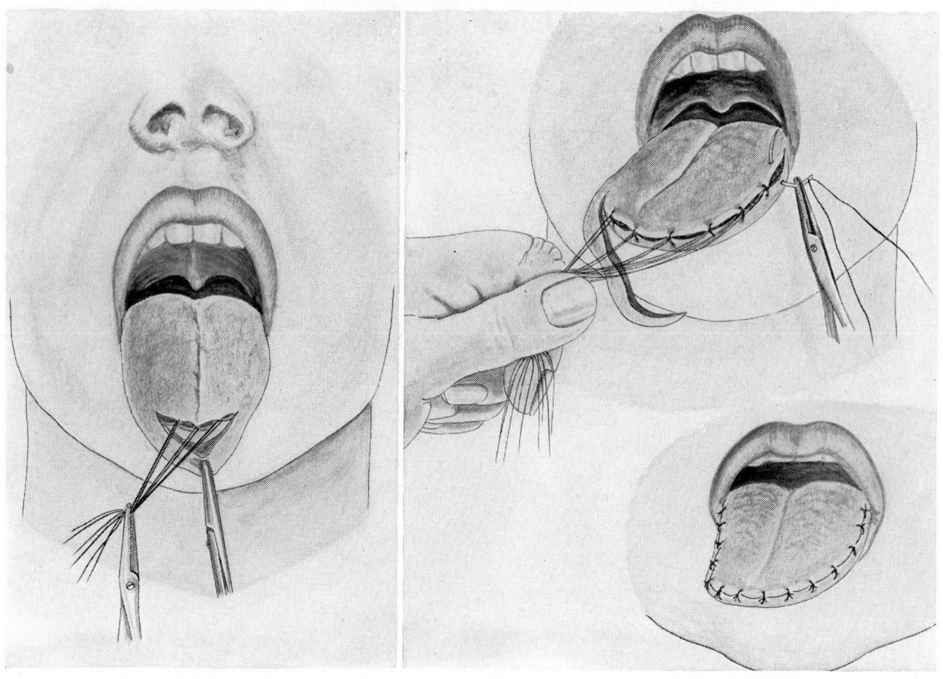

Fig. 282 Fig. 283 Fig. 284

Fig. 282. Butlin's operation for marginal resection of the tongue, first step.
Fig. 283. Butlin's operation, second step.
Fig. 284. Butlin's operation, completed.

tongue should be resected through the mouth and the submaxillary and cervical lymph nodes, the submaxillary gland as well as the surrounding and adjacent fascial tissues on the affected side, removed at a later date.

When a half-tongue resection is being done, the lingual artery of the affected side may be ligated in the usual manner (which see) and the lymphatic and salivary nodes, etc., removed when the mouth and diseased part of the tongue are in a comparatively clean condition; if foul and septic, the latter part of the operation should be deferred.

Step 1. Insert a mouth gag between the jaws; separate the blades and draw the tongue forward.

Step 2. Introduce two stout silkworm ligatures, one into each half of the tongue, an inch or so behind the tip; tie each in the form of a loop about 6 inches long. One of these is grasped by the assistant who manipulates the tongue by this means, throughout the operation.

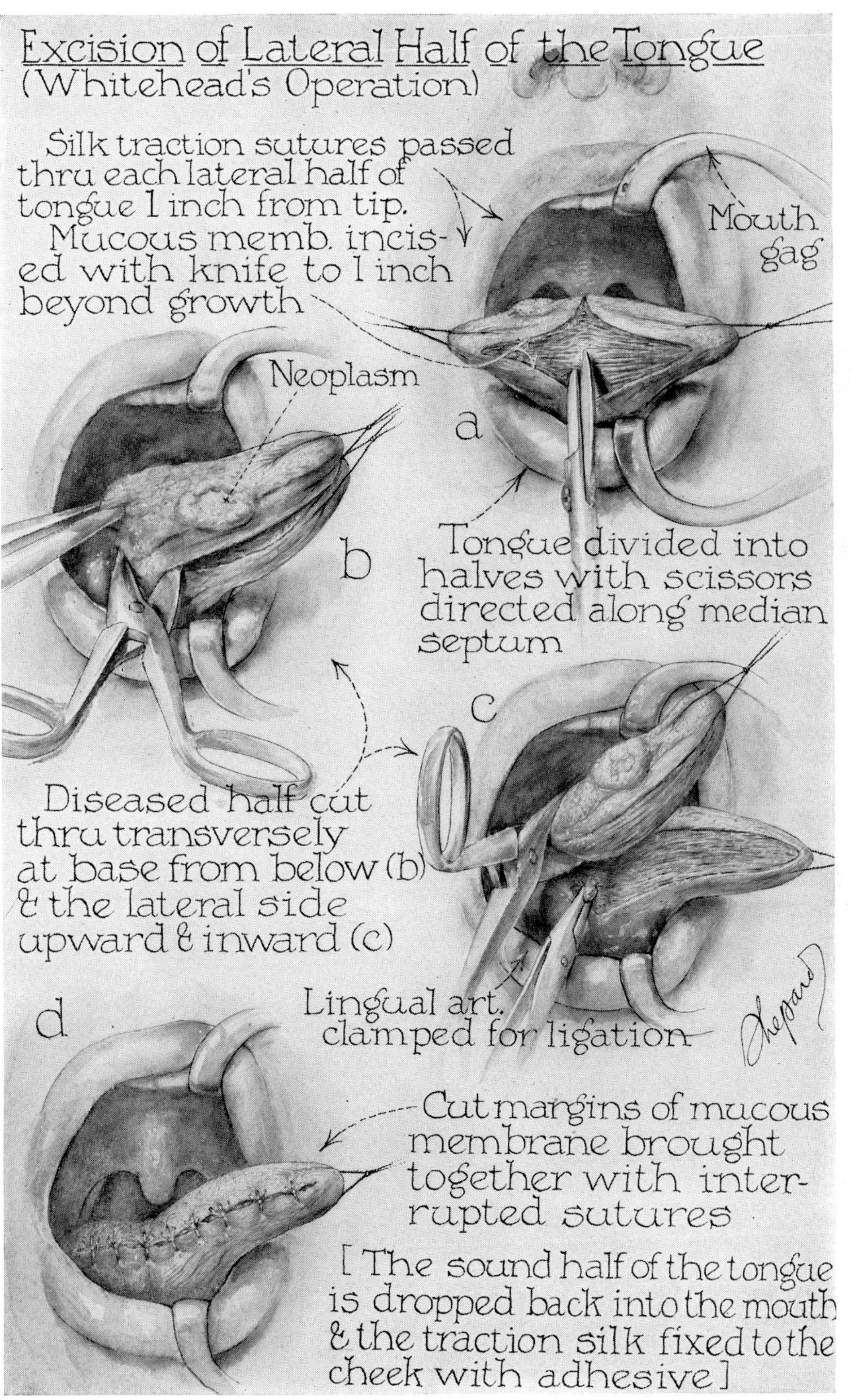

FIG. 285. Excision of lateral half of tongue.

Step 3. With a scalpel or diatherm knife make an incision in the midline through the mucous membrane on the lower and upper surfaces of the tongue. While traction is exerted laterally by means of the ligatures, the median septum is defined at the tip of the tongue by a few snips with the scissors. The surgeon now separates the two halves of the tongue as far back as necessary by pulling on the ligatures, and dividing the tongue. (Fig. 285 a.)

Step 4. Hold both halves of the tongue toward the unaffected side and, with scissors, cut the diseased half through transversely at its base from without and below, upward and inward. The lingual artery which lies near the lower aspect is picked up with pressure-forceps when it comes into view, and, if not already ligated, it is doubly ligated now. Any other bleeding points are also picked up, and ligatures applied to them. (Fig. 285 b and c.)

Step 5. Attend to hemostasis. Join the cut margins in the anterior part of the mucous membrane with catgut. Permit the stump of the tongue to fall back into the mouth; the silkworm gut ligature which has been passed through the unaffected half may be fixed to the cheek with a piece of strapping, if it is considered advisable. This ligature enables the tongue to be readily drawn forward, if hemorrhage occurs as a result of the slipping of ligatures. (Fig. 285 d.)

Operation for Removal of the Whole Tongue Through the Mouth

The operation for removal of the whole tongue through the oral cavity by means of scissors is often referred to as Whitehead's operation. Strong, straight blunt-pointed scissors, gag, large needle and sponge-holders are required.

Step 1. The patient is placed in the usual dorsal position. The mouth-gag is introduced on the least affected side, and held firmly open by the assistant at the head. A strong ligature is passed through the anterior portion of the tongue, at the junction of the anterior with the middle third. This is left long, and serves as a retractor to pull the tongue forward.

Step 2. The tongue is drawn forward and upward toward the roof of the mouth and the anterior pillars of the fauces are divided. This enables the surgeon to pull the greater part of the tongue out of the mouth, and thus gives a better view of the parts which are being operated upon.

Step 3. The soft parts of the tongue are divided if possible, one inch beyond the limits of growth, by a series of snips with the scissors from without inward and directed toward the middle line. One or two small arteries will be divided; they are picked up by the pressure-forceps and ligated. The lingual arteries, when they have not been ligated in the neck, are looked for in the anterior part of the incision, on each side of the median line, and nearer the inferior surface of the organ than the dorsum. When they are seen they are seized with pressure-forceps, and divided on the distal side.

Step 4. Next, the remainder of the tongue is cut through with scissors, and the entire organ removed. Care must be taken to carry the incision well beyond the limits of the disease. The lingual arteries are ligated; the cut surface of the base of the tongue is sponged, and any other bleeding points sought and tied.

Step 5. The base of the tongue may be hooked forward by passing the index-finger into the upper part of the pharynx and exerting forward traction.

This procedure is of considerable value in the temporary arrest of hemorrhage from the lingual arteries, if they have been divided before being seized with pressure-forceps. The vessels are compressed against the posterior aspect of the lower jaw.

Step 6. Before the operation is finished, a loop of strong silk should be passed through the stump of the tongue. This is brought out through the mouth, and fixed to the cheek with a piece of adhesive plaster. It will serve to pull the stump of the tongue forward, and help in the control of hemorrhage, should it occur.

Step 7. When all hemorrhage from the base of the tongue and the floor of the mouth has been arrested, the incised surfaces are sponged dry, and, if possible, portions of the divided mucous membrane of the floor of the mouth in front and laterally, and the base of the tongue behind are joined together by the insertion of chromicized catgut. The unsutured portion is packed with gauze and the operation is completed.

Comment. Excision of the entire tongue through the mouth is the more usual operation practiced for extensive carcinoma, since this method permits complete removal of the diseased organ, and does not leave a visible scar. It must be borne in mind, however, when deciding upon the adoption of this method, that in all cases where malignant disease (carcinoma) has been present for some time, the muscles of the tongue are frequently the seat of carcinomatous infiltration, and in order to completely remove all affected tissues, certain muscles must be removed down to their attachments to the hyoid bone and the styloid process. This free removal of the muscles gives rise to considerable limitation of movement of the stump of the tongue at the floor of the mouth. The lymph vessels in some instances appear to have been the seat of carcinomatous invasion. Usually, however, the carcinomatous elements are carried direct to the lymph-nodes in the neck, and are not arrested in the course of the lymphatic vessels.

In all cases the cervical operation must also be carried out on one or both sides according to the method already described on page 246. Whenever a carcinomatous growth of the tongue extends to the middle line of the tongue or beyond, the lymph structures on both sides will probably become affected with the disease. Operation on both sides will then be necessary, but only one side at a time should be operated upon, the side of the affected portion of the tongue being selected first. When the carcinomatous growth of the tongue is in a septic and foul condition, it is better not to ligate the lingual artery in the neck when the tongue is removed but to remove the submaxillary and cervical lymph-nodes and fascial tissues at a second operation. In septic cases of this kind, suppuration in the cervical wound is liable to occur. This may be followed by serious consequences, such as cellulitis in the fascial planes of the neck and secondary hemorrhage from the lingual artery.

Excision of the Tongue with Median Incision of the Lower Lip and Division of the Symphysis of the Lower Jaw

Step 1. Make a vertical incision through the soft tissues of the lower lip and the submental region (Fig. 286) beginning at the midline of the lower lip and

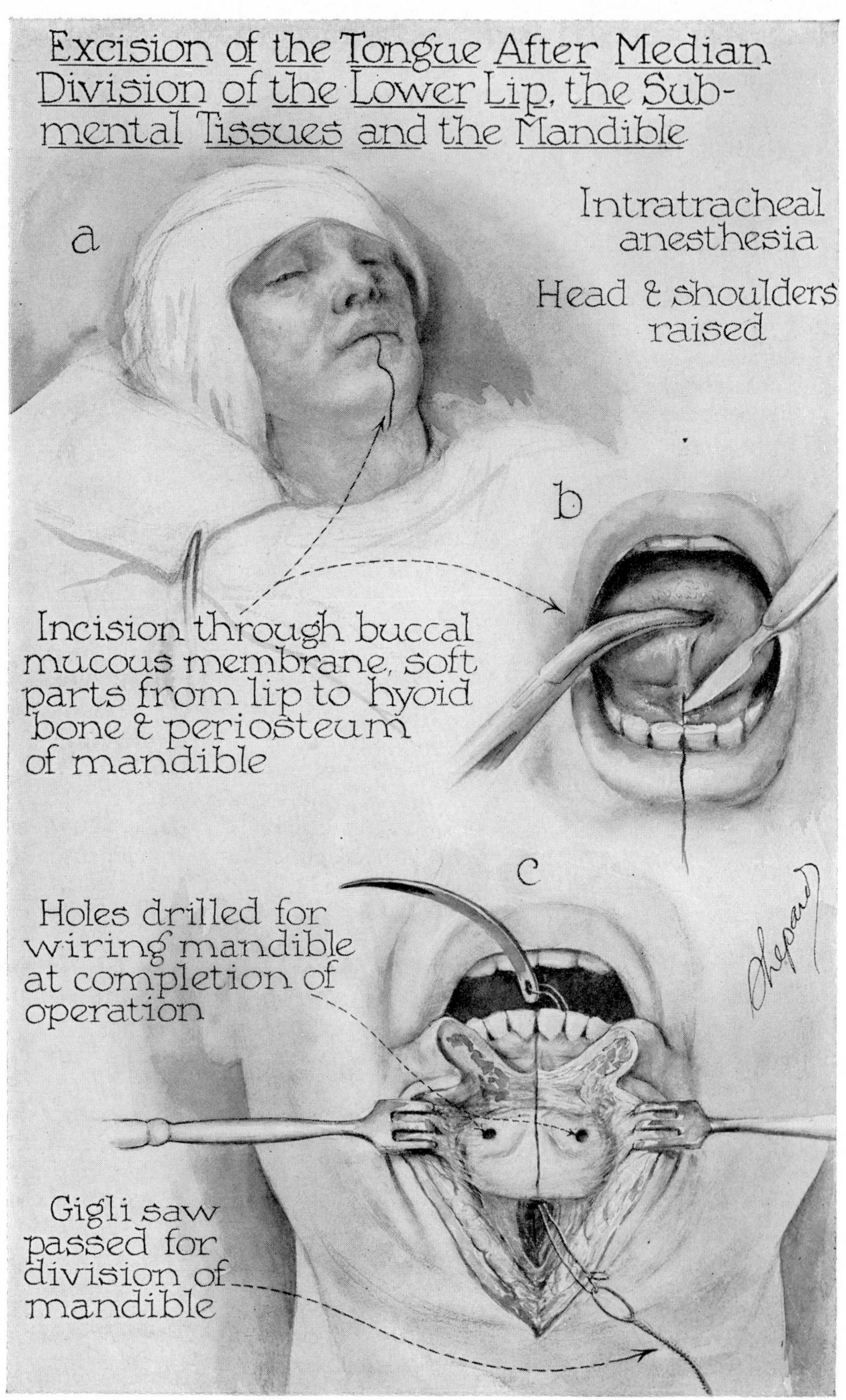

FIG. 286. Excision of the tongue.

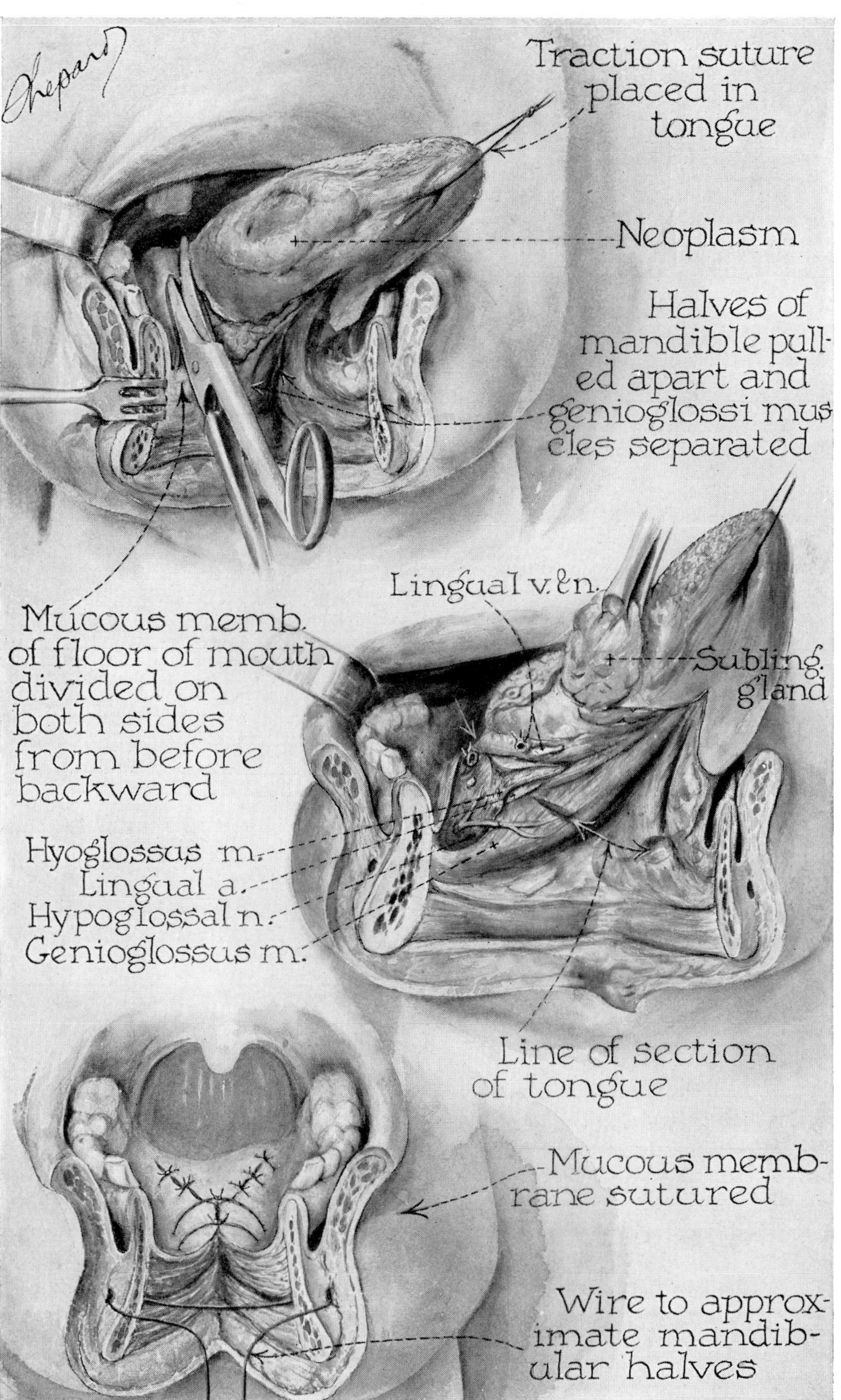

FIG. 286 (continued). Excision of the tongue.

extending downward to immediately above the upper border of the body of the hyoid bone. (Fig. 286 a.)

Step 2. Cut through the soft tissues of the lip, including the internal mucous membrane, and the periosteum on the external aspect of the lower jaw. (Fig. 286 b.)

Step 3. While the jaw is being supported by an assistant, make drill openings in the jaw on each side, one-quarter of an inch from the midline; these are to be used later for the insertion of a wire suture.

Step 4. Extract one central incisor tooth, if necessary. Saw through the bone at the symphysis menti with a Gigli saw, being careful not to lacerate unduly the structures on the deep aspect of the mandible. Pull the two halves of the jaw apart; the geniohyoid and geniohyoglossi muscles are separated, thus bringing to view the lower aspect of the tongue and the floor of the mouth. (Fig. 286 c.)

Step 5. Pass a loop of strong silk through the anterior portion of the tongue and pull the tongue with this in a forward direction and toward the sound or least affected side.

Step 6. With strong scissors divide the mucous membrane of the floor of the mouth on each side from before backward carrying the line of section as wide of the diseased area as possible. The lingual vein is now exposed as it lies upon the hyoglossus muscles and the lingual nerve on the inferior and lateral margin of the tongue under the mucous membrane. The hypoglossal nerve lies deeper upon the external surface of the hyoglossus and sends branches forward to the geniohyoglossus, which should be preserved if they can be avoided with safety so that the mouth may be left in as satisfactory a condition as possible. If, however, the margins of the carcinomatous growth render this impossible, the surgeon should not hesitate to divide them in order to prevent recurrence.

Step 7. Pick up and ligate the lingual artery which will be seen lying between the hyoglossus and the geniohyoglossus as it passes upward.

Step 8. Cut through the hyoglossus and pull the tongue further forward; divide the mucous membrane on its dorsum with the scissors. It may be necessary, in order to carry the incisions well beyond the diseased area, to encroach upon the adjacent parts of the soft palate, the tonsil, and the lateral wall of the pharynx. Make similar incisions on the other side; cut through the base of the tongue and remove the organ. (Fig. 286, cont. p. 261.)

Some surgeons prefer to section the substance of the tongue with the thermocautery, because of the small amount of hemorrhage which follows and the lessened probability of recurrence. Hemorrhage, however, is not of any great importance, since with the tongue pulled well forward, each bleeding artery can be picked up and ligated.

Step 9. Attend to thorough hemostasis. Pull the tongue forward and suture, if possible, the divided mucous membrane on the dorsal and lateral aspects to the margins of the wound in the floor of the mouth. This method of fixation helps prevent the tongue falling back; it hastens union, and enables the patient to swallow more easily.

Step 10. Bring the sewn surfaces of the mandible together by means of a silver-wire suture which is introduced through the holes already drilled:

tie the wire sutures. Drain and pack the wound; close the incision in the lip and neck.

Step 11. Introduce an ample rubber drainage-tube into the lower part of the wound from the neck, and pack the surrounding parts with strips of gauze. The wounds of the divided lip and neck are sutured with silkworm gut with the exception of the lowest portion which is left open for the exit of the lower end of the rubber tube. Dressings are then applied.

Excision of the Tongue After Splitting the Cheek and Division or Resection of a Portion of the Lower Jaw

This operation is especially applicable in those cases of carcinoma of the tongue which extends backward and infiltrates the region of the fauces, the floor of the outer portion of the buccal cavity, and the adjacent portion of the lower jaw. This method of operation gives very free exposure of the diseased areas, and enables the surgeon to take away all the infiltrated tissues. Some surgeons object to the operation on account of the deformity which results, and also to its increased mortality by reason of the development of septic processes in the neck. The first objection has been very much overrated, since little deformity results if care be taken to suture together exactly the divided portions of the cheek. Concerning the increased mortality from septic causes, this will not usually be the case, provided each patient is well looked after for the first week and efficient drainage is provided in the lower portion of the wound so as to avoid any accumulation of septic discharges.

Usually it will be found best to have the anesthetic administered by the intratracheal method, but in occasional cases it may be necessary to perform a preliminary laryngotomy, and afterward to plug the pharynx with a sterile sponge plug.

The operation can most conveniently be divided into the following four steps:

Step 1. **Skin Incision and Splitting the Cheek.**—The assistant grasps the cheek on the affected side so as to control the circulation, and then the surgeon makes an incision which commences at the angle of the mouth, extends horizontally backward to the anterior margin of the masseter whence it is continued downward parallel to the anterior margin of this muscle as far as the inferior margin of the horizontal ramus of the lower jaw, and then onward to the anterior margin of the sternomastoid muscle in the submaxillary region, whence it is curved inward, forward, and upward for about one inch in the direction of the symphysis menti. This incision is made to divide all the tissues of the cheek, and to expose the lower jaw and the anterior margin of the sternomastoid muscle. In the outer part of the incison over the ramus of the jaw or on the anterior margin of the masseter, the external maxillary (facial) artery will be divided and will require ligating. Other vessels requiring ligature are the coronary arteries in the region of the angle of the mouth. The flap thus formed by the cheek and tissues of the neck is next dissected downward and forward, so as to expose fully the horizontal ramus of the lower jaw and the structures in the submaxillary triangle.

Step 2. **Division or Resection of a Portion of the Lower Jaw.**—When it is not necessary to remove a portion of the lower jaw, on account of its freedom from disease, it is sawn through immediately behind the last molar tooth.

The anterior segment is then drawn forward and toward the opposite side, while the other part is pulled forcibly outward and backward. By these means the lateral aspect of the tongue, the floor of the mouth and the region of the fauces are laid bare. When, however, a portion of the jaw is involved in the disease, the limits of the infiltrated bone are exactly defined and the tooth at each extremity of the affected portion is removed. With a small saw, the ramus of the jaw is now sawn through in front of and behind the region of the infiltrated portion. Great care must be taken to make the section of the bone wide of the disease. When the bone has been sawn through, the separated portion is removed and the two segments pulled aside so as to give a full exposure of the interior of the buccal cavity and the extent of the disease.

Step 3. Removal of the Tongue.—This having been accomplished the mucous membrane of the floor of the mouth is cut through one inch beyond the margins of the diseased area; if necessary, the pillars of the fauces are divided, and the tongue is cut through well behind the infiltrated or ulcerated portions. When only one-half of the tongue is involved the mucous membrane should be divided along the midline on the dorsal and ventral aspects, and the organ split backward into halves. These cutting operations can be most easily done with strong curved scissors. In cutting through the substance of the tongue, especial care should be taken, when the ventral aspect is being reached, to ascertain the position of the lingual arteries, and, when seen, these should be seized with pressure forceps before sectioning. The sublingual-nodes can generally be removed at the same time as the tongue.

Step 4. Closure of the External Wound.—If possible, the margins of the mucous membrane on the dorsum of the stump of the tongue should be approximated to the cut margins of the mucous membrane of the floor of the mouth by a few sutures. This facilitates healing and tends to prevent the stump of the tongue falling back over the upper aperture of the larynx. In those cases in which the lower jaw has been divided, and no portion taken away, the two fragments are brought in apposition, drilled with some form of bone perforator, and then fixed in close connection by the insertion of a suture of silver wire. When, however, a segment of bone has been removed, after all hemorrhage has been arrested, the cavity of the wound is packed with strips of gauze. Finally, the margins of the wound are fixed close together by the insertion of a series of interrupted silkworm-gut sutures. Especial care should be taken to secure exact coaptation at the angle of the mouth. The lowest and most dependent portion of the wound should be left unsutured, and through it either a strip of gauze or a drainage tube brought out.

When the operation has been completed, the laryngotomy tube is removed, and the external incision covered by a dressing. Before removing the tube, care must be taken to remove the sponge plug from the upper portion of the pharynx and to sponge all the air-passage free from blood clots.

EXCISION OF THE CERVICAL LYMPH-NODES, SUBMAXILLARY SALIVARY GLANDS AND FASCIAL STRUCTURES OF THE NECK IN CONNECTION WITH OPERATIONS FOR CARCINOMA OF THE TONGUE AND FLOOR OF THE MOUTH

Step 1. Place the patient in the dorsal posture, the head being turned toward the opposite side and the shoulders slightly raised in order to throw the head somewhat backward. The surgeon stands on the side of the patient which is to be operated upon, and his assistants opposite him.

Step 2. Make a semilunar incision as far back as possible in the natural fold or crease of the neck, extending from the anterior border of the sternomastoid a little below the level of the apex of the mastoid process downward and forward to the middle line of the neck, about halfway between the mental process and the body of the hyoid bone. From the convexity of this in-

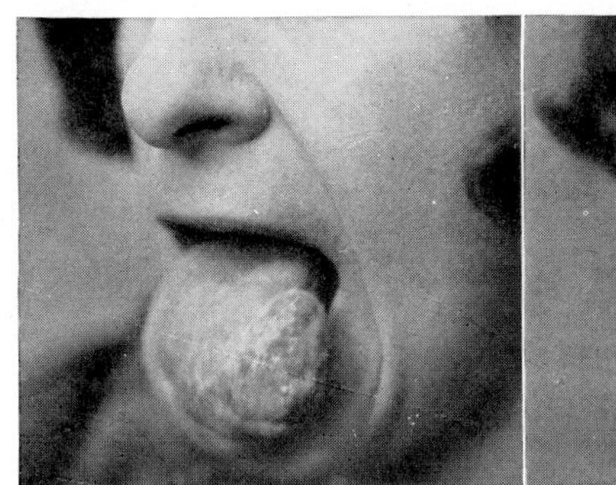

Fig. 287. Hemangioma of tongue; patient 20 years of age. Photograph taken November, 1924.

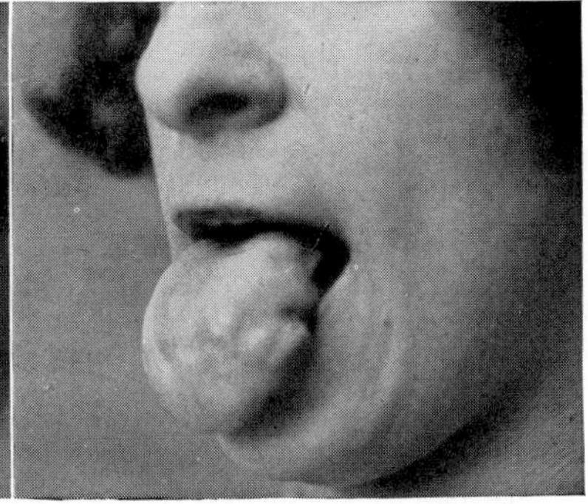

Fig. 288. Same patient treated with radium; over two years later. (Courtesy of Dr. F. E. Simpson.)

cision and a little in front of the anterior margin of the sternomastoid, make a second incision downward to the level of the cricoid cartilage, or even lower, according to the extent of the lymphnodal infection. Some surgeons recommend prolonging the lower limb of the incision as far back as the upper border of the sternoclavicular articulation, but in most cases, this is not necessary.

Step 3. Dissect free three flaps of skin and subcutaneous tissues—one upward, one outward and one inward.

Step 4. Beginning at the angle below, dissect upward a triangular-shaped flap of fascial tissues and attached lymph nodes and vessels, until the horizontal ramus of the lower jaw is reached. Careful and meticulous dissection is necessary in order to separate all the cervical lymph-nodes along with the fascial tissues, and to avoid injury to the contents of the carotid sheath.

Step 5. Recognize and ligate the external maxillary (facial) artery in the upper part of the dissection before it enters the groove in the submaxillary gland. Isolate the salivary gland from its deep connections; ligate its duct. Remove the entire mass of cervical lymph-nodes, submaxillary salivary gland and fascial tissues by cutting through the upper attachments in the region of the horizontal ramus of the lower jaw. During this division the external maxillary (facial) artery is again cut and ligated as are also a number of facial veins.

Step 6. Sponge the entire space carefully so that the surgeon may be enabled to detect and ligate with catgut any small bleeding points.

Step 7. Bring the margins of the flaps, consisting of skin and subcutaneous tissues, into exact apposition and secure them with interrupted sutures of

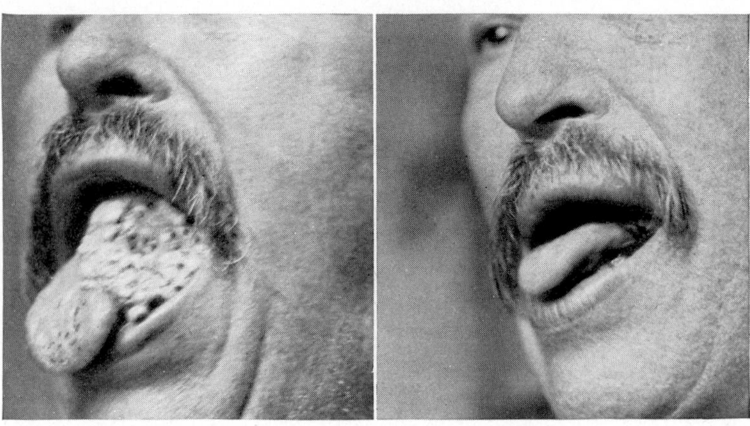

FIG. 289. FIG. 290.

FIG. 289. Carcinoma of the tongue, July 7, 1921.
FIG. 290. Same patient as in preceding illustration. Clinically well over 5 years. Died of acute pneumonia, 1927. (Courtesy of Dr. F. E. Simpson.)

dermal suture. Insert a small rubber drainage tube into the deep part of the wound in the submaxillary region, thus preventing an accumulation of blood and serum which might cause trouble later.

Comment. In view of the remarkable progress made in the treatment of tumors of the lips, mouth and tongue by the use of radium, this chapter would be incomplete without calling attention to the striking results obtained from the use of radium in some well-selected cases of carcinoma of the tongue. The accompanying illustrations emphasize the point clearly. (Figs. 287, 288, 289, 290.)

CHAPTER 13

SURGERY OF THE SALIVARY GLANDS

INJURIES

A buccal fistula, the result of a recent injury is of slight importance. It is different when an external salivary fistula results. The divided ends of the duct should be promptly united wherever possible, using chromic catgut. The jaw should be immobilized, and feeding done through a tube.

ACUTE INFECTIONS

SUBLINGUAL GLAND

An abscess here is incised through the mouth in the long axis of the gland. Leave the wound open or drain.

SUBMAXILLARY GLAND

Acute suppurations here should be dealt with promptly by surgery. The tendency of the infection to extend may result in its invading the fascial planes in the neck and may cause rapid edema of the glottis calling for prompt tracheotomy.

The incision should run parallel with and just below the ramus of the mandible; it should be ample; divide the deep fascia to relieve tension and aim to avoid, if possible, the facial artery, coursing at the posterior border of the gland (Fig. 291). In case the artery is divided, secure the divided ends and ligate them.

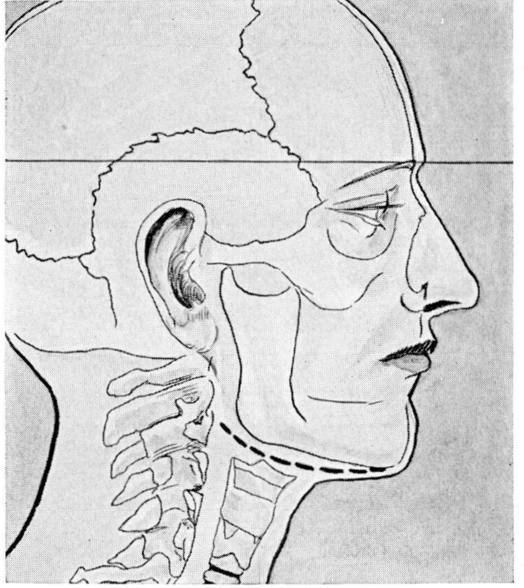

Fig. 291. Incision for abscess of the submaxillary gland.

PAROTID GLAND

Here suppurations should be met with by incisions over the most prominent portion of the swelling in the line of the course of the facial nerve fibres. Purulent collections in this situation are usually deep seated and should be attacked at an early date by penetrating the structures overlying them. (Figs. 292 and 293.)

CALCULUS OF THE SALIVARY GLANDS AND DUCTS

SUBLINGUAL DUCT

When the calculus is not firmly imbedded here it may be removed from the duct; if it is, it is best to remove the concretion together with the gland. In the former case, after infiltration anesthesia, the sublingual duct is incised over the palpable stone or the long axis of the gland (stereo-x-ray studies will aid in orientation) and the stone is extracted, preferably in toto. Insure hemostasis. Leave the wound open. Avoid injury to the lingual nerve.

Where the gland also is to be removed, recall that the gland rests on the mylohyoid muscle; mesially to it is the lingual nerve and Wharton's duct (submaxillary).

REMOVAL OF SUBMAXILLARY GLAND

Step 1. General anesthesia (tracheal insufflation). Insert a mouth gag; retract the tongue to the opposite side.

Step 2. Divide the mucous membrane and separate it from the gland by blunt dissection. Expose the gland. Pressure by an assistant from under the jaw will aid in making the gland prominent.

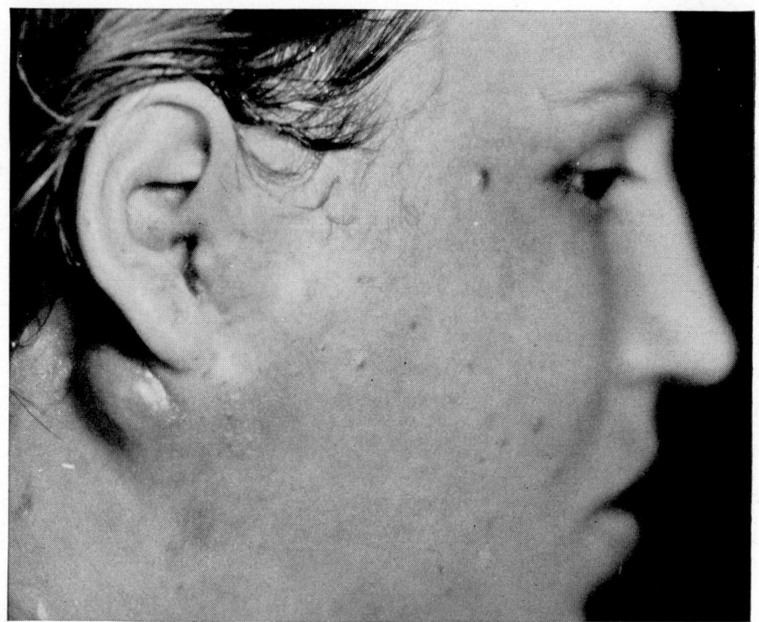

Fig. 292. Suppurative parotitis discharging through external auditory meatus.

Step 3. Enucleate the gland from its surroundings with curved scissors. If the lingual nerve is injured there will be loss of sensation of the anterior half of the tongue. Avoid cellulitis by leaving the wound open. Injury to Wharton's duct is not of much significance.

REMOVAL OF STONE FROM WHARTON'S (SUBMAXILLARY) DUCT

The duct is superficial in situation, about 2 inches in length, and its walls are thin. The lingual nerve crosses the duct at the anterior border of the hyoglossus muscle.

Use infiltration anesthesia. Incise directly over the stone in the long axis of the duct in order to avoid injury to the lingual nerve. Extract the calculus. Leave the wound open.

Removal of the stone and submaxillary gland by the external route is the operation of choice where no coexistant abscess is present. In the latter case free drainage is of utmost importance.

Step 1. Make an incision parallel with the lower border of the mandible. Divide the tissues; expose the gland.

Step 2. Have an assistant place his gloved finger at the floor of the mouth and push the structures downward, thus making them accessible to operative manipulations.

Step 3. Enucleate the gland by blunt dissection. Lahey forceps may be used to pull the gland forward. The divided Wharton's duct is permitted to remain behind. Do not perforate the mucous membrane at the floor of the mouth. Drain (rubber tube or cigarette drain).

CALCULUS OF THE PAROTID DUCT

Buccal Portion. The buccal portion of the parotid duct is from ½ to ¾ in. long. It extends from the edge of the masseter muscle, through the buccinator, to the opening on the buccal surface of the cheek opposite the second upper molar tooth (Fig. 294).

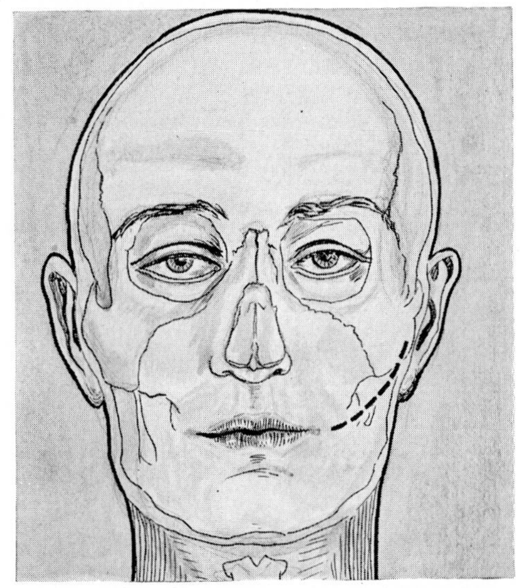

FIG. 293. Incision for parotid abscess.

Step 1. Make counter-pressure on the outside of the cheek; inject the anesthetic in the buccal tissues directly over the calculus.

Step 2. The incision is made in the long axis of the duct down to the calculus; extract it. Leave the wound open. If an internal salivary fistula forms at the site of incision, it is of no consequence; as a rule it will close spontaneously.

Masseteric Portion. The masseteric portion of the parotid duct runs from the anterior edge of the parotid gland, lying on the masseter muscle, as far as its anterior edge and is about 1½ in. long. In its posterior portion it receives the duct of the accessory parotid gland. The course of the duct corresponds approximately to the middle third of a line drawn between the lower portion of the external auditory meatus and the middle of the upper lip. Its diameter is about ⅛ in. The facial nerve has branches both below and above it.

Step 1. Make an incision through the skin and superficial fascia in the line of the duct and through the duct wall to the calculus. Seize the stone with forceps and extract it.

Step 2. Ascertain the presence of stricture in the proximal or distal part of the duct. If present, dilate it with probes of increasing caliber. Coapt the edges of the divided duct with fine chromic catgut sutures which are not permitted to penetrate the lumen. Bring the skin and superficial fascia together accurately with sutures. Immobilize the jaw for several days. Feed the patient through a tube. Inaccurate coaptation of the divided edges of the duct or faulty union from necrotic edges may result in the formation of an external salivary fistula. Should this occur, sufficient time should be given for wound contraction, in the hope that the fistula will gradually close, before resorting to any of the plastic procedures described below.

X-ray, as a therapeutic measure, is, in these cases, of distinct value.

When the **calculus is imbedded in the glandular portion of the parotid,** such stones are removed in a manner similar to that employed for those found in the masseteric portions of the duct with the difference that the gland tissue over the duct is separated before the latter is incised. Remember while operating, that the facial nerve filaments perforate the parotid.

Step 1. Use tracheal insufflation. Make a skin incision over the calculus cutting parallel to the course of the facial nerve fibers.

Step 2. Deepen the incision through the gland until the calculus is exposed; remove it with appropriate forceps. If the stone is firmly imbedded, remove

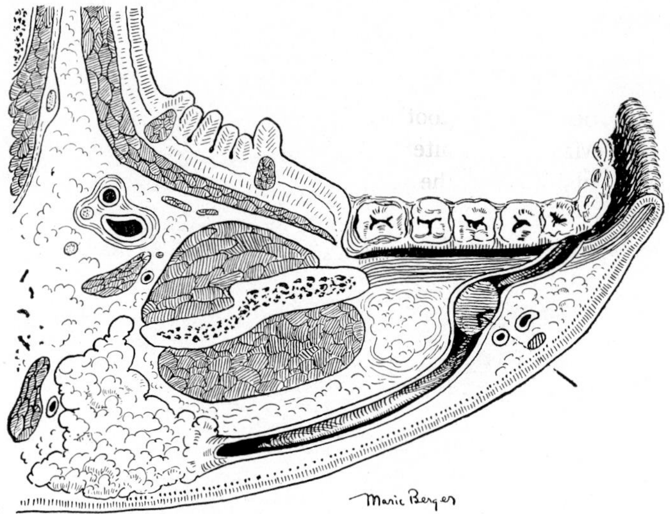

Fig. 294. Salivary calculus in Stensen's duct. Arrow points to impacted stone in duct.

a little of the surrounding parotid tissue by careful scalpel dissection. When no inflammatory involvement of the parotid exists, the wound may be closed without drainage; the gland tissue is approximated by deep sutures preventing the development of dead spaces where salivary puddles might form. Unite the skin carefully to avoid salivary fistula.

TUMORS OF THE PAROTID GLAND

BENIGN TUMORS

Step 1. When the parotid tumor is of large size (Fig. 295), make an incision (Fig. 296) over its most prominent part along the course of the facial nerve fibers.

Step 2. Separate the capsule of the gland from the surrounding glandular tissue by blunt dissection. Ligate each bleeding point separately as encountered. Control oozing with lap-pads wrung out of hot salt solution.

Step 3. Enucleate the tumor and secure a dry field. Do not use approximating sutures through the gland tissue or the capsule. The neighboring parotid tissue crowding into the opening left by the removal of the tumor will obliterate much of the space created by the removal of the tumor.

Step 4. Carefully unite the skin edges together with the subcutaneous fatty tissue with silk sutures. Apply moderate pressure. The skin sutures had best be left in, if possible, for 8 to 10 days, and light pressure with bandages kept up for another week. For cosmetic reasons, a subcuticular suture may be used. It is important to bring the whole of the subcutaneous fatty layer in apposition over the wound in the gland.

Since large benign tumors tend to grow downward and outward, a curved flap incision is best made for their exposure.

Step. 1. The incision is begun slightly anterior to the lobule of the ear and follows the posterior and inferior borders of the ascending and horizontal

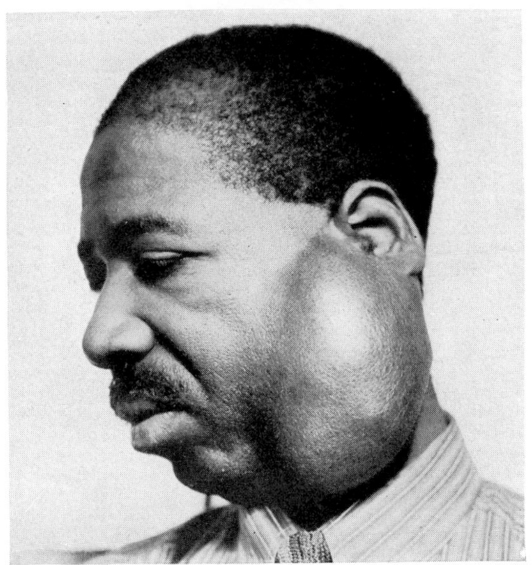

Fig. 295. Benign parotid tumor 18 years duration. Note displacement of lobule of ear.

rami of the jaw. The flap is reflected on the cheek while the skin and subcutaneous fatty layers are dissected upward leaving the facial nerve fibers on the parotid or on the growth.

Step 2. The location of the capsule of the tumor is determined and the parotid gland tissue pushed away from it by blunt dissection. This is followed by careful hemostasis.

Excision of the Parotid Gland

Step 1. Fig. 297 shows the type of incision which should be made through the skin over the region of the gland. Reflect the skin so as to expose the whole parotid covered by its fascia.

The anterior (horizontal) part of the incision begins midway between the mastoid process and condyle of the mandible and extends to the anterior border of the masseter muscle. The posterior (vertical) portion may commence just beneath the anterior border of the sternomastoid muscle. Avoid injury to the internal jugular vein. Walter E. Sistrunk's method of avoiding injury to the facial nerve during the removal of the parotid gland is depicted in Fig. 298.

Step 2. Mobilize the anterior edge of the gland and tumor. Ligate the blood vessels as encountered, as well as Stensen's duct. Separate the gland and tumor from the masseter muscle working from the front.

Step 3. Further mobilize and separate the lower edge of the gland from its surroundings by blunt dissection ligating and dividing all important vessels, as encountered.

Step. 4. Expose the upper end of the anterior portion of the sternomastoid muscle; open its sheath and retract the muscle backward.

Step 5. Expose the external carotid artery working from below upward and elevating the lower edge of the gland. Ligate the artery doubly and divide it. Mobilize the tumor and gland up to the level of the styloid process of the temporal bone.

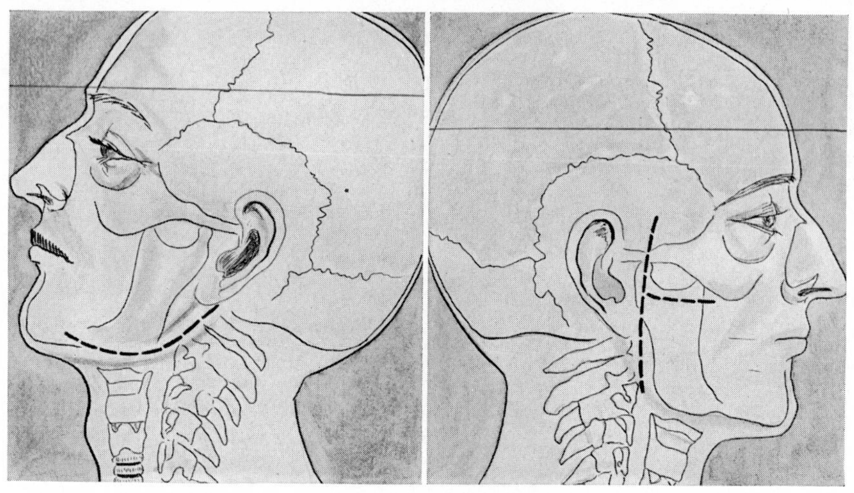

FIG. 296 FIG. 297

FIG. 296. Incision for large benign tumors of the parotid.
FIG. 297. T-shaped incision for the removal of the parotid gland.

Step 6. Separate and sever all connections between the tumor and the temporomaxillary joint by blunt dissection. Ligate the temporal vessels at the level of the zygoma and divide them.

Step 7. Pull the gland, etc., back; the numerous veins which run along with the internal maxillary artery from behind the neck of the lower jaw into the gland are thus exposed. This group of vessels is now ligated and divided.

Step 8. Separate the posterior and pharyngeal connections of the gland by blunt dissection. Take care not to injure the internal jugular vein.

Step 9. Attend to hemostasis by packing the wound. Suture the wound after providing for drainage.

Note. If there are any enlarged lymph nodes near the parotid they should be removed at the same time. The operation is a difficult one and calls for experience.

Zarraga's operation[1] is essentially as follows:

[1] Described in the *Revista del Hopital Juarez,* (Mexico), T. I. No. 5, May, 1912 and summarized in the Journal de Chir., Paris, Sept., 1912.

Step 1. Make an incision downward extending from the tip of the mastoid process, continuing along the anterior border of the sternomastoid muscle to a point a little below the angle of the lower jaw. Continue this incision forward immediately below and parallel to the mandible until the anterior border of the masseter is reached; continue the incision upward along the anterior edge of the masseter and terminate it on the zygoma.

Step 2. Reflect the skin flap thus outlined, upward, exposing the sternomastoid muscle, the facial nerve, the parotid, the masseter muscle and the lower jaw in front of it, also the facial artery and the zygoma. With the elevator and knife expose the bone of the lower jaw just in front of the masseter and divide it with a Gigli saw. Divide the masseter muscle at its zygomatic insertion as well as Stensen's duct.

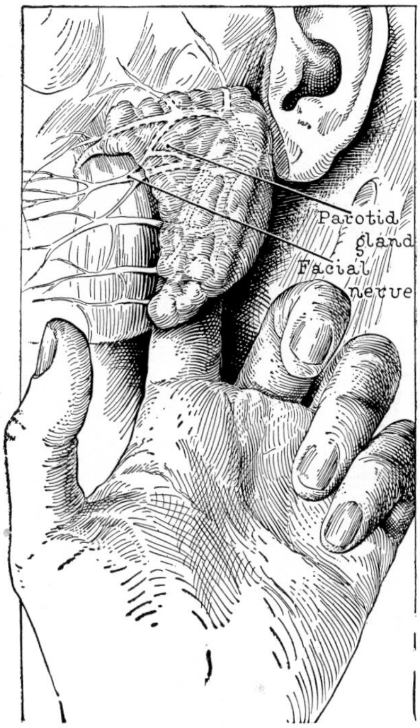

Step 3. Grasp the ascending ramus of the jaw with lion forceps and dislocate it outward and backward; at the same time divide the internal pterygoid muscle, ligate the inferior dental vessels and divide the tendon of the temporal muscle. Ligate the external carotid artery immediately before it enters the parotid gland. Ligate the internal maxillary as it passes behind the condyle of the inferior maxilla; ligate also the superficial temporal and the posterior auricular arteries.

Step 4. Remove the parotid gland and the ascending ramus of the jaw together. Investigate now whether or not the pharyngeal prolongation of the parotid gland is adherent to the carotid packet; if so, separate the adhesions. Close the wound.

FIG. 298. Method sometimes used in trying to prevent injury to the facial nerve. The facial nerve has been exposed and separated from the anterior portion of the parotid gland. A finger is kept in front of the nerve while the tumor is being removed. (Walter E. Sistrunk, Surg. Cl. N. Am., W. B. Saunders Co.)

GUTIERREZ[1] METHOD OF TOTAL PAROTIDECTOMY UNDER LOCAL ANESTHESIA

In all parotidectomies executed by Gutierrez, the parotid gland is removed under local anesthesia. The skin is first infiltrated following the line of the operative incision. (Fig. 300.)

Step 1. Divide the auricular nerve, ligate the external jugular vein, exposing and mobilizing the posterior border of the parotid gland which exposes the anterior edge of the sternocleidomastoid muscle (Fig. 299).

Step 2. The upper part of the incision exposes the mastoid apophysis at which level a small quantity of anesthetic solution is infiltrated deeply to block the facial nerve. (Figs. 301, 302, 303.)

[1] Revist. de Cirug. Buenos Aires, May, 1936.

Step 3. In the lower part, following exposure of the posterior belly of the digastric muscle, a small quantity of anesthetic solution is infiltrated at the

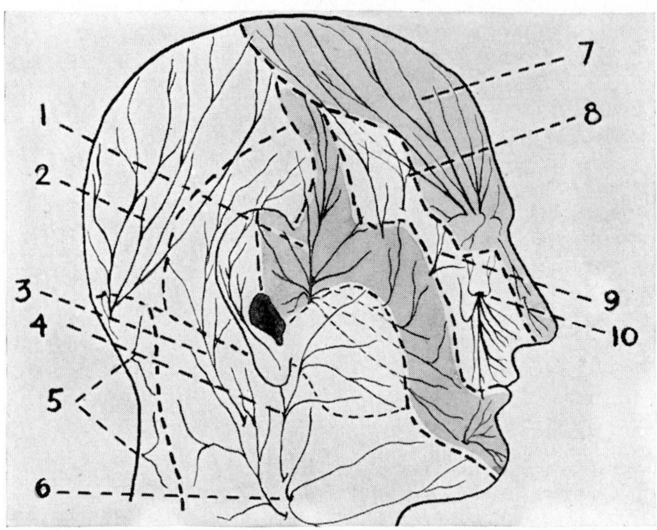

FIG. 299. Distribution of sensory nerves of head (after Krause). Dark areas designate first and third branches of the trigeminus, 1. auricular temporal, 2. great occipital, 3. lesser occipital, 4. great auricular, 5. posterior cervical (dorsal), 6. lateral cervical (ventral), 7. ophthalmic nerve, 8. temporo zygomatic, 9. facial zygomatic, 10. infra-orbital.

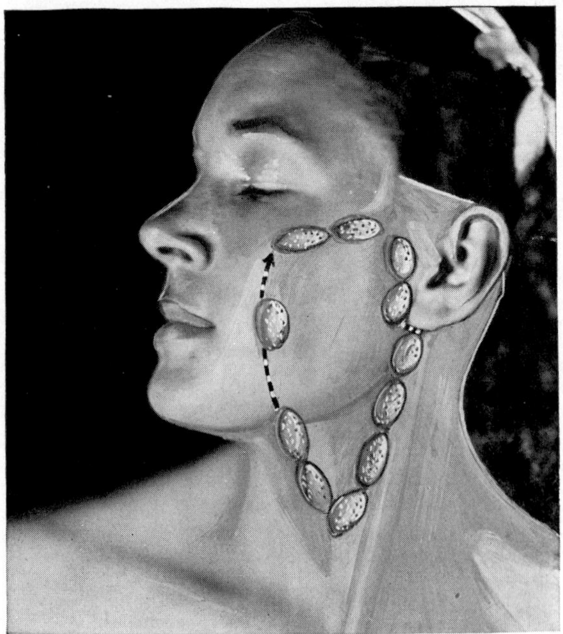

FIG. 300. Infiltration of the skin following the line of the operative incision. (Gutierrez.)

digastro-sterno-mastoid muscle; the external carotid artery is freed below the digastric and ligated.

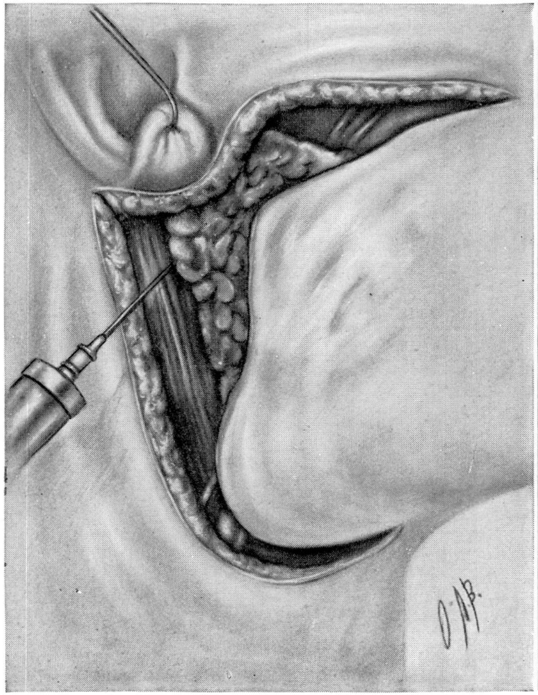

Fig. 301. Blocking of facial nerve. (Gutierrez.)

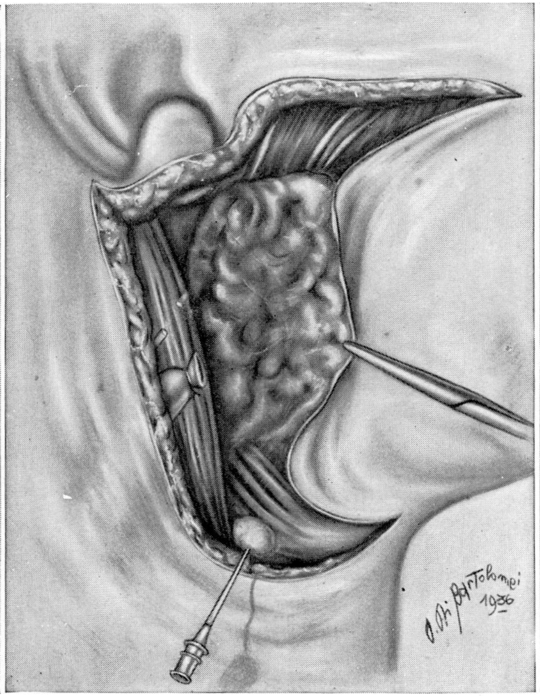

Fig. 302. Blocking of the zone in which the external carotid artery is to be ligated.

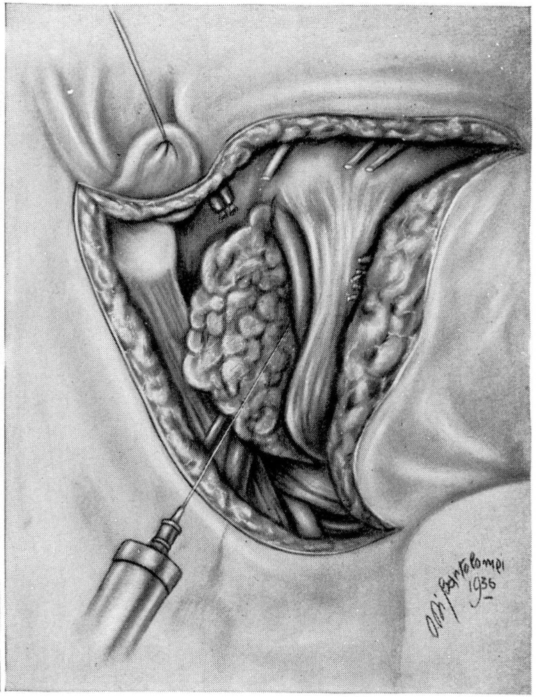

Fig. 303. Blocking of zone in which the internal maxillary vessels run.

Step 4. Free the parotid gland from the pavilion of the ear. Displace the deep-lying blocked facial nerve; expose the temporal vein and block the auriculo-temporal nerve.

Step 5. The liberation of the parotid gland at its anterior extremity is continued. The vasculo-nervous elements, Stensen's canal and branches of the facial nerve have been blocked at the commencement of the cutaneous anesthesia. The gland is freed from the masseter muscle as far as the posterior border of the inferior maxilla. Here a small quantity of anesthetic solution is injected and the liberation of the gland continued until the internal maxillary vessels are exposed. These vessels are ligated and the gland is totally freed.

Note. An exact knowledge of the technic is necessary in order that the blocking of the nerves may be effected at the precise time of the freeing of the parotid gland.

SALIVARY FISTULAS

Salivary fistulas may be connected with the parotid gland or its duct. In the vast majority of cases, they may be divided into two groups: (a) glandular fistulas and (b) fistulas of Stensen's duct.

In recent injuries involving the cheek, locate Stensen's duct, if possible. Fix it immediately in position so that it will discharge into the mouth.

TREATMENT OF GLANDULAR FISTULAS

Immobilization of the Jaws. Pietri reports 38 cases cured by this method. The method consists of holding the jaws together, sometimes preventing the jaws from opening for several months by such devices as intermaxillary ligatures, splints, or bandages. During the period of immobilization, only liquid nourishment is allowed and speaking is forbidden.

Dieulafé believes that many cases will heal spontaneously without immobilization of the jaws and that the fistula persists just as often in those who have been subjected to immobilization as in those who have not had the jaws closed.

Cauterization. Chemical cauterization with silver nitrate or with the actual cautery should be tried in fistulas of the glandular type. The cautery should be applied directly to the fistulous tract every few days. X-rays have of late been lauded in the treatment of glandular fistulas.

Avulsion of the auriculo-temporal nerve (running between the temporal artery and the ear) may be tried. The purpose is to diminish the secretion of the gland. Good results have been reported by the use of this method by Leriche, Deupes, Dieulafé, Tromp, Ianni and others. (Fig. 299, p. 274.)

Morestin considers extirpation of the fistulous tract the method of choice.

Extirpation of the entire gland should not be attempted until all other methods have failed.

Submaxillary glandular fistulas are very rare as compared with those of the parotid. Here, extirpation of the gland is the operation of choice.

FISTULAS OF STENSEN'S DUCT

Many operations have been devised for the relief of fistula of Stensen's duct. The object of this multiplicity of procedures is to divert the flow of saliva into the mouth, instead of discharging on the surface.

These operations vary with the position of the fistula: (A) where the fistula is anterior to the masseter muscle; (B) where the fistula is in the masseteric portion of the duct.

Fistulas Anterior to the Masseter Muscle

VON LANGENBECK'S OPERATION

Step 1. Pass a probe through the fistula. Make an incision on the surface as shown in Figure 304.

Step 2. Dissect the fistula and Stensen's duct from its masseteric bed, from the fistula to the gland, leaving it attached to the gland.

Step 3. Perforate the buccal mucous membrane with a delicate pointed knife, at a convenient point.

Step 4. Pull the free end of the mobilized duct into the mouth through the perforation in the mucosa and suture it in place here. The stab-wound should be made in such a position that there will be no tension on the duct when sutured to the mucous membrane inside the mouth.

Step 5. Close the wound on the cheek.

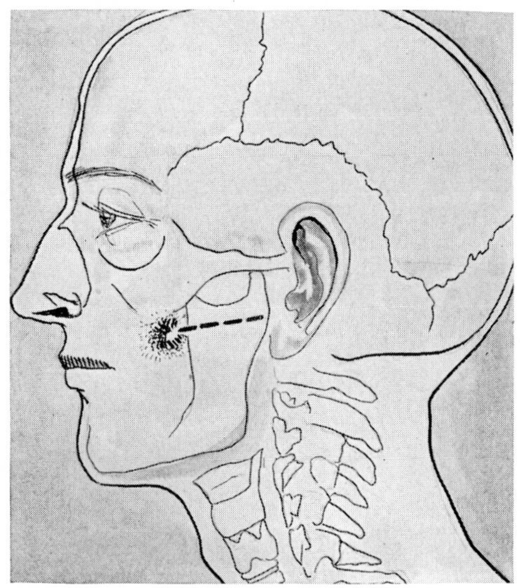

FIG. 304. Incision in von Langenbeck's operation for salivary fistula.

The object of this, von Langenbeck's operation, is to convert an external into an internal fistula. This is the operation of choice when the duct is anterior to the masseter muscle; unfortunately, however, the fistulas are usually found much farther back.

DEGUISE'S OPERATION

Step 1. A puncture is made through the fistula, opening obliquely backward and inward to the inner surface of the cheek; through it is passed one end of a leaden wire.

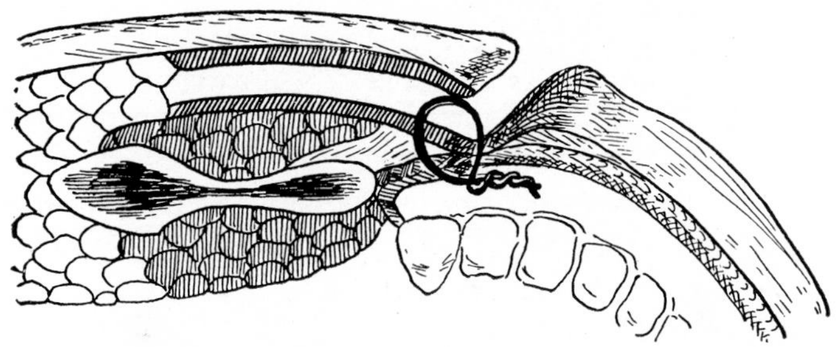

FIG. 305. Deguise's operation for fistula of Stensen's duct.

Step 2. A second puncture is then made through the same external opening, but directed obliquely forward to the inner surface, through which the other end of the wire is passed into the mouth and united snugly with its fellow by twisting. The parotid secretion promptly follows the leaden guides into the mouth, and the external opening quickly heals. Silver wire, silk or an elastic ligature may be used instead of lead wire (Figs. 305 and 306).

KAUFMAN'S OPERATION

This procedure, like the two above described, is devised for the purpose of converting an external into an internal fistula.

Step 1. A small rubber tube about 3 mm. thick is passed into the mouth through an opening made by pushing a trocar through the tissues of the cheek from the external fistula. The rubber tube is withdrawn in two or three weeks or when epithelialization of the tract has been well begun.

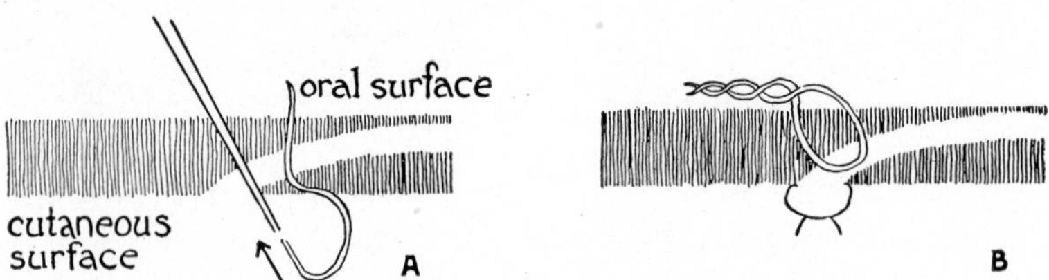

Fig. 306. A. Introduction of the wire. B. wire on oral surface twisted; cutaneous surface closed by suture.

Step 2. The aperture of the external fistula is then freshened and its edges sutured. The rubber tubing (heavy silk cord may be substituted) may be secured in place by using a small safety pin which is passed through the outer opening. This is covered with sterile adhesive plaster to keep it attached to the skin of the cheek.

Fistula Situated in the Masseteric Portion of Stensen's Duct

Von Langenbeck's (p. 277) operation may be used if the duct is long enough and can be brought through a transverse incision in the masseter muscle to the buccal mucous membrane. The methods of Kaufman and Deguise may also be used, but the masseter should not be punctured and the ligature or rubber drain should be passed through a tunnel burrowed between the masseter and the skin.

BRAUN'S OR KÜTTNER'S OPERATION

In this method a new duct is formed by a plastic procedure.

Proceed as is shown in Figures 307-308-309-310.

Step 1. Mobilize the fistulous orifice by dissecting it free from the skin. The incision should penetrate all the tissues of the cheek except the mucosa and the masseter muscle. Retract the edges of the wound, exposing the outer surface of the mucosa. (Figs. 307-308.)

Step 2. Construct from the buccal mucosa a flap with its pedicle at the edge of the masseter. The flap should be of sufficient length to reach from the masseteric edge to the fistula.

Step 3. Suture the upper and lower edges of the flap together in such a manner as to form a tube lined with epithelium. (Figs. 309-310.)

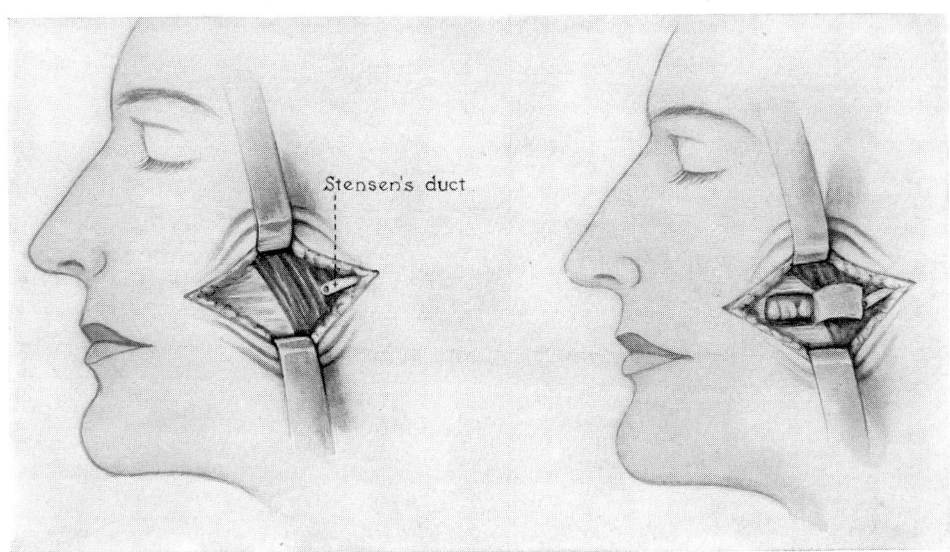

FIG. 307 FIG. 308

FIG. 307. Divided end of Stensen's duct dissected free, shown resting on the masseter muscle.

FIG. 308. Flap of mucous membrane of the cheek dissected and displaced backward.

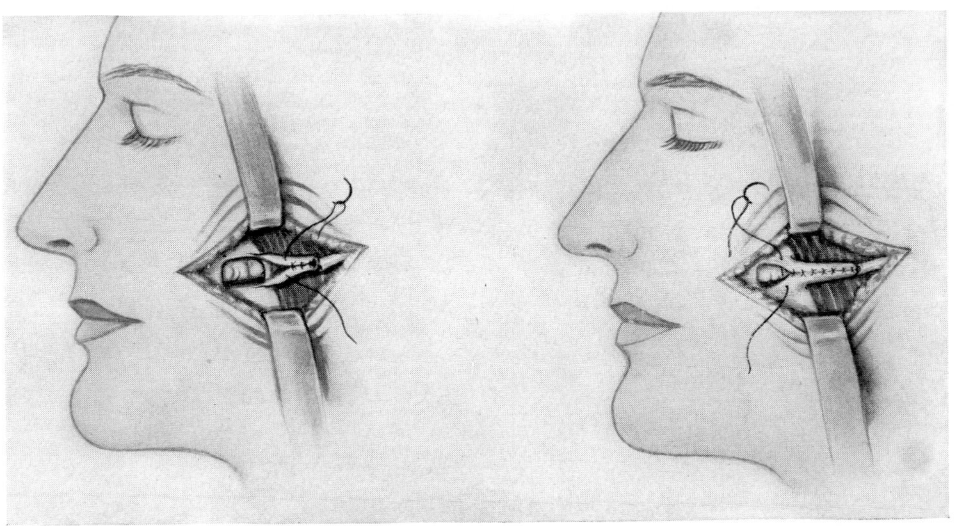

FIG. 309 FIG. 310

FIG. 309. Flap of mucous membrane shown in preceding figure sutured after being folded on itself to form a tube.

FIG. 310. Tube formed as shown in preceding illustration ready to be united to end of Stensen's duct. After this is accomplished, the rest of the structures are so united as to cause the saliva to be discharged into the mouth.

Step 4. Close the cutaneous wound.

Crouse's Operation. This operation is much the same as that of Braun.

Parotid-Submaxillary Anastomosis

In cases in which lesions of Stensen's duct seriously interfere with the secretion of the parotid, Ferrarini[1] demonstrated the possibility of establishing drainage through a submaxillary anastomosis between the parotid and submaxillary glands in the following manner:

Step 1. Expose the submaxillary gland by an incision running parallel to and below the horizontal ramus of the inferior maxilla. Continue the incision back to and around the angle of the jaw, freely exposing the lower part of the parotid, the capsule of which is opened. Mobilize the submaxillary gland by blunt dissection.

Step 2. Isolate and mobilize the lower end of the parotid behind the angle of the jaw.

Step 3. Incise or resect corresponding portions of the two glands.

Step 4. Suture the raw surface of one gland to the raw surface of the other.

Step 5. Close the external wound. Dress the wound.

Ligation of Stensen's Duct

It is an established fact that when scar tissue obliterates Stensen's duct in close proximity to the gland, the gland will atrophy. Morestin takes advantage of this fact, and in cases where other methods fail he dissects the stump of the duct free with all the surrounding tissue and then ligates it at its origin. The soft tissues are then mobilized and closed without drainage. This obliteration of the duct causes rapid atrophy of the parotid. Morestin reports gratifying results from this procedure.

[1] Zentrbl. f. Chir. 13, June, 1914.

CHAPTER 14

SURGERY OF THE JAWS, UPPER LIP AND CHEEK

OPERATIONS ON THE UPPER JAW

The superior maxilla may be removed (Figs. 311-312) partially or as a whole for the following conditions:

1. Benign Tumors.
2. Malignant Tumors.
    a. Sarcoma.
    b. Carcinoma (squamous celled or columnar celled).
    c. Epithelioma terebrant of Reclus.
3. Carcinoma of the nasopharynx.
4. Necrosis of the maxilla.
5. Odontomas.

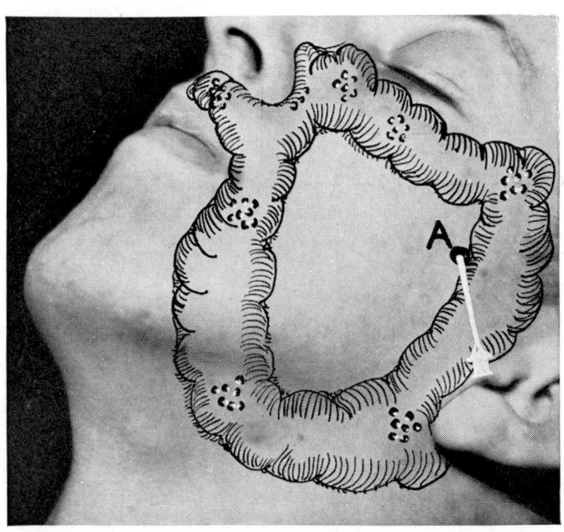

FIG. 311. Resection of upper jaw. Wheals show extent of subdermal infiltration. A. Point of entrance of the needle for blocking the maxillary branch.

In removal of the superior maxilla, Kocher recommends preliminary ligation of the external carotid artery (see under ligation of arteries). His reason for this preliminary step is that removal of the upper jaw is often accompanied by excessive loss of blood or followed by aspiration pneumonia. The advice is therefore sound and has many supporters. The writer also subscribes to it. It will repay in time saved and render the operation cleaner.

EXCISION OF THE UPPER JAW

Fergusson's Operation

Either one or both halves of the upper jaw may be removed by this technic.

While there are a number of other surgical procedures for the removal of the upper jaw, this operation is very suitable when the skin is not involved.

Step 1. Kocher's, Fergusson's or Dieffenbach's incision may be used. (Figs. 313-314.) Make a median incision beginning about 1.3 cm. below the inner canthus of the eye; continue it downward in the nasofacial groove, following the convexity of the ala nasi and passing along the margin of the nostril to the midline of the lip and thence through the center of the upper lip. Make a horizontal incision passing from the beginning of the median incision along the lower border of the orbit to end over the malar bone beyond the outer canthus.

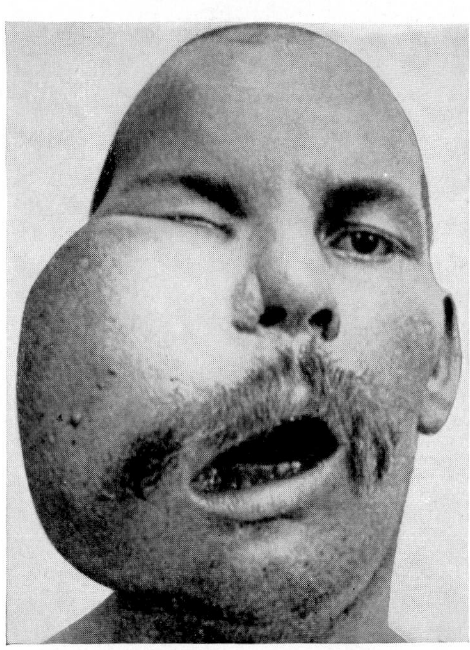

Fig. 312. Sarcoma of upper jaw. Total resection of upper jaw of man 31 years of age (Trendelenburg).

While incising from the inner canthus to the septum nasi and from the inner canthus to the malar bone, compress the facial artery over the inferior maxilla. Just before dividing the upper lip, compress it on either side of the median line and, when it is severed, ligate the superior coronary arteries while still compressed. In making these incisions several arteries must be divided and ligated.

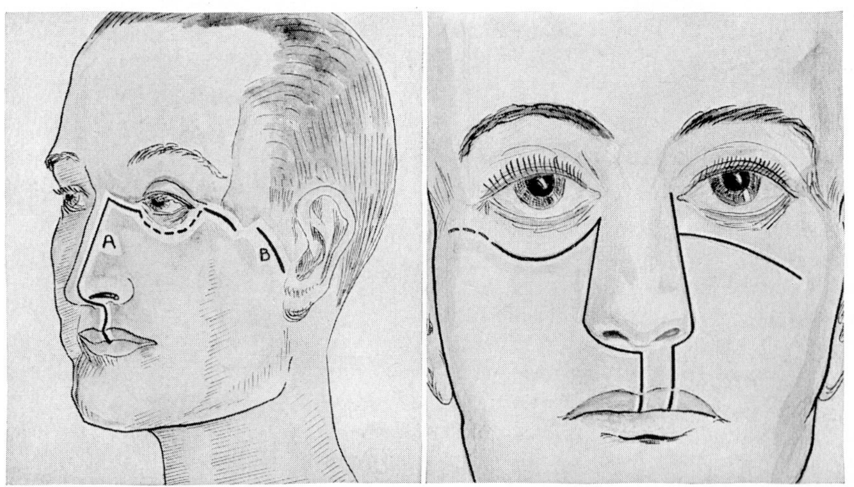

Fig. 313 Fig. 314

Fig. 313. A. Incision for removal of the upper jaw. B. Incision for excision of the condyle of the mandible.

Fig. 314. Incisions for removal of the upper jaw. Right side, Fergusson's incision; left side, Kocher's incision.

Step 2. The flap thus outlined is dissected up. Clear the surface of the superior maxilla as completely as possible but not subperiosteally. The infraorbital artery is now divided.

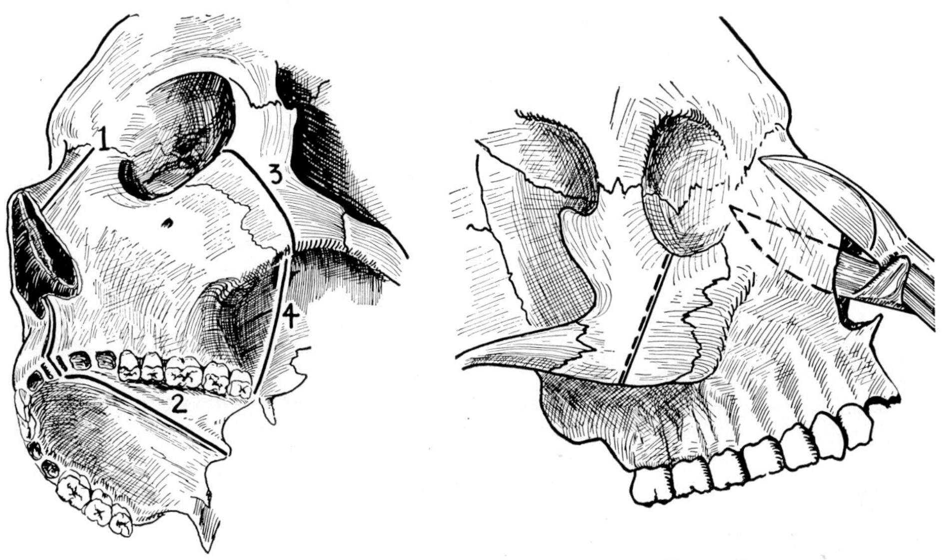

Fig. 315 Fig. 316

Fig. 315. Resection of superior maxilla. Lines indicate positions of bone division.
Fig. 316. The bone cutting forceps divides the ascending process of the upper jaw, while the line indicates the point of section of the malar bone.

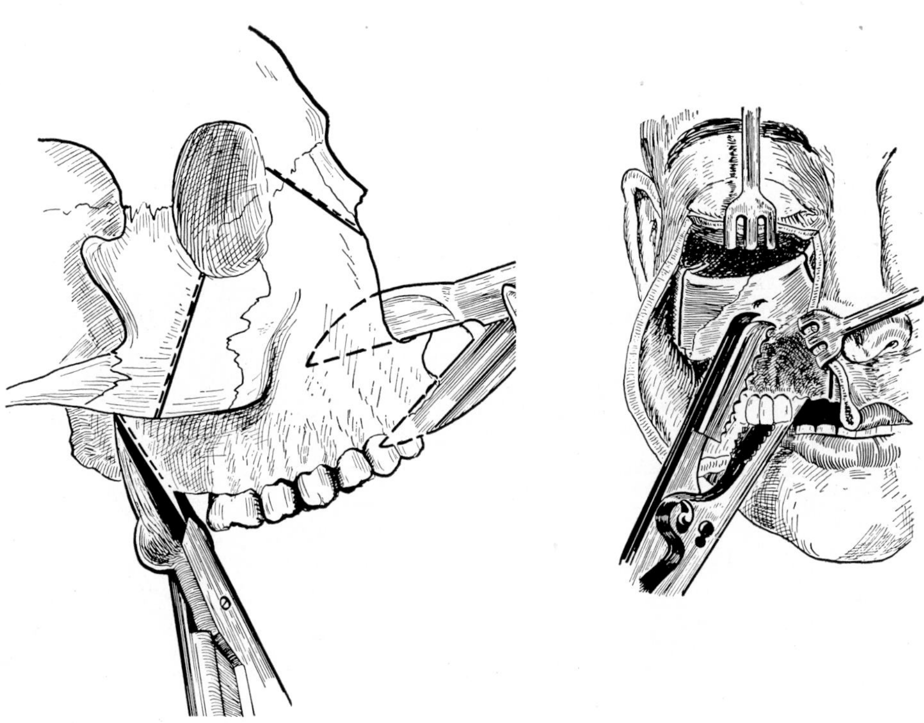

Fig. 317 Fig. 318

Fig. 317. Illustrating method of division of the palatine vault and pterygomaxillary disjunction.
Fig. 318. A Faraboef forceps removes the completely detached upper jaw.

Step 3. Detach the nasal cartilages from the bone. Divide the nasal process of the superior maxilla from the junction of the nasal process with the lower border of the nasal bone, to the margin of the orbit. Raise the periosteum from the floor of the orbit (including the origin of the inferior oblique muscle) and retract these upward. Chisel obliquely across the orbital plate to the anterior end of the sphenomaxillary fissure. The orbital and external surfaces of the malar bone are now cleared. The malar bone is divided obliquely through its middle with a Gigli saw, from the anterior end of the sphenomaxillary fissure downward and outward to the center of its free border (Figs. 315-316-317).

Step 4. Extract the central incisor tooth of the involved side. Divide the muco-periosteal covering of the hard palate in the median line along the intermaxillary and the interpalatal sutures from the alveolar process to the posterior nasal spine. Similarly divide the muco-periosteal covering of the floor of the nose, cutting as near the septum of the nose as possible from the posterior to the anterior nasal spine. Make a transverse incision across the roof of the mouth at the junction of the hard and soft palates and separate these. With a fine saw, chisel or scissors, divide the horizontal plate of the palate and palatal and alveolar portions of the superior maxillary bone, as nearly in the middle line as the septum nasi will allow.

Step 5. Grasp the superior maxilla with a large bone forceps and gently move it from side to side to determine the position and extent of its remaining attachments. The two remaining bony connections are part of the orbital plate and the union between the pterygoid processes and superior maxilla. These are divided with bone forceps. (Fig. 318.)

Step 6. The inferior maxilla is depressed, the outer and posterior surfaces of the superior maxilla are freed and, by means of angular bone-cutting forceps introduced within the mouth and passed up behind the maxillary tuberosity, the superior maxillary bone is separated, taking care that the soft palate is held out of the way. A number of arteries will have to be divided and ligated.

Step 7. All bleeding vessels are secured and hemorrhage is controlled by tamponade. The wound is sutured throughout. Particular care is to be taken in suturing the skin to avoid disfigurement. Drainage is established through the mouth.

Note. Preservation of branches of the facial artery is important.

Dangers. 1. Hemorrhage. This is prevented by preliminary ligation of the external carotid artery.

2. Aspiration Pneumonia. This is forestalled by preliminary laryngotomy and plugging of the pharynx.

3. Shock. Administer the usual shock-treatment before and after the operation.

4. Secondary Hemorrhage. Be on the lookout for its occurrence and treat it accordingly, should it eventuate.

OPERATIONS ON THE LOWER JAW

In resection of the lower jaw, certain structures must be kept in mind: the auriculo-temporal, the inferior dental and lingual nerves, and the nerve to the internal pterygoid muscle; the external carotid artery; and the stylo-maxillary ligament. (Fig. 319.) The lines of incision, depending upon the extent of bone to be removed, are those indicated in Figure 320.

Points of injection and direction of the needle as well as general directions for infiltration anesthesia in resection are depicted in Figure 321.

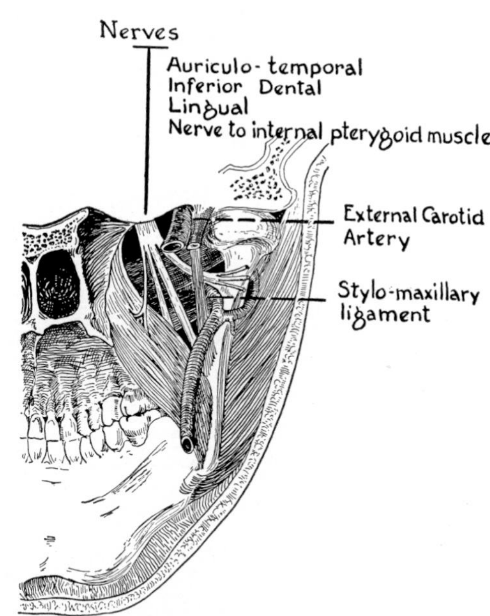

FIG. 319. Important structures concerned in temporo-maxillary resection and disarticulation of the mandible.

TEMPORO-MAXILLARY ANKYLOSIS

Murphy's Operation

This consists of a typical arthroplasty on the temporo-maxillary joint using a pedicled flap composed of aponeurosis of the temporal muscle and fat. The procedure is carried out as follows:

Step 1. Make an L-shaped incision above the zygoma and in front of the ear as shown in Figure 322; or a modified incision may be used as depicted in Figure 323. In the former the perpendicular incision begins just in front of the ear and extends from 1½ inches above the zygoma in the hair-line downward to the lower border of the zygomatic arch.

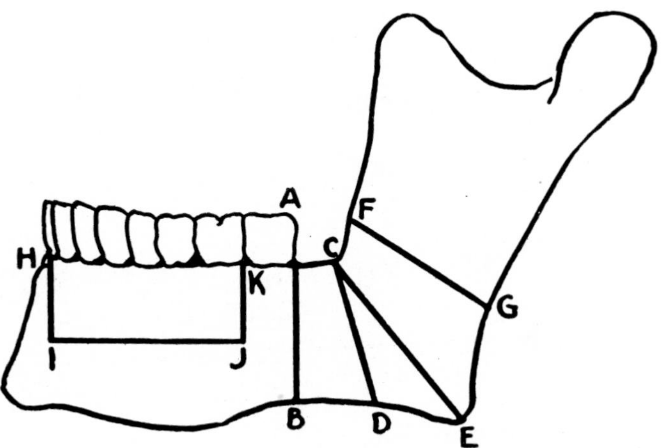

FIG. 320. Lines of incision in resection operations upon lower jaw.

The incision then curves forward on the superior margin of the zygoma for a distance of about ¾ of an inch, then curves slightly upward to avoid injuring the temporal and orbicular branches of the facial nerve. This incision has much to commend it; it affords better access to the joint than does a perpendicular incision and is certainly superior to the incisions practised heretofore in exposing the temporo-maxillary articulation. The cicatrix resulting from this operation is slight, its greater part being hidden in the hair line.

Step 2. Expose the neck of the mandible and divide it with a Gigli saw. (Fig. 324.) Separate the divided ends by traction. While there are other methods devised for dividing the head and neck of the mandible at the line of the bony ankylosis (chisels, electrically driven olive-tipped dental burrs), the Gigli

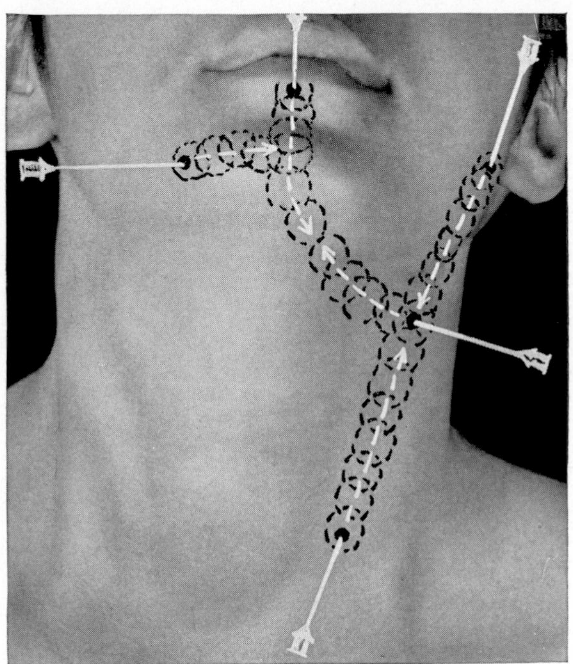

Fig. 321. Resection of the lower jaw. Lines of skin infiltration in removal of the lower jaw. Black circles indicate area to be infiltrated; black dots, the entrance of the needle point; white arrows, the direction of the infiltrated fluid. The masseter and particularly the buccinator nerve must be thoroughly infiltrated. The deep structures are blocked as for the removal of cervical glands (Fig. 274, p. 248). Sufficient anesthesia should be deposited in the mental foramen. It is advisable to block the nerves at the lingula before infiltration in the neck is made. The mucosa of the floor of the mouth should also be infiltrated. If the entire half of the jaw is to be taken away, the third branch should be thoroughly blocked at its exit from the foramen.

saw method is best. Caution should be exercised in using the chisel or burr lest injury result to the internal maxillary artery or even the brain, which is in close proximity. It is well to recall that the brain is separated from the head of the mandible only by a very thin, transparent plate of bone.

To frustrate such injuries, Murphy devised some special periosteotomes. The tip of such a periosteotome passes directly beneath the neck of the mandible and the internal maxillary artery. One periosteotome is placed in position from each side and all the bone lying in front of these instruments may be removed without danger. Expose the joint-surface with the periosteotomes which push the tissues away all around the anterior surface of bone-union and then around the posterior surface. When the bone has been bared, pass the two periosteotomes behind the neck of the bone on each side, completely encircling the neck of the mandible behind, hugging close to the head during the removal of the bone.

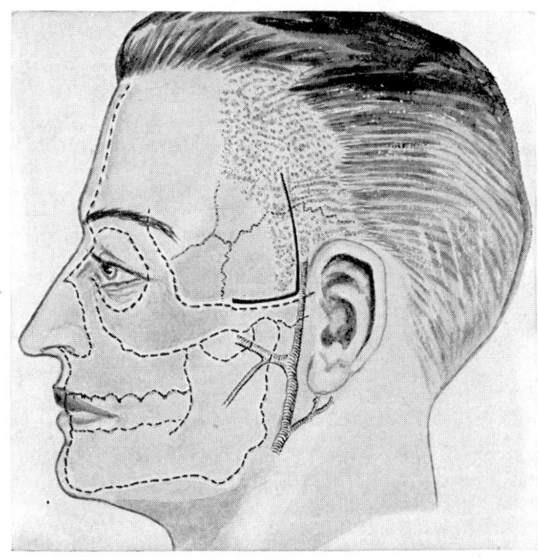

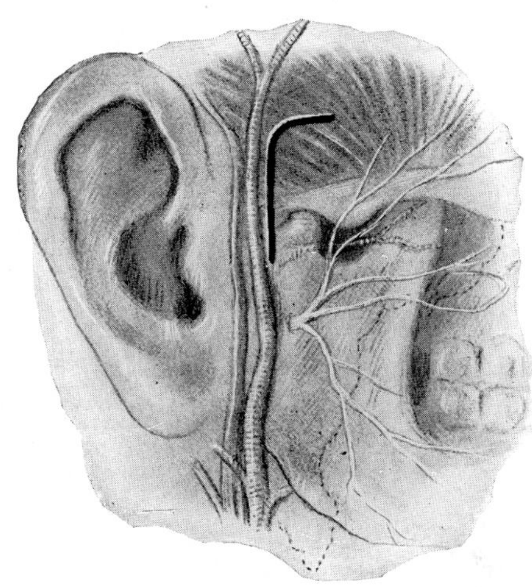

FIG. 322 FIG. 323

FIG. 322. Murphy's temporomaxillary arthroplasty. L-shaped skin incision above the zygoma and in front of the ear, so placed to avoid injury to the facial nerve. Note the relation of the external carotid, the temporal, and internal maxillary arteries to the field of operation. The last-named vessel, in passing inward behind the neck of the mandible, lies close to the bone and must be carefully protected from injury during the operation, especially at the time when the neck of the mandible is divided.

FIG. 323. Incision for temporomaxillary arthroplasty modified from Mayo Clinic (Davis, Applied Anatomy).

These minutiae must be observed if success is to be attained. Remove about ½ inch of bone clear across the neck of the mandible. The periosteum

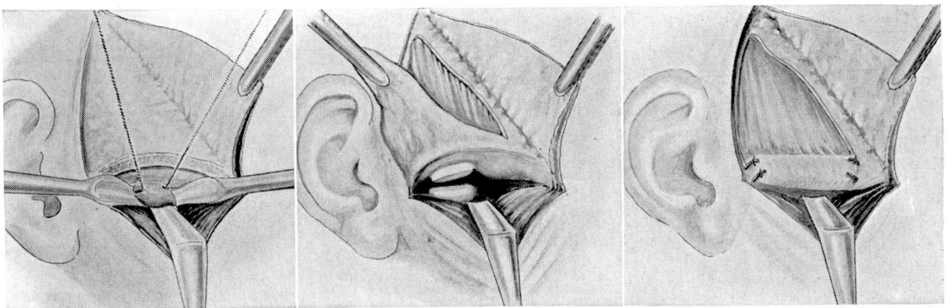

FIG. 324 FIG. 325 FIG. 326

FIG. 324. Murphy's temporomaxillary arthroplasty. Dividing the neck of the mandible with a Gigli saw. (In actual operation the saw is not allowed to make so acute an angle as shown in the illustration, because of its great tendency to break when sharply bent.)

FIG. 325. Murphy's temporomaxillary arthroplasty. The pedicled fascia and fat flap is dissected out from the temporal fascia, and the free end of the flap is turned inward between the divided ends of the mandible and sutured securely in place with tacking stitches.

FIG. 326. Murphy's temporomaxillary arthroplasty. The fascial flap is now placed in position and the wound is ready for closure.

must be excised with it and enough space created for the interposition of the fascial and fat pad. A small rongeur is an aid to remove smaller fragments of bone. With careful work the Gigli saw may be substituted effectually by a chisel of proper size.

Step 3. A pedicled flap of fat and fascia is dissected from the temporal region and turned downward and inward between the separated ends of the mandible. The flap is sutured in place. This flap is U-shaped and taken from the temporal fascia and should be about 2 inches long and an inch wide. Its base should be at the upper margin of the zygoma. Its dissection is started from above downward; it is folded over the zygoma and packed into the gap created by the removal of the bone described. It is retained in place by a few catgut sutures at its anterior and posterior basal angles. (Figs. 325-326.)

Step 4. Replace the skin-flap and suture it in place. Dress. A dental splint such as Blair's modification of the Gunning splint may be used advantageously to keep the jaws apart. (Fig. 344, p. 298.)

Comments. During the time of the operation no special effort should be made forcibly to spread the jaws, because it is important that the mandible should remain steady on the unaffected side. Hence a wooden block inserted on the operated side maintains wide separation of the molar teeth until the flap has securely healed in its new position. By all means, avoid hematoma formation. If it occurs it may frustrate the results aimed at.

Complications. If the internal maxillary artery is inadvertently injured the external carotid must be ligated opposite the corner of the hyoid bone. Injury to the branches of the facial nerve may be avoided by using the incision described and by careful operating. No attempt should be made to clean out the glenoid fossa. Remember that the base of the skull will surely be penetrated if the ankylosis is divided in the line of the original articulation.

Rochet's Operation

Where the experience of the surgeon is limited and he wishes to avoid operative complications incident to such operations as just described, and to safeguard the facial nerve and other important structures from injury, etc., Rochet's operation may be substituted.

Step 1. Make an incision at the border of the angle of the jaw; extend it along the lower edge of the horizontal ramus and about an inch along the posterior edge of the ascending ramus of the mandible. Through this incision, expose the inferior insertion of the masseter muscle. With an elevator, detach the muscle from below upward, thus exposing the external surface of the mandible. Similarly expose the inner surface of the bone by separating the insertion of the pterygoid muscle.

Step 2. Divide the mandible with a Gigli saw, or chisel, along the lines indicated in Figure 324 and remove the section of bone between the lines shown. It is better to remove a rather larger section of bone than too little.

Step 3. From the deep surface of the masseter muscle, dissect a flap about one and one-half inches long with its pedicle above, consisting of about half the thickness of the muscle. The free end of this flap is pulled through the breach in the bone and sutured to the pterygoid muscle. (Fig. 327.) In case the flap from the masseter is insufficient to accomplish the object of the operation, a subsidiary flap is taken from the pterygoid.

Step 4. Close the wound.

Comment. Figure 328 depicts a patient in whom the resection of the coronoid process, etc., was rendered hazardous by reason of excessive callus formation and displacement of the corresponding parts. I performed the

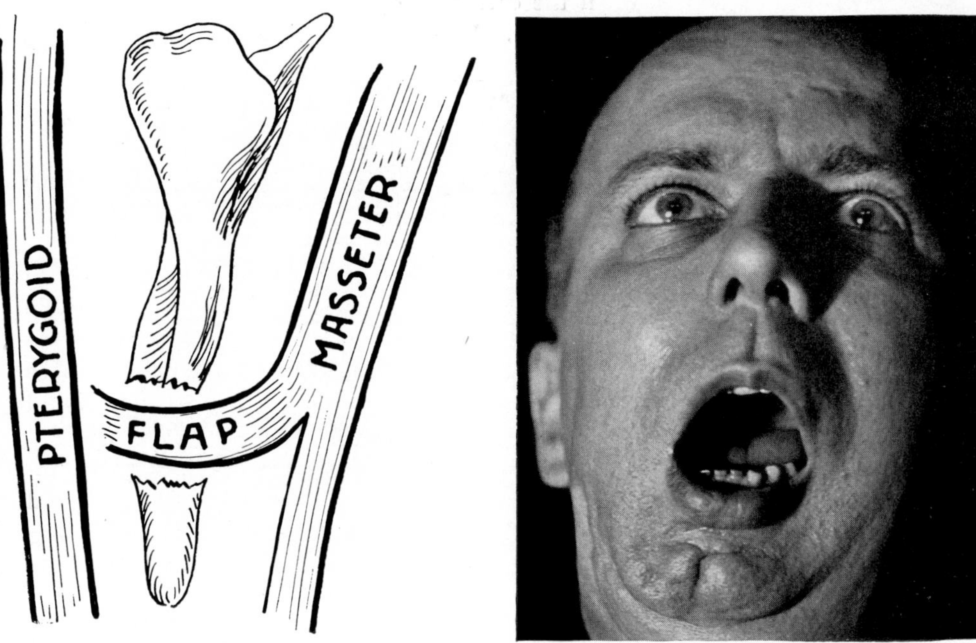

Fig. 327 Fig. 328

Fig. 327. Rochet's operation (after Monod and Vanwerts).

Fig. 328. Resection of mandible by Rochet's method. Patient 17 years after operation.

Rochet operation on this patient. The photograph taken 17 years later depicts the range of mobility of the jaw. He enjoys perfect control of his masticatory apparatus.

DISLOCATION OF THE JAW

Disengage the coronoid process in front of the malar bone; depress the jaw, then push it backward. It should be kept in mind that simply pushing the chin upward only results in further displacement of the condyle and that the mouth cannot be closed nor its hinge-like movements regained until the condyle is reinstated in its cavity.

Treatment. Place the patient in a sitting position. Stand directly in front of him. Have an assistant hold the patient's head securely. Protect your thumbs from injury when the jaws suddenly come together by wrapping them in several thicknesses of gauze. (Fig. 329.)

With palms down, place your thumbs in the patient's mouth while your fingers take a firm hold along the exterior outline of the mandible. With the hands in this position, exert firm pressure downward and backward maneuvering the dislocated condyle back into its socket, aided by the action of the masseter and temporal muscles.

In some cases, especially those of long standing, it is advisable to effect reduction under anesthesia.

SUBLUXATION OF THE JAW

This condition results when the cartilages of the joint slip backward causing the condyles to be thrust forward. Individuals who frequently have a dis-

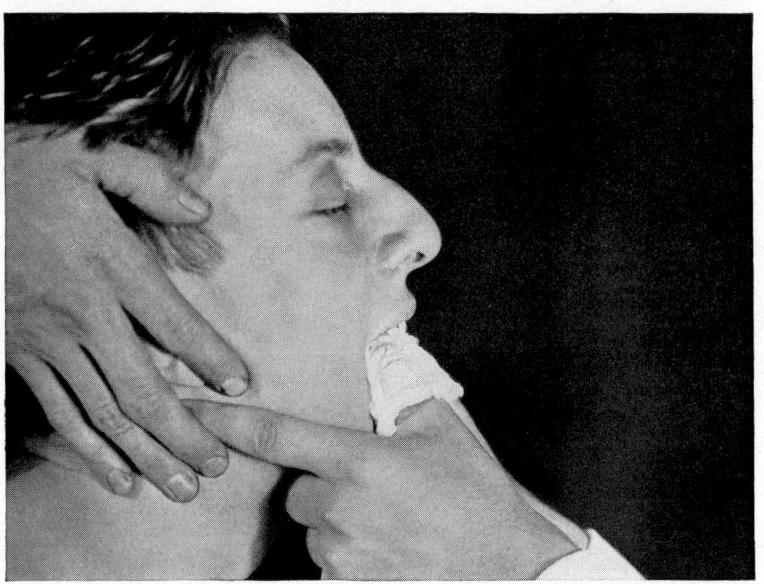

FIG. 329. Method of reduction of dislocation of jaw. Have fingers protected to avoid accidental bites from the patient.

location of this kind are able to reduce it without assistance. If the case, however, is more difficult than usual, force the mouth open by means of a wedge of wood or bone while an assistant mobilizes the jaw.

After reduction is accomplished, apply a Barton or four-tailed bandage. Retain it in place for about a fortnight. Instruct the patient to be especially cautious in opening his mouth for about three weeks or until the injured capsule is completely healed.

Irreducible Dislocation

Under general anesthesia, make an incision immediately under the zygoma. Introduce a McGraw's hook just over the edge of the sigmoid fossa. While an assistant firmly holds and elevates the symphysis menti, bring the condyle back into its socket with the aid of the hook.

FRACTURE OF THE LOWER JAW

Two methods of immobilization are used: (a) **indirect fixation,** consisting of keeping the broken fragments of the mandible in their proper relation to the sound jaw and (b) **direct fixation** by means of dental splints, wire or bone plates. (Fig. 330.)

Indirect Fixation

To Dr. Thomas L. Gilmer, of Chicago, we owe the simple but extremely effective device, the soldered dental band, which consists of a band of thin metal made to conform to the circumference of the crown of a given tooth which is cemented in place and to which may be soldered a ring, tube or a bar. When properly applied, these bands cause no damage to the teeth, and will remain in place rather indefinitely. The adjustable band, which dates back to the early part of the last century, can be applied and tightened with an appropriate special wrench. These may be obtained from the dental supply houses under the name

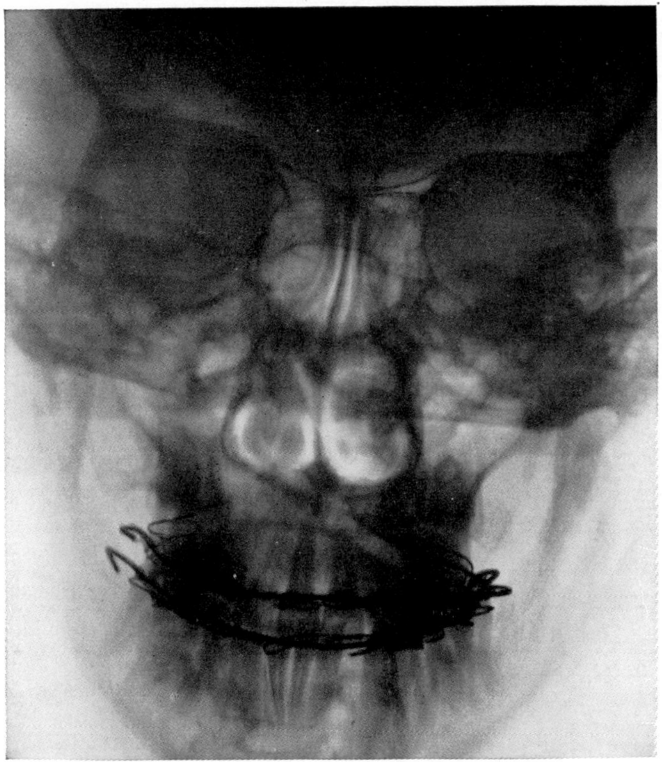

Fig. 330. Fractured mandible treated by direct fixation (wiring).

of Angle's fracture bands. They come in two sizes, one to fit the cuspid and bicuspid and the other for the molar teeth.

Dr. Gilmer first advocated direct fixation of the lower to the upper jaw by means of the teeth as a treatment of fracture of the mandible (1887). Where applicable, this is a very simple and efficient procedure and has a broader field of usefulness than any other means at the disposal of either surgeon or dentist. Fixation may be done by dental bands (Fig. 331) or by wires fastened directly to the necks of the teeth (Fig. 332).

If bands are used, the jaws are fixed by silk or fine wire ligatures that extend between the bands, each band having a lug or button on its outer surface for this purpose. The use of bands has certain points in its favor over the direct wiring of the teeth, but the latter is the more practical method; the materials required are nearly always at hand, and can be applied by any surgeon with a pair of artery forceps, a pair of scissors or wire cutters.

The disadvantage of this method is that in order to open the mouth the wires have to be cut, and if it is found desirable to continue the fixation, the whole procedure may have to be repeated on teeth already sore from traction. However, Blair states that "if one will refrain from the exercise of unwarranted curiosity, the necessity of reapplying the wires will not often arise." Blair counsels a soft iron wire that can be obtained on spools from the hardware shop, or in rolls at any florist, using No. 24 for the molars and cuspids, and No. 26 for the incisors. This iron wire is very pliable and does not stretch, but if it cannot be obtained, a soft brass, copper, or silver wire may be substituted. The wire is cut into

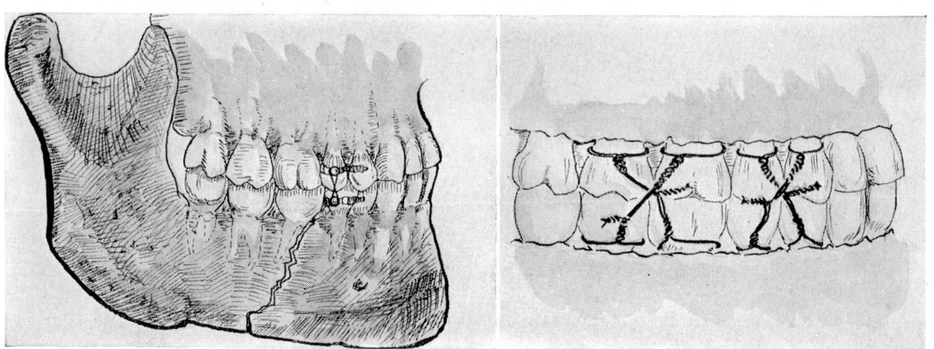

FIG. 331 FIG. 332

FIG. 331. Diagram showing fracture treated by wiring the lower to the upper jaw by means of Angle's fracture bands.

FIG. 332. Gilmer's method of treating a fracture of the jaw by fastening the lower to the upper jaw by means of wires passed around the necks of the teeth.

lengths of about 45 cm. each, is bent in the middle, and by means of forceps is passed from the lingual surface through the interdental spaces on each side of the tooth to be ligated. An assistant holds the intra-oral loop of the wire well down on the neck of the tooth, while the operator, having obtained a firm grasp on each end, makes a twist of two full turns. This is the most important part of the application of the wire ligature. It should grasp the neck of the tooth so firmly as to preclude any motion. The ligature can be tightened with forceps, but it is better to get the tension while the first twist is being made. The serrations on the jaws of the forceps weaken the wire wherever they grasp it. The upper wires are being twisted together with the lower and the teeth should be held in occlusion by pressure from below the chin. It is also very important that the teeth be held in occlusion while the wires are being tightened.

Wiring of a Fractured Mandible

DIRECT FIXATION

Step 1. Make an incision about 2 inches in length, or longer if need be, extending along the lower border of the jaw. Avoid injuring the **facial nerve** while working in its vicinity (posterior border of the ramus of the jaw at the level of the lower border of the lobe of the ear). Deepen the incision to the bone.

The facial artery and vein will, of course, have to be divided between two ligatures. Insure hemostasis.

Step 2. Raise the soft tissues covering the jaw, except the periosteum, on both surfaces of the mandible. Freely expose the site of the fracture. Separate the insertions of the masseter and internal pterygoid muscles from the bone. Drill holes in the bone at either side of the fracture at the most advantageous points, while steadying the bone with bone forceps. Pass appropriate wires through the drill holes. The wire when placed should cross the line of fracture at right angles. While drilling the bone have an assistant hold a flat retractor on the opposite side of the mandible to prevent the drill from injuring contiguous soft structures. Immediately after a hole is drilled the wire should be passed through it; this will avoid trouble in finding it later. The drill holes should be large enough to admit a doubled wire. Blair recommends an admirable method of inserting a No. 20 piece of silver wire; this is shown in Figure 333. Tie wires.

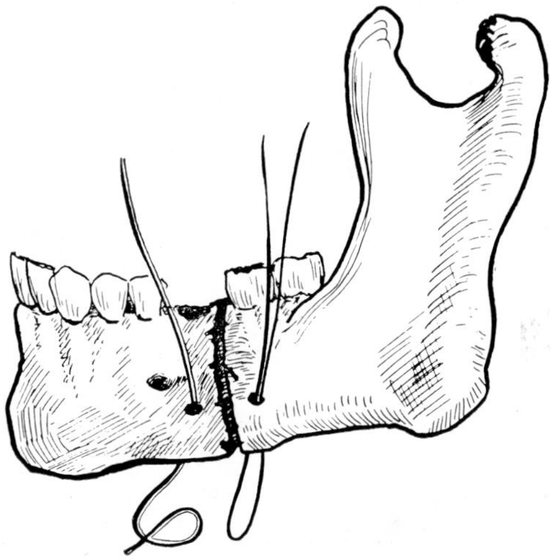

FIG. 333. Blair's method of passing a wire from the deep surface of the bone. The silver wire is passed through the first hole from the external to the mesial surface. A loop of another wire is passed through the second hole in the same manner and the first wire is caught in the loop of the second and drawn through the second opening.

Step 3. Close the superimposed soft structures with silkworm-gut sutures. Provide for drainage.

Comments. **Lane plates of proper size (2 cm. long, 2 mm. thick and 5 mm. wide) may be used. Dental splints may also be used to advantage.**

RESECTION OF THE ALVEOLAR PROCESS

Step 1. Make an incision of the inner periosteum around the portion to be excised.

Step 2. Remove the affected area with chisel and mallet; or, if the growth is small, with a rongeur forceps. Have an assistant support the chin while you remove the growth. Where the lesion demands more extensive resection two vertical incisions may be made with a finger saw. (Fig. 334.) The lower ends of the vertical incisions are joined by a horizontal one made with a chisel.

PARTIAL RESECTION OF THE HORIZONTAL RAMUS OF THE LOWER JAW

Step 1. Make an incision through the skin down to the bone along the inferior border of the mandible.

Step 2. Separate the soft tissues from both the inner and outer surfaces of the jaw. In necrosis, preserve the periosteum; in tumor, sacrifice it.

Step 3. Remove the teeth overlying the segment of bone to be removed. With a Gigli or finger saw make vertical incisions outlining the segment to be removed. Remove the segment between the two vertical incisions. Wherever possible leave a ledge of lower jaw behind. (Figs. 335-336.)

Step 4. Close the wound. Drain. Metal splints (Lane plates) or tibial grafts may be used to bridge the gap. (Fig. 337.)

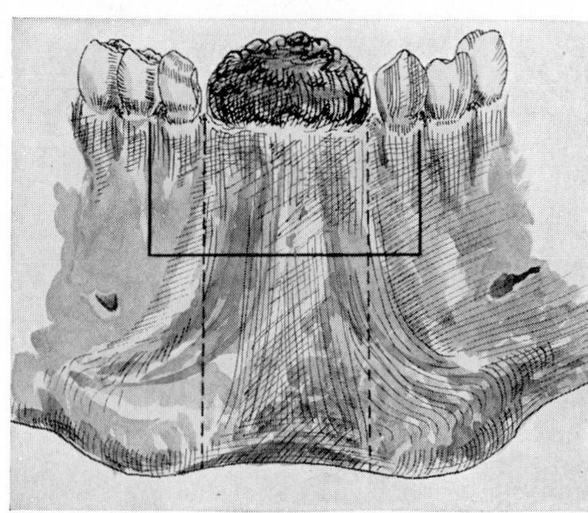

FIG. 334. Partial resection of the alveolar process of lower jaw in a case of epulis. The dotted lines indicate a complete resection of the median portion of the inferior maxilla.

RESECTION AND EXARTICULATION OF THE LOWER JAW

The resection may be unilateral or bilateral.

Indications. Partial Removal: (a) epulis (Fig. 338); (b) epitheliomas arising at the floor of the mouth and extensively invading the gum; (c) epithelioma or myeloid sarcoma of the mandible; (d) necrosis of the mandible (Figs. 339-340).

Step 1. Begin the incision in the middle of the chin (Fig. 341); continue it down in front of the chin, thence along the lower border of the mandible and upward along the posterior border of its ascending ramus, ending about opposite the center of the ascending ramus. Along its entire extent the incision is carried through skin, fascia, the platysma myoides muscle and periosteum to the bone except over the facial artery where the skin alone is incised, the artery itself being exposed, doubly ligated and cut. (Fig. 342.)

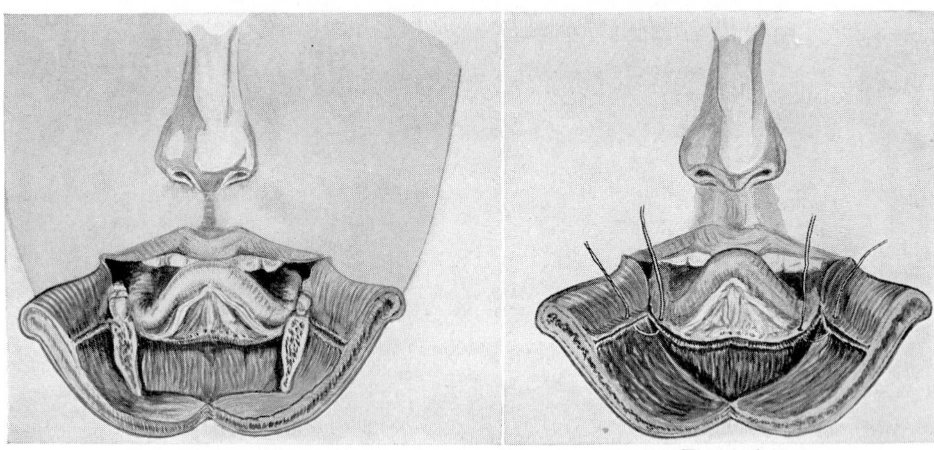

FIG. 335 FIG. 336

FIG. 335. Partial resection of median portion of lower jaw. The median portion of the mandible has been resected. Note the divided surface of the bone on each side; also the lines of section of the lingual and gingival mucous membranes.

FIG. 336. Suture of lingual to gingival mucous membrane. The divided surface of the maxilla has already been covered by the suture.

Step 2. Raise the structures covering the outer surface of the lower jaw subperiosteally, working from the free border of the bone toward its alveolar

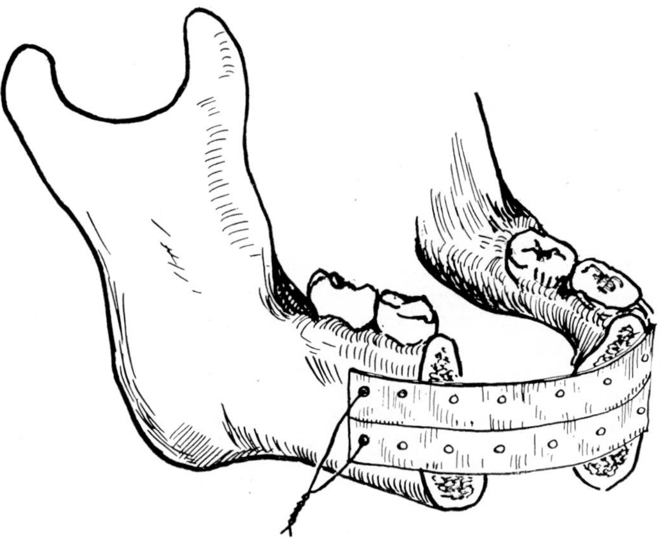

FIG. 337. Metal splint used after resection of the mandible.

margin and from the symphysis menti toward the angle and upward along the ascending ramus of the mandible. Divide the mental vessels and nerves

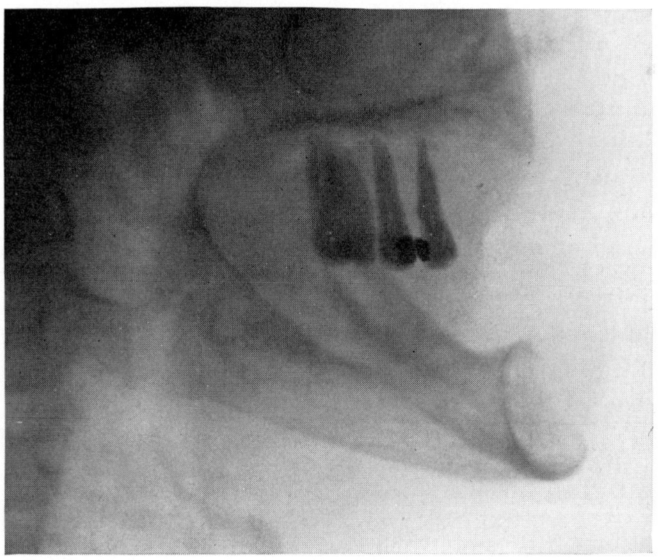

FIG. 338. X-ray appearance of an epulis invading extensively the midportion of the lower jaw.

at the foramen. The clearing is continued as high up the ascending ramus as possible.

Step 3. Separate subperiosteally the structures attached to the inner aspect of the horizontal ramus of the mandible.

Step 4. Divide the mucous membrane along the alveolar margin on the outer and inner sides of the maxilla; free the muscles from both aspects of the bone, saving as much of these as possible.

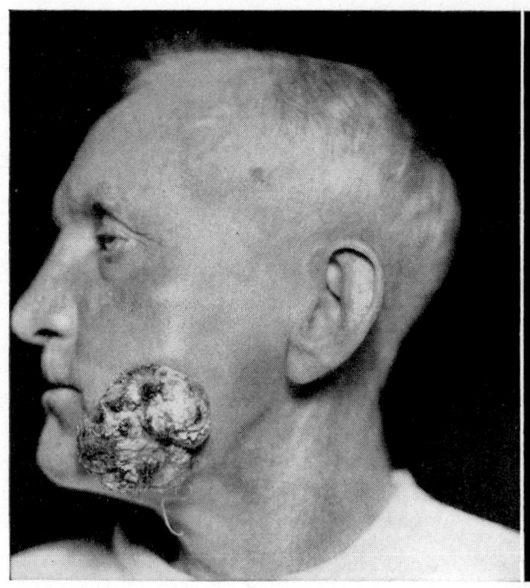

FIG. 339

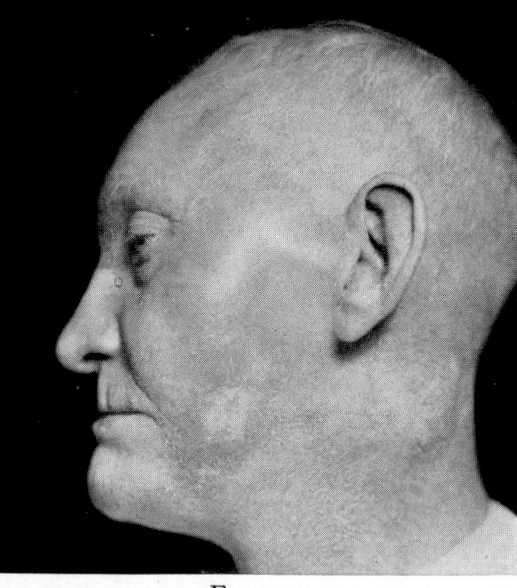

FIG. 340

FIG. 339. Extensive epithelioma of alveolar crest with extension through face. Controlled by means of actual cautery—surgical diathermy and radium. Repair through pedicle flap from neck. (Service of Cook County Hospital, Chicago, patient of Dr. T. E. Schaeffer.)
FIG. 340. Same patient after treatment.

Step 5. Seize the anterior end of the severed mandible, draw it outward; detach all remaining structures from its inner aspect. If not already done, the mylohyoid muscle and the posterior part of the mucous membrane of the mouth are now separated.

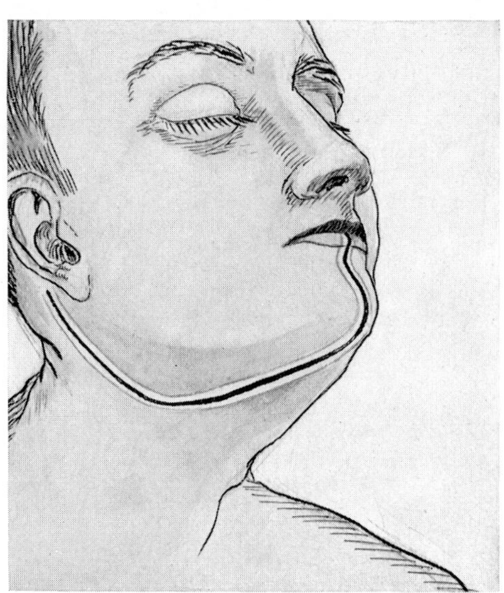

FIG. 341. Kocher's incision for excision of the mandible.

Step 6. Firmly depress the anterior portion of the inferior maxilla. (Fig. 343.) With blunt scissors, detach the temporal muscle from its insertion. Render the coronoid process as accessible as possible. Approach it from before rather than from behind. Care should be exercised to avoid injuring the important structures near the upper half of the posterior border of the ascending ramus of the mandible.

Step 7. Free the insertion of the external pterygoid muscle with elevator or blunt scissors by following along the upper and inner aspect of the condyloid process. Divide the joint capsule and disarticulate the head of the bone forward. Sever any remaining ligaments and adhesive bands of fascia.

Step 8. Drain the wound temporarily through the posterior portion of the incision. Suture the skin carefully to avoid scarring.

Note. This operation may at times necessitate a preliminary ligation of the external carotid artery or a preliminary tracheotomy or division of the entire thickness of the lower lip. Both halves of the inferior maxilla may be simultaneously removed by a repetition of the above procedure.

Partsch, after removing a segment of the lower jaw, used a perforated metal plate held in place by wire sutures to keep the ends of the bone in correct position. (Figs. 337 and 344.) The metal plates are protected with rubber tubing. The mucous membrane of the floor of the mouth and cheek is sutured together below the metal plate so that the plate lies exposed in the oral cavity. The temporary plate is removed as soon as a proper dental prosthesis can be substituted. Berndt uses a celluloid prosthesis where half of the mandible has been removed. Macewen implanted a piece of rib between the divided ends of the jaw. If expertly performed, free transplantation of bone is the method of choice. The transplant is obtained from a portion of rib, tibia, ilium, spine of scapula or metatarsal bone.

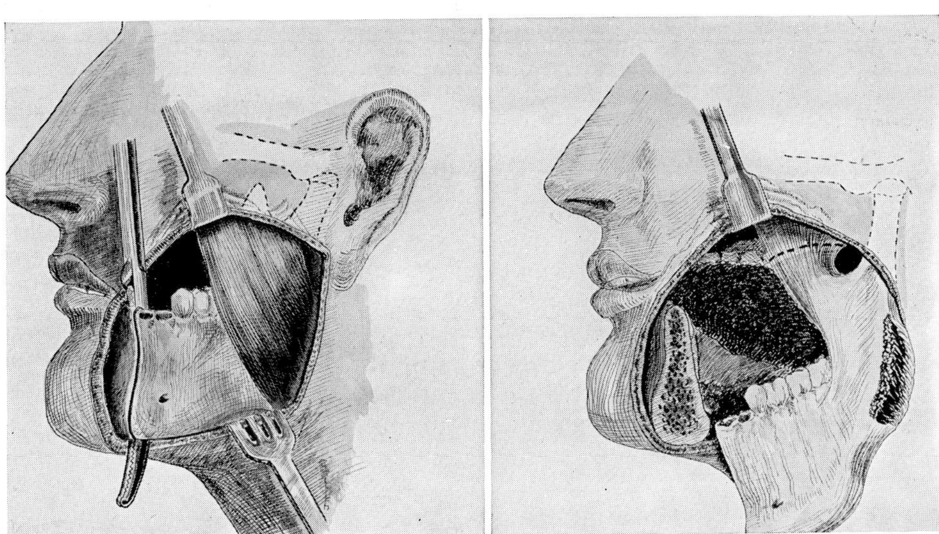

FIG. 342 FIG. 343

FIG. 342. Unilateral resection of inferior maxilla. A curved forceps is passed behind the bone to protect the soft parts from the saw.

FIG. 343. Unilateral resection of inferior maxilla. The bone, divided in the middle, is now almost detached. The tendon of the temporal muscle is seen.

NERVE ANASTOMOSIS FOR FACIAL PARALYSIS

Historical Notes. The first operation for nerve anastomosis was performed by Ballance and Purves in 1895. Fauré operated in 1898 and in 1900 Robert Kennedy divided the facial nerve in a case of severe facial spasm. He then united the proximal extremity of the distal portion of the facial to the partially divided spinal accessory nerve. A perfect result was obtained. Cushing successfully operated in 1903.

Anatomic Considerations. The facial nerve is deeply seated in the stylomastoid foramen from which it emerges. Its course from here is downward, outward and forward, finally winding round the styloid process; it then runs forward horizontally until it crosses the posterior auricular artery into the parotid gland. The horizontal portion of the nerve is found about ¾ inch below the lower border of the zygomatic arch at the level of the tip of the lobule of the ear.

The hypoglossal nerve leaves the skull through the anterior condylar foramen and lies on the inner side of the deep cervical vessels. As it descends, the nerve comes forward between the internal carotid artery and jugular veins to the lower border of the digastric muscle where it curves forward round the origin of the occipital artery, the sternomastoid branch of which turns downward over the nerve. From this point the nerve runs forward above the hyoid bone, passes under the tendon of

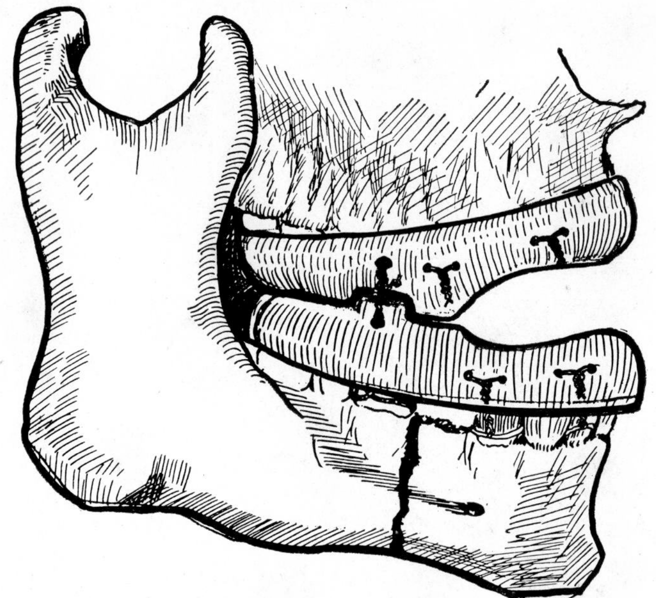

FIG. 344. Modified Gunning splint, applicable in instances where the jaws are to be kept apart. The splint consists of two pieces fixed together after each half of the splint has been put in place. Its application is much simpler than the original Gunning splint (Blair).

the digastric, the lower end of the stylohyoid and the mylohyoid muscles, and crosses the external carotid and lingual arteries.

The external, spinal or surgical portion of the spinal accessory nerve runs through the jugular foramen from the skull and then passes downward, outward and slightly backward in front of (in a few instances behind) the internal jugular vein, between it and the occipital artery which it crosses perpendicularly. Its course is now between the transverse process of the atlas and the posterior border of the digastric. The nerve next passes behind the posterior border of the parotid and enters the sternomastoid 2 inches below the apex of the mastoid process.

Anastomosis Between the Facial and Spinal Accessory Nerves

Step 1. Make an incision along the anterior border of the sternomastoid muscle. Begin above in the groove between the external ear and the mastoid process at the level of the tragus and terminate the incision at a point about 5 inches lower.

Step 2. Retract the ear forward. Divide the fibrous tissues covering the mastoid process in order to gain access to its anterior border. Expose the anterior border of the sternomastoid.

Step 3. By blunt dissection, penetrate between the parotid gland and the anterior border of the mastoid. Move the dissecting instrument horizontally, not vertically, in an endeavor to avoid injuring the facial nerve. According to Marion, the nerve should be found at a depth of a little less than ½ an

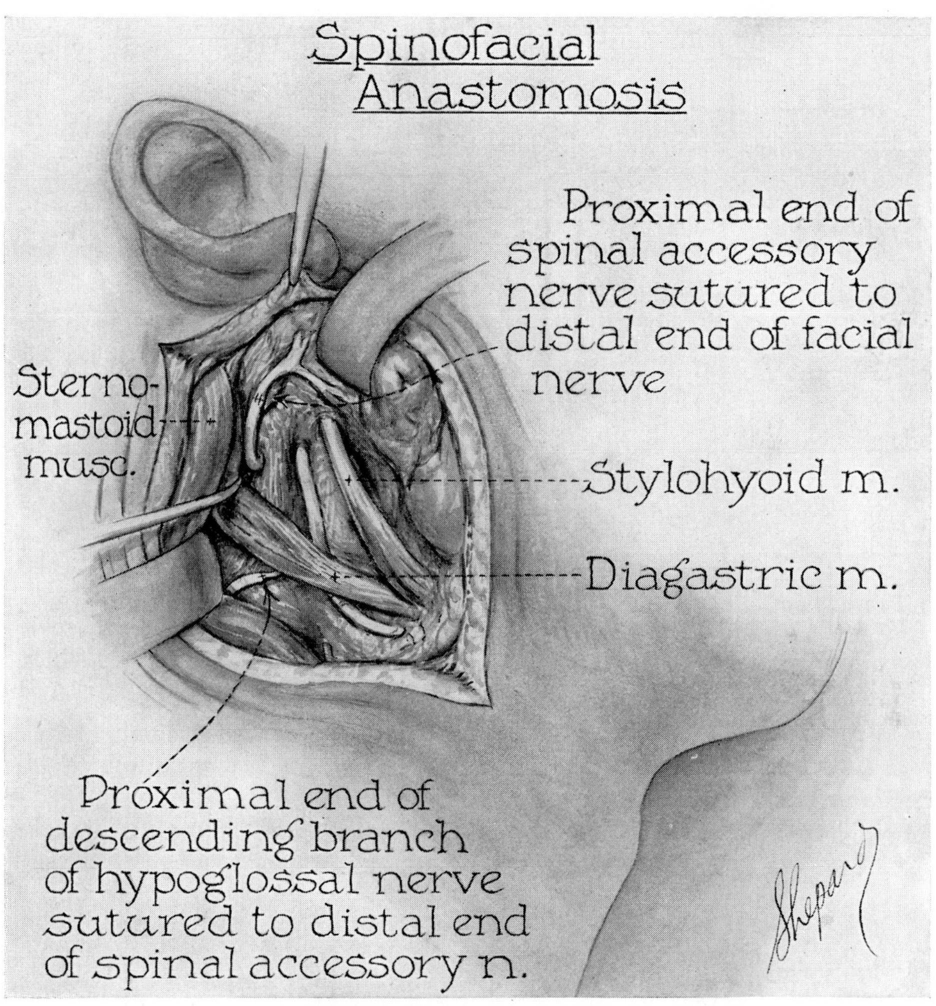

FIG. 345. Spinofacial anastomosis.

inch from the surface of the mastoid process at the junction of its lower and middle thirds. The nerve is isolated and divided as far back as possible.

Step 4. Open the sheath of the sternomastoid muscle longitudinally. The transverse process of the atlas should be recognized about ½ an inch below the mastoid process; it should be clearly exposed by bluntly dividing the fibrous tissues covering it. The posterior belly of the digastric muscle in front of the atlas is recognized. The spinal accessory nerve lies between the transverse process of the atlas behind and the digastric muscle in front. The nerve is isolated.

Step 5. Divide the nerve at its entrance into the sternomastoid muscle. Do an end-to-end anastomosis between the proximal segment of the spinal accessory and the distal segment of the facial nerve. Instead of completely dividing the spinal accessory nerve, an opening may be made in its side and the facial nerve implanted into this aperture (end-to-side anastomosis). End-to-end anastomosis is preferred. (Fig. 345.)

Step 6. Bury the line of nerve suture in the belly of the digastric muscle after incising the muscle for this purpose.

Step 7. Close the wound.

Anastomosis Between the Facial and Hypoglossal Nerves

Step 1. Make an incision in the groove between the external ear and the mastoid, from a point on the level of the tragus. Carry this incision downward along the anterior border of the sternomastoid muscle to a point a little below the angle of the jaw. Continue the cut horizontally forward for about one inch on the level of the hyoid bone. (Figs. 345-346.)

Step 2. Expose and divide the facial nerve as described above in discussing anastomosis between the facial and spinal accessory nerves.

Step 3. Open the sheath of the sternomastoid muscle anteriorly in the lower part of the wound. Retract the muscle backward. Divide the deep layer of the sheath of the muscle at the level of the greater cornu of the hyoid bone. The hypoglossal nerve is to be found either posteriorly where it crosses the external carotid artery or anteriorly between the greater cornu of the hyoid bone and the posterior belly of the digastric muscle.

Step 4. Free the nerve very gently from its surroundings. Divide the nerve sufficiently far forward so that enough isolated nerve trunk is left to be turned upward and forward to be united without tension to the distal segment of the divided facial nerve. Complete the anastomosis as in Steps 5 and 6 of the preceding operation.

Comments. When, during an operation, the surgeon has the misfortune to divide the facial nerve completely, an attempt should be made to unite the divided ends at once. If, for some reason, this is not practicable, one of the forms of anastomosis described above should be done as soon as possible.

When in doubt, wait. If within six months recovery does not ensue, one must consider operation.

When the facial muscles are atrophied and no longer respond to the faradic current, operation will probably prove futile. If the muscles respond to faradic stimulation, operation is indicated.

In facial palsy from "cold" or middle ear disease, the prognosis without operation is usually favorable. If after four to six months the facial muscles are still almost completely paralyzed and reaction of degeneration is pronounced, Spiller recommends anastomosis.

Treatment of Facial Paralysis by Muscle Transportation

Jianu, in 1910, endeavored to relieve facial paralysis by taking a flap from the sternomastoid muscle, with its pedicle situated above, and suturing it to the angle of the mouth. The results were satisfactory.

Jonnescu, following Jianu's principle, exposed the masseter muscle by a curved incision following the edge of the inferior maxilla (both ascending and

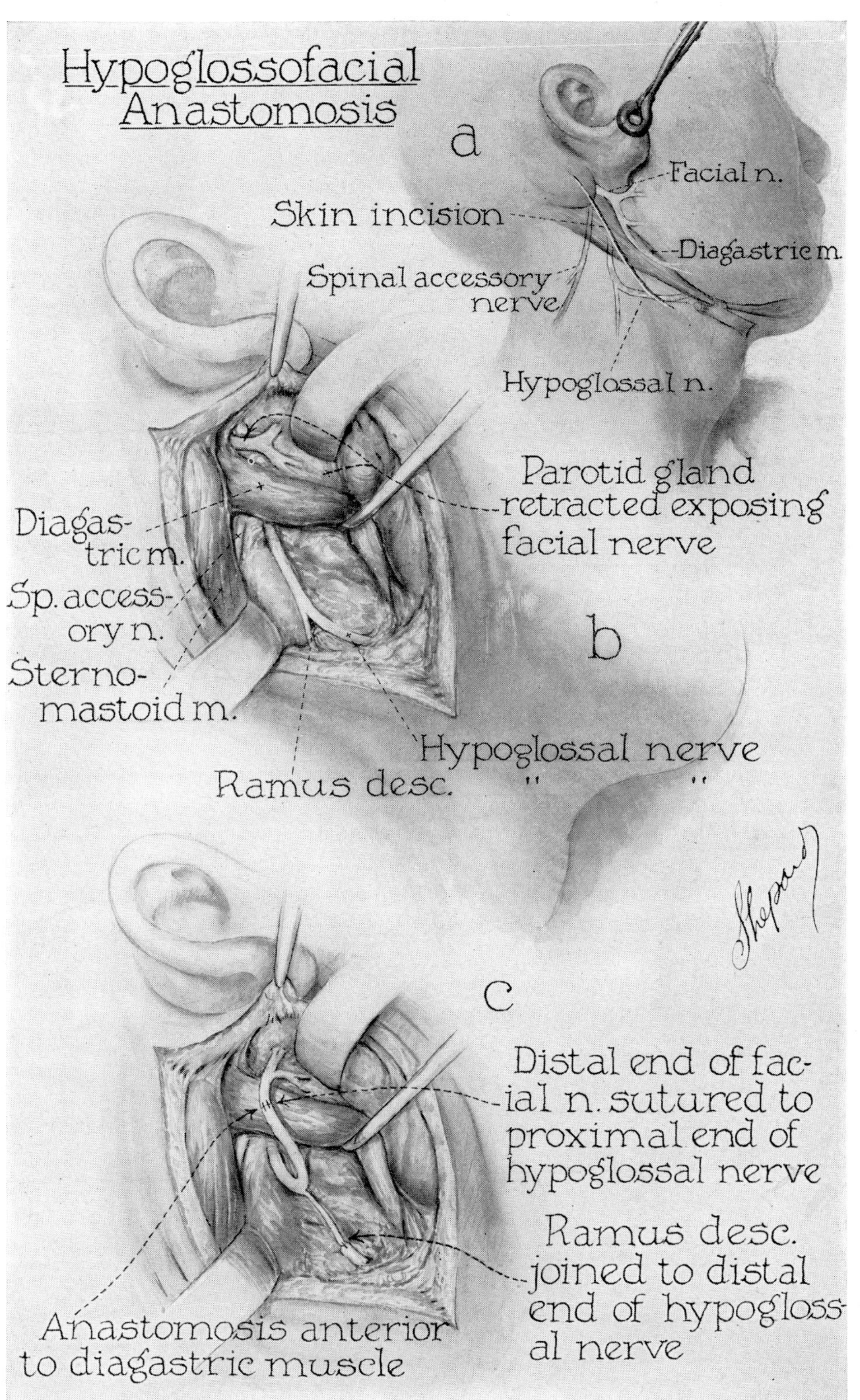

FIG. 346. Hypoglossofacial anastomosis.

horizontal rami); he then split the masseter in the direction of its fibers, separated the anterior portion of the muscle from its insertion into the jaw, and thus formed a muscular flap attached to the zygoma. This flap he sutured to the angle of the mouth. This resulted in correction of the deviation of the mouth, prevention of the escape of saliva, and ability to move voluntarily the angle of the mouth.

Cuneo states that Jianu's operation should be reserved for cases of total facial paralysis and to those in which nerve anastomosis has failed, and that when

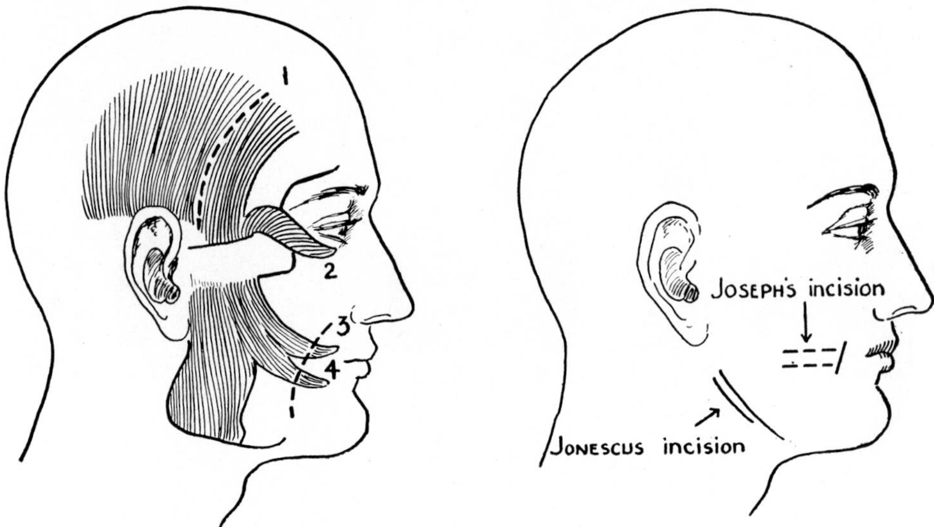

Fig. 347 Fig. 348

Fig. 347. Lexer's operation for facial paralysis: 1. incision of temporal muscle, 2. flap of temporal muscle implanted in lower eyelid, 3. incision in cheek, 4. flaps of masseter muscle implanted in musculature of upper and lower lip.

Fig. 348. Operation for facial paralysis.

performed, it should be supplemented by some operation on the eyelids such as angular tarsorrhaphy.

Lexer, on the suggestion of Wredes, operated in 1908 as follows:

An incision was made in the naso-labial fold. From this point he undermined the skin of the face to the masseter muscle bluntly. A flap about the width of a finger was dissected from the anterior border of the masseter muscle. The free end of this flap was split into two segments as shown in the illustration. (Fig. 347.)

Overcorrection is aimed at; as time goes on the stretching of the flap brings the mouth into proper position.

As stated, Jonnescu operated in a similar manner and reported good results. Jonnescu's incision is shown in Figure 348. This incision permits better dissection of the masseter muscle. Joseph made another small incision at the angle of the mouth (Fig. 348) and from this point he undermined the skin of the cheek to the point of the first incision. From this point on, the flap of the masseter was brought up subcutaneously to the angle of the mouth to which it was sutured. Studies made by Joseph, together with Friedl, indicated that failures were due to an improperly placed incision which divided terminal branches of the masseteric nerve which supplies that part of the masseter which is used for implantation at the angle of the mouth. This happens when the usual incision is used. However, if the incision (outlined in Fig. 349) is made, the nerve is avoided. The incision must not extend too high. A study of the diagram here explains the rationale for the placing of the incisions. A study of these anatomic factors will tend to avoid failures.

KATZENSTEIN'S OPERATION

Katzenstein's procedure consists of lengthening the temporal flap, recommended by Lexer, by using the temporal fascia in conjunction with the muscle.

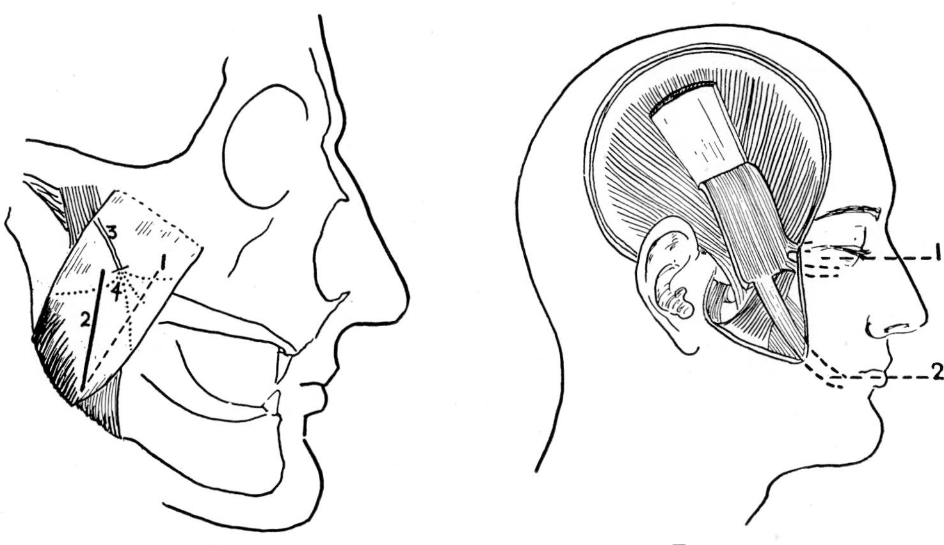

Fig. 349 Fig. 350

Fig. 349. Course of masseteric nerve and incisions in masseter muscle (after Joseph and Friedl): 1. wrong incision, 2. right incision, 3. nerve before entering masseter muscle, 4. course of principal nerve fibers in muscle.

Fig. 350. Katzenstein's operation for transplantation of temporal muscle and fascia: 1. fascial flaps from temporal muscle for closing the eye, 2. fascial flaps for elevating angle of mouth.

The strips of fascia thus obtained were implanted in the upper lip and eyelid. In one case Katzenstein used a free fascial transplant. The technic is simple.

Step 1. A small longitudinal incision is made in the region of the hairy scalp overlying the temporal muscle, which is exposed. A muscle flap is now formed which is brought down toward the orbit (Fig. 350); two smaller incisions are now made, one on the upper and the other on the lower eyelid, and a third incision at the upper lip. These incisions are about 1 to 2 cm. in length.

Step 2. The overlying skin is tunneled with an appropriate pair of forceps which is introduced through the temporal wound and extends to the orbit and lip. The free fascial transplant which is much recommended by Katzenstein is taken from the fascia lata; it is brought into position by the forceps and sutured to the upper lip and eyelid. The other end is thoroughly united with sutures to the muscle flap made from the temporal muscle. Overcorrection is aimed at because as time goes on the fascia relaxes somewhat.

Such overcorrection is particularly desirable at the upper lip and should be carried to the point at which the patient gives the impression of laughing.

ROSENTHAL'S OPERATION

Rosenthal believes that neurotization can take place. His mode of operation follows: (Fig. 351)

Step 1. A curved incision is made in the temporal region above the hair line. After dividing the fascia of the temporal muscle, a sufficiently long flap of temporal muscle of about the thickness of the thumb is mobilized. Injury to the temporal nerve, which springs from the third branch of the trigeminus, is hardly possible because these nerves approach the muscle from behind

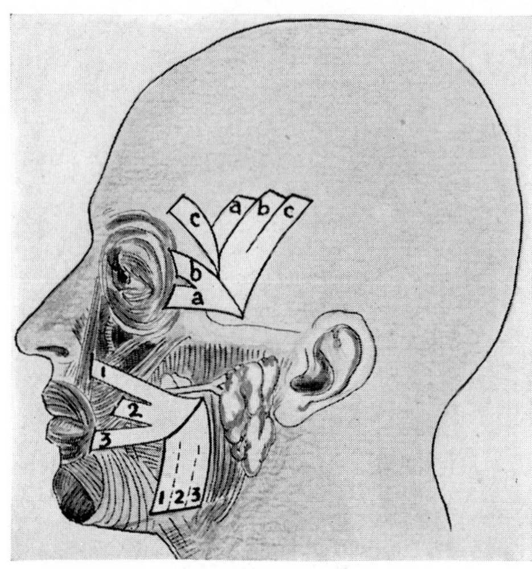

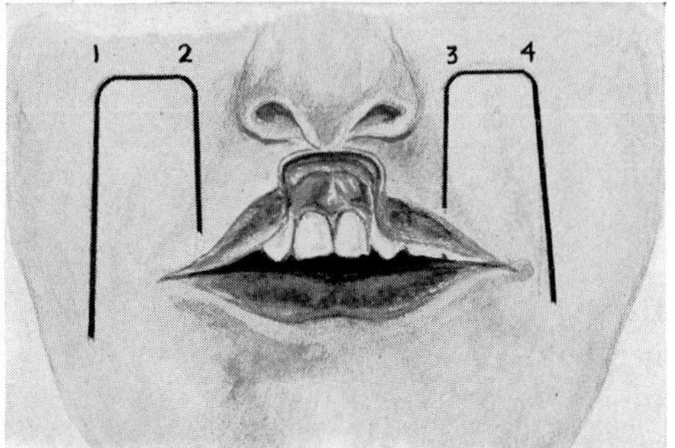

FIG. 351 FIG. 352

FIG. 351. Rosenthal's muscular neurotization operation in facial paralysis.

FIG. 352. Dieffenbach's operation: flaps 1-2 and 3-4 on each side are made up of the whole thickness of the tissues of the cheek; after freeing these they are rotated inwards so that 1-4 and 2-3 are sutured.

and below. A second incision is now made at the margin of the orbit encircling the latter above and below to about half of its extent; the atrophied remnants of the orbicularis oculi muscle are thus exposed. The flaps fashioned from the muscle and their method of attachment are shown in the illustration. Only the finest catgut should be used in suturing.

Step 2. A similar operation is performed a little later at the angle of the mouth. A flap of masseter muscle is taken and mobilized upward and implanted into the angle of the mouth as depicted in the drawing. The muscles elevating the angle of the mouth are exposed by a naso-labial incision; the implantation of sections of muscle are shown in the diagram. Injury of the nerve is rare because of the approach to the nerve from behind. The approximation must attempt to unite muscle to muscle. This is of cardinal importance.

Comment: After the lapse of three or four months, the first signs in a successful case are fibrillatory twitchings about the eye which occur synchronously with masticatory attempts and the appearance of better tone in the cheek.

SURGERY OF THE UPPER LIP

Small defects in the upper lip may be repaired by triangular freshening as is the case in resections of the lower lip (which see). The direction of the triangle is reversed. Larger defects resulting from the removal of tumors are to be repaired by

Dieffenbach's Operation

Outline a quadrilateral flap on each side of the defect, the base of each flap being at its lower end. The whole thickness of the cheek as outlined by the flaps being mobilized, the flaps are turned inward (in the opposite direction to the base) and sutured into place so that the defect is covered. (Fig. 352.)

HARELIP AND CLEFT PALATE

Harelip is a congenital deformity making its appearance as a fissure or cleft in the lip. Usually the upper lip is affected. The condition is liable to be complicated by an alveolar or velopalatine fissure. (Figs. 353-354-355-356.)

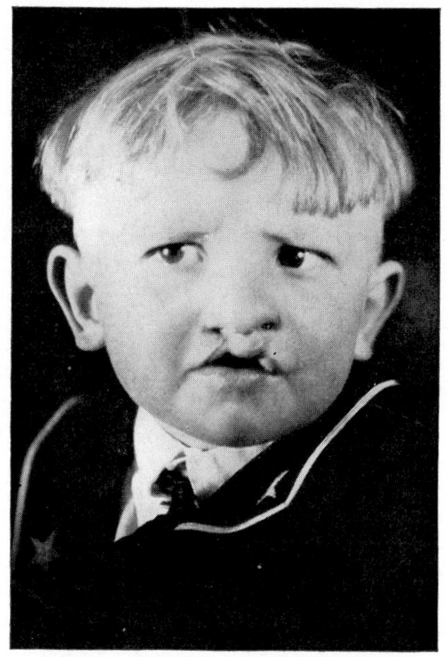

Fig. 353. Double bilateral harelip.

Cleft palate is a congenital defect in the palate consisting of a fissure running in an anteroposterior direction, frequently involving the uvula, the soft or hard palate or both. **His** has shown that up to the end of the second or beginning of the third month of fetal life the tongue lies above the free palatine margins, which later ascend to unite above the tongue. Sometimes the same individual will have a harelip with a divided velum or posterior portion of the hard palate, the intermediary segment of the palate being intact.

Varieties of Harelip

Incomplete Harelip. Here a fissure does not extend into the nostril.

Complete Harelip. A fissure extends into the nostril.

Median Harelip.

Incomplete Harelip:

(a) **Single (unilateral) Harelip.** The nostril may or may not be widened. The palate may or may not be involved.

(b) **Double (bilateral) Harelip.** The nostrils may or may not be widened and flattened. The palate may or may not be involved.

Complete Harelip may be subdivided into

(a) **Single (unilateral) Harelip.** This form is often associated with cleft palate.

(b) **Double (bilateral) Harelip.** This is often associated with cleft palate.

(c) **Double Complete and Incomplete Harelip.** Complete on one side, and incomplete on the other.

In the Infant. If cleft palate exists, it may be operated on before the harelip is corrected because the gap in the lip gives better access to the palate. Some surgeons believe that after restoration of the lip, the cleft in the palate becomes narrowed in the course of a few months so that the operative procedure for closure of the palate becomes relatively easy.

The defect should be repaired as early as possible (from six weeks to four months). Some advise that a child, if undernourished, should receive the benefit of a building up régime. Others again (Blair, Brophy, Lane) advocate operating on cases of cleft palate within a few hours after birth. The consensus of opinion is that it is better to wait until the lip closure is effected. I subscribe to this latter view.

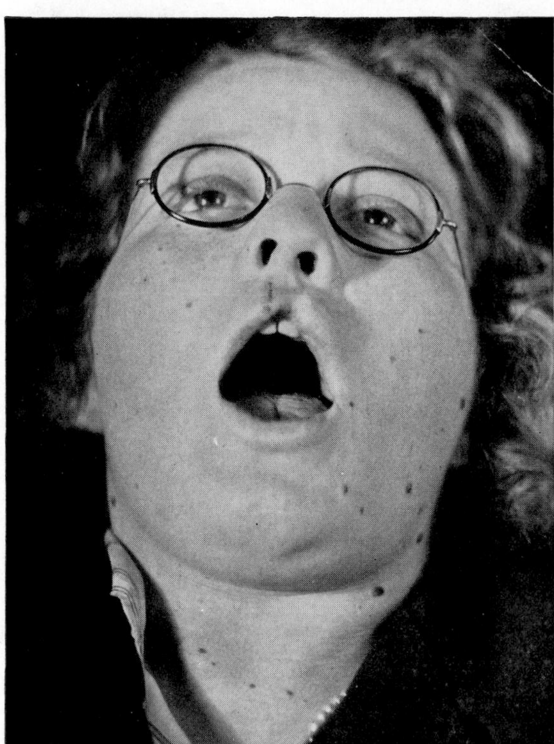

FIG. 354. Harelip and cleft palate. The harelip had been repaired with only partial success before any attempt was made at closure of the defect of the palate.

Adults with harelip or cleft palate should be afforded the benefit of operative relief. Successful closure of the palate in these cases will probably cause little improvement in the speech, but closure of the lip, when associated with a complete cleft palate, will change a repulsive person into a fairly normal looking individual. (Figs. 357-358.)

Anesthesia. General anesthesia is necessary in operating for harelip and cleft palate. **Ether** (warmed) is administered either through a nasal tube or through a tube in the mouth gag. In older children intratracheal anesthesia is of much benefit and eliminates the danger of aspiration pneumonia.

Position of the Patient During Anesthesia. Many surgeons prefer to have the patient held in a sitting position during the operation for harelip and cleft palate. My preference is to have the patient lying down with the head supported by a well-padded circular head-rest attached to the table. In cleft palate operations **Rose's position** (see p. 240) should be given preference.

Preparation of the Part. The lip and adjacent portions of the face should be washed with ether or benzine and then painted with one-third strength tincture of iodine. The field should be isolated with properly applied sterile drapings.

"How much relief of tension should one obtain?" the surgeon often asks himself. The answer is: "Until the edges of the cleft in the lip join in the midline freely without lateral pull, when approximated with tenacula." (Figs. 359-360.)

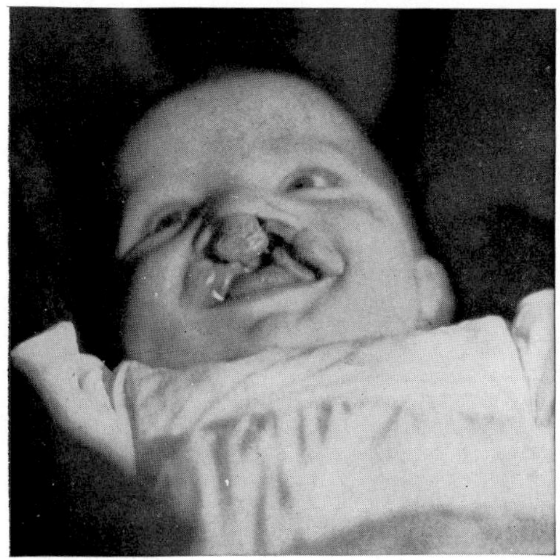

Fig. 355. Double harelip and cleft palate.

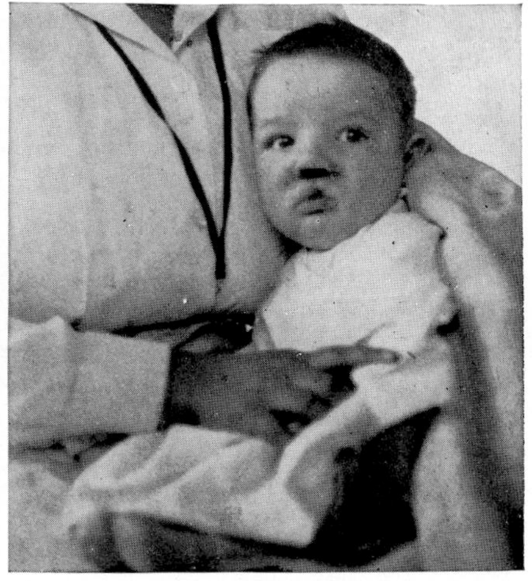

Fig. 356. Patient shown in Fig. 355, after operation.

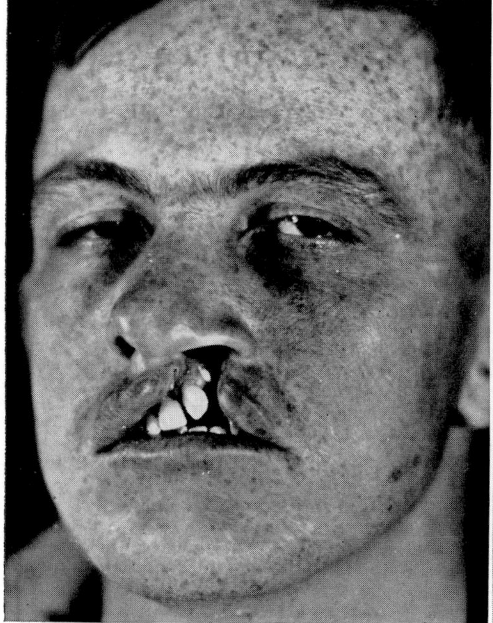

Fig. 357. Harelip and cleft palate before operation.

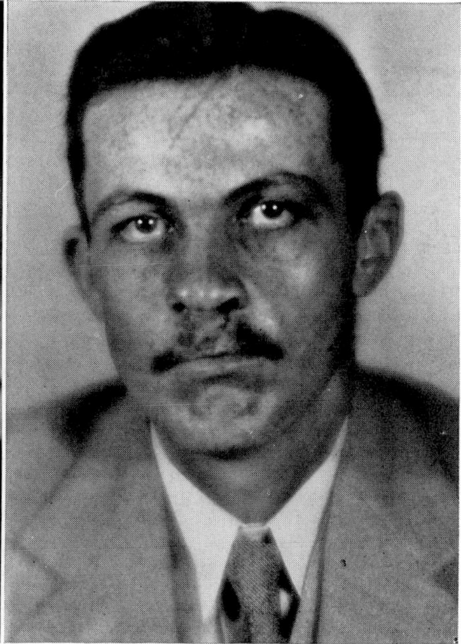

Fig. 358. Same patient after operation.

Three important steps comprise almost all forms of operative procedures for harelip, viz.:

1. **Tension of the flaps must be relieved** by freely separating the lip, and where necessary the cheek, from their attachment to the bone, at either side.

Restraining alae of the nose should also be separated from their bony attachments. Figs. 359 and 360.)

2. **Planing and paring of the borders** of the cleft with a sharp pointed knife or scissors. (Fig. 361.)

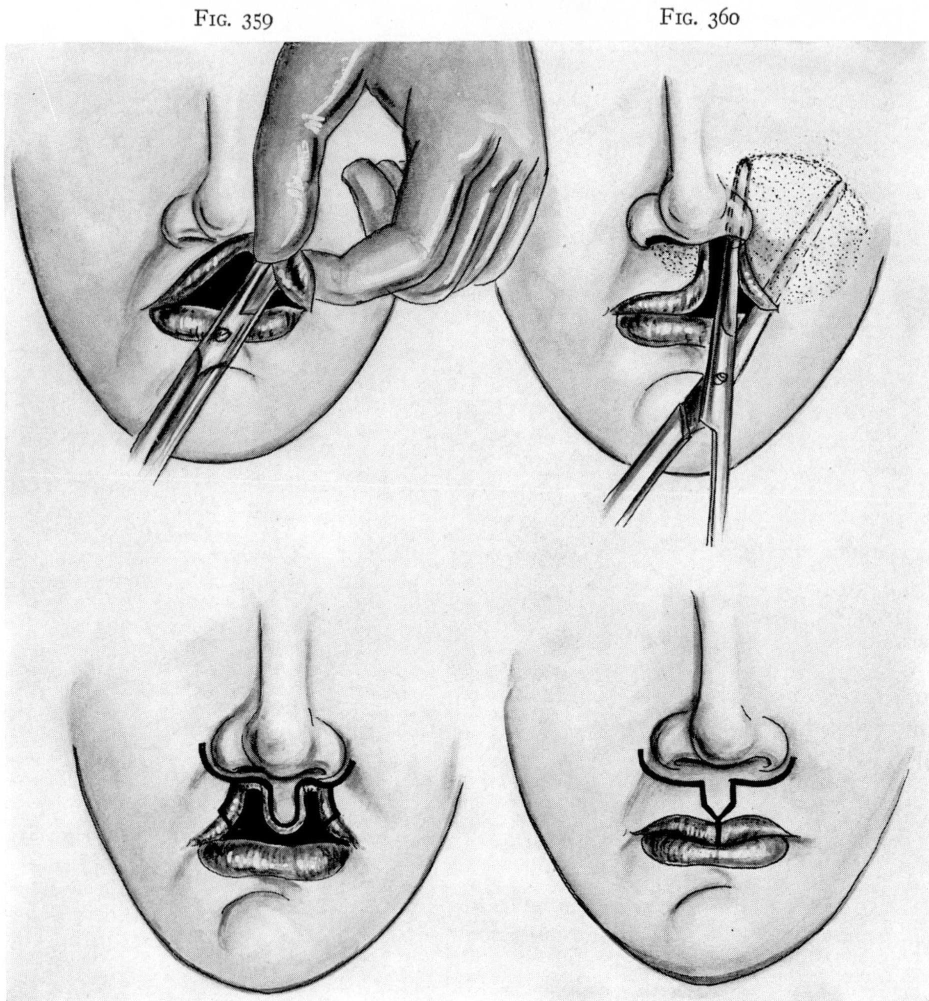

Fig. 359 Fig. 360 Fig. 361 Fig. 362

Fig. 359. Operation for simple harelip. Introduction of the scissors to loosen the lip from its attachments.

Fig. 360. Same operation. The dotted area represents the extent of detachment usually done to render the lip sufficiently mobile.

Fig. 361. Operation for simple bilateral harelip. Outline of incision.

Fig. 362. Same operation. Free liberation and coaptation of flap.

3. **Approximation of the freshened surfaces** of the cleft. Careful union of the vermilion border of the lip. (Fig. 362.)

Comment. The lip line must reach from one side of the newly formed lip to the other in an uninterrupted curve. The mucous membrane on either side of the line of suture must be of equal depth. The newly formed lip should be lengthened sufficiently to cover the gums. The nostril should be

of the same size and made to the same contour as the normal nostril. The nose should not be flattened on the affected side.

If the gap is wide and the controlling muscles active, and the cleft takes in all of the soft palate or part of the hard palate, it may be necessary

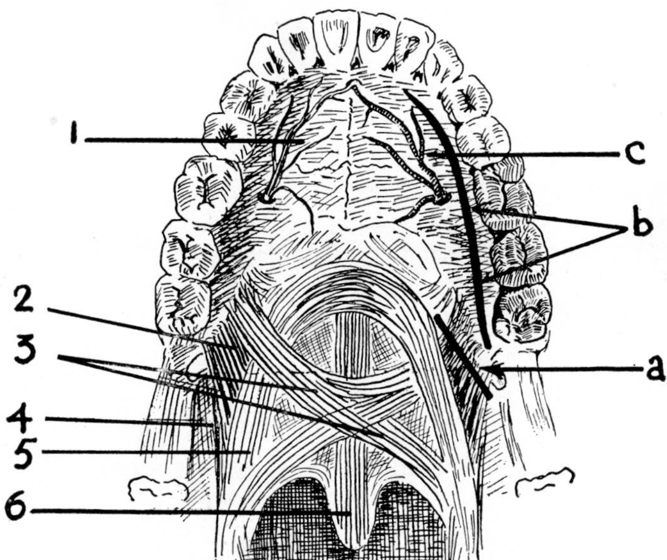

FIG. 363. Muscles of the soft palate: a. line of division of muscle, b. line of incision, c. palatine vessels; 1. anterior palatine muscle, 2. pharyngopalatine muscle, 3. levator veli palatine muscle, 4. hamulus pterygoideus, 5. thyropalatine muscle, 6. azygos muscle.

to overcome muscular influence before uniting the cleft by dividing the contracting muscles (tensor- and levator-palati, the palato-glossi and palato-pharyngei). If these are incorrectly divided the velum will remain flabby

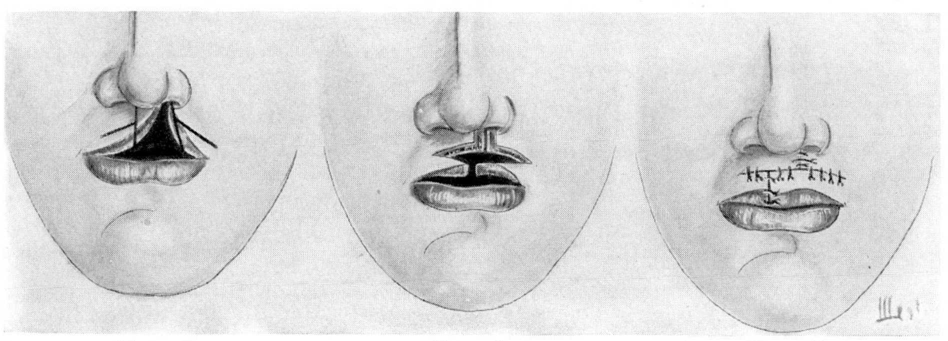

FIG. 364 FIG. 365 FIG. 366

FIG. 364. König's operation for harelip: outlining the flaps by incision.
FIG. 365. Flaps mobilized.
FIG. 366. Flaps sutured.

and motionless. Their relations to the adjoining tissues are shown in Fig. 363.

By dividing the posterior pillars of the fauces, of which they form the principal part, the palato-pharyngeal muscles may be cut with a pair of blunt-pointed scissors. The palato-glossi muscles, which include the anterior pillars, may be divided in the same manner. After passing a silk thread through the velum on each side of the cleft at points corresponding to the origin of the uvula, looping the ends of the threads and making the velum firm with a tenaculum, the remaining muscles are divided. (Fig. 363.)

The Tensor Palati. The hook-shaped process around which the tendon of the tensor palati runs is located a little behind and internal to the upper posterior molar tooth. The segment of velum is made rigid by a traction suture and the point of a narrow-bladed knife is introduced a little below and at the inner side of the process with the cutting edge upward; the knife is carried upward, backward and inward until the point is visible through the gap. The entire width of the velum together with most or all of the tendon of the tensor palati is divided.

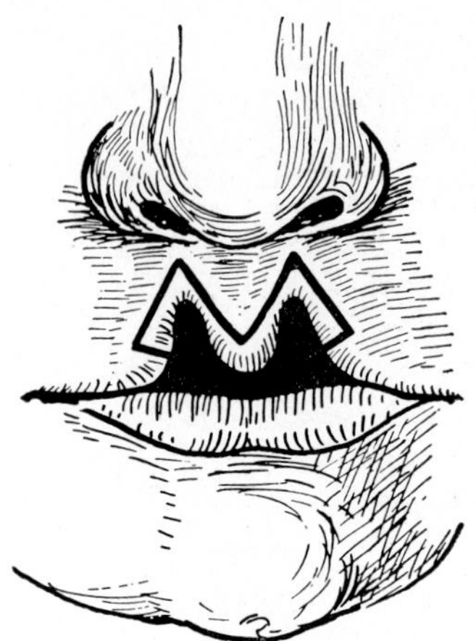

Fig. 367

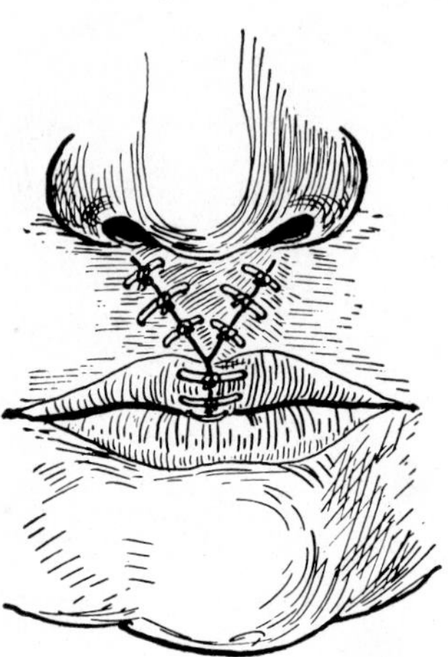

Fig. 368

Fig. 367. Simple bilateral harelip. Outlining the incision.
Fig. 368. Same operation. After loosening the flaps they are united as shown.

The Levator Palati. Many of the lower fibers of this muscle will be divided during the above procedure. However, if greater section is required, the handle of the knife is depressed and carried outward making an oblique incision on the posterior surface of the velum as it is withdrawn.

König's Operation for Single Harelip

Step 1. Two more or less vertical incisions are made parallel to the borders of the cleft and passing through the entire thickness of the halves of the lips, from the upper limit of the cleft through the vermilion border. (Fig. 364.)

Step 2. Auxillary incisions are now made above the borders of the lips slanting from the more vertical incisions slightly downward. The incision at the outer side of the cleft is somewhat the longer. As a result of these incisions the vertical and horizontal openings shown in Figure 365 result.

Step 3. Pull the flaps downward and after thorough mobilization suture them as shown in Figure 366.

Operation for Simple Bilateral Harelip

Step 1. Freshen the central portion of the defect on both sides.
Step 1. Make lateral flaps with their attachments below at the outer borders.
Step 3. Separate the connections of the lips.
Step 4. Approximate the freshened flaps (Figures 369-370-371).

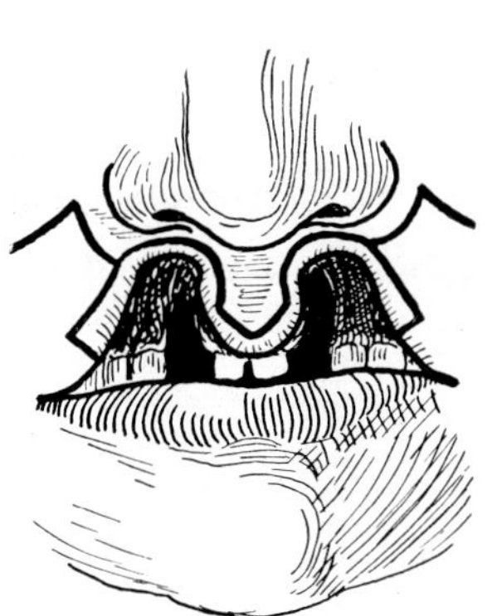
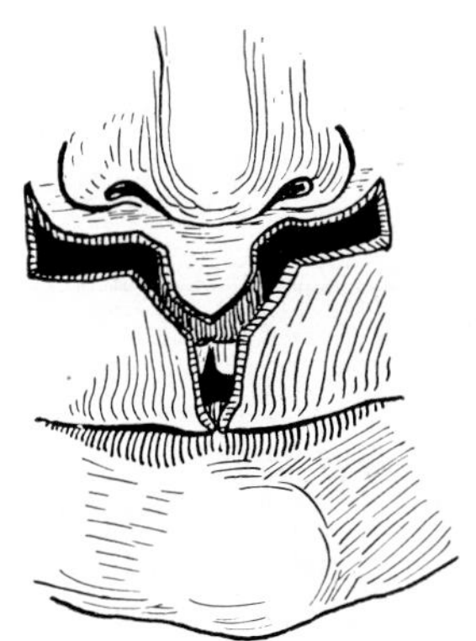
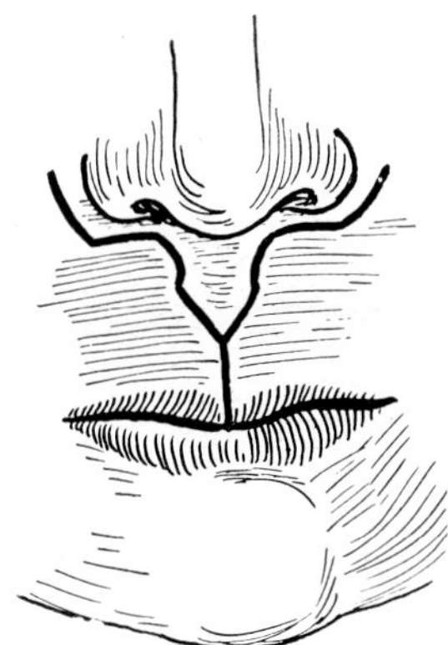

FIG. 369 FIG. 370 FIG. 371

FIG. 369. Doyen's operation for simple bilateral harelip. Outlines of complementary incisions in case of excessive shortness of the lateral flaps.
FIG. 370. Same operation. Freshening of edges completed. Reconstruction of lip.
FIG. 371. Same operation completed.

Malgaigne's Double Flap Method

Figures 372-373 dipict the incision, flap formation and suture of this procedure.

Ferdinand C. Lee ably discusses the principles underlying the repair of double harelip.[1] He stresses that the important points in the operation are: (a)

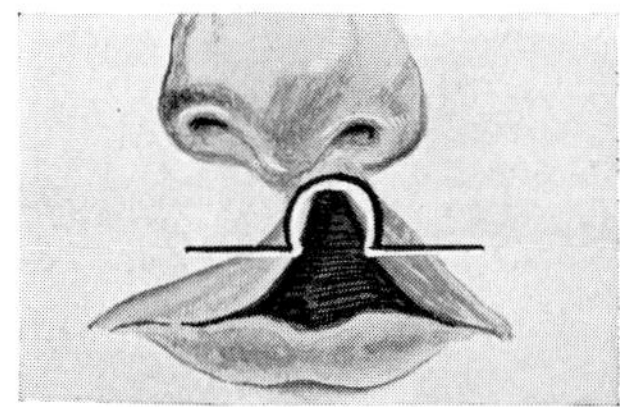
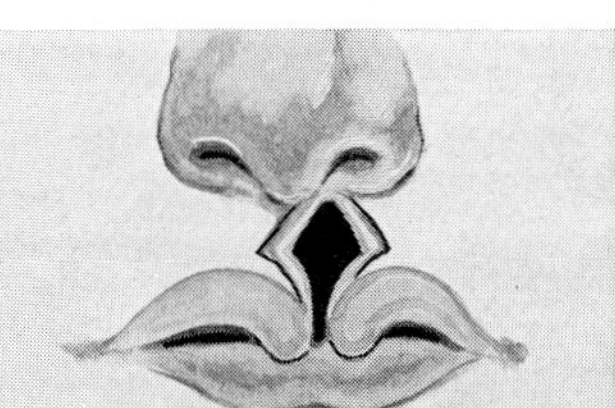
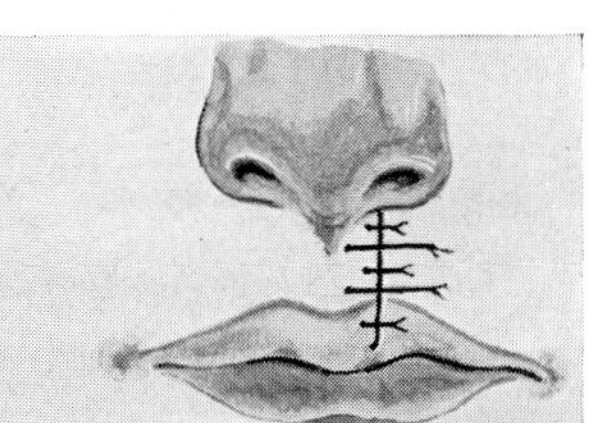

FIG. 372 FIG. 372a FIG. 373

FIG. 372. Malgaigne's operation: outlining flaps.
FIG. 372a. Freshening edges.
FIG. 373. Suturing complete.

the preservation and utilization of the tissues at hand; (b) the symmetrical approximation of the two lateral flaps, with an abundance of orbicularis oris muscle; (c) the careful suturing of the denuded surfaces with almost three rows of sutures; (d) the approximation of muscular tissue in the midline and the ample use of sedatives to insure complete rest for the wound. Lee feels that by this method a surgeon with relatively little experience in plastic surgery may achieve satisfactory results in double harelip operations.

[1] Jour. of the Med. Assoc. of Georgia, October, 1934, No. 10.

Projecting Intermaxillary Bone

A variety of methods have been suggested to remedy this condition. (Fig. 374.) Blandin counseled free removal of a properly estimated triangular-shaped section of the vomer. (Fig. 375.) Hemorrhage and frequent failure of union caused many surgeons to seek recourse to **subperiosteal resection** which is easily accomplished by raising the periosteum together with the superimposed mucous membrane with a delicate periosteotome through incisions placed along either side of the edge of the vomer.

Rose made a single vertical incision through the bone, following denudation. Bardeleben, following denudation, divided the bone for about ¾ inch. He then

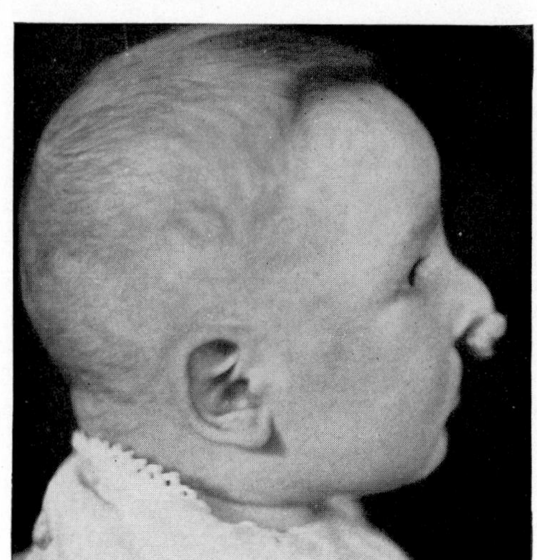

Fig. 374

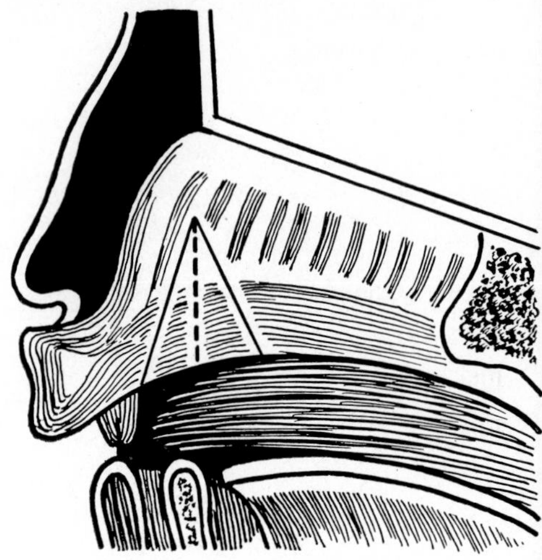

Fig. 375

Fig. 374. Projecting intermaxillary process.
Fig. 375. Operation for projecting intermaxillary bone. Triangular incision, Blandin's operation; dotted line, Rose's operation.

reduced the deformity resulting in an overlapping of the borders of the vomer; this is followed by union of the opposed surfaces. Some surgeons advise complete removal of the projecting process. In this I do not concur. Doyen pointed out that the removal of a triangular section is followed, after reposition, by an awkward, inward displacement of the incisor teeth; this is obviated by quadrangular resection. (Figs. 376-377-378-379.)

Step 1. Retract the divided tissues.
Step 2. Remove the triangular section with strong scissors.
Step 3. Force the projecting portion into place.
Step 4. Proper intranasal and supralabial support keep the soft parts in position.

OPERATIONS FOR CLEFT PALATE

(Uranoplasty, Staphylorrhaphy)

Historical Notes. The first successful cleft palate operation was executed by von Graefe in 1816. In 1825, Roux reported 112 such operations. Dieffenbach made large lateral incisions on the palate. Fergusson divided the muscles of the palate while Krimer was first in 1824 to perform an operation for cleft in the hard palate by making wide lateral flaps of mucous membrane and uniting these in the middle. Other names prominently connected with the further development of the operation

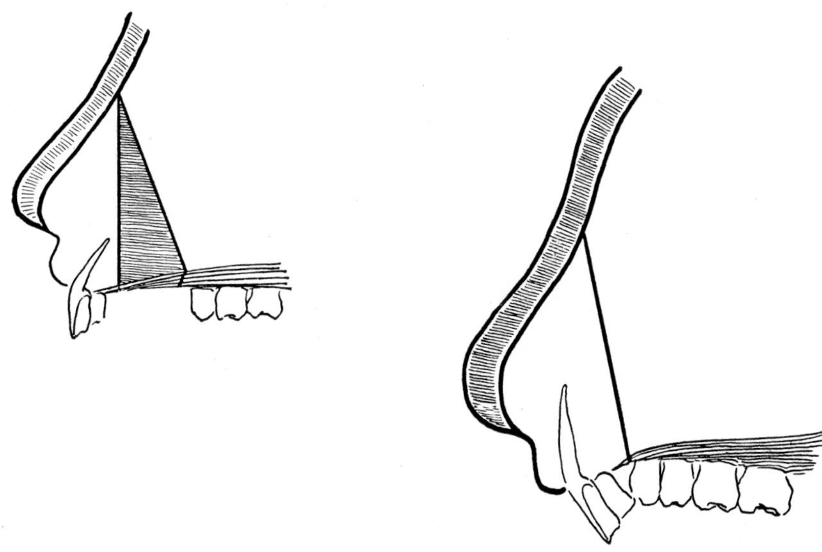

Fig. 376 Fig. 377

Fig. 376. Exaggerated projection of incisive tubercle. Defective resection of nasal septum in double harelip.

Fig. 377. Backward deviation of incisor teeth after triangular resection of nasal septum in double harelip.

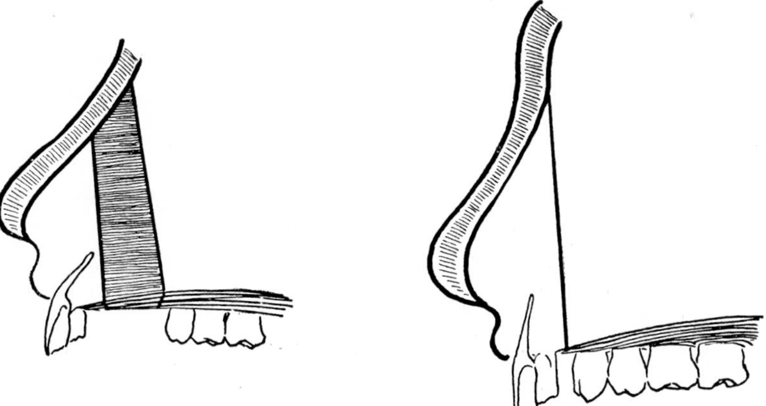

Fig. 378 Fig. 379

Fig. 378. Outline of quadrangular resection of the nasal septum suitable for reduction of the incisive tubercle in bilateral harelip.

Fig. 379. Reduction of incisive tubercle to normal position after resection of nasal septum in bilateral harelip (after Doyen).

are: von Langenbeck, Brophy, Lane, Codirilla, Lexer, Lorenz, Moskowitz, Shoemaker and others.

The best time for operating on cleft palate is between the second and fifth years. The operation may be followed by serious consequences. Binnie maintains that the proper time to operate for cleft palate is when the patient is less than three months of age.

The Brophy method of operating for cleft palate is inapplicable in children over six months old; it should be done before closing of an accompanying harelip.

Brophy's Operation

Step 1. Place a traction suture in the anterior end of the tongue.

Step 2. Pare the bony edges of the cleft in the palate; either pare or horizontally split the edges of the cleft in the soft-palate.

Step 3. Thread a Brophy needle with a strong silk or celluloid hemp-suture. Pass the threaded needle through the superior maxilla from without inward

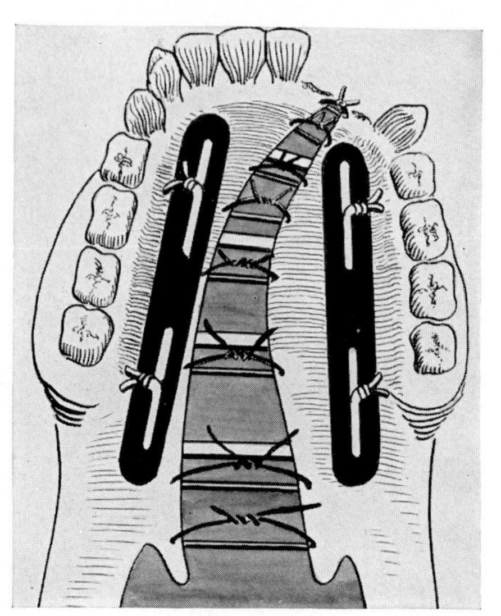

Fig. 380

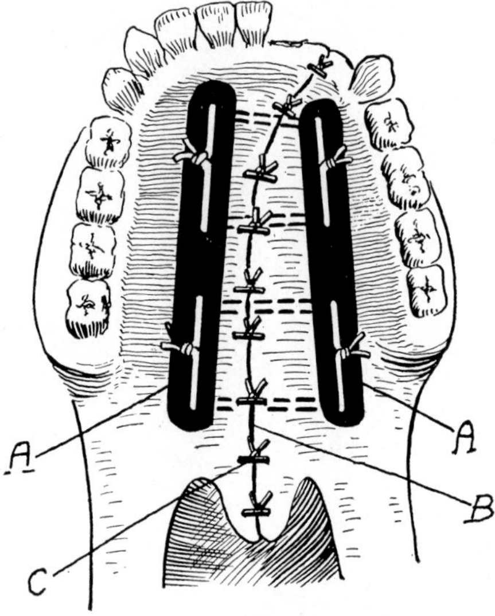

Fig. 381

Fig. 380. Brophy's operation. Method of inserting tension sutures and application of lead plates.
Fig. 381. Brophy's operation showing approximation of edges of cleft by means of increased tension on silver wires: A-A. lead plates, B. closed palate, C. coaptation sutures.

at a point just back of the malar process and above the palate; when it appears in the cleft, pick up the thread and withdraw the needle. Pass a threaded needle through the corresponding part of the opposite bone in the same way, this second loop of thread being passed through the first and both pulled out. By means of this thread, pull a strand of very strong silver wire through the same track.

Step 4. In the same way pass one or two other silver wires through the anterior portion of the maxilla above the level of the palate.

Step 5. Pass the ends of the silver wire through holes in lead plates which have been molded to fit the convexity of the buccal surfaces of the bones, then draw the wires tight and twist them together. Press the two maxillary bones together until the cleft is completely closed, twisting the wire sufficiently so as to hold the bones firmly together. (Figs. 380-381.)

Berry and Legg's Operation

Step 1. Detach the mucoperiosteal structures of the palate from the oral surface of the bony palate. (Fig. 382.) Make a small incision near the alveolar border. Insert into this opening a raspatory or periosteal elevator. By a to-and-fro motion and with the back of the instrument against the bone, the instrument is made to advance until its tip emerges at the margin of the cleft through which it is pushed. Withdraw the raspatory. Introduce an ordinary aneurysm-needle through the opening at the inner aspect of the cleft and work it backward and forward until the necessary amount of mucoperiosteal

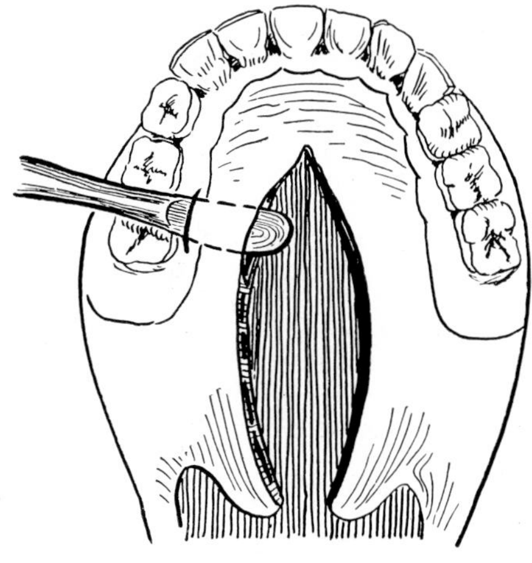

Fig. 382

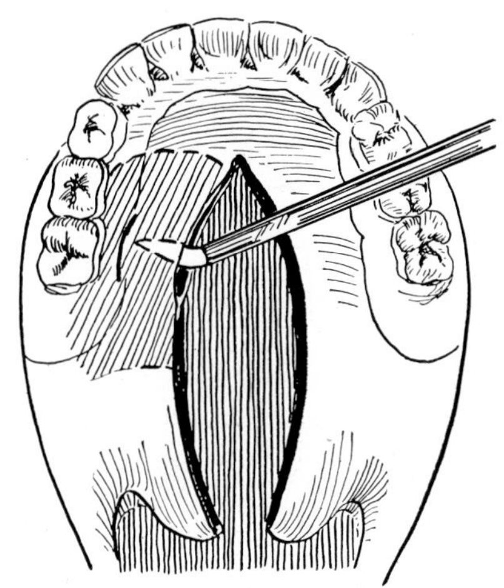

Fig. 383

Fig. 382. Berry and Legg's operation for cleft palate. Position of first incision and manner of passing a periosteal elevator between the mucoperiosteal flap and the surface of the hard palate.

Fig. 383. Berry and Legg's operation for cleft palate. Passing of blunt instrument (aneurysm needle) into the wound at the edge of the cleft palate. Shaded area indicates the extent to which the mucoperiosteum is detached from the bone.

tissue is separated from the hard palate. (Fig. 383.) Repeat the same procedure on the opposite side. Temporary pressure arrests bleeding. Insert into the wound at the edge of the cleft a rectangular knife and extend the incision in a posterior direction to the point of junction of the soft and hard palates.

Step 2. The authors consider this step the most important one of the operation, stressing that, if not properly and completely accomplished, closure of the cleft in the soft palate without undue tension will become impossible.

To accomplish this, insert one blade of a pair of sharply curved blunt scissors into the space between the inferior surface of the hard palate and the mucoperiosteal flap where the hard palate joins the soft palate. (Figs. 384-385.) The other blade of the scissors is introduced over the nasal surface. In doing this the length of the incision should not be too large in order to avoid injury to the **posterior palatine artery.**

Step 3. This consists of paring of the margins of the cleft and is performed by grasping with appropriate forceps, the edge of the cleft opposite the erstwhile junction of the soft and hard palates—now separated. Thrust a very fine, sharp scalpel through the whole thickness of the soft palate, transfixing it as far as the notch. Withdraw the scalpel and reinsert it somewhat posterior to the forceps at the same distance as the first and continue the incision toward the uvula.

Step 4. This consists of suturing the pared edges. An appropriate needle armed with Pagenstecher linen has served me well in this step of the operation. The needle is passed about 4 mm. from the freshened edge, and made to emerge on the nasal side and enter on the same side on the opposite flap. The tie is to be made in such a manner that eversion toward the buccal side results. Tenacula steady all flaps while the sutures are placed. They should be only approximated and not too tightly tied—lest strangulation

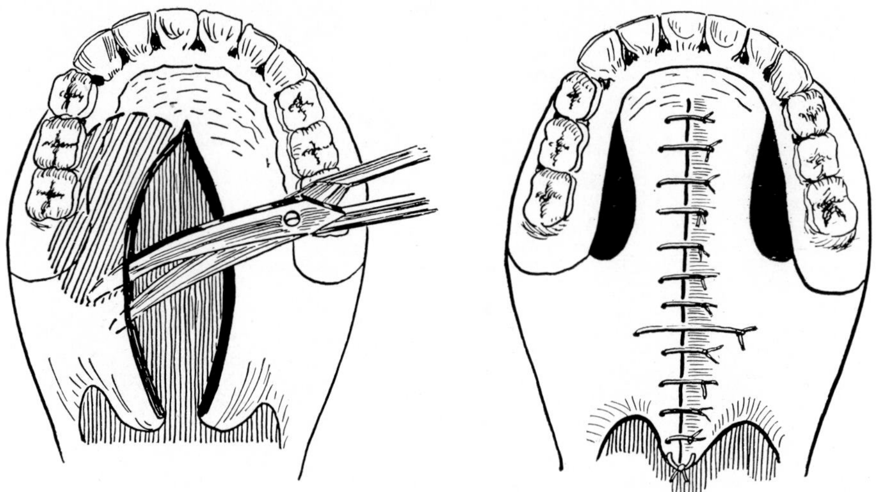

Fig. 384 Fig. 385

Fig. 384. Berry and Legg's operation. Introduce curved scissors and detach the soft from the hard palate.

Fig. 385. Berry and Legg's operation. Union of freshened edges of flaps. Dark areas indicate the incisions to relieve tension.

with marginal necrosis result. A tension suture here and there may be of value.

Step 5. Make lateral incisions to relieve tension wherever deemed advisable. These should be made somewhat in front of the junction of the hard with the soft palate near the alveolus and internal to the posterior palatine foramen; these incisions must not be too long, too much to the front or toward the middle line.

Von Langenbeck's Operation

(Fig. 386)

Step 1. Pare the margins of the cleft. Grasp the uvula with an appropriate tenaculum forceps. With a fine sharp pointed knife begin the freshening behind the tenaculum and excise a strip along the soft and hard palates in such a manner that a slanting, wide, freshened margin results. Begin the resection at the hard palate to be finished at the uvula with fine scissors. Treat the opposite side in the same manner. Clear the nasopharynx of accumulated blood. Tampon the cleft with gauze.

Step 2. Make lateral incisions through the hard-palate and extend these as shown in Fig. 387.

Step 3. Detach the mucoperiosteal flap from the hard palate as described in the Legg and Berry operation. This is followed by separating the soft palate from the horizontal portion of the palate-bone at the margin of the cleft, but laterally it is left attached to the bone. Next, approximate the two halves of the soft palate by blunt dissection. The mucoperiosteal flaps must be detached sufficiently to allow apposition of their mucous surfaces. These

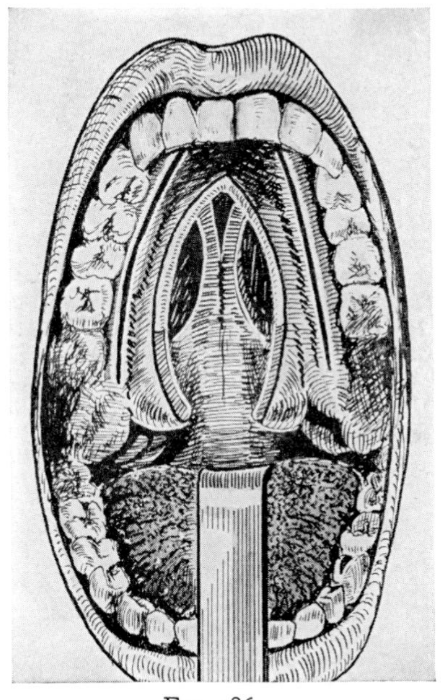

Fig. 386

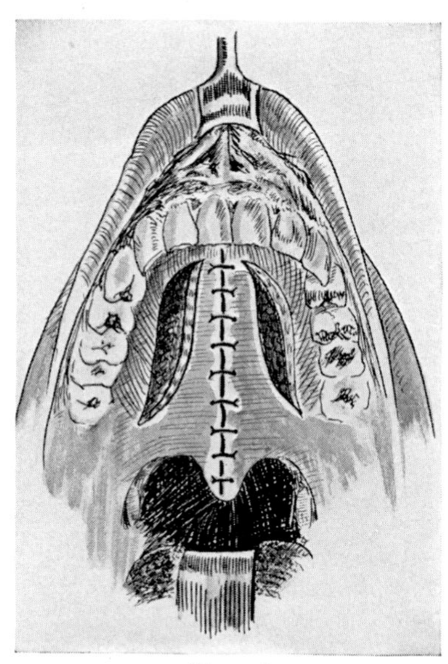

Fig. 387

Fig. 386. Von Langenbeck's operation for cleft palate. Lateral incision and freshening of edges.
Fig. 387. Von Langenbeck's operation for cleft palate. Note lateral incisions and approximated freshened edges thus covering the cleft.

must meet without tension. Treat the opposite side in exactly the same manner.

Step 4. Union of the pared edges. Use fine silk or Pagenstecher linen. Interrupted sutures are simplest and easiest to place. Pack lightly.

The Davis-Coley Operation

Step 1. Make a triangular-shaped flap comprising all of the soft parts taken from the wider part of the hard palate. The apex of the flap is situated behind the insertion of the incisor teeth; the base of the flap should extend inward and backward from the border of the alveolus of the last molar tooth to near the border of the cleft of the soft palate close to its attachment to the bone.

Step 2. Make a somewhat similarly shaped flap at the other side of the cleft, the inner border of which remains continuous with the soft parts at the border of the defect.

Step 3. With an elevator, raise the flap last formed from the bone, and turn it over, across the cleft while remaining attached at its inner border by a hinge of mucoperiosteal tissue.

Step 4. Join this flap by means of two or three catgut sutures to the freshened opposite border of the defect.

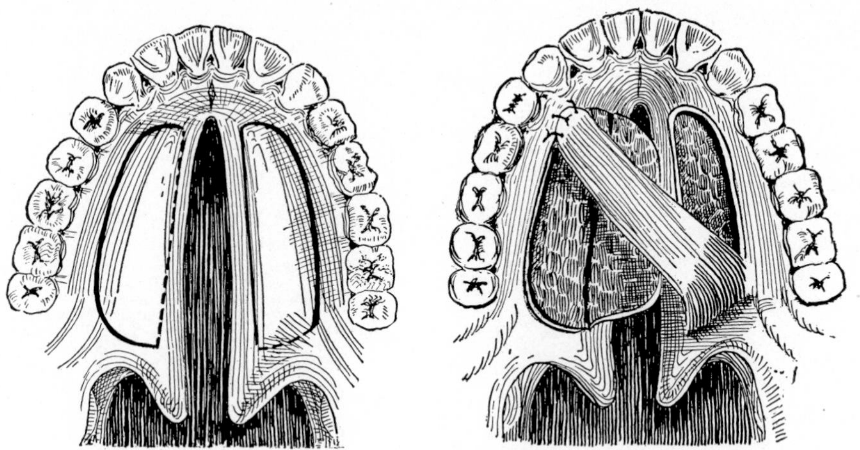

Fig. 388 Fig. 389

Fig. 388. Davis-Coley operation for cleft palate. Flaps marked out.
Fig. 389. Same as before. Flaps sutured.

Step 5. Similarly, lift the first flap and bring it across to the opposite side joining its apex with the outer margin of the opposite gap by two or three silver-wire or silkworm-gut sutures. (Figs. 388-389.)

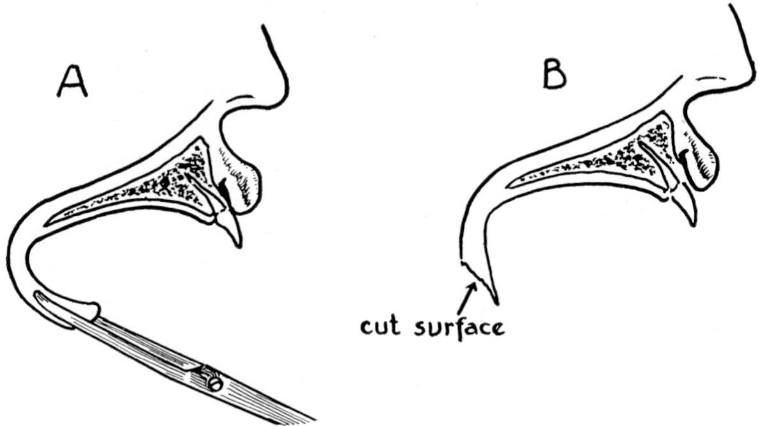

Fig. 390. Uvulectomy: A. uvula grasped with forceps and slightly tensed, B. redundant portion removed.

Comment. This procedure is less severe than the other operations described; it is accompanied by less hemorrhage, pressure of the tongue against the roof of the mouth is less harmful, while necrosis and a possibility of septicemia are not so pronounced.

Sir Arbuthnot Lane's Operation

is an adaptation of the **Davis-Coley** method. It is an ingenious procedure and beset with many technical difficulties to be surmounted only by the hands of the expert. It should not be attempted by surgeons who have no special training in this work. For the general surgeon the methods described above will suffice in the vast majority of well-selected cases.

Elongated Uvula

Have the patient withdraw his tongue aided by a dry towel. Grasp the end of the elongated uvula with appropriate forceps, pull it forward and remove the desired segment with scissors. (Fig. 390.) The slight discomfort following the operation may be relieved by the application of a novocaine solution.

CHAPTER 15

SURGERY OF THE ORBIT AND EYE

OPERATIONS ON THE ORBIT

INCISION FOR ORBITAL CELLULITIS

This results from the breaking of an abscess located in a contiguous space (frontal, maxillary, ethmoidal or sphenoidal sinus) into the orbital cavity.

Operation. Use general anesthesia. Govern the incision by the probable location of the collection of pus—often a most difficult task. Hug the wall of the orbit closely thus avoiding injury to important structures. Drain.

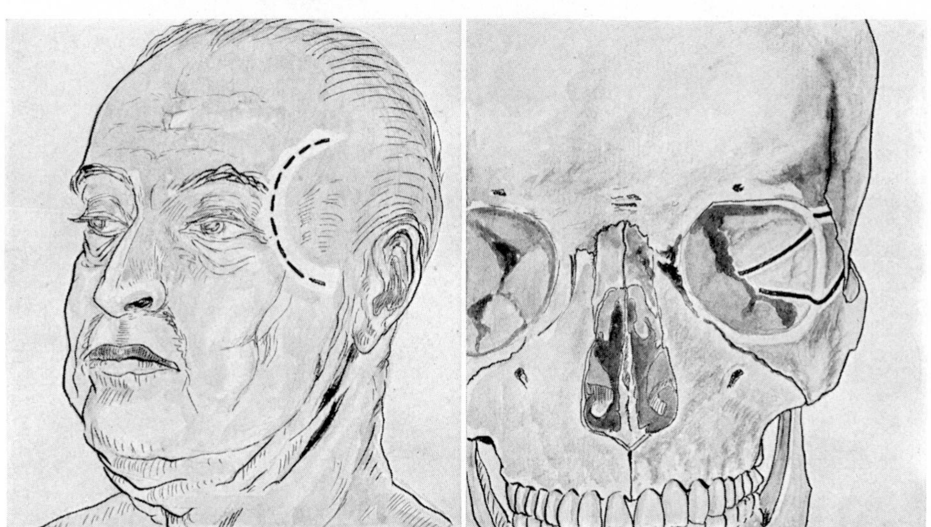

Fig. 391 Fig. 392

Fig. 391. Skin incision in Krönlein's operation on the orbit.
Fig. 392. Bone incision in Krönlein's operation.

Usually the pus collection results from extensions, the result of ethmoiditis or frontal sinusitis. These obviously are located on the nasal side where important structures may be injured with the scalpel, viz., superior and inferior oblique muscles and levator palpebrae superioris; ptosis then results. The prognosis in these cases is usually grave. Orbital suppuration may best be reached through an external fronto-ethmoidal operation.

OSTEOPLASTIC RESECTION OF THE OUTER WALL OF THE ORBIT

Krönlein's Operation (Franke's Modification)

The object of this operation is to remove orbital neoplasms, particularly retrobulbar tumors without sacrifice of the eyeball. The operation may also be used in cases of foreign bodies in the orbit. The principles of the operation consist of removing a large portion of the orbital wall with the attachments of the soft tissues. The detachment is not made complete, however, the soft parts acting as a hinge. After the operation is completed, the structures are sewed back in position.

Step 1. Make an incision below the level of the eyebrow, corresponding to the external half of the upper margin of the orbit. (Figs. 391-392.) Continue the incision downward along the outer margin of the orbit to a point near the lower orbital margin. From this point carry the incision backward on the malar bone to the middle third of the zygoma.

Step 2. (a) Divide the zygoma subperiosteally near its middle.

(b) Beginning at the upper and outer part of the orbital rim, divide it with a chisel, also subperiosteally, backward and downward to the inferior orbital fissure.

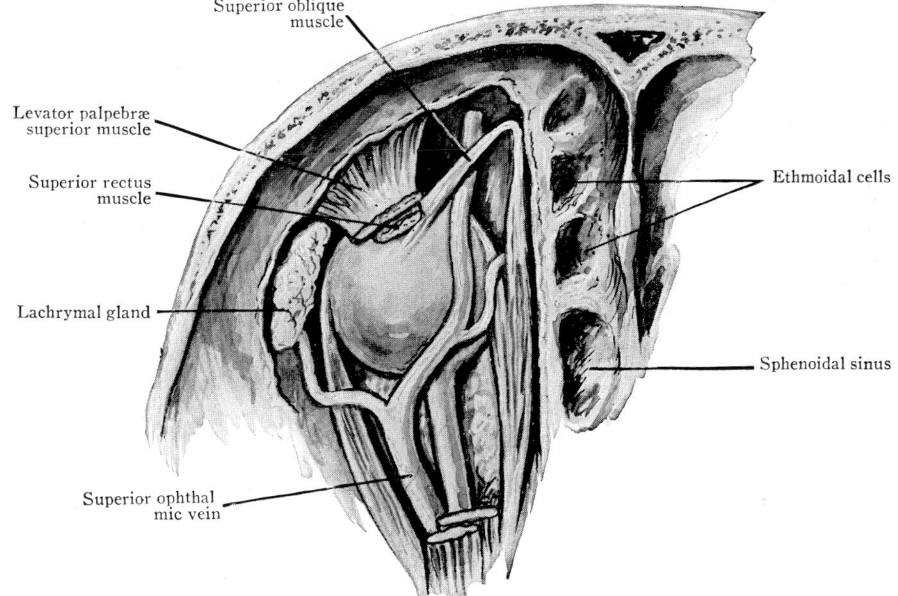

Fig. 393. The roof of the orbit has been removed, showing the contents. (Davis, Applied Anatomy.)

(c) Similarly (subperiosterially), beginning at the lower and outer part of the orbital rim, divide the malar bone backward, to the inferior orbital fissure and to the origin of the masseter muscle.

Step 3. The bone flap thus formed is reflected. Any portions of the external orbital plate which form an obstruction should be removed and the orbital fat exposed.

Step 4. Perform the particular operation indicated.

Step 5. Replace the bone flap. Suture the skin. Suture of the bone is unnecessary.

Resections of the upper and median portion of the orbit may also be performed under certain conditions.

OPERATIONS ON THE EYE

Anatomic Considerations. (Figs. 393-394.) The eyeball has three main coats, viz.: a fibrous outer coat called the sclerotic; a vascular middle coat, the choroid; and a nervous inner coat, the retina.

The sclerotic coat forms a firm protective covering or case for the delicate retina within. It is continuous posteriorly with the fibrous coat or dura of the optic nerve, which is a continuation of the dura mater of the brain. At the optic foramen, the dura mater splits into two layers; the outer layer forms the periosteum, while the inner forms the dural coat of the optic nerve. This nerve also, like the brain, has an arachnoid and a pial membrane. The sclerotic coat is continued forward over the front of the eye as the cornea. It is essentially a membrane intended to be protective in its function.

The choroid or vascular coat of the eye contains the pigment or color of the eye. It is continued forward as the ciliary body (or processes) and iris. Being a

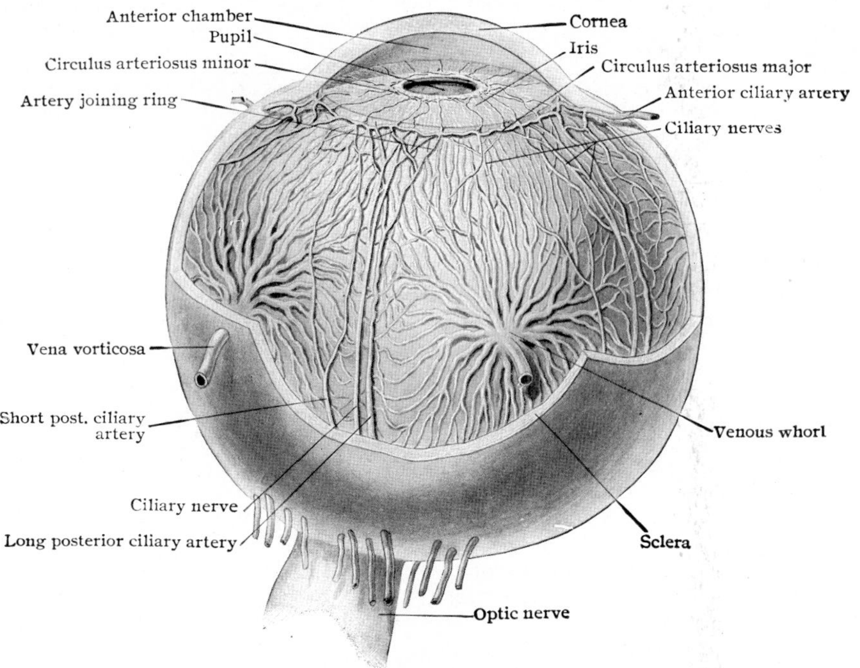

FIG. 394. Injected eyeball, showing arrangement of ciliary arteries and of choroidal veins. ×3. Drawn from preparation made by Professor Keiller.

vascular tissue, its diseases are inflammatory. If the choroid is affected we have choroiditis; if the ciliary region is inflamed, it is called cyclitis; and if the iris is inflamed we have iritis.

The retina or nervous coat of the eye is concerned in the function of sight and it, like other nerves, may be affected with inflammation, called retinitis. Sometimes it becomes loosened from the choroid beneath by a hemorrhage or rapid stretching of the sclera, constituting a detachment of the retina. Outside the disk is the macula lutea and fovea centralis or region of distinct vision.

Filling the interior of the eye is the jelly-like transparent vitreous humor, enclosed in the hyaloid membrane. In front of the vitreous humor is the lens; and the clear, limpid liquid between the anterior surface of the lens and the posterior surface of the cornea is the aqueous humor.

The lens, immediately behind the iris, is suspended in its capsule from the ciliary processes by its suspensory ligament or zonule of Zinn. Between the ciliary processes and the sclera lies the ciliary muscle which regulates the accommodation or focussing power of the eye. The ciliary processes are formed of convoluted blood vessels supported by connective tissue and covered by the pigmented extension of the retina. This ciliary region is an exceedingly sensitive one and a serious wound of it usually means a loss of the eye.

The iris is the continuation of the choroid through the ciliary body, and extends down to the pupil, its free edge resting on the anterior surface of the lens. The iris is composed of a vascular and fibrous anterior portion, and a muscular and pigmented posterior portion. In consequence of its vascularity, the iris is the frequent site of inflammation. When inflamed it pours out lymph which may cause it to adhere to the lens behind, forming a posterior synechia. An anterior synechia occurs when, because of perforation of the cornea, the iris washes forward and becomes attached to the cornea in front.

The circular muscle fibres surrounding the pupil are anterior, and form the sphincter pupillae muscle; it contracts the pupil. The radiating muscular fibres, which lie slightly posterior to the sphincter pupillae dilate the pupil. The dark pigment layer is on the posterior surface of the iris, and after an attack of iritis, as the adherent iris is torn loose from the lens, it leaves patches of pigment adhering to the anterior capsule.

The iris, as it rests at its pupillary margin on the lens, divides the space anterior to the lens into two parts. The part between the posterior surface of the iris and the anterior surface of the lens forms the posterior chamber. The anterior chamber lies between the anterior surface of the iris and the posterior surface (Descemet's membrane) of the cornea. The two chambers communicate through the pupil. The anterior surface of the iris toward its periphery is of the nature of a coarse mesh work, the spaces of which are the spaces of Fontana. They communicate with a venous or lymph canal which passes around the eye at the sclerocorneal junction (canal of Schlemm).

The aqueous humor is of the nature of lymph. It is secreted by the ciliary processes and posterior surface of the iris. It passes through the pupil to the anterior chamber, and enters the spaces of Fontana to empty into the canal of Schlemm. The canal of Schlemm empties its contents into the anterior ciliary veins.

The optic nerve reaches from the optic chiasm to the eyeball, a distance of about 5 cm. (2 in.). It enters the apex of the orbit through the optic foramen at the upper inner angle, in company with the ophthalmic artery. The artery crosses the under surface of the nerve from its inner to its outer side. The optic nerve has as its covering a prolongation of the membranes of the brain. The dura mater when it reaches the foramen splits and gives one layer to form the periosteum lining the orbit and the other to form a fibrous sheath of the nerve. This arrangement prevents pus, forming in the orbit, from passing through the optic foramen into the skull. The arteria centralis retinae enters the nerve on its under side and passes through its center to the interior of the eye. The nerve itself is covered with a fine pial membrane and an arachnoid separating it from the dura thus forming subdural and subarachnoid spaces. As these membranes and spaces are continuous with those of the brain, hemorrhage or serous effusions occurring within the brain can thus find their way into the sheath of the nerve.

As the nerve enters the eye, it is contracted and forms the optic disk or papilla. It is readily seen with the ophthalmoscope as a round spot somewhat lighter in color than the surrounding eye-ground. Coming from a depression or cup in the disk, called the porus opticus, are the retinal arteries and veins.

The Muscles and Nerves of the Orbit. Directly under the periosteum of the roof of the orbit is found the levator palpebrae superioris which draws the upper eyelid upward and backward. It is supplied by the oculomotor nerve by means of the internal rectus and external rectus. The combined action of the superior rectus and the inferior oblique results in the direct elevation of the eyeball; direct depression is brought about by the inferior rectus and the superior oblique. The fourth (trochlear) nerve supplies the superior oblique and the sixth (abducent) nerve the external rectus. The third cranial or oculomotor nerve supplies the ciliary muscle, the sphincter of the iris and the remaining ocular muscles.

The dilator fibers of the iris, the unstriped muscle of the upper eyelid, and the unstriped muscle of Müller, which bridges the sphenomaxillary (inferior orbital) fissure are supplied by the cervical sympathetic. If this nerve is paralyzed, constriction of the pupil, slight ptosis and recession of the eyeball take place according to Horner's syndrome.

The two divisions of the **lacrimal gland** are known as the orbital and palpebral. The orbital is found on a fossa on the frontal bone and the palpebral extends downward beneath the upper eyelid, to the superior fornix of the conjunctiva. The ducts from both portions of the gland open into the superior fornix. Tears reach the puncta lacrimales by crossing the conjunctiva. These tiny openings are found on the very top of the lacrimal papillae which occupy the margins of the eyelids close to the inner canthus of the eye. The puncta enter the lacrimal canaliculi at first running vertically and then turning abruptly inward to open by a common canal into the outer part of the lacrimal sac. Normally, the puncta are placed opposite the conjunctiva, but the lower punctum may be everted causing the tears to flow over the lower lid onto the cheek (epiphora). Obstructions of the lacrimal passages often found where the lacrimal sac and naso-lacrimal duct join also cause this condition.

The lacrimal sac is formed by the dilatation of the upper extremity of the naso-lacrimal duct. Its upper end is found back of the internal tarsal ligament and is covered by some of the fibres of the orbicularis palpebrarum muscle. When abscesses form in this sac, they are likely to discharge through the skin below the internal tarsal ligament, if unrelieved, and may be opened in this situation.

The naso-lacrimal duct is about ¾ inch long, extending downward and slightly backward within a bony canal and opening into the inferior meatus of the nose. By extending a line from the inner canthus to the front of the first molar tooth, its course may be indicated on the surface. The lower eyelid is everted and the lower punctum identified when a probe is passed along the lacrimal passages. The probe is inserted through the lower punctum and is directed first vertically and then horizontally toward the inner wall of the sac; then it is turned downward vertically and slightly backward toward the inferior meatus.

The eyelids are composed of five layers which from the exterior to the interior are: (1) the skin, (2) the subcutaneous tissue, (3) the muscular layer, (4) the tarsal plates, and (5) the conjunctiva.

The skin of the eyelid is very fragile. The subcutaneous tissue is loose in texture, quite elastic and free from fat. Oedema accompanying inflammation of the orbit and surrounding structure is generally quite noticeable in the eyelids. The muscular layer is comprised of the orbicularis palpebrarum in ring-like combinations and some involuntary muscle which is discerned more clearly in the upper lid than in the lower.

The tarsal plates are two very thin layers of dense fibrous tissue found in the border of their respective lids and connected to the palpebral ligaments at their extremities. The Meibomian glands resemble sebaceous follicles in structure and lie between the tarsal plates and the conjunctiva. Upon everting the eyelid, the ducts may be seen through the conjunctiva as thin yellowish streaks running out freely. A Meibomian cyst appears on the deep surface of the eyelid and is likely to become quite large before it is noticed. The glands of Moll which resemble modified sweat glands and the glands of Zeiss which resemble sebaceous glands lie along the free border of the eyelids. If the glands of Zeiss become obstructed or infected a sty (hordeolum) results.

The Conjunctiva. The ocular surface of the lids is lined with the palpebral portion of the conjunctival sac while the adjacent surface of the sclerotic is covered with the bulbar portion. The palpebral is firmly attached over the tarsal plates but is loose and moveable elsewhere upon the lid. The bulbar conjunctiva continues uninterrupted with the palpebral part along the conjunctival fornices and is firmly adherent at the limbus but is quite loosely attached to the sclerotic.

Blood which has collected within the orbit, usually resulting from fractures of the anterior cranial fossa is noticed first under the conjunctiva of the globe near the corneal border. Later, it may reach under the upper eyelid and continue upward beneath the skin. The palpebral fissure is formed by the eyelids between the inner and outer canthus; they enclose, at the inner canthus, the lacus lacrimalis in which lies the caruncle which appears as an oval elevation, and the plica semilunaris, which appears on the outer side of the caruncle as a vertical crescentic fold and designates the end of the bulbar conjunctiva (Piersol).

ANESTHESIA IN EYE OPERATIONS

Local anesthesia is used for most operations upon the eye.

Some operations such as for enucleation of the eyeball, acute glaucoma, etc., often call for general anesthesia. Voluntary movement of the eye under local anesthesia is of great aid to the surgeon. Butyn, 1 per cent, instilled into the conjunctival sac is excellent. Such an instillation is made every five minutes. To accomplish complete anesthesia, from six to eight instillations are required. Butyn does not cause drying of the corneal epithelium or produce dilatation of the pupil as does cocaine. (Other anesthetics that may be used are cocaine, novocaine, eucaine, stovaine, alypin, etc.). These are sufficient for intraocular operations such as cataract, corneoscleral trephine and operations on the cornea and conjunctiva.

In **operations on the eyelids** a solution of one to one hundred of novocaine or procaine crystals injected along the orbital margins of the lids is efficacious. In operations on the extraocular muscles a similar solution, to which a few drops of adrenalin are added, injected subconjunctivally will answer the purpose well.

REMOVAL OF FOREIGN BODIES FROM THE EYE

Conjunctiva

The eye is anesthetized with a freshly made solution of butyn (1½ per cent) or novocaine (5 per cent), introduced into the conjunctival sac; wait a few minutes; give the anesthetic an opportunity to act. Occasionally there is no foreign body but simply an **abrasion of the corneal epithelium**; pain and lacrimation are, in these cases, usually marked. A drop of 2 per cent fluorescin solution introduced into the eye will stain an abraded area of the cornea bright green while the conjunctiva will assume an orange-yellow hue.

A dark room is best for the removal of foreign bodies. Focal rays of light directed on the eye are best for the purpose.

Retract the eyelid. Locate the foreign body. Attempt to wipe it away with a piece of absorbent cotton on an applicator. If this fails the point of a needle is used to remove the foreign body.

Cornea

To dislodge foreign bodies from the cornea is often a more difficult task than those in the conjunctiva. Instill butyn (1 per cent). A good oblique light or focal illumination is essential. The patient is seated and the surgeon stands behind him. The lids are held apart with a proper lid-retractor. Use a fine curet or cataract needle to gently dislodge the foreign body. The instrument is kept parallel to the cornea and the head of the patient is kept steadied to avoid movements which may cause inadvertent injury. In more difficult cases, transfix the cornea over the foreign body and divide the cornea from without inward, after which the foreign body is readily removed. Care should be exercised to prevent traumatic ulcers or pushing the foreign body from the cornea into the anterior chamber of the lens.

Some metal particles may be removed with an ordinary magnet. Deeply imbedded foreign bodies of metal are extracted with an electromagnet. (Fig. 395.) If the foreign substance is in the iris, or anterior chamber or the lens, the point of entry must be enlarged and the foreign body extracted with an appropriate forceps. If it is impacted in the iris and the magnet is ineffective, the segment of iris carrying the foreign body should be removed; its dislodgement

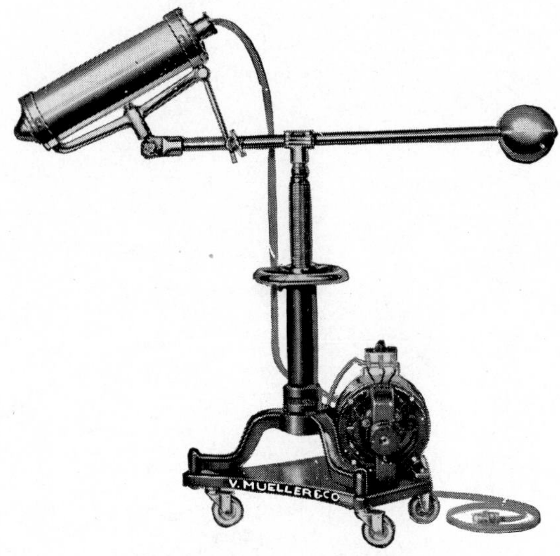

Fig. 395. Victor giant magnet.

from the lens is difficult. A traumatic cataract is frequently encountered; it should be extracted.

Crystalline Lens

Make an incision in the cornea with a keratome. Introduce a delicate forceps and remove the foreign body.

A magnet inserted in the anterior chamber will often extract metal bodies. The chemistry of the lens being neutral, foreign substances lodged there cause no ill effects and it is often advisable to leave them alone until the lens loses its transparency when it is removed. However, iron, steel and copper bodies should be removed at once.

Vitreous, Choroid and Retina

Foreign bodies in the posterior portions of the eye are treated as follows:

Ascertain the exact position of the foreign body (ophthalmoscope, x-ray, Sweet localizer, etc.) Its extraction entails operative maneuvers. It should not be attempted in inadequate surroundings or with improper training. If your experience is limited, keep the conjunctiva clear by irrigations, aseptic dressings, etc., until a specialist performs the necessary procedure. The duty of the general surgeon is to avoid infection from ensuing.

OPERATIONS ON THE CONJUNCTIVA

Pterygium

Pterygium (wing) is a triangular fold of thickened conjunctiva resulting from exposure to the wind, sun and dust. It is more common on the nasal side of the cornea than on the temporal side, but may appear on both sides. The apex is referred to as the head; a small adjoining part is called the neck; and the wing-like expansion is termed the body. As growth takes place, the head advances from the corneal margin toward the center of the cornea, causing a cosmetic disfigurement and endangering the sight.

The treatment consists in excision or transplantation, and the operation of McReynolds gives the most satisfactory results. Very few recurrences follow the proper performance of this procedure.

(a) The following is the least complex operation for removing a pterygium:

Step 1. The conjunctiva is anesthetized with cocaine or butyn-solution and the neck of the tumor is grasped with a small forceps at the corneal margin. The tumor is detached from the cornea with a pterygium, cataract or some other very sharp knife. (Fig. 396 A.) Great care should be exercised so that

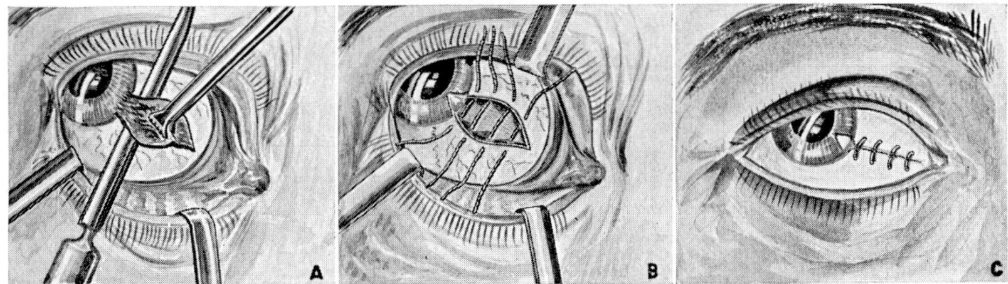

Fig. 396. A. Operation showing pterygium grasped with forceps and detached from cornea with a very sharp knife, B. sutures placed, C. suture of the conjunctiva.

the head of the pterygium and all loose tissue is removed without injuring the corneal stroma.

Step 2. The surface of the cornea should be cauterized with the actual cautery where the head of the pterygium has been excised. A wedge-shaped piece of the attached conjunctiva is excised with a fine scissors after the head and neck have been detached with a knife.

Step 3. The edges of the wound may be undermined for a short distance before closing. (Figs. 396 B and C.)

(b) When the pterygium is of such size that cutting away its conjunctival pedicle is likely to result in excessive shrinkage of the conjunctiva, the following operation is offered as an alternative: The pterygium, instead of being excised, is transplanted under the conjunctiva a short way from the cornea and healthy, new conjunctiva is brought up to the stripped margin of the cornea. Sliding flaps of many kinds have been offered for use in this procedure.

Benign Tumors of the Conjunctiva

Pinguecula. This is a tiny, fatty growth appearing on the conjunctiva; it is about the size of the head of a common pin and of a reddish or saffron hue.

It should be cut away in such a manner that only one suture need be required to unite the edges of the wound.

Lipoma. This condition occurs rather infrequently beneath the conjunctiva. The tumor is shelled out following an incision in the conjunctiva and the edges of the wound sutured.

Angiomas. The most successful procedure in this case is complete excision of the angioma by means of a small surgical knife after which the veins are ligated at the surface. Galvanocauterization may be instituted as an auxiliary remedy.

Polypi. These growths are sometimes referred to as pediculate papillomata and are generally excised, the wound sutured and cauterized with the galvanocautery.

Cysts. These are of a serous or dermoid nature. Great care should be exercised when detaching them from the conjunctiva so that they may be completely enveloped when lifted out. The transparent qualities of cysticerci cause them to be readily identified if present in the conjunctiva. The same procedure is followed as in the case of lipoma. Great care must be taken so that the entire cyst wall is removed in order to prevent its return.

Malignant Tumors of the Conjunctiva

Epithelioma. The margin of the cornea is very often the starting point of primary epithelioma of the conjunctiva. Excision should be promptly prescribed. Electrosurgical destruction or radium give better results than scalpel surgery.

Malignant Encanthis. This condition is also referred to as epithelioma of the caruncülus lacrimalis. The treatment prescribed is thermocoagulation or radium. When an epithelioma of the eyelid or lacrimal passage becomes enlarged it is usually identified as secondary epithelioma of the caruncülus and calls for the same treatment as malignant encanthis.

Sarcoma: Melano-Sarcoma. This is, generally speaking, a primary sarcoma of the choroid. Great skill on the part of the surgeon is required in dealing with this serious affliction. The treatment is complete enucleation of the eyeball supplemented by thermocoagulation to the retrobulbar structures, followed by radium.

OPERATIONS OF THE EYELIDS

Hordeolum (Stye)

Operation is performed for infection of the glands of Zeiss. A local anesthetic solution is injected. Incise the skin parallel with the border of the eyelid; avoid injury to the tarsus, for such injury may eventuate in cysts or chalazions.

Chalazion (Meibomian Cyst, "Hailstone")

A chalazion is in intimate relationship with the tarsal cartilages. It may become reabsorbed after an incidental inflammatory condition. Its removal may be accomplished through an intermarginal incision, a conjunctival incision, or a cutaneous incision.

THE INTERMARGINAL METHOD (AGNEW'S PROCEDURE)

This method is preferred by many and it is particularly applicable if the chalazion is situated near the border of the eyelid.

Anesthetize (novocaine) the eye and affected lid. Make an incision along the margin of the eyelid between the cutaneous and mucous surfaces of the lid. Enter the cyst. Express and curet out its contents and destroy its walls. Apply a compression dressing. Union by suture of the conjunctival margins is unnecessary. Avoid hematoma formation.

THE CONJUNCTIVAL ROUTE

Step 1. Grasp the eyelid with a chalazion forceps, placing the spatula blade over the chalazion on the skin side. Evert the lid by a simple rotation of the handle of the forceps. Make an incision in the conjunctiva either perpendicular to or parallel with the lid margin (Fig. 397). (If a parallel incision is made it should not extend beyond the limits of the chalazion to prevent the destruction of adjacent meibomian glands.) This incision should extend through the chalazion.

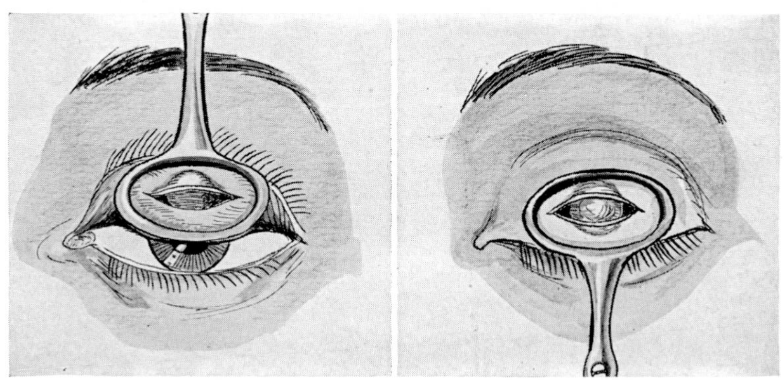

FIG. 397 FIG. 398

FIG. 397. Extirpation of a chalazion by the conjunctival route. Luxate the eyelid with a Desmarres' forceps, the spatula of which supports the cutaneous surface.

FIG. 398. Extirpation of a chalazion by the cutaneous route. The spatula of the Desmarres' forceps is introduced into the superior conjunctival culdesac.

Step 2. The contents can now be removed and the cyst wall completely destroyed with a chalazion curet. It is unnecessary to unite the wound edges with sutures. The space where the chalazion was removed will immediately fill with blood, but this will soon resorb.

THE CUTANEOUS ROUTE

Excessive size of the chalazion calls for this method. Inject the anesthetizing solution. Make an incision running parallel with the margin of the lid extending down to the chalazion (Fig. 398). Dissect it out of its bed. Curet the bed, if necessary. Secure hemostasis. Unite the wound edges of the skin with a few interrupted Pagenstecher linen sutures.

Blepharospasm

FUNCTIONAL

This is occasioned by contractions of the orbicularis palpebrarum muscle. It may be a purely reflex manifestation (conjunctivitis, acute or chronic). The treatment is removal of the cause. Partial resection of the orbicularis has been recommended by some. Where narrowing of the palpebral fissure resulted, external canthoplasty (which see) is indicated.

ESSENTIAL

This consists of tonic and clonic contractions of the orbicularis muscle such as is observed in tic douloureux. Treatment consists of resection of the infra-orbital nerve or, if this fails, intracranial resection of the ophthalmic branch of the trigeminus.

Blepharoptosis (Drooping of the Eyelids)

Ptosis of the ocular muscles through affection of the nerve supplying the muscle is caused by an underdevelopment of the levator muscle, or paralysis. Mechanical ptosis is due to dragging down of the upper lid (tumors, trichiasis). The following procedures are used to correct the condition, though success is not always attained.

1. Excising the skin to shorten the lid.
2. Advancing the point of insertion of the levator palpebrae muscle.

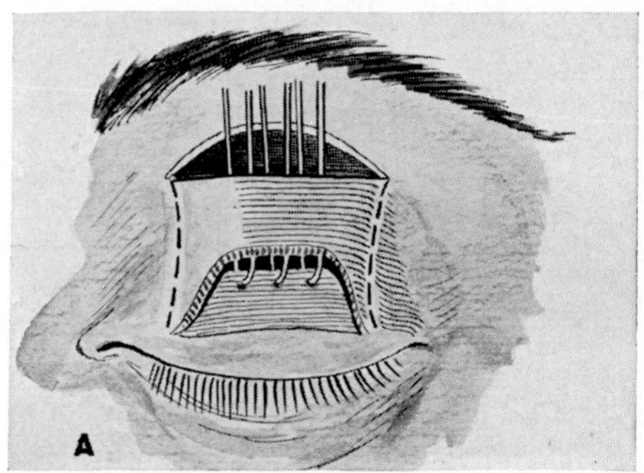

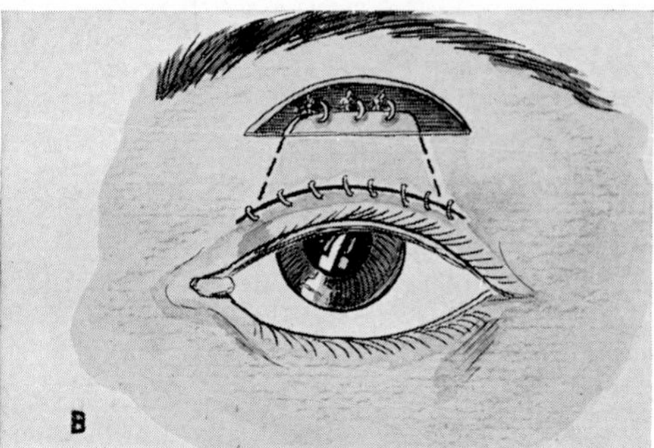

FIG. 399. Paralytic ptosis: A. the epidermis is detached from the cutaneous flap. Note the introduction of 3 suture loops which are passed beneath the musculocutaneous bridge. B. The palpebral-cutaneous flap drawn under the musculocutaneous bridge, is now united to the occipitofrontalis muscle. Suture the wound in the upper eyelid.

3. Substituting the action of the frontalis muscle for that of the levator palpebrae superioris.
4. Combining the two methods just mentioned.
5. Substituting the action of the superior rectus muscle for that of the levator palpebrae.

SUTURE OF A CUTANEOUS FLAP FROM THE UPPER EYELID TO THE FRONTALIS MUSCLE

Step 1. Put the eyelid on the stretch. Dissect from its upper surface a quadrilateral flap with its base directed downward. Detach the cutaneous surface down to the tarsal cartilage (Fig. 399 A).

Step 2. Make a horizontal incision extending along the entire length of the superior border of the eyelid exposing the fibers of the frontalis and corrugator supercilii muscles.

Step 3. Mobilize the bridge of skin between the two openings. The cartilaginous flap now divested of skin is sutured to the muscle as shown in the illustration.

Step 4. Unite the edges of the upper and lower cutaneous wounds with interrupted sutures (Fig. 399 B).

Claiborne removes a rectangular-shaped piece of tarsus (12 to 15 mm. long and 2 to 3 mm. wide) together with the conjunctiva. The wound is closed with a central suture of stout thread and placement of two sutures of finer thread on either side of it; four lateral stitches are then introduced.

Cicatricial Ectropion

WHARTON JONES' OPERATION

Step 1. Make a V-shaped flap, governing its size by the everted lid, including the scar tissue (Fig. 400 A).

Step 2. Extend the convergent incisions downward forming a Y-shaped flap which is dissected up in its lower part.

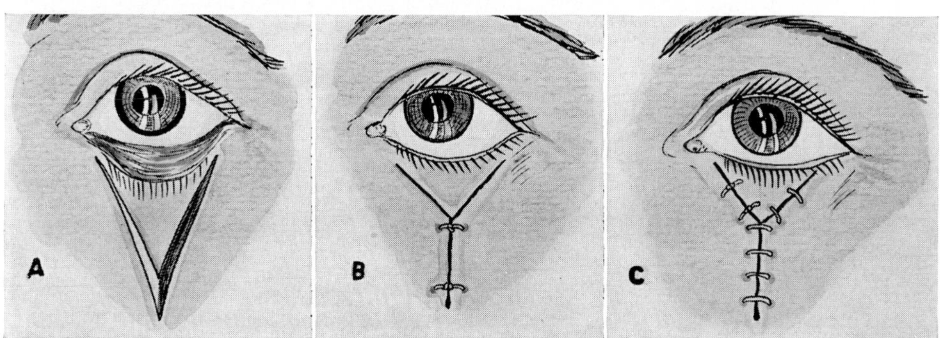

Fig. 400. A. Wharton Jones' operation for ectropion of the lower eyelid. (V-shaped incision). B. After mobilization of the flap, suture of the wound in the form of Y. C. Appearance of the suture complete.

Step 3. Suture the lower part vertically in such a manner that the tension upon the ectropion is relieved (Fig. 400 B).

Step 4. Suture the upper parts of the margins to those of the Y-shaped flap which has been drawn back (Fig. 400 C).

Atonic Ectropion

DIEFFENBACH'S OPERATION

Step 1. This consists of tracing and excising a small triangle, the base of which is directed upward forming an outward prolongation of the external commissure (Fig. 401 A).

Step 2. Resect the exuberant portion of the free margin of the lower eyelid.

Step 3. Reunite the edges of the denuded triangular surface as shown in the illustration (Fig. 401 B).

Step 4. Repair the conjunctiva and skin.

Entropion

Entropion is an inversion of an eyelid. The eyelashes are turned toward the eyeball. The condition is frequently associated with trichiasis.

Canthotomy

This is performed under local anesthesia, the object being to make the palpebral opening larger.

Make a horizontal incision with one blade of a pair of blunt-pointed scissors inserted in the conjunctival sac and divide the canthal ligament and conjunctiva simultaneously. The wound may or may not be sutured.

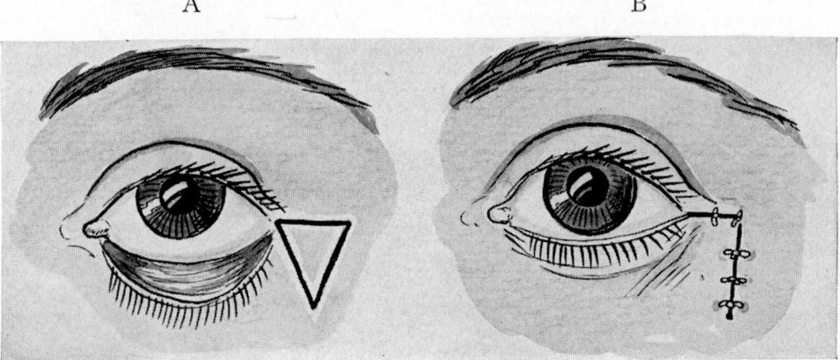

FIG. 401. Dieffenbach's operation for atonic ectropion.

Canthoplasty

Step 1. Incise the external commissure horizontally from within outward for about 10 to 15 mm. dividing the skin, orbicularis oculi muscle and soft tissues, to the bone (Fig. 402 A).

Step 2. Reunite the conjunctiva at the external angle of the incision (Fig. 402 B).

Step 3. Unite by interrupted sutures of the conjunctiva to the respective upper and lower cutaneous wound (Fig. 402 C).

Tarsorrhaphy and **blepharorrhaphy** are synonymous terms designating the shortening or complete closing of the palpebral fissure which may be partial or total, temporary or permanent.

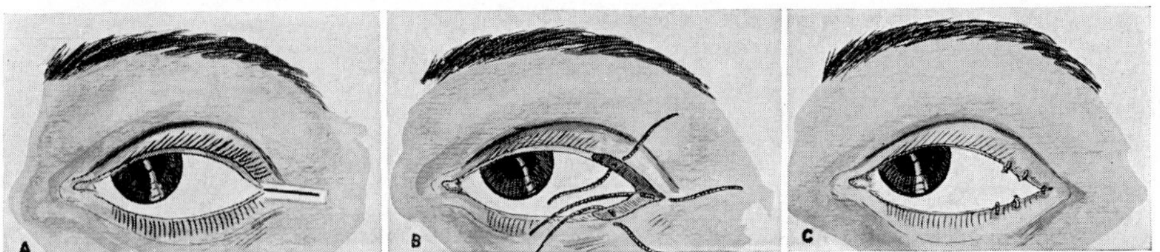

FIG. 402. A. External canthoplasty. The horizontal incision divides the skin and conjunctiva. B. Placing of the first three sutures to unite the new palpebrocutaneous commissure. C. Suture completed.

Comment. Total tarsorrhaphy is objectionable because of retention of secretions of the eye and because of the difficulty of reopening the external canthus. Median tarsorrhaphy is more adequate.

Ankyloblepharon signifies partial or complete junction of the eyelids, It may be congenital or acquired.

Symblepharon is an adhesive process between the conjunctiva of the eyeball with that of the eyelid.

Blepharoplasty

This signifies repair of defects of the eyelids. For total blepharoplasty the integrity of the conjunctiva and the fibro-cartilaginous framework of the eyelids is a sine qua non. Four methods are applicable.

1. French Method (sliding flaps).
2. Indian Method (pedicled flaps transposed by torsion or rotation).
3. Italian Method (pedicled flaps from distant parts—arm).
4. Grafting.

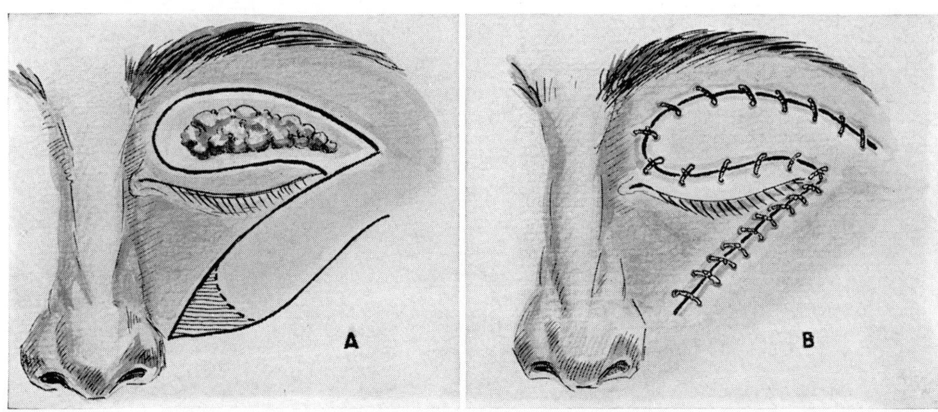

FIG. 403. A. Extirpation of a neoplasm or scar from the upper eyelid. B. Transfer the flap into its new position. Suture in place. Obliterate the denuded area by approximating the borders of the cutaneous wound.

BLEPHAROPLASTY OF THE UPPER EYELID

Step 1. Dissect out the scar; mobilize the surrounding margins (Fig. 403 A).

Step 2. Mobilize the autoplastic flap.

Step 3. Suture the flap after shaping it, into its proper place (Fig. 404 B).

Step 4. Repair the bed whence the flap was taken. Dress the wound.

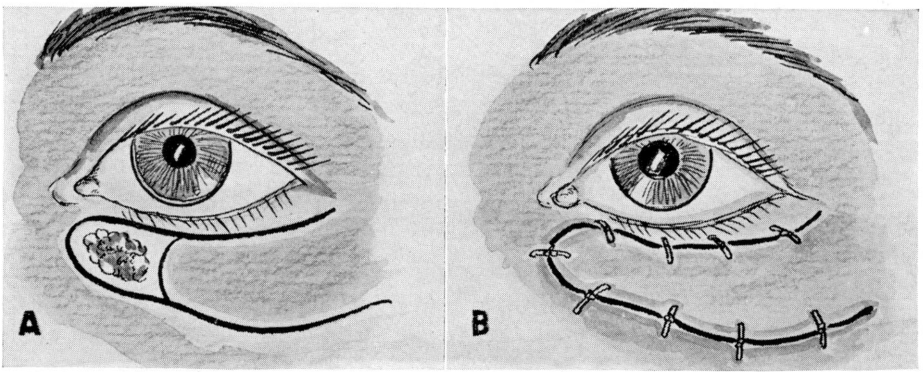

FIG. 404. A. Extirpation of a small tumor from the lower eyelid. A sliding flap is used. B. Operation completed.

BLEPHAROPLASTY OF THE LOWER EYELID

Step 1. Make a tongue-shaped incision around the defect; remove it (Fig. 404 A).

Step 2. Make a second similar incision beginning at the same point as the first, thus creating a flap which is sutured into the bed left by the excised and freshened defect (Fig. 404 B).

Operation for Symblepharon

Symblepharon signifies scar formation between the conjunctiva of the eyeball and the conjunctiva of the eyelid. Partial symblepharons are characterized by adhesions consisting of single cords while complete symblepharons consist of adhesions of broad bands which have been known to completely obliterate the cul-de-sac.

Arlt's procedure which is indicated when not more than a third of the eye is affected, is performed under cocaine analgesia.

Step 1. The adhesions may be seized with a forceps or a suture-tractor may be used. The apex of the symblepharon is severed from the cornea with a sharp knife; the remainder with a blunt curved scissors.

Step 2. The scar-tissue is dissected from the symblepharon by two incisions reaching from the apex to the base. The flap which results is placed in the lid-aperture which is left after excising the symblepharon.

Step 3. For mobilization purposes, the borders of the conjunctival wound are undercut and sutured.

Operations for Trachoma

Trachoma is a condition characterized by chronic conjunctivitis accompanied by an abnormal increase in the size of the conjunctiva and follicular formation.

THE USE OF ROLLER FORCEPS IN EXPRESSING TRACHOMA BODIES: KNAPP'S TECHNIC

General anesthesia should be used.

Step 1. Evert the edge of the upper eyelid; grasp it with the Knapp's roller-forceps (Fig. 405) and pull the lid upward, exposing the fornix.

Step 2. Insert one cylinder of the roller forceps into the upper fornix while the other cylinder is made to roll over the tarsal region of the conjunctiva.

Step 3. Press the blades of the instrument together causing the cylinder to exert pressure in expressing or "milking" out the secretion and granules. This procedure may be repeated several times until the conjunctiva is smooth; the procedure is practiced also on the conjunctiva of the lower eyelid. Following the expression, apply cold compresses. When the exudation has ceased, apply a 2 per cent silver nitrate solution daily.

PARTIAL EXCISION OF THE TARSUS AND CONJUNCTIVA
CLAIBORNE'S CLAMP-OPERATION FOR TRACHOMA

The clamp used in this operation resembles that of Desmarres' (Fig. 406); it consists of a metal plate upon which descends a fork of five prongs which fit into fenestrae when the instrument is closed.

Step 1. Lift up the middle of the eyelid with the fingers or forceps. Introduce the right prong of the instrument under the lid followed by the left; screw the fork on the lid by means of the ratchet. Reverse the clamp, thus exposing the conjunctival surface of the lid. The curve of the prongs serves as a guide for the incision. Because of tension, the tarsus when incised springs away from the subjacent tissue.

Step 2. In order to lessen the tension when the conjunctiva is sutured to the lid, the tarsus and conjunctiva over it are dissected up and the conjunctiva of the fornix is loosened. The sutures should be about ten inches long, double-armed, and inserted parallel to the inferior margin of the tarsus, the middle stitches being inserted first. Excise the tarsus above the suture line; remove the clamp and continue the suturing.

No blood is lost during this operation and it may be performed in a short time (10 or 15 minutes). It differs from other methods in that the middle sutures

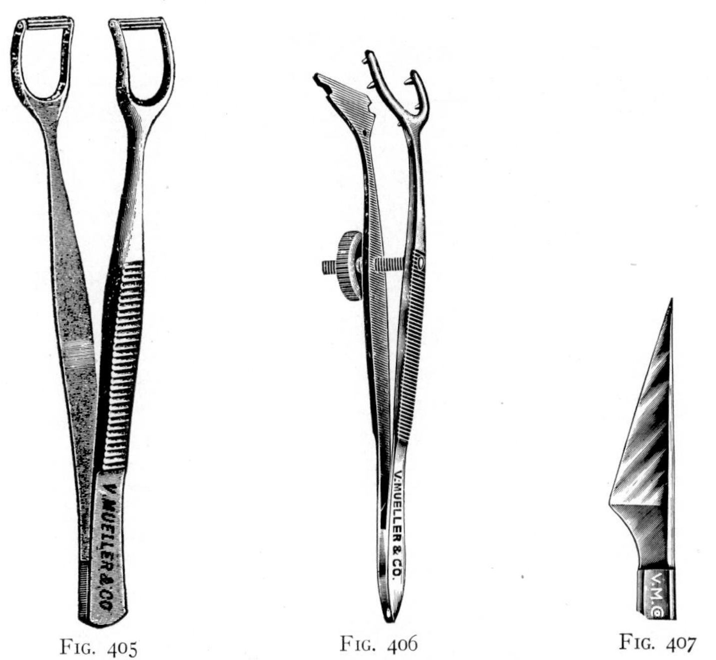

Fig. 405 Fig. 406 Fig. 407

Fig. 405. Knapp's trachoma forceps.
Fig. 406. Claiborne's lid clamp for removal of tarsus in old trachoma.
Fig. 407. Beer's knife.

are placed at a greater distance from the ciliary area, thus insuring a deeper fornix and avoiding tucking of the lid in the center.

Operations for Pannus: Peridectomy

This operation consists of excising the conjunctiva all around and very close to the cornea; after excision the area is cauterized with nitrate of silver. The vessels on the cornea are scarified by means of a Beer knife (Fig. 407).

Peritomy

is a modification of the above procedure and consists of incising the conjunctiva all around the cornea as near the limbus as possible; the larger vessels, if exposed, are seared with a hot electrode after which the eye is cleansed with hot boric-acid solution and dressed. These operations are indicated where superficial ulcers or corneal vascularity exist (trachomatous pannus, etc.)

Operations for Removal of the Lacrimal Gland

RESECTION OF THE PALPEBRAL PORTION OF LACRIMAL GLAND

Cocaine anesthesia.

Step 1. Evert the upper lid and draw same up forcibly with forceps; have the patient look down; the gland can now be seen. Apply a pledget of cotton saturated with a solution of adrenalin (1-1000) for a minute or so.

Step 2. Make an incision over the gland (Fig. 408 A). Hold the wound open with forceps or strabismus-hook. Free the gland by blunt dissection, first above, then below (Fig. 408 B). After the lobes are well dissected out, draw the gland down and cut it off with scissors from the nasal side out. Control hemorrhage by clamping, styptics or pressure.

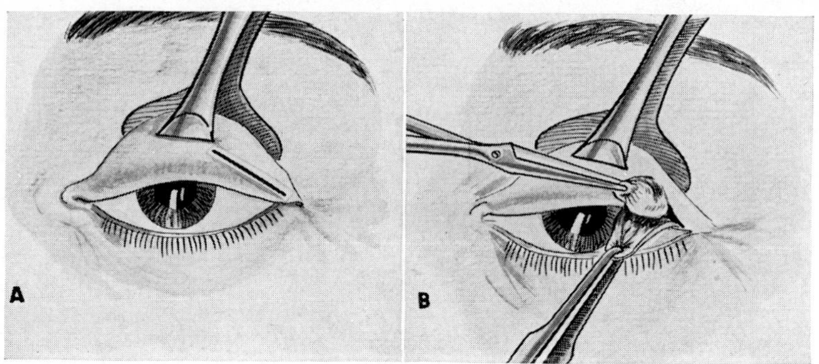

Fig. 408. A. Resection of palpebral portion of lacrimal gland. Conjunctival incision. B. Dissection of gland almost completed.

EXCISION OF THE ORBITAL OR SUPERIOR LACRIMAL GLAND

It has been shown that if conditions necessitate the removal of the orbital or superior lacrimal gland for such conditions as cysts, epiphora or fistula, the remaining glands of the eye (Krause's meibomian, etc.) are sufficiently capable of lubricating the eyeball.

General anesthesia. Shave the eyebrow.

Step 1. Make a curved incision parallel to the outer half of the orbital border through the skin and subcutaneous tissues down to the periosteum. Do not carry the incision too far forward mesially.

Step 2. Expose the lacrimal gland by drawing the edges of the wound apart. Grasp the gland with appropriate forceps and remove it by blunt dissection and delicate scissors.

Step 3. Ligate the lacrimal artery; suture the tarso-orbital fascia with catgut.

Step 4. Close the skin with Pagenstecher linen.

Probing the Lacrimo-Nasal Duct

In the presence of a stricture of the canaliculus or nasal duct, an attempt at dilatation with a probe introduced into the canaliculus and nasal duct may be followed by success (Fig. 409). To eliminate the pain incident to the procedure a few drops of novocaine solution are instilled into the culdesac and lacrimal sac. In probing, caution should be exercised not to penetrate the lacrimal bone or the wall of the sac or duct during the manipulations.

Incising a Canaliculus or Lacrimal Duct

This procedure is indicated in some form of stricture, displaced puncta lacrimalia and dacryocystitis. It is contraindicated as a preliminary procedure to probing the lacrimal duct unless absolutely necessary. Its benefits are temporary. Gas or local anesthesia should be used. **Weber's** or **Agnew's** canaliculus knife is well adapted for the purpose.

Step 1. Evert the lower eyelid.

Step 2. Introduce the knife into the punctum in a vertical direction. (Fig. 410 A.) Put the lid on the stretch away from the tendo oculi and hold in slight eversion. Introduce the knife in such a manner that its cutting edge is directed upward and backward so that the incision will come in contact with the conjunctiva of the globe when the lid is released. Be sure that the end of the knife is in contact with the conjunctiva of the globe when the lid is released; also that the end of the knife is in contact with the interior of the nasal wall of the sac—then the incision should be made. (Fig. 410 B.)

Step 3. After the incision is made, introduce a probe of appropriate size and leave it there for a few minutes.

Dilate the channel for four or five days and continue catheterization for as long as is deemed necessary. (Fig. 410 C.) Incisions may be made in other directions and into the nasal duct as shown in the illustrations. (Fig. 410 D.)

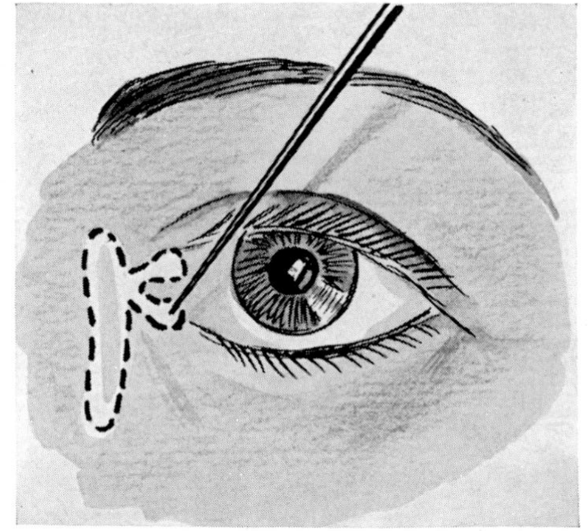

Fig. 409. Introduction of conical stylet into the inferior lachrymal punctum.

Note. The canaliculus should never be cut unless it cannot be opened by means of blunt probes; cutting renders it functionless.

Extirpation of the Lacrimal Sac

Anesthesia. General or local. The superficial injection of the analgesizing solution is made under the skin along the anterior crest of the lacrimal groove. The deep injection into the tissues is made by introducing the hypodermic needle 4 mm. above the inner canthus and carrying the point of the needle straight back to the tissues above the dome of the sac. In usual cases the needle should be inserted about 6 mm. (¼ in.) entering the skin at a point where the lower border of the orbit and the upper anterior portion of the lacrimal bone join, and following a downward, backward and inward path to penetrate the neck of the lacrimal sac. When the anesthetizing solution is forced into the sac it generally causes the fluid already in the cavity to enter the canaliculus along with the anesthetic. Further injections are unnecessary as the solution already injected is sufficient to bleach and anesthetize the canaliculi, the mouth of the nasal duct, the sac wall and adjacent tissues.

Step 1. Make the incision along the entire length of the anterior crest of the lacrimal groove beginning at a point 3 mm. above the canthal ligament and 3 mm. to the nasal side of the inner canthus and ending at the mouth of the duct.

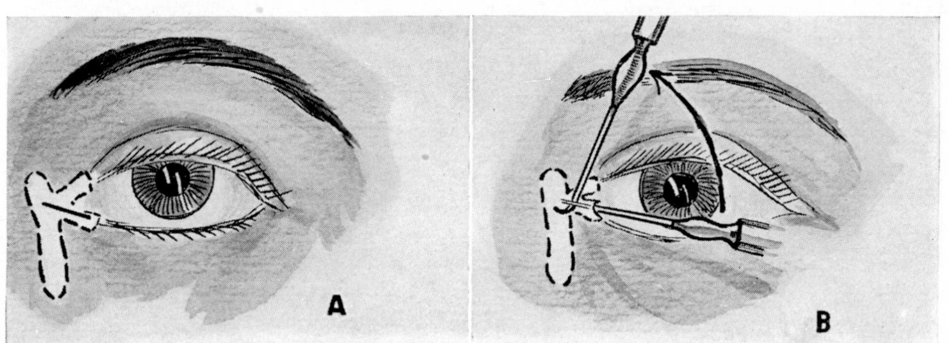

Fig. 410. Incising a canaliculus or lacrimal duct: B. Weber's knife has been introduced into the sac, the arrow indicates the arc of rotation; A. Appearance of completed incision of the inferior canal after cicatrization.

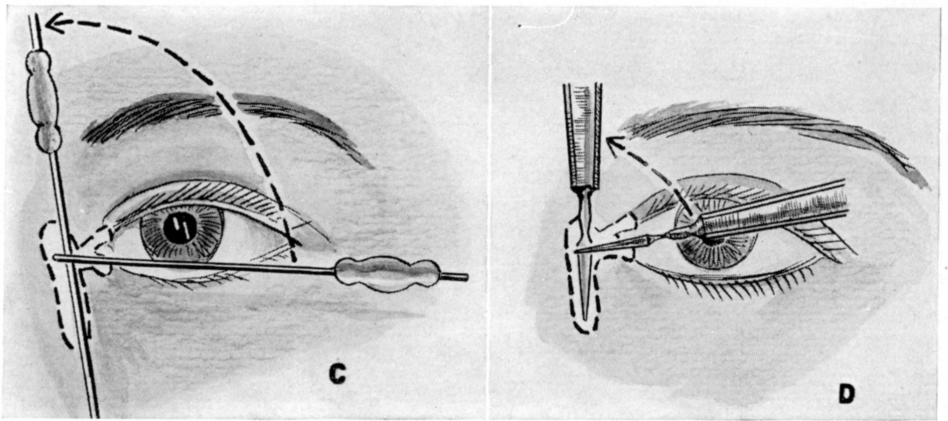

Fig. 410 (continued). Incising a canaliculus or lacrimal duct: C. catheterizing the nasal duct with Bowman's sound. The sound is introduced into the lachrymal canal until it comes into contact with the wall of the lachrymal sac. Its free end is then raised so as to point in the direction of the nasal duct; D. operation for stricture of the nasal duct, with Stilling's knife. The blade of the knife, the extremity of which is blunt, is introduced horizontally as far as the internal wall of the lacrimal sac. It is then raised, as in using Bowman's sound, till it takes the direction of the nasal duct.

Step 2. With a tooth forceps and scissors detach the skin from the canthal ligament and the adjoining orbicularis muscle; introduce a Müller's speculum.

Step 3. Expose the canthal ligament by making an incision parallel to its fibers on the upper and lower borders.

Step 4. Incise the canthal ligament backward and inward about 2 mm. from its nasal extremity; separate the orbicularis fibers along the anterior crest, from the upper to the lower end of the first incision. The deep fascia around the lacrimal sac is thus exposed.

Step 5. Incise the deep fascia behind the stump of the canthal ligament exposing the front wall of the lacrimal sac which is more flabby and of a different color than the tough fascia surrounding it.

Step 6. Separate the fascia along the anterior crest of the lacrimal groove. (The incisions in the orbicularis muscle and the deep fascia should fall immediately behind the first incision and be of the same length; complete exposure of the sac facilitates extirpation.)

Step 7. Dissect the deep fascia from the sac-wall with a mouse-tooth forceps and scissors; extend the dissection to the posterior crest of the lacrimal groove.

Step 8. Dissect the sac from the periosteum with the aid of forceps and scissors and extend the dissection from the dome of the sac to the mouth of the duct. After cutting the connective-tissues at the dome and grasping the upper part of the sac wall, drawing it gently out of its bed, the adhesions along the posterior crest are divided with scissors.

Step 9. While drawing the sac upward, the mouth of the duct is divided with scissors as far down as possible. Curetting and probing are unnecessary if the sac has been entirely removed. Irrigate with boric acid solution or swab with weak tincture of iodine.

Step 10. With fine catgut, suture first the ligament, then the skin so that the temporal flap is slightly elevated to prevent ectropion and proptosis of the lower lid which is likely to follow.

Comment. The Toti-Mosher operation for chronic dacryocystitis consists of approaching the lacrimal sac through an external incision and creating a communication between the sac and nasal cavity. This can also be accomplished by West's operation, the approach being from the inside of the nose.

OPERATIONS ON THE CORNEA

Wounds of the Cornea

Ordinary wounds without prolapse of the iris require no suture. In prolapse of the iris, snip off the herniated portion. Apply dressings after closing the lid. Suture of the sclera is accomplished with a fine curved needle and 00 catgut. The sutures are interrupted and tied lightly. Do not pass the needle through the entire thickness of the sclera—only the conjunctiva and superficial layers of the cornea are sutured. In injury to the posterior chamber Lejars recommends using a needle on each end of the catgut sutures, both entering the wound from within outward. Give a guarded prognosis.

Paracentesis of the Cornea

Retract the lids with a speculum. Steady the eye. Insert a von Graefe knife or a paracentesis needle at the lower end of the vertical meridian of the cornea; the instrument is withdrawn slowly as soon as it enters the anterior chamber of the eye. If necessary, the iris is replaced and the eye dressed.

Guthrie-Saemisch's Operation for Corneal Ulcer

KERATOTOMY

This operation is performed to avoid destruction of the cornea. Steady the eye with fixation forceps. Hold the lids apart with a speculum. Insert a v. Graefe knife on the temporal surface of the horizontal meridian of the cornea. By drawing it outward it will divide the ulcer. Remove all affected tissue. Irrigate the eye with warm salt-solution. Dress. Serious postoperative complications sometimes follow this procedure. It is performed only in the hope of saving an eye that might otherwise be lost.

KERATECTOMY

KNAPP'S OPERATION FOR STAPHYLOMA

Bulging of the cornea is often occasioned by penetrating (knife) injuries, ophthalmia neonatorum, etc., and results in total blindness.

Step 1. Place a mattress-like suture on the nasal side of the vertical meridian and another on the temporal side of the eye.

Step 2. Steady the eye with a fixation forceps. Introduce a Beer knife at the temporal end of the horizontal meridian; hold it flat and carry it downward

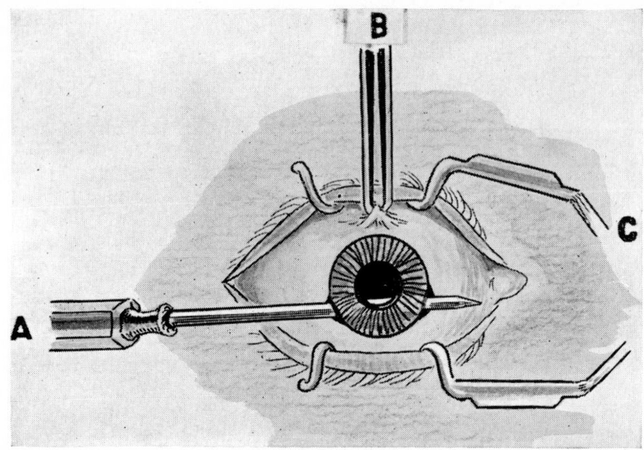

FIG. 411. Paracentesis of the anterior chamber: A. von Graefe's knife transfixing the lower part of the anterior chamber, B. fixation forceps, C. lid retractor.

and outward along the base of the staphyloma until half of it is dissected; grasp the detached part with a mouse-tooth forceps, draw it upward and divide it with scissors along its upper attachment in accordance with the dissection made below. The lens and vitreous may not always be saved.

Step 3. Tie the mattress-like sutures.

This operation is performed principally for esthetic reasons. The surgeon has the choice of removing the eye or excision of the staphyloma. Beer recommends leaving the wound open and the eye dressed.

Transplantation of the Cornea

The transplant is usually obtained from an eye that has just been removed. Many of these corneas unite with the surrounding structures satisfactorily. However, the ultimate result is not very satisfactory; the transplant often loses its transparency. This operation should be attempted only by a specialist well versed in corneal transplantation.

In partial keratoplasty the Descement membrane and the posterior transparent layer of the cornea are omitted. In total keratoplasty the entire thickness of the cornea is used.

OPERATIONS ON THE SCLERA

Paracentesis of the Sclera

This is indicated in detachment of the retina; the subretinal fluid is withdrawn.

Step 1. Novocainize the eye; draw back the eyelid and steady the eyeball with fixation forceps; draw a portion of the conjunctiva to one side with a forceps and see to it that the puncture point will not be made directly over that in the sclera. (Fig. 411.)

Step 2. Insert a von Graefe knife into the sclera and choroid withdrawing it so that the scleral fibers are separated.

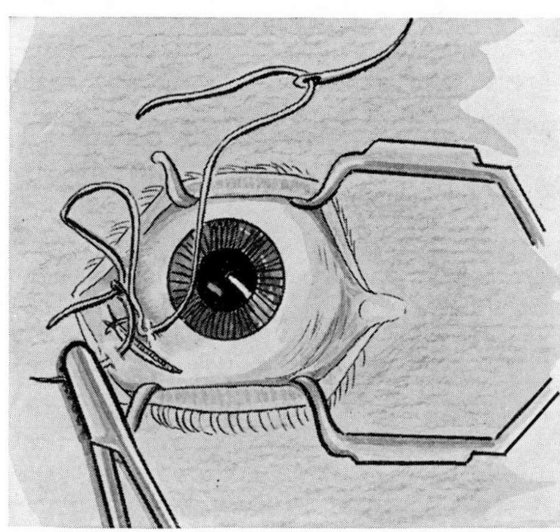

FIG. 412

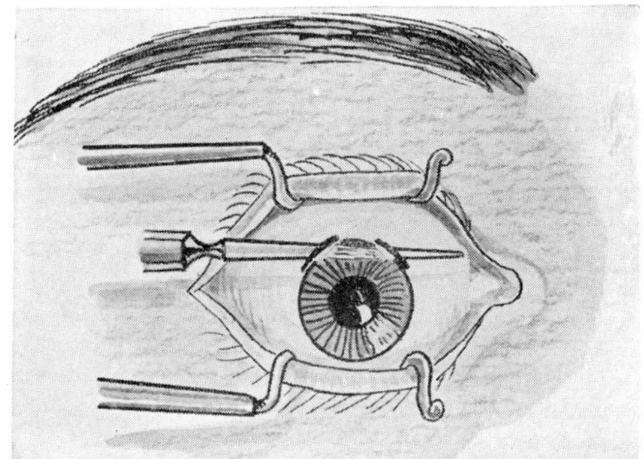

FIG. 413

FIG. 412. Suturing a wound of the sclera. Note that two needles are used. Observe that one end of the suture has just passed through the conjunctiva and outer layer of the sclera from within outward.

FIG. 413. Anterior sclerotomy. The von Graefe knife is manipulated in such a manner as to leave a superficial sclerotic bridge.

Step 3. Insert a cataract knife to the posterior retinal-sac, exercising care so as not to injure the retina; raise the conjunctiva slightly permitting the retinal fluid to escape. Instill atropine; dress the eyes and permit the patient to remain in bed for several days.

Wounds of the Sclera

Wounds of the sclera are repaired by suture as shown in Fig. 412.

Anterior Sclerotomy

This operation is performed to relieve tension within the eye. A filtering scar is created in the anterior chamber of the eye which will permit the escape of aqueous humor.

Step 1. Use a narrow bladed von Graefe knife. With its edge directed upward, penetrate at a point 1 mm. outside the margin of the superior-external quadrant of the cornea entering the anterior chamber and emerging at a point directly opposite the point of entrance (Fig. 413).

Step 2. With a see-saw motion of the knife, the superior sclero-corneal bridge is incompletely divided leaving a thin lamella of the sclerotic at its middle.

Posterior Sclerotomy

In this operation the vitreous space is punctured through the sclera. Often, iridectomy is performed immediately following this operation which is rendered much easier due to the softer globe resulting from the escape of vitreous. The benefit derived from this operation is only temporary.

Sclerectomy and Sclerecto-Iridectomy

Sclerectomy is occasionally indicated where the tension is increased at intervals, caused by chronic glaucoma; sclerecto-iridectomy is used in instances of chronic glaucoma where the increased tension is constant. A partially closed incision is made with the object of creating a cystoid filtering cicatrix, thus diminishing tension. Sclerectomy consists of excision of part of the sclera; in sclerecto-iridectomy, sclerectomy is followed by an iridectomy.

Trephining of the Sclera

This is used in glaucoma and is accomplished by inserting a trephine on the limbus, creating an aperature in the sclero-corneal line for filtration purposes.

OPERATIONS ON THE IRIS

Injury to the Iris

The iris is rarely injured without injury to the crystalline lens. A hernia of the iris through the corneal wound usually results. If there is no inflammation, an attempt should be made to replace the iris; resection of the protruding iris is usually done.

Iridectomy

Local or general anesthesia may be used. The procedure consists of incising the anterior chamber of the eye, usually through the sclera but occasionally through the cornea (Fig. 414A); the iris is grasped with a forceps which is introduced through this opening, drawn out and severed (Fig. 414B, C, and D).

This operation is done for the purpose of forming an artificial pupil, for diminishing intra-ocular tension and as an accessory to the operation for cataract.

In adhesions of the iris an attempt may be made to destroy these with the help of a properly constructed instrument introduced through a small incision in the cornea. This, however, is usually unsuccessful.

Iridotomy

Insert a scissors through an incision in the cornea, one blade entering in front, the other behind the iris. The blades of the scissors are brought together dividing the inner peripheral side opposite the cornea.

Extraction of the Crystalline Lens for Cataract

An opacity of the crystalline lens is spoken of as cataract. Structurally, three kinds of cataract are recognized, (a) lenticular, (b) capsular and (c) capsulo-lenticular. They may be either primary or secondary. They are referred to according to their density as soft, hard and fluid. There may be either a complete or partial covering of the lens. The condition may be stationary or progressive.

In extracting the lens affected in cataract a linear incision is made with a keratome or a flap incision is made with a v. Graefe knife. In the case of simple extraction, the lens is removed without removing the iris; in other instances a portion of the iris is removed with the lens. The combined procedure is used more

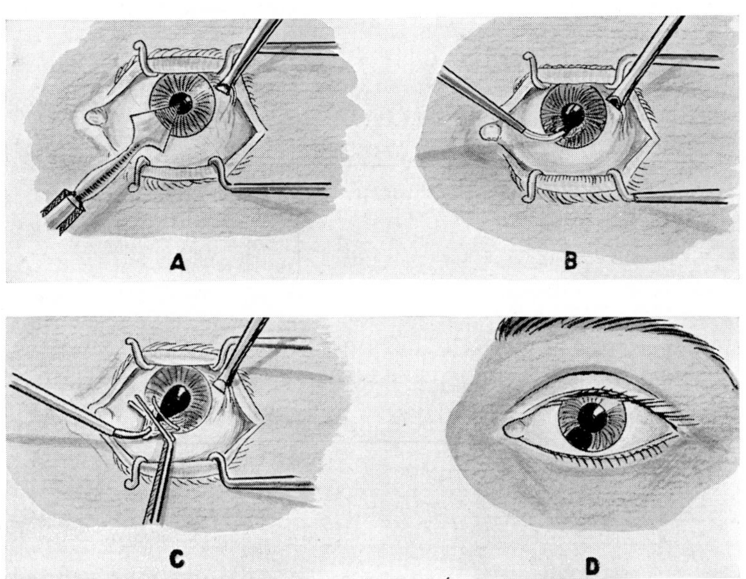

FIG. 414. Optical iridectomy: A. incision of the cornea, B. iris seized with iridectomy forceps along one of its radii, C. iris drawn out and divided with de Wecker scissors, D. iris reduced; appearance of the artificial pupil.

often; however, it is a matter of choice and judgment to be decided in individual cases.

ASPIRATION FOR SOFT CATARACT

Soft, non-nucleate cataracts of young subjects and recent traumatic cataracts may be evacuated by aspiration. Use a hypodermic syringe having a canula about 1 mm. in caliber. Plunge it into the crystalline lens, the needle taking an oblique direction.

Simple Extraction of the Lens for Cataract in its Capsule

EXTRACAPSULAR EXTRACTION FOR SENILE CATARACT

A preliminary iridectomy as described above may be done some weeks or months before the cataract is removed. Preliminary resection of the iris (iridectomy) simplifies the procedure.

Step 1. Cocaine analgesia. Introduce an eye speculum. Fix the eye with proper forceps. Grasp the conjunctiva below the transverse diameter of the cornea. Ask the patient to look downward. Introduce a v. Graefe knife at the junction of the cornea with the sclera. Pass it horizontally across the anterior chamber of the eye and allow it to emerge at an exact point opposite that it entered—

a flap is thus produced as shown in the illustration. (Fig. 415A.) At this juncture, aqueous humor escapes and often a herniation of the iris takes place.

Step 2. An adequate sharp pointed instrument is introduced, taking care while so doing that no injury is inflicted to the iris, and the capsule of the cataract is torn open. When this is effectually accomplished the lens projects into the anterior chamber. Remove the forceps which steady the eye (Fig. 415B).

Step 3. This step consists in extracting the lens. Have the patient look downward. Depress the upper lip of the incision with the curet (Fig. 415C) while pressure is being exerted with a blunt instrument from below upwards, thus the lens is dislodged. Should difficulties in dislodging the lens be encountered at this stage of the operative procedure do an iridectomy. When the lens has been removed, take away the retractor; have the patient close the eye.

Step 4. If there be remaining cortical fragments, express these gently into the anterior chamber of the eye by friction on the lower segment of the globe, whence they are brought out with appropriate forceps.

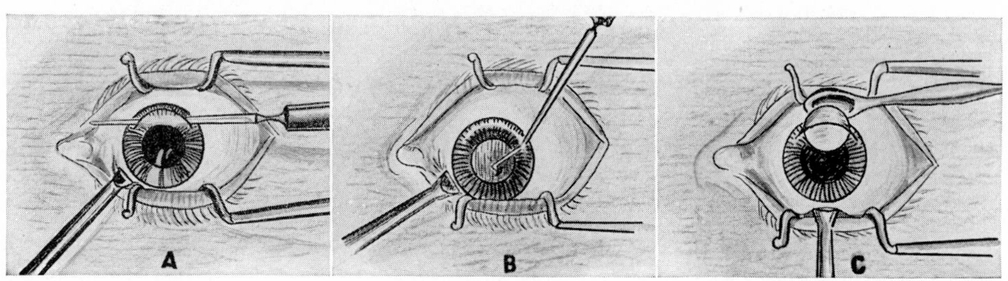

Fig. 415. Operation for cataract: A. Extraction by small superior flap. Incision of the cornea. B. Incision of the capsule with cystotome. C. Extraction of the crystalline lens. The upper lip of the incision is depressed with a blunt curet, while the forceps acts from below upwards for expulsion of the lens.

Step 5. Reduce the iris with a spatula. Doyen, at this stage of the operation, directed the patient to close the eyelid gently. A tampon of cotton is soaked in ice-cold boric acid solution and applied to the closed lid. This is to produce prompt contraction of the iris and to diminish the risk of "entanglement of the wound." Before applying the cold tampon, warn the patient to remain perfectly still to frustrate brusque movements of the eyelid.

Step 6. Instill 1:200 eserine salicylate into the conjunctival sac. See that the corneal flap is properly coapted. Delicate squares of fine absorbent cotton soaked in boric acid solution are applied over the closed eyelid; over this place an oil-silk dressing and over all a voluminous dressing. The opposite eye is also permitted to remain covered with a bandage applied prior to the operation.

Comment. Change the dressings in a dark room when called for—usually about the fourth day. Boric acid dressings are used the following day. The patient should remain in a darkened room until all conjunctival irritation has receded. He should wear smoked glasses and avoid winds and drafts. Proper glasses should be fitted after 6 or 8 weeks.

Operative Accidents

(a) Wounds of the iris, if small, need be of no concern.

(b) Luxation of the lens into the vitreous, demands immediate iridectomy and removal of the lens. If the quantity of escaped vitreous is one-third of its total, the condition is not considered irremediable.

(c) Locking of the iris should be remedied by resecting it at the first dressing.

Intracapsular Extractions

EXPRESSION OR SMITH-INDIAN METHOD

Corneal Incision. Iridectomy. Pressure on lower limbus with Smith expression hook dislocates the lens by breaking the zonular fibers. If the fibers of the

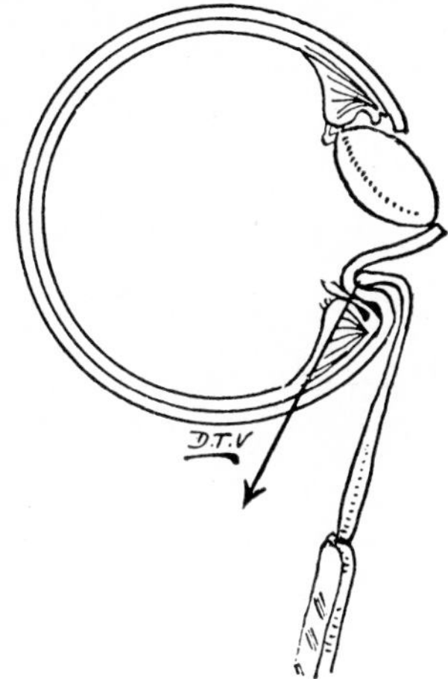

FIG. 416. Intracapsular extraction. Lower edge is presented first due to breaking of zonular fibers. (Vail.)

zonule break at the top of the lens near the incision the lens will be delivered in the upright position but if the zonular fibers below break first, the lens will turn over and the lower edge of the lens will present first (Fig. 416). The latter is the best method.

TRACTION METHOD

Forceps Operation. The lens capsule is grasped with a toothless forceps and by gentle traction the lens is extracted from the eye (Fig. 417A and B).

Vacuum Operation. A vacuum cup is placed over the anterior capsule of the lens; a vacuum is created by means of a vacuum pump (being connected to the cup by means of a rubber hose) and the cataract is extracted by a gentle pull of the cup, either lifting the lens out of the eye in the upright position or by tumbling.

Combined Traction and Expression Method. This method is employed to the best advantage. Either the capsule forceps or the vacuum cup is used for traction and a Smith hook or Nugent's utility forceps is used for expression (Fig. 418).

OPERATIONS ON THE OCULAR MUSCLES

These operations have for their object to increase, decrease or modify muscle-functions. If an increase is desired the muscle is shortened or advanced; if a decrease, it is set back either by tenotomy or recession. Lateral displacement of the muscle insertions is used to correct any defect regarding the direction of the muscle-pull.

Strabismus (squint) may be either convergent or divergent depending in which direction the eyeball turns—in or out; the former is usually the more common type, particularly in children. The underlying principles for the correction of strabismus rests on the (a) weakening of the rectus muscle by tenotomy; (b)

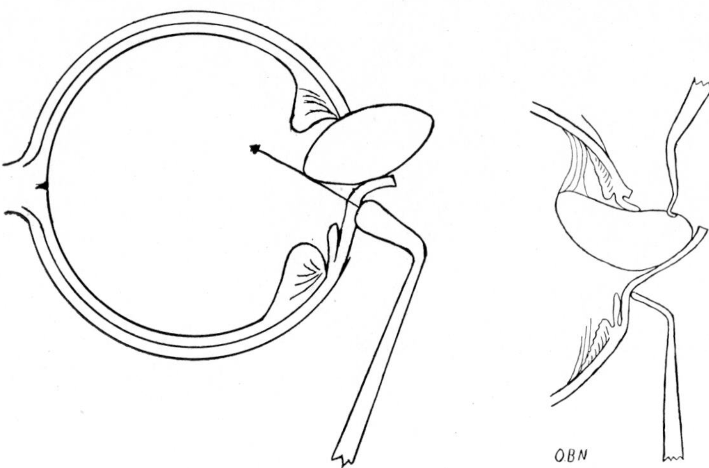

Fig. 417A Fig. 417B

Fig. 417. A. The lens capsule is grasped with a toothless forceps and gently extracted from the eye (after Nugent).
Fig. 417. B. Same as preceding.

by strengthening an opposing muscle by advancement of its insertion or resection of a portion of the muscle.

In advancement the tendon is divided and its insertion carried forward from its normal position toward the cornea. Numerous methods have been described—the aim of all advancement operations is to increase the power of a comparatively weak muscle.

Internal (Open Method)

TENOTOMY OF THE RECTUS MUSCLES (OPEN METHOD)

Step 1. Expose the muscle to be divided through an incision in the conjunctiva made with a strabismus scissors (Fig. 419).

Step 2. Expose the margin of the muscle by blunt dissection.

Step 3. With the aid of a strabismus hook draw out the muscle and sever it with a scissors between the hook and insertion of the muscle (Fig. 420A and B).

Irrigate the eye with boric-acid solution and examine it to determine the degree of correction accomplished. If under-corrected expose other muscle fibers with the strabismus hook and divide them. If over-corrected insert a suture into Tenon's capsule, the muscle and the episcleral tissues thus shortening the muscle slightly. When the desired correction is accomplished the wound is sutured and the eye dressed.

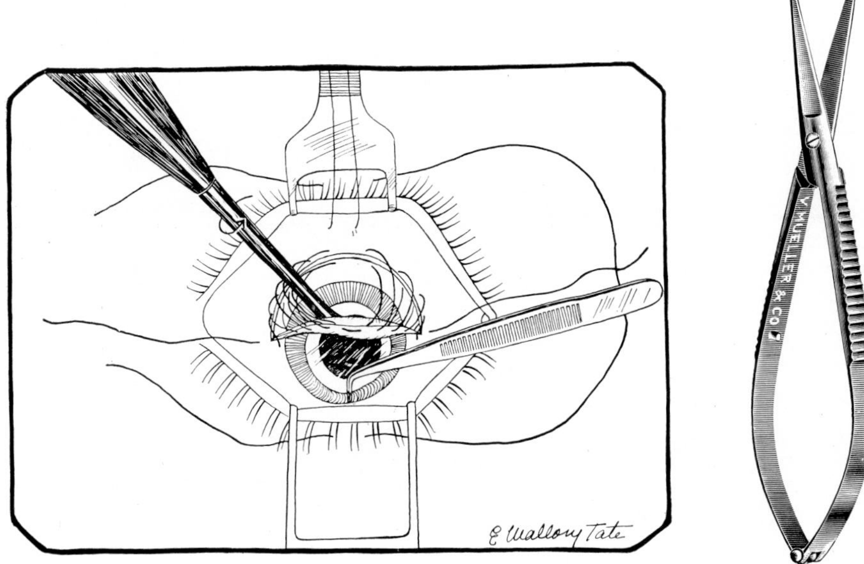

FIG. 418 FIG. 419

FIG. 418. The forceps being used as an expression instrument to aid in the delivery of the lens.
FIG. 419. Westcott's strabismus and general purpose scissors.

This operation is superior to subconjunctival tenotomy. Hemorrhage is checked by the adrenalin contained in the novocaine solution. Use a dull-pointed

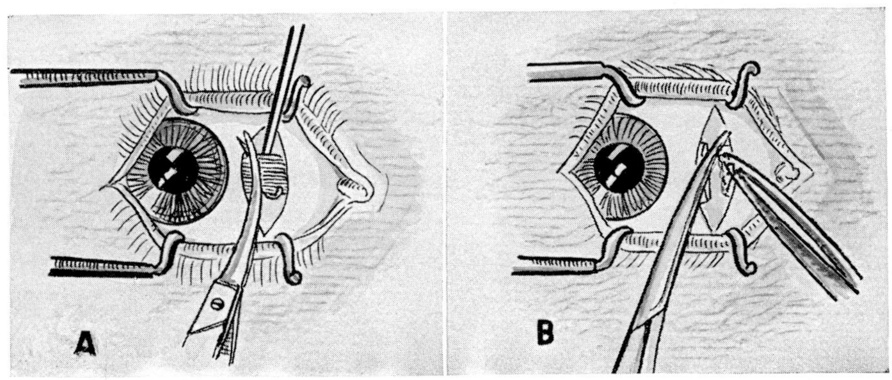

FIG. 420. A. Tenotomy of the tendon of the internal rectus muscle; the tendon of the internal rectus muscle is raised on a blunt hook. Division of the subconjunctival aponeurotic expansion of the tendon. B. Completion of operation.

scissors in dividing the tendon in order to avoid injury to the sclera. Suture the retracting end of the severed muscle to the sclera if it draws back too far. The eyeball may protrude from Tenon's capsule if incised too freely.

EXTERNAL RECTUS

Tenotomy of the external rectus is done in the same manner, only it is slightly less difficult; the same procedure may also be applied to the superior and inferior recti muscles, but in this instance the procedure is more difficult (Fig. 421 A, B and C).

Recession Operation with Control-Suture

NUGENT'S OPERATION

Nugent has devised an operation for use in almost every type of strabismus, in which a control suture is used giving the operator a chance to readjust the muscle on the second or third postoperative days. This provides a means of securing better results in a larger percentage of cases.

Cocaine or novocaine anesthesia (Figs. 422A and B).

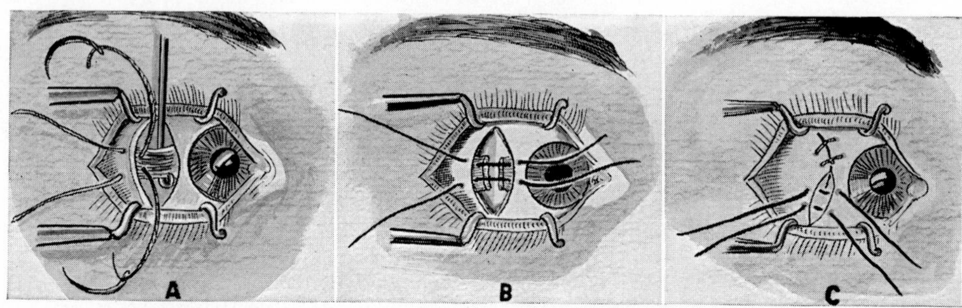

FIG. 421. Muscular advancement of the external rectus muscle: A. introduction of the two principal sutures into the conjunctiva and the peripheral end of the respective tendon; B. after the tendon has been divided the sutures are passed through the conjunctiva close to the corneal margin; C. the suturing is nearly completed.

Step 1. Make a vertical conjunctival incision 10 mm. long directly over the attachment of the strong muscle (Fig. 422C).

Step 2. Pick up the capsule of Tenon and incise it with scissors just above and below the attachment of the muscle.

Step 3. Pass a strabismus hook under the muscle (Fig. 422D).

Step 4. Secure the muscle in the clamp and cut off the tendon.

Step 5. While the muscle is still on the clamp, place a double armed silk suture through the muscle, capsule of Tenon and conjunctiva, 2 mm. apart near the center of the muscle from behind forward. Pass each needle back through, one at the upper edge and one at the lower edge of the muscle and attach by passing the needles through the cut tendon stump from behind forward including the conjunctiva (Fig. 422E); form a surgeon's knot.

Note. There should now be an overcorrection; if this does not produce it, there should be some form of advancement operation performed on the opposite muscle. The surgeon's knot is now tightened sufficiently to straighten the eye and the long ends of the suture are fastened on the forehead with a piece of surgeon's adhesive (Fig. 423). The conjunctiva is now sutured (Fig. 422E, F). The capsule of Tenon must be left free. The next day if there is an over- or undercorrection, the surgeon's knot can be tightened or loosened. No eye-patches are used but the patient must wear proper correcting lenses instead.

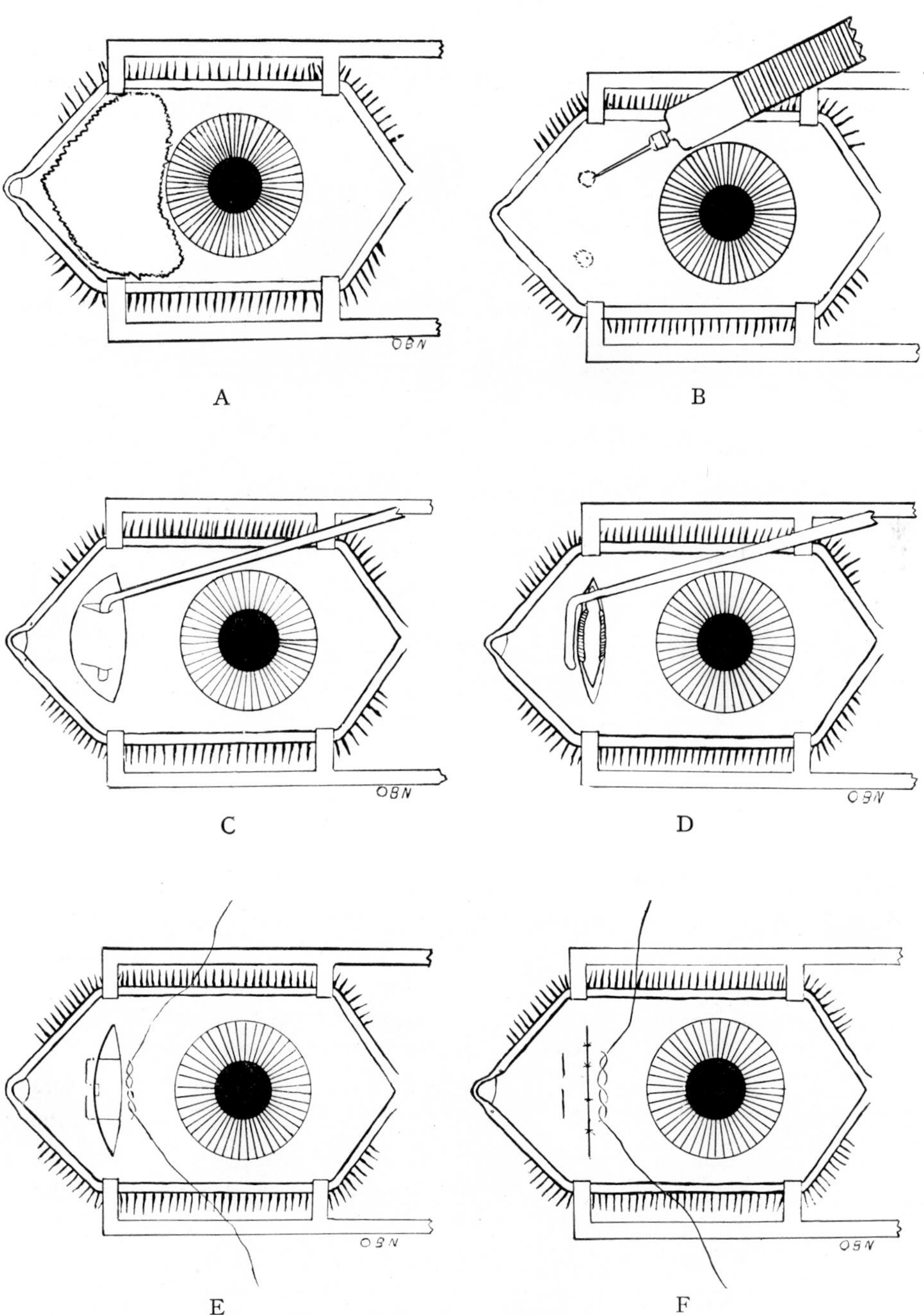

FIG. 422. Recession operation with control suture (after Nugent). A. and B. Injections of cocaine and novocaine are used for anesthesia. C. Strabismus hook is passed under muscle. D. Muscle is secured by clamp and tendon is cut off. E. Suturing of wound. F. Conjunctiva is sutured and capsule of Tenon left free.

Enucleation of the Eyeball

This operation consists of completely excising the eyeball from Tenon's capsule and is indicated in cases of malignancies, conditions threatening the sight of the opposite eye and incurable loss of vision accompanied by much pain and in irremediable damage the result of trauma.

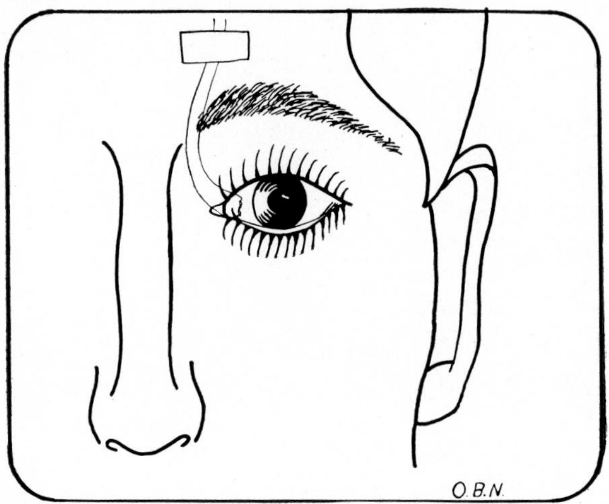

FIG. 423. Recession operation with control suture (after Nugent). Long ends of suture are fastened on the forehead with a piece of surgeon's adhesive.

Step 1. Irrigate the eye with boric acid solution. Instill 1:1000 adrenalin for hemostasis. General anesthesia. Introduce appropriate eye speculum. Where the anterior portion of the eyeball is badly lacerated, sew up the wound with silk or linen sutures. Leave the ends of these sutures long; they will act well as a tractor.

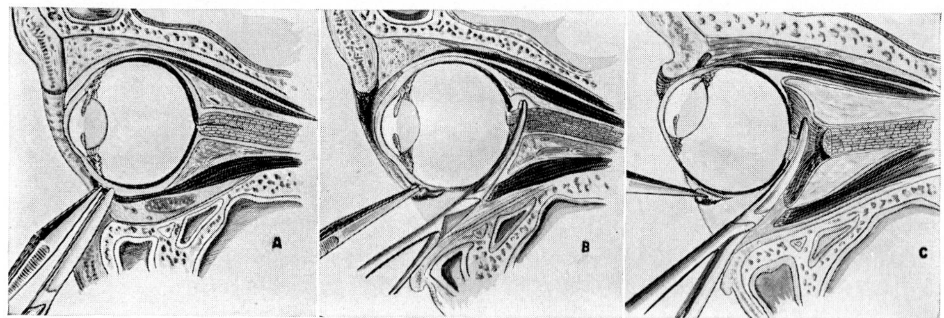

FIG. 424. Enucleation of the eyeball: A. first stage, section of the conjunctiva and of the tendon of the external rectus muscle; B. second stage, section of the optic nerve; C. third stage, luxation of the eyeball.

Step 2. If no traction-sutures are used, grasp the conjunctiva with mouse-tooth forceps, incise it near the cornea with a pair of small curved scissors and dissect it free from the cornea all the way around. Dissect all conjunctival and subconjunctival structures from the globe backward, and expose the insertion of the rectus tendons (Fig. 424A). Pick up the tendons with a strabismus hook and divide them.

Step 3. Force the globe of the eye forward by traction. Pass the blades of the dissecting scissors behind the globe; divide the optic nerve at its ocular extremity (Fig. 424B). This will permit the eye to come freely forward.

Step 4. Dissect and divide the tendons of the superior muscles as close to the sclerotic as possible. Divide the inferior muscles and conjunctiva below the cornea. Free all further attachments (Fig. 424C).

Step 5. Tampon and arrest all bleeding. Suturing of the conjunctiva is optional. Dress the wound daily until it is healed.

Modified Enucleation Operations. There are a number of variations of this procedure.

(a) Evisceration; this consists of dissecting the contents of the eyeball and leaving behind the sclera with its connecting muscles;

(b) Operations where, following enucleation, an artificial eye is placed in Tenon's capsule or into the sclera following evisceration.

The introduction of adipose tissue into the cavity after removing the eyeball has been used effectually; the abdomen or thigh usually furnishes the fat. No doubt some of the fat is absorbed, but enough adipose tissue remains for a good stump.

BARRAQUEZ-LAUBER METHOD

As each rectus muscle is severed during the process of enucleation, a mattress-suture of catgut is placed in each end with the loop within. A fat-transplant is placed in Tenon's capsule, spaced so as not to overfill it, the ends of the four recti muscles being brought together over it in the form of a cross. Tenon's capsule is joined over the muscles with catgut-sutures and the conjunctival borders are sutured with silk.

Evisceration of the Eyeball Followed by Insertion of an Artificial Globe Within the Scleral Sac (Mules' Operation)

After the eyeball is removed in the usual manner, a hollow globe is placed in the scleral sac and the sclera and conjunctiva are sutured over it. Later (about 10 to 14 days after operation), a cup-shaped artificial eye is placed between the conjunctiva and the eyelids. This must be carefully fitted into the cavity so as not to injure the conjunctiva causing granulation and scar tissue formation. The conjunctiva and lacrimal sac should be scrutinized if the artificial eye seems to cause pain. An infected lacrimal sac should be treated or removed; in cases of inflamed conjunctiva, do not remove the eye until the conjunctivitis is cured. Granulation tissue should be ablated with a scissors, followed by cauterization with a lunar caustic pencil. Excessive contraction of scar-tissue sometimes renders the retaining of an artificial eye impossible. This condition usually follows injury to the conjunctiva or an improperly performed enucleation. In cases of complete obliteration of the conjunctival culdesac a new one is formed with skin grafts. The restoration of eye sockets by this method is difficult and not always satisfactory especially if the levator palpebrae superioris is injured or a new upper culdesac has to be made.

CHAPTER 16

SURGERY OF THE NOSE

RHINOPLASTICS

LOCAL ANESTHESIA FOR NOSE OPERATIONS

Shrinking Solution

This is made up of 1 per cent of cocaine hydrochloride; to each ounce of this solution is added sixty drops of 1:1000 epinephrine solution. The solution is very potent and must be used with caution.

As a rule, the turbinate tissue will shrink down in a few minutes after a small amount has been sprayed into the nostril. This facilitates a thorough examination of the nasal chambers owing to the contraction of the tissues produced by the cocaine-epinephrine.

Block Anesthesia

The points of injection are indicated in Fig. 425.

Preparing the Nasal Chambers for Operation with Cocaine

Combine 2 drams of a 10 per cent solution of cocaine with 2 drams of 1:1000 epinephrine. Anesthesia should take place 5 or 10 minutes after this has been applied with cotton pledgets. Two pledgets about 3 inches long and a half inch wide are used for each side of the nose, one inserted as far up in the nose as possible and placed so that it covers much of the mucosa.

COCAINIZING THE PHARYNX

After instructing the patient not to swallow, spray a small amount of a 5 per cent cocaine solution into the pharynx, the excess of which is held in the mouth for a few minutes and then expectorated. This is repeated twice within 5 minutes.

COCAINIZATION OF THE LARYNX FOR DIRECT EXAMINATION

First cocainize the pharynx as above; with a laryngeal applicator paint the root of the tongue with a mixture of 20 per cent cocaine and adrenalin. The epiglottis is then covered with the cocaine on the applicator and the applicator passed into each pyriform sinus. This is done with the aid of a laryngeal mirror. Next, the solution is applied to the arytenoids, vocal cords and interior of the larynx by means of the applicator.

COCAINE ANESTHESIA FOR BRONCHOSCOPY AND ESOPHAGOSCOPY

Cocainizing the pharynx suffices in cases of esophagoscopy. The larynx is anesthetized as described above in cases of bronchoscopy. (Imperatori advises spraying a small amount of 10 per cent solution when the bronchoscope is inserted, just before its beak reaches the carina tracheae.) One cc. of 1 per cent cocaine is dropped between the vocal cords into the trachea.

Anesthesia is unnecessary for children under five years of age. General anesthesia may be employed for those between the ages of five and fifteen who are difficult to handle.

When frequent examinations of the bronchi and esophagus become necessary, patients frequently request that no anesthesia be given.

TAMPON OF NASAL CAVITIES FOR NASAL HEMORRHAGE

In attempting to check bleeding from the nose, simple measures should first be given preference. There are certain dangers connected with nasal tamponade,

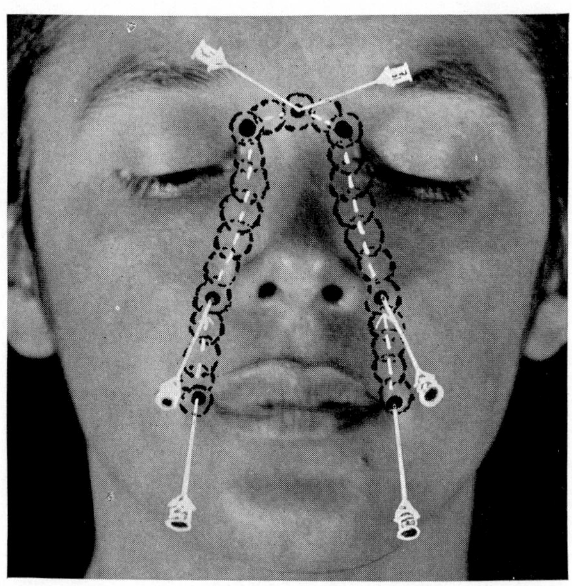

FIG. 425. Points of blocking and areas of injections of anesthetizing fluid in operations of the nose.

viz.: injury to the intranasal structures; sepsis introduced into the nasal cavities or accessory sinuses, and in some cases into the Eustachian tubes and middle ear.

Determine whether the hemorrhage issues from (a) a capillary or telangiectatic vessel or (b) whether a systemic condition is the causative factor.

Among the simple measures which may be mentioned are: a spray of adrenalin solution 1:1000 projected into the nostril or applied to the bleeding point with a cotton-covered applicator; a piece of ice pressed against either ala of the nose and another piece pressed against the neck. (Hot saline solutions may sometimes check the bleeding.) When the bleeding-point is located, exert direct pressure against it.

When all simple measures fail, tamponade of the nasal cavities is resorted to.

(a) **Tamponing the Anterior Nares.** Pack the nostril with strips of sterile or medicated gauze (adrenalin, tincture of benzoin compound, etc.) through a nasal speculum. The tampon should be introduced back of the bleeding point; otherwise the oozing will continue into the nasopharynx.

Bernay's compressed cotton sponges are often useful. They are introduced into the nostril and fed sterile saline solution through a medicine dropper until the sponge swells sufficiently to compress the nasal walls and fill the nostril, thus causing the arrest of the bleeding.

Packing the Posterior Nares by Postnasal Tampon

This procedure is done without anesthesia as local application is valueless in the presence of extensive bleeding. Insert a small soft rubber catheter into the nostril. This will be seen in the pharynx, coming down behind the palate. Grasp the end with a hemostat and bring it through the mouth. This is repeated on the other side. A postnasal tampon consists of a roll of gauze or cotton of a size that will fit into the postnasal space. Attached to the center are three linen strings about nine inches long. Two of these are attached to the projecting catheters. (Fig. 426A.) The nasal ends of the catheters are pulled forward, drawing the postnasal tampon into the nasopharynx; the finger is used to wedge the pack firmly into the nasopharyngeal space. The third string is brought out of the mouth and attached loosely to the cheek with adhesive. The purpose of this string is to facilitate the removal of the tampon.

The anterior nares is then packed with small strips of vaseline gauze, which are placed firmly against the postnasal tampon. (Fig. 426B.) While the anterior packing is being done the strings holding the postnasal tampon should be held taut by an assistant. When the anterior nares is packed sufficiently to control the bleeding, the strings should be tied together, with a small strip of gauze to protect the columella.

The tampon should not be left in place longer than 48 hours, as there is a grave danger of causing an acute otitis media or an acute purulent sinusitis. If bleeding occurs upon removing the tampon a fresh one should be inserted.

Historical Notes. Repair of the nose by plastic measures is an ancient procedure. Ancient India and Italy contributed much to its progress. As early as 1492 Benedictus contributed his experience with plastic procedures. Tagliacozzi, in 1597, paved the way to further endeavors which while dormant for some centuries was resumed enthusiastically toward the end of the eighteenth century. Dieffenbach of the moderns did much pioneer work in this field. He was first to attempt to substitute, by plastic means, an entire nose. He used only the skin from the forehead or arm to accomplish that end. Contraction of the tissues marred the final result. Two important factors were lacking in Dieffenbach's procedure: First, a lining for the interior of the nose, and second a support for the tegumentary appendage. Efforts to accomplish the first were made by Dieffenbach, Dilpech, von Langenbeck and Lapat. Supports made of metals (gold, platinum and lead) were not satisfactory. Leisnick was successful in 1877 in implanting a support made of light amber in a case of saddlenose. The credit of attempting to create flaps of skin and periosteum belongs to von Langenbeck. These were not successful. It was Ollier who, in 1861 supported the skin, periosteal-flap with bone. Following Ollier's advice von Langenbeck elaborated the method. König, in 1886, made much progress with his operation by using skin, periosteum and bone-flap taken from the forehead. A host of observers followed with contributions as the decades rolled on; among these the following form a partial list: Rosenstein, Carpeie, Bozer, Dubois, Leis, v. Graefe, Balfour, Warren, Roux, Blandin, Serre, Jobert, Joseph, Post, Pancoast, Buck, Roberts, Prince Israel, Nélaton, Keegan, Roe, Kolle, Reverdin, Smith, Krause, Thiersch, Gersury, Lexer, Carl Beck of New York and many others.

TOTAL RHINOPLASTY

may be divided into the following five surgical groups:

1. The Indian Method (Flap from the Forehead).
2. The French Method (Flap from the Cheek).
3. The Italian (Tagliacotian) Method (Flap from the Arm).

4. The Finger Method.
5. The German Method (Flap from the Chest).

The Indian Method

KEEGAN'S OPERATION

This procedure is advocated in cases where the nasal cartilages, alae, septum and columnae cannot be saved but in which the bones of the nose and the skin covering them are in sound condition.

Step 1. With a pencil outline a flap on the forehead, the size and shape of which corresponds with the area of tissue to be replaced. In order to avoid including any of the scalp, the flap must be taken diagonally across the forehead, not vertically. The pedicle is attached to the internal angle of the orbit and great care should be exercised that the angular artery, which nourishes the flap, is not injured. (Fig. 427A.)

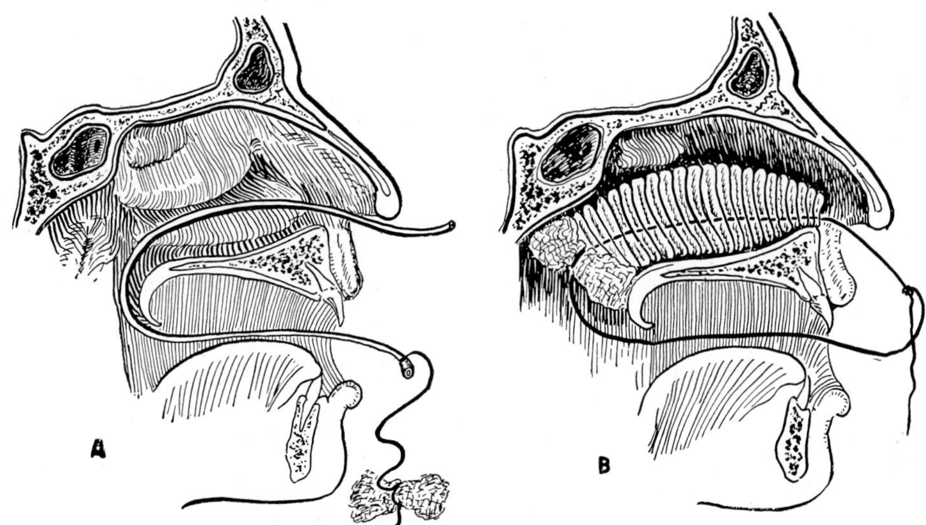

FIG. 426. A. Plugging of nasal fossae for epistaxis. Tampon attached to end of catheter. B. Posterior and anterior tampons in place.

Step 2. Freshen the edges of the defect and prepare the lining of the nose. Make two convergent incisions at a point a little outside the roots of the alae of the nose, extending upward to two points about ¾ in. apart. A horizontal incision is now made slightly above the border of the defect, from the center of which incision another perpendicular incision is made, reaching downward to where the nasal bones are joined by the cartilages. Thus two quadrangular flaps are formed; these are placed in such a position that the nasal cavity is lined by their skin surfaces; the remaining edges of the defect are now freshened. (Fig. 427B.)

It will now be seen that the triangular pieces overlap when the flaps are folded down. Keegan recommends that these pieces be removed and transplanted into the wound on the forehead. Smith does not cut away these two pieces but splits the old septum, suturing the edges of the triangular pieces into the wound, in this manner making a septum and columna.

Step 3. The outline-incision of the flap is now deepened by cutting down to but not through the periosteum. The flap is detached from the forehead and twisted down over the nose with as little manipulation as possible. The fact that the hinge has been made oblique, being higher on one side than the other, makes the twisting much easier.

Step 4. The two raw surfaces now lie apposed. Suture together the inferior margins of the quadrangular nasal flaps and the forehead flap. The part of the flap fashioned for the purpose is fitted into the former site of the old columna which was previously prepared when the edges of the defect were freshened. The two converging incisions made first are now deepened

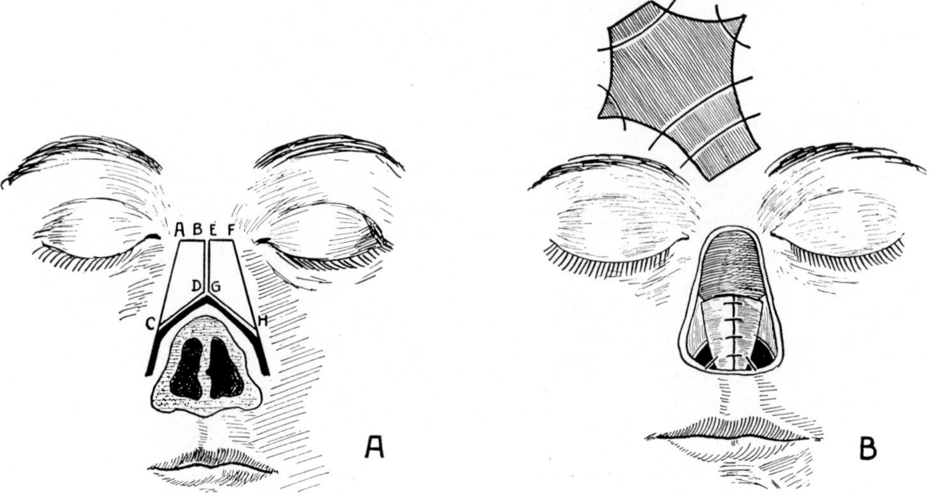

FIG. 427. A. Keegan's operation (Indian method) of rhinoplasty. Formation of nasal flap, B. Nasal cavity lined.

and are beveled for the purpose of suturing them to the lateral margins of the flaps.

Step 5. Approximate the sides of the wound on the forehead.

Step 6. Drainage tubes are inserted into each newly formed nostril and boric acid-ointment dressings applied over the lateral margins of nose and cheek.

Step 7. About two weeks after the first operation the pedicle is divided. A wedge-shaped segment of tissue taken from the forehead is implanted into the frontal defect.

Although this method has been modified and improved upon, it is generally agreed that a flat nose results where there are no nasal bones to support the transplanted substance. For this reason, pieces of bone and cartilage are transplanted with the flap.

NÉLATON'S OPERATION

Stage 1

Step 1. Expose the entire length of the costal cartilage of the eighth rib.

Step 2. Excise the rib and trim it down to 2.5 cm. long by 3 mm. wide.

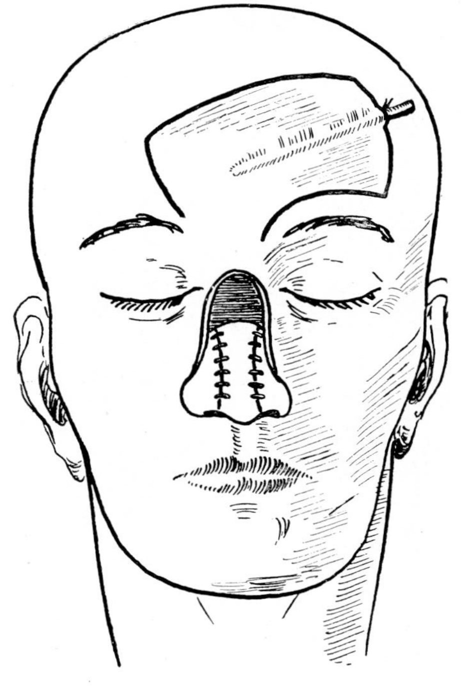

Fig. 428

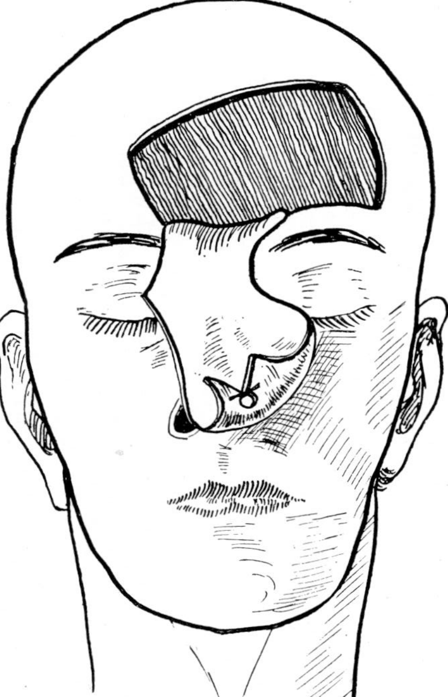

Fig. 429

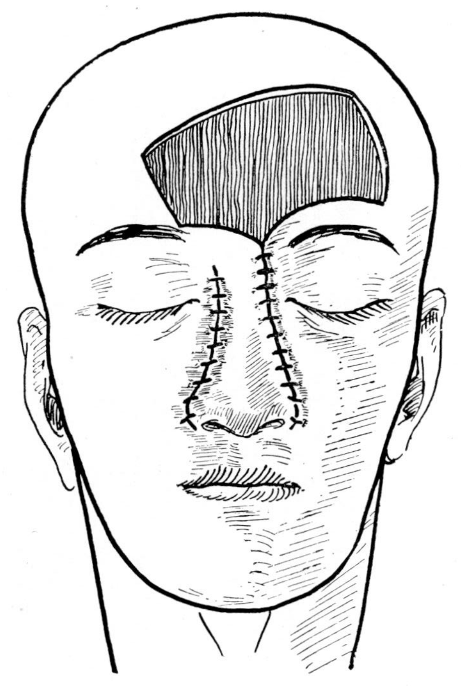

Fig. 430

Fig. 428. Nélaton's rhinoplasty operation for total loss of the nose. Stage 1.
Fig. 429. Nélaton's rhinoplasty operation for total loss of the nose. Stage 2.
Fig. 430. Nélaton's rhinoplasty operation for total loss of the nose. Stage 3.

Step 3. Cut a notch where the point of the nose is to be formed by this cartilage, that is, about 0.5 cm. from the end nearest to the base of the forehead pedicle.

Step 4. Outline a flap on the forehead.

Step 5. Incise the base of this flap down to the bone for about 0.5 cm. and make a tunnel to fit the strip of cartilage.

Step 6. Introduce the strip of cartilage with its notch toward the skin incision so that it rests between the frontal bone and its periosteum. (Fig. 428.)

Step 7. Close the skin-periosteal incision.

Stage 2

Step 8. Two months later make an incision about the nasal defects in such a manner that two lateral and one upper central flap will result.

Step 9. Turn these over so that the skin surfaces will look into the cavity of the nose.

Step 10. Stitch these in place with catgut so as to retain them in position.

Step 11. Cut the flap on the forehead with its pedicle toward the opposite inner corner of the eye over which the flap is situated (as shown in Fig. 429). It will be remembered that the flap contains the cartilage of the rib previously introduced. The periosteum also is part of this flap.

Step 12. The flap is now turned downward over the previously turned flaps fashioned from the margins of the defects. Fashion the flap into a sort of a tip of a nose by bending the cartillage where the notch had been cut in it, thus resulting in a columella.

Step 13. Suture the parts into place.

Step 14. Close the defect in the forehead either by skin grafts or sliding flaps. Joseph Beck states that the defect in the forehead can be covered much better by sliding the skin and making counter release incisions in the hairy portion of the scalp.

Stage 3

Step 15. One week later cut the pedicle, trim it and implant it into the defect at the root of the nose (Fig. 430).

Step 16. Further cosmetic readjustments are done subsequently.

SEDILLOT'S OPERATION

Step 1. A tongue-shaped flap is formed from the upper lip, not including the mucous membrane which has its pedicle at the nasal floor.

Step 2. A forehead-flap is made with especial attention being given to forming a longer median flap for making the columella.

Step 3. The edges of the nasal defect are freshened.

Step 4. The frontal flap is brought down and sutured laterally. In forming the columella the central flap is sutured to the little flap from the lip so that there is a cutaneous surface on the outside as well as in the nose, one over the other.

The French Method

The outstanding characteristic of this method is that the flaps used in forming a new nose are taken from the cheeks. Because the newly formed nose is flattened to almost the level of the face by the resulting contraction of the cicatricial tissue, this method is not advocated.

SYME'S OPERATION

Step 1. Form a flap from each cheek with its pedicle at the root of the nose (Fig. 431A).

Step 2. The inner edges of the flaps are united down the center line and the outer edges are brought together with the freshened edges of the defect with sutures (Fig. 431B).

Step 3. Close the wounds in the cheek by means of skin grafts or sutures. Insert a tube into each nostril.

The Italian Method

The restoration of a nose by means of a flap of skin taken from the arm is an operation of Italian origin, Gaspard Tagliacozzi (or -cotti) being the first

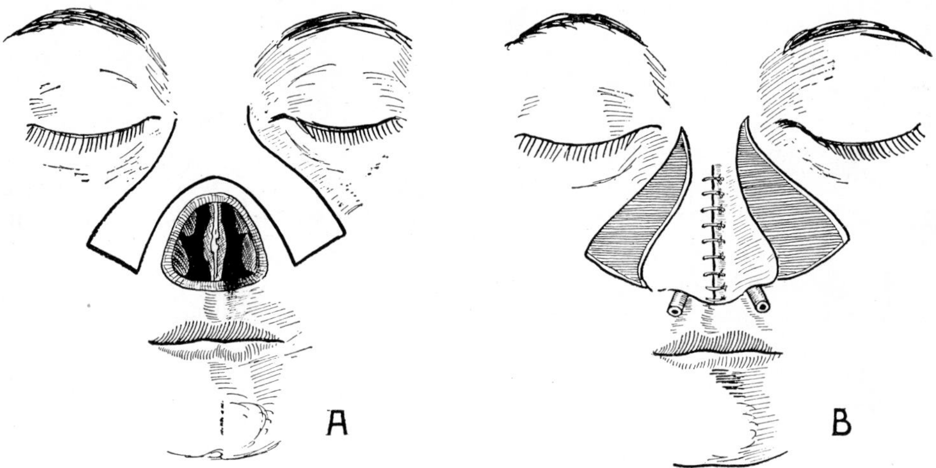

FIG. 431. A. Syme's rhinoplasty operation (French method), stage 1. B. Syme's rhinoplasty operation (French method), stage 2.

to use it in 1597. Fabricius used the method later. The special feature of this operation is that the pedicle, which is left when the flap of skin is raised from the upper arm, is not divided until after the free portion of the flap has united with the nose. This method is now only used when there is no available tissue on the face; or when the operator wishes to avoid further scarring of the face. The method is also shunned because of the inconvenience the patient experiences by reason of his constrained position in a plaster cast.

MacCormac describes the operation as follows:

Step 1. Provide a means whereby, with the minimum of inconvenience, the patient's arm may be kept in the needful position for the requisite period. This takes from 1 to 3 weeks.

Step 2. Make a gutta-percha model for the nose and from this pattern the flap to be taken from the arm; this should include skin and subcutaneous fat and be twice the size required, thus allowing for shrinkage. At the same time arrange for a piece of tissue to be used for the septum, using the anterior surface of the left upper arm near the elbow (Fig. 432A).

Step 3. After the flap, together with the piece for the septum, has been designated on the arm, it is lifted from the underlying tissues throughout its whole length remaining attached only by the two ends. Sterile rubber tissue strips are placed under this bridge and the surfaces allowed to granulate, careful attention being given to asepsis meanwhile. Thus the tissues of the flap thicken and circulation is reëstablished before the flap is attached to the face.

Step 4. Detach the upper end of the flap from the arm, make a slightly curved incision parallel to the border of the defect on the right side and suture the edge of the flap into this incision. Apply an adhesive retention dressing as shown in Fig. 432B. Remove the sutures after about ten days and apply a complete immobilization plaster cast (Fig. 432C). Protect the eyes while

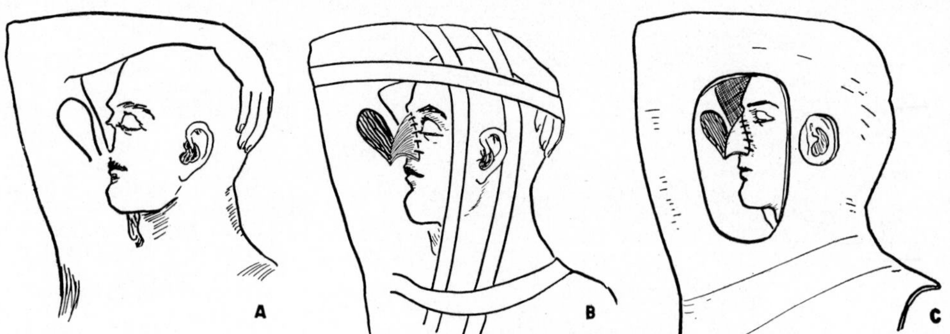

FIG. 432. Italian (Tagliacozzi) method of rhinoplasty: A. Formation of flap from arm, B. Suturing flap into place. C. Plaster of Paris encasement.

putting on the cast, then cut out windows to expose the eyes, ears and mouth. Allow the cast to remain until the parts are healed.

Step 5. After 3 weeks the flap is cut from the arm, and the septum and the other side of the flap are sutured into the freshened edges of the nose.

Step 6. It may be necessary to supplement this with additional minor procedures to perfect the aesthetic requirements of the case.

ISRAEL'S OPERATION

In this procedure, the flap is derived from the forearm instead of the arm. The arm and forearm are placed in a position to conduce to greater comfort of the patient. The arm is immobilized as in the Tagliacozzi method. The steps of the operation are as follows:

Stage I

Step 1. Make a symmetrical incision on both sides of the ulnar edge of the left forearm, resulting in a trapezoid skin flap (Fig. 433A), the lesser portion of the trapezoid (pointing toward the wrist), being about 5 cm. from the styloid process.

Step 2. With a chisel, outline a bone-flap from the ulna connected with the partially dissected skin; this should be about 6 cm. long and ¾ cm. wide.

Step 3. With a fine saw partially disengage the section of bone from the ulna, taking care that it remains integral with the skin flap and attached to the upper end of the ulna. Interpose iodoform or paraffined gauze to prevent reunion.

Stage 2

Step 4. A few days later break the bridge of bone at the point where it is proposed to make the tip of the nose. Dress. Wait another four or five days to allow greater thickening to take place.

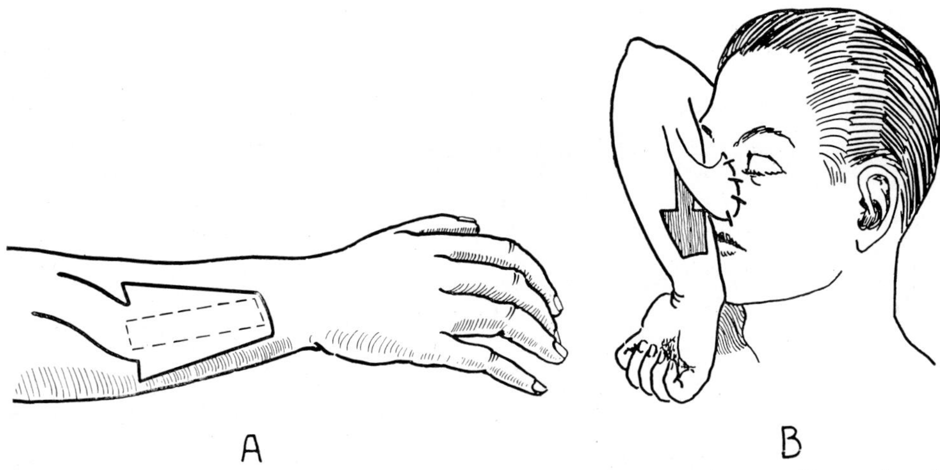

FIG. 433. Israel's operation for loss of nose: A. flap fashioned from forearm, B. suturing of flap into position.

Step 5. After freshening the edges of the nasal defect, transplant the flap of the forearm into it and fix in place with interrupted sutures. Immobilize in a plaster of Paris jacket (Fig. 433B).

Stage 3

Step 6. Two weeks later sever the pedicle consisting of bone and skin and shape the tissues to form a nose. The bone should be united with the spine of the nose at the floor of the nose. The skin is sutured about the sides of the nose.

Step 7. The nostrils and columella are fashioned from the remaining skin flaps.

Finger Method

WOLKOWITSCH'S OPERATION

Stage 1

Step 1. Incise the dorsal surface of the fourth finger of the left hand mesially through the skin and underlying tissue. The incision should extend from the metacarpophalangeal joint to the nail, both sides being dissected freely (Fig. 434A and B).

Step 2. Remove the fingernail, care being taken that the entire matrix is removed with it. Do not disturb the tendon.

Step 3. The skin is removed from the end of the finger in front to be used later at the root of the nose.

Step 4. Make a median incision at the root of the nose through the skin and subcutaneous tissue to the bone. Separate freely the remaining borders of the apertura pyriformis and the tissues on either side of the incision.

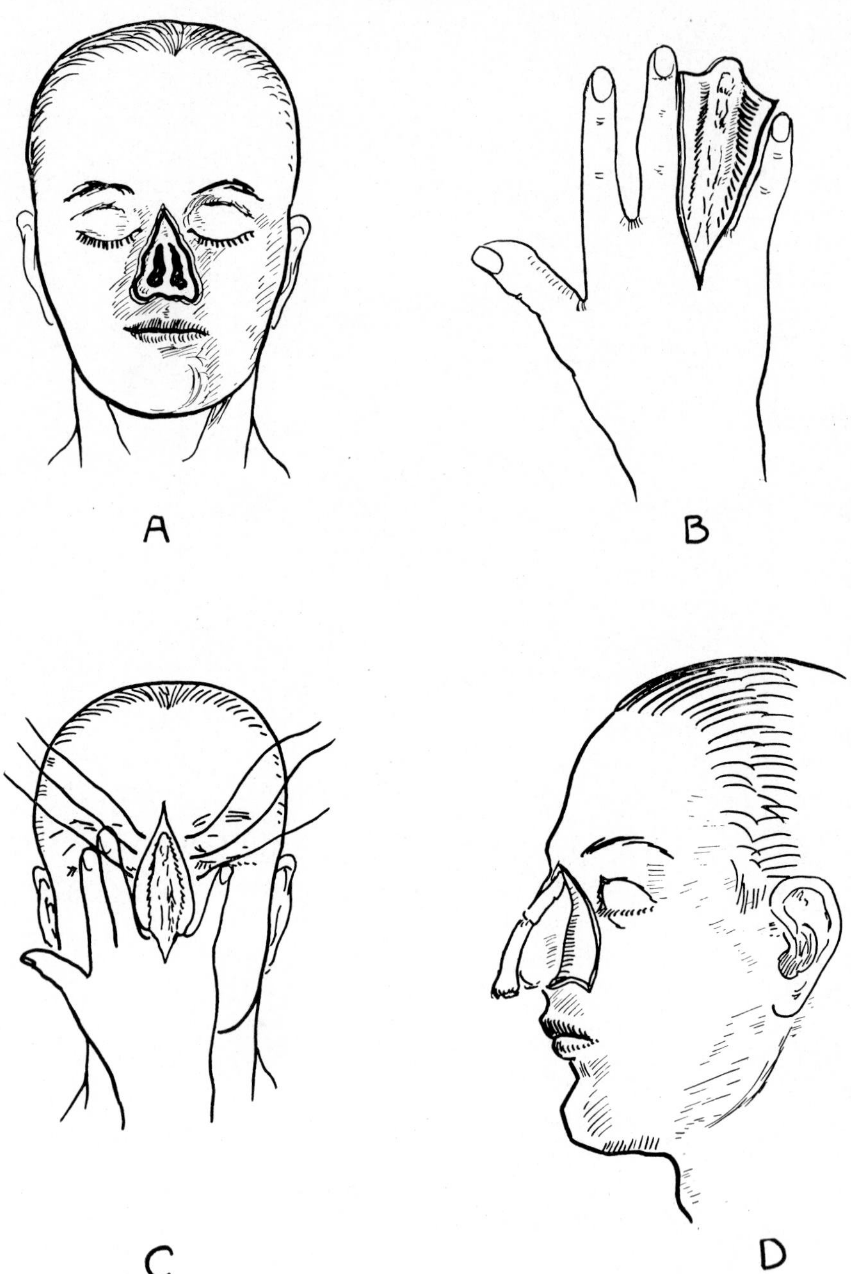

FIG. 434. Wolkowitsch's operation for total loss of the nose.

Step 5. To avoid a noticeable hump at the root of the nose, a dent is made in the bony structures with a gouge into which the tip of the finger may be inserted.

Step 6. The finger is brought to the area of the nose made ready for it; its skin flaps are inserted below the dissected lateral flaps close to the apertura pyriformis, the tip of the finger being fitted into the hollow space at the root (Fig. 434C).

Step 7. The finger is sutured at the root while its skin flaps, which are inserted beneath the skin of the nose defect, are joined by two mattress sutures on either side.

Step 8. The median incision at the root of the nose is brought together as far down as possible over the finger and a fairly large amount of marly (Scotch-gauze) is inserted below the finger, to sustain it in the shape of a nose, and a dressing placed over the surface. A fixation bandage is applied in accordance with the usual Italian operation.

Stage 2

Step 9. Nine days later remove the sutures and extend the incision over the back of the hand exposing for excision the entire metacarpophalangeal joint.

Step 10. Divide the skin laterally and incise it on both sides but not in front.

Stage 3

Step 11. During the next five days separate the skin pedicle and disarticulate the metacarpophalangeal joint, at two different sittings.

Step 12. Cover the defect in the hand anteriorly with the remaining skin as in the usual disarticulation procedure.

Step 13. Shape the attached finger into the form of a nose. Insert a new supply of Scotch-gauze under it and allow it to remain for three more days so as to become more firmly joined to the surrounding tissue.

Step 14. Bend the finger between the first and second phalangeal joints in such a manner that the first phalanx may be inserted into the nasal cavity.

Step 15. Prepare the floor of the nose and if perchance a piece of septum is left, remove all mucous membrane so that its bony surface is exposed.

Step 16. After the skin and granulations have been removed from the disarticulated end of the finger, it is placed in the floor of the nose against the raw surfaces provided for it (Fig. 434D).

Step 17. Dissect the lateral borders of the apertura pyriformis downward to the point of formation of the alae and tuck under the remnants of the skin flap of the finger and once more fasten these on either side with one mattress suture.

Step 18. A Krause or any other flap is taken from either the forehead or arm and placed over the denuded surface of this bony reconstruction. Minor readjustments such as forming the nostrils and covering the columella are done later.

SUBTOTAL RHINOPLASTY

Nélaton's Operation for Subtotal Loss of the Nose

Ch. Nélaton devised a most ingenious operation for complete rhinoplasty which is applicable to all cases where a nasal stump remains having a protuberance of at least 7 to 8 mm.

Step 1. The surgeon takes his position on the left side of the patient and starts the incision at a point on the right cheek which is located a finger's width from the nasal fossa on a line extending from the anterior nasal spine to the lobe of the ear. Following the nasogenial furrow, the incision is brought upward, passing 6 mm. inward of the lacrimal caruncle to the eyebrow which is divided vertically at its inner end. The incision is continued directly up-

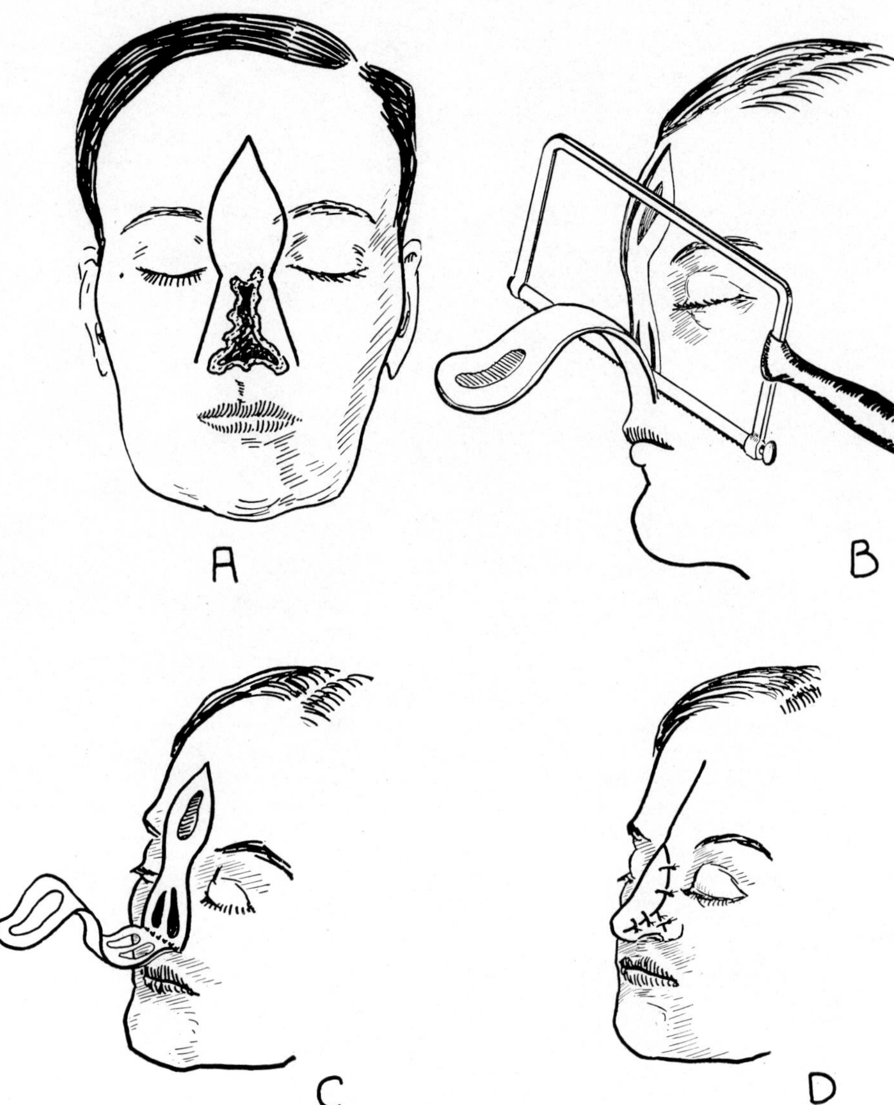

Fig. 435. Nélaton's operation for subtotal loss of nose.

ward for a short distance after passing the eybrow and is then slanted inward to the edge of the hairy scalp in the middle line. This is repeated on the left side from below upward ending near the edge of the scalp at the same point. Thus a horseshoe-shaped flap has been cut entirely around the defect caused by the destruction of the nose (Fig. 435A).

Step 2. The frontal flap is separated from the bone at its upper extremity and edges, leaving only a long middle strip of the bone attached to the flap from the upper end to the level of the frontal sinus. A side of the flap that has been detached is turned back by an assistant permitting the surgeon to trace a groove upward with a chisel through the external layer of the bone, extending from the frontal sinus to a point near the end of the flap. The same course of action is followed on the opposite side and an attempt made, with a fine flat chisel, to dissect the thin external layer of the bone from above downward. This strip is attached to the flap for a breadth of about 3 cm. and is entirely detached from the bone near the frontal sinus. The bony structure at the root of the nasal bones is exposed for about 6 or 8 mm., according to the size of the stump, by the dissection which is continued downward from the region of the frontal sinus.

Step 3. The ascending process of the superior maxilla is dissected by means of a saw passing from above downward being directed in a line starting 1 cm. in front of the anterior nasal spine and extending toward the second molar and ending 6 to 7 mm. in front of and below the infraorbital foramen. If the course of the saw has been clearly revealed and the soft parts freely incised, the bones can be divided easily (Fig. 435B).

Step 4. A gouge introduced on either side after the saw is withdrawn, is used to fracture the root of the ascending process. Great care must be exercised here. The surgeon completes the fracture, in lowering the flap and nasal structures, in such a manner that the ascending process is left loosely attached to the body of the maxilla connected slightly by some bony fibers (Fig. 435C and D).

Step 5. The soft tissues are then properly sutured into place.

SIMPLE RHINOPLASTY

Israel's Operation for Saddleback Nose

Step 1. Make an incision 2 cm. long on the outside of the saddle; separate the sides subcutaneously so that when the tip of the nose is pulled upon, a normal appearance is obtained.

Step 2. Chisel off from the anterior border of the tibia, a piece of bone 3 cm. in length; make sharp points at each end.

Step 3. By means of dissection, the originally separated tunnel is located from the inside of the nose; the fragment of bone is inserted so that the upper end comes in contact with the nasal bone and the soft tissues over it are closed.

Hump Nose

KOLLE'S OPERATION

Step 1. Make a longitudinal incision over the most conspicuous portion of the hump dissecting the skin and the periosteum to either side until full exposure is obtained (Fig. 436A).

Step 2. The hump is removed with a chisel, being careful not to tear away the mucous membrane or enter the interior of the nose. If, by accident, a tear is made, it should be sutured at once (Fig. 436B).

Step 3. If, in taking away the hump, a broad bone defect results, a sharper ridge may be obtained by pressing the margins together with a heavy forceps.

Step 4. Closure is effected by means of Halsted's subcuticular periosteal suture. The operation may also be done by the intranasal route (Ballinger).

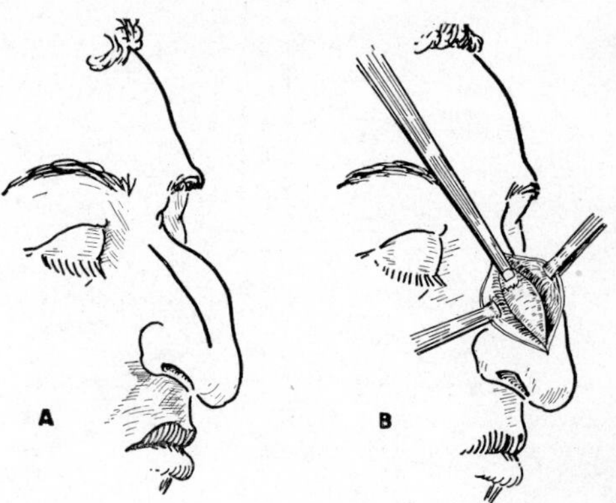

FIG. 436. Kolle's operation for "hump nose": A. skin incision, B. chiseling off "hump."

INTRANASAL OPERATION (AUFRICHT TECHNIC)

Step 1. Make an incision on the inner surface of the lateral side of the nasal vestibule. Direct the blade of the cutting instrument upward and outward until it emerges immediately under the skin and perichondrium of the nose.

The columellar incision (either through the center or across the columella) leaves an almost invisible scar, not casually visible at all since it is along

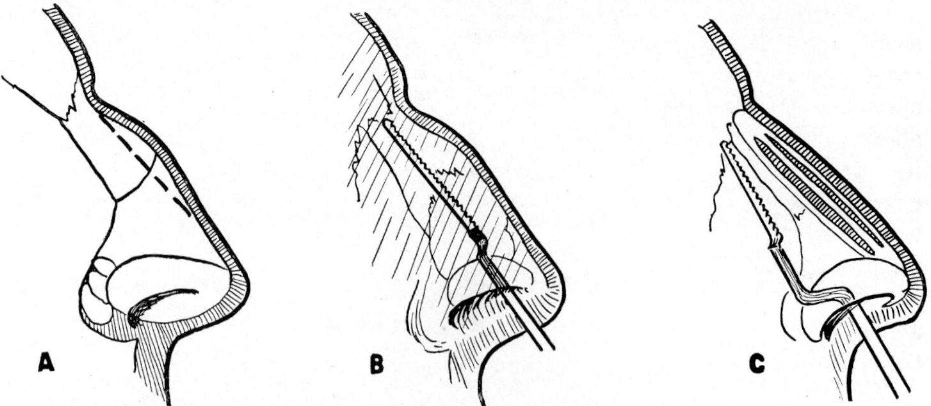

FIG. 437. Submucous resection: A location of the saw cut for removing the "hump," B. the saw in position for removing the "hump," C. sawing through the nasomaxillary junction, the "hump" already having been removed leaving the nasal chambers temporarily open anteriorly.

the base or line of the columella, and is easier for the inexperienced operator than the intranasal approach. It is closed with horse-hair sutures (Fig. 437A).

Step 2. Dissect away the skin and subcutaneous tissues from the bone and cartilage of the nose by means of a blunt-pointed side-cutting knife introduced into the incision and directed over the bridge of the nose to the opposite side and ending on the tip of the nose.

Step 3. Insert a right-angled saw into the wound until the teeth of the instrument lie over the hump (Fig. 437B).

Step 4. Guided by the finger of the left hand, the hump is detached and withdrawn by means of forceps introduced through the original wound (Fig. 437C).

Step 5. Saw entirely through the lateral nasomaxillary connection of each bone of the nose.

Step 6. Bring the bones of the nose toward the midline to the width desired.

Step 7. Form a splint by molding dental compound material over the nose, holding it in place with adhesive tape.

Pirogoff's Operation to Lengthen the Nose

In this operation a short nose is made longer by means of an inverted V-shaped incision, the point of which should appear in the midline about the level of the canthi and the limbs between the cheek and nose above the alae (Fig. 438A). When the adhesions are loosened and the flap is lifted up, the lips of the wound are brought together in the form of an inverted Y (Fig. 438B). This procedure is not recommended when the nose is too wide. Satisfactory results depend upon a normal condition of the tissues.

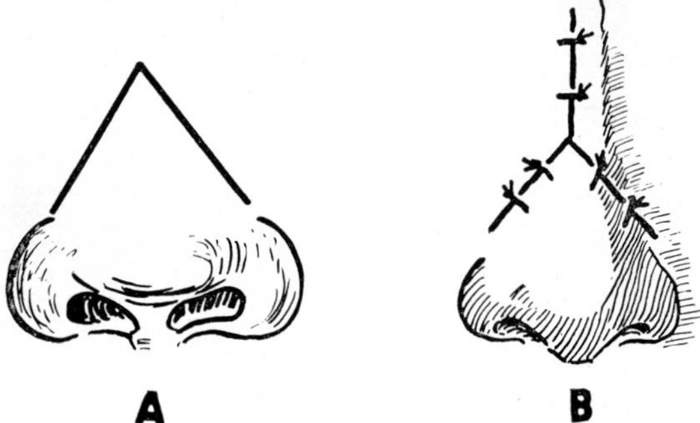

FIG. 438. Pirogoff's operation to lengthen nose: A. outlining incisions, B. after mobilizing the flaps the freshened edges are united as shown here.

Szymanowski's Operation to Narrow the Nose

A piece of tissue in the shape of a wide triangle is removed from the upper lip, its apex at the midline, slightly above the vermilion border and its base reaching the inner edges of the alae from one side to the other. After the alae are loosened, the incision is brought together in the midline by means of a traction suture through the base of the nose.

If a triangular-shaped piece of tissue is removed from under each nostril and a strip of skin left between, the same results may be obtained with less injury to the upper lip.

Rhinophyma (Acne Hypertrophica)

General anesthesia.

Step 1. To prevent the influx of blood, introduce gauze strips through the anterior nares, plugging the posterior two-thirds of the nose and leaving the anterior portion free. The same results may be obtained by plugging the posterior nares.

Step 2. The forefinger of the left hand is introduced into one nostril, as a guide. An incision down to, but not into the cartilage of the nose is made, circumscribing the growth from the middle line outwards. Be sure to leave as much skin as possible near the opening of the nares to avoid subsequent constriction (Fig. 439).

Step 3. The mid-portion of the tumor-mass is seized with forceps and held out of the way. Remove all of the diseased tissues within the circle of the incision with knife or scissors. Attend to hemostasis (Fig. 440).

Step 4. Steps 3 and 4 are repeated on the opposite side.

Step 5. The nasal plugs are removed. Short drainage tubes are introduced into each nostril. The wounds are covered with gutta percha tissue or silver foil. Apply compressive dressings.

SUBMUCOUS RESECTION OF THE NASAL SEPTUM

This operation is indicated in cases of septal abnormalities which interfere with respiration.

An incision is made in the mucous membrane of the septum; through this incision a portion of the bone and cartilage of the nasal septum are removed submucoperichondrially (Figs. 441 and 443).

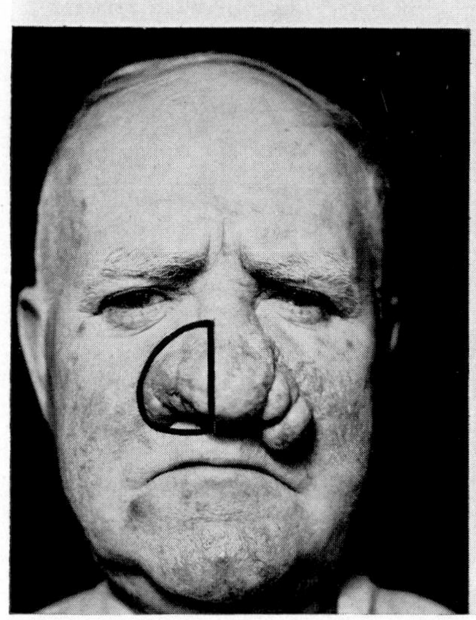

FIG. 439. Operation for rhinophyma: outline of incision. (Cook County Hospital, Chicago.)

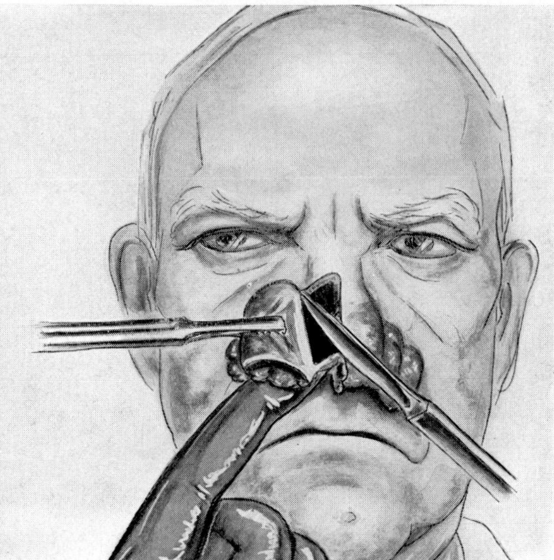

FIG. 440. Technic of operation. (Cook County Hospital, Chicago.)

Step 1. Cut the vibrissae even with the mucosa. Irrigate the nostrils with boric acid solution several times during the 24 hours preceding operation. The skin and mucosa of the region may be painted with tincture of iodine.

Step 2. Local anesthesia is applied as previously described. General anesthesia may be used (Fig. 442).

Step 3. Make a curvilinear incision on the convex side of the septum, its extent and direction varying with the nature of the deformity (Fig. 443 left). The Freer knife should not penetrate beyond the mucous membrane and perichondrium.

Step 4. With an appropriate instrument (some surgeons prefer a sharp and others a blunt one) raise the mucoperichondrium and mucoperiosteum from the involved cartilage and bony structure intact. Avoid injury to the soft parts—this is important (Figs. 441 and 443).

Step 5. If the first incision is made where the mucous membrane of the septum joins the skin of the vestibule, make a similar incision in the septal cartilage with a short knife; a finger inserted in the opposite nostril serves as a guide to determine the extent of the incision. If the first incision is made along the anterior border of the septal cartilage, no second incision is necessary.

Step 6. Separate the cartilage and mucoperichondrium on the opposite side with a sharp elevator, following the same procedure as in detaching the first side of the nasal septum (Fig. 442B).

Step 7. Retract the mucous membrane on either side of the nasal septum with a nasal retractor or speculum, exposing the cartilage. This is cut with a Ballenger's swivel knife (Figs. 443-444) or some other sharp instrument and removed in one piece with a forceps.

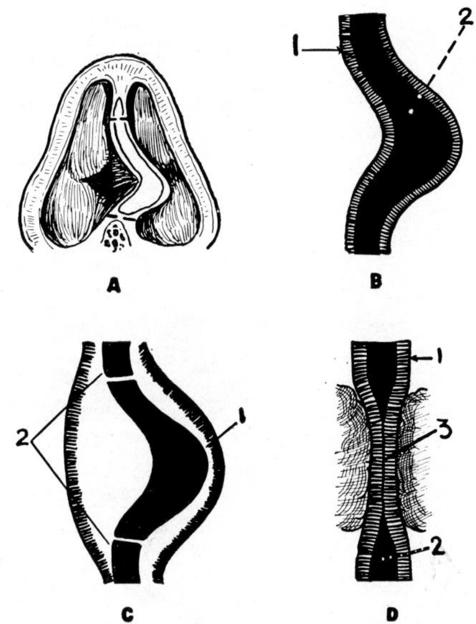

FIG. 441. Submucous resection of the nasal septum: A. points of incision, B. 1. 2. deviated septum mucous membrane and cartilage, C. mucous membrane elevated, cartilage incised, D. mucous membrane after septum is removed, approximated by intranasal packings.

Step 8. While the tissues are still retracted, the portion of the perpendicular plate of the ethmoid to be removed is grasped by a Foster-Ballenger forceps and removed in bites; lateral twisting or wrenching should not be resorted to as unnecessary damage is likely to ensue.

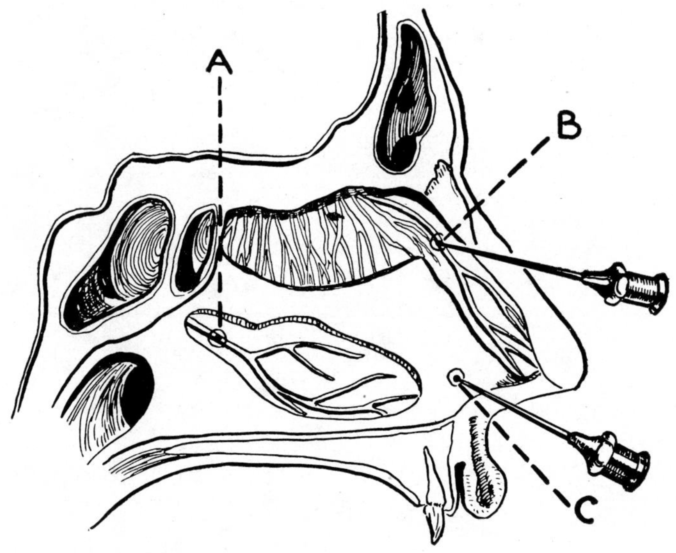

FIG. 442. Local infiltration anesthesia for submucous resection of the septum. A, B and C are points of injection. A. Nerus nasopalatinus superior, B. nerus ethmoidalis anterior.

Step 9. In excising the deflected part of the vomer, Hurd's reversible septal-ridge forceps are introduced into the incision while the tissues are retracted and the desired amount of the vomer is bitten off. Ballenger's or Hajek's chisel may also be used to accomplish this step (Fig. 443C).

Step 10. Carefully examine the wound to make sure all corrections have been made. Hemostasis is attained by using gauze pledgets saturated with adrenalin solution. Repair with sutures any inadvertent openings which have been made in the soft flaps.

Step 11. Not all surgeons suture the wound; some leave it open to drain. If suturing is done, use a Reverdin or small, curved needle. In dressing the

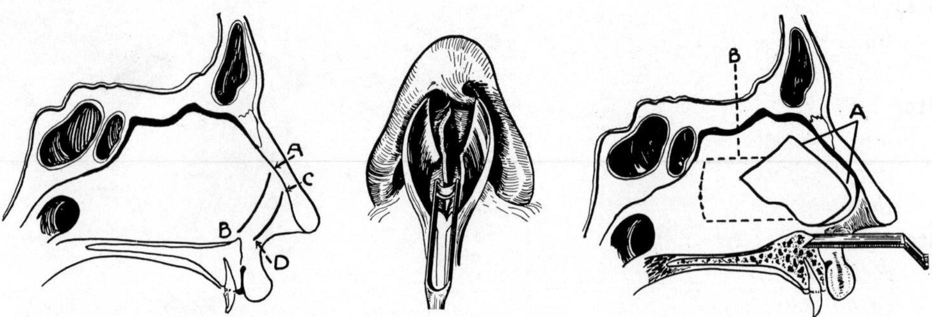

Fig. 443. Submucous resection of the nasal septum: Left. The incision is made on the convex side of the septum from A to B. If the free end of the quadrilateral cartilage is displaced from behind the cutaneous part of the septum, and presents in one nostril, then the incision is made from C to D. Center. Nasal speculum is inserted between the mucopericondrium on either side of the septum showing the use of Ballenger's swivel knife. Right. Removal of maxillary crest with chisel. A. Portion of cartilaginous system removed. B. Portion of bony septum taken away.

wound, endeavor to bring the raw edges of the wound together; prevent hematoma formation. To accomplish this, insert one or two Simpson-Bernays cotton sponge-tents in each nostril and drop sterile water on them until the desired expansion is reached. Todd's splint may also be used and the nostrils left open. After removing the splints, irrigate the nose with a mild antiseptic.

Comment: To prevent the bridge from sinking, do not remove the cartilage too close to it; leave a quarter inch or more attached. Avoid mutilating the mucosa during the operative manipulations and hematomas from forming.

ABSCESS OF THE NASAL SEPTUM

This condition follows either trauma to the nose or is a postoperative complication of submucous resection. It is usually the result of infection of a hematoma of the septum.

Step 1. Make a vertical line with 70% phenol over the more swollen side of the septum. Make a vertical incision through this line, cutting through the mucous membrane only.

Step 2. Remove all the necrotic cartilage from between the flaps of mucous membrane.

Step 3. Remove a large triangular section of mucous membrane from the side that has been incised. Do not pack the nares.

Comment: It is important to warn the patient that a saddle nose may result, as a result of destruction of cartilage. This can later be repaired. The drainage of the abscess should be done as early as possible to minimize the amount of deformity that results.

TUMORS OF THE NOSE

Operation for Removing Nasal Polypi with a Snare

Step 1. After thoroughly anesthetizing the tissues as described, introduce the wire snare so that it is vertical to the floor of the nose.

Step 2. Direct the snare along the side of the polyp until its lowest portion comes immediately below the margin of the polyp where it is manipulated until the polyp drops through it.

Step 3. While encircling the growth, the loop of the snare is directed toward the middle meatus. Endeavor to insert the tip of the cannula into the meatus (Fig. 445).

Step 4. Grip the shaft of the snare with the finger, tightening the wire loop, and pull down the cannula.

Step 5. With the snare firmly grasping the polyp, it is detached from its bed by a quick forward movement.

Step 6. If the polyp is not withdrawn with the snare, instruct the patient to blow the nose with force; if this does not suffice, the growth is removed with suction or forceps.

Comment. Polypi appearing in the posterior part of the nose are removed in a similar manner and may be brought forward by the patient blowing the nose or by means of suction. As a rule, there is little bleeding connected with this operation and any oozing is taken care of by means of cotton pledget compression.

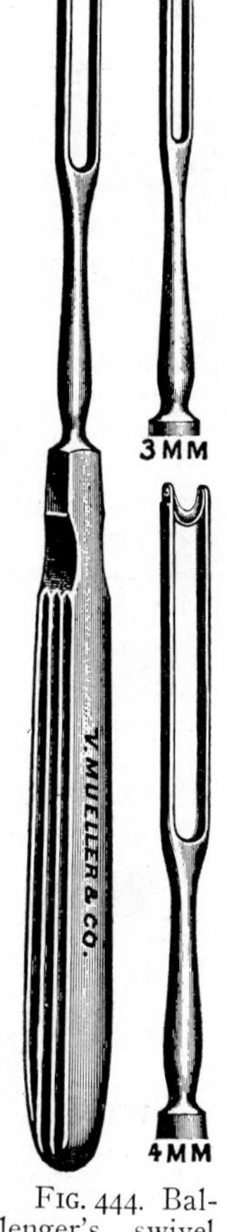

FIG. 444. Ballenger's swivel knife.

Denker's Transmaxillary Excision of Intranasal Malignant Tumors

Step 1. Pull up the angle of the mouth and upper lip with blunt hooks. Make a slightly curved upward incision through the gum of the upper jaw to a point near the frenum of the upper lip, beginning opposite the wisdom tooth. Separate the soft parts of the upper jaw with a periosteal elevator. Expose the bone nearly to the lower margin of the orbit laying bare the pyriform aperture of the nose.

Step 2. Separate the mucous membrane from the outer wall of the lower and middle sinuses of the nose and partly from the floor of the nose beginning at the pyriform aperture. This separation is continued backward to the posterior limits of the antrum of Highmore. If the lower turbinate bone is not involved in the tumor, it is removed with strong scissors. Hemostasis is obtained by temporary packing with gauze.

Step 3. Remove the external bony wall of the antrum of Highmore with a chisel and hammer. If the mucosa lining the inner surface of this wall is unaffected, incise it freely so as to gain free access to the sinus. If it is involved in the neoplasm, remove it together with the growth. Remove the bone completely and also the mucosa of the inner or nasal wall of the antrum of Highmore.

Step 4. With scissors or probe pointed knife remove the mucosa of the already separated outer wall of the nose (See **Step 2**). If the tumor originated from the middle sinus of the nose it generally will follow with the removal of the

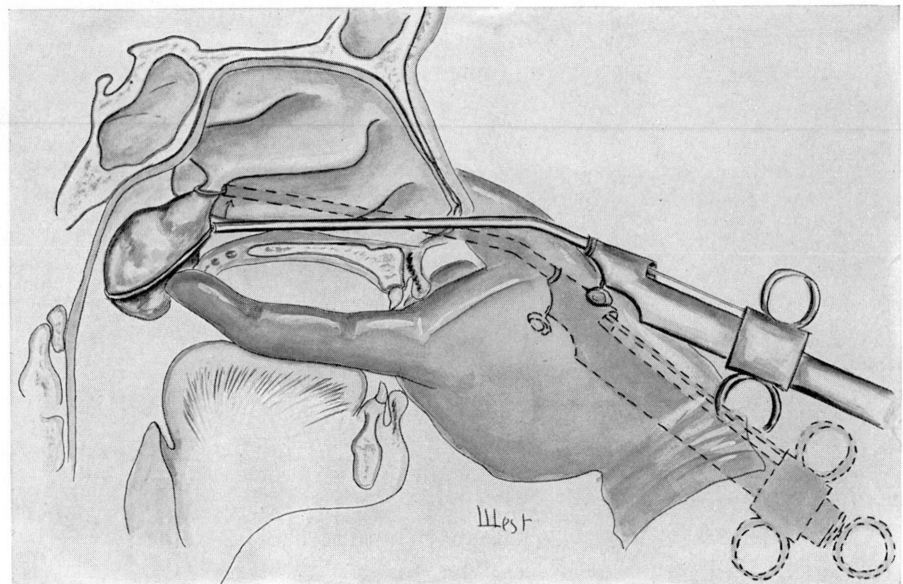

FIG. 445. Removal of nasal polypi with a snare.

nasal mucous membrane. The ethmoidal and sphenoidal sinuses are now accessible and may be taken care of as need be.

Step 5. Pack the wound with gauze. Suture the wound in the mouth. Insure oral asepsis with mouth washes. After three or four days the pack is removed. Tumors arising from the nasopharynx, retro-maxillary or pterygopalatine fossae are not amenable to the above procedure.

Comment. Malignancies on the cutaneous surface in the region of the nose may at times be treated successfully with radium (Fig. 446A and B). Proper prosthesis yields satisfactory results (Fig. 447A and B).

FOREIGN BODIES IN THE NOSE

Children are the usual patients who introduce foreign bodies into the nasal chambers. These usually consist of nuts, peas, beans, etc., which tend to swell and give rise to difficulties.

If anterior rhinoscopy fails to reveal the foreign body, one may await further developments. Where a child is suffering from a chronic, unilateral nasal discharge (purulent or muco-sanguinous) or if there is a dermatitis of the nostril the presence of a foreign body may be assumed. If the case is recent, anterior

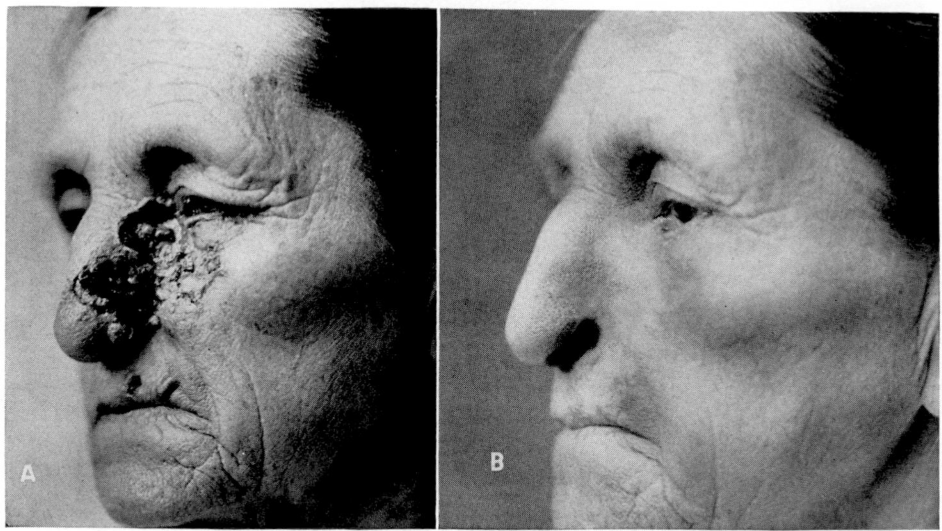

FIG. 446. A. Epithelioma of the nose. B. Same patient after radium treatment.

rhinoscopy is likely to reveal it; but, if of long standing, the swelling of the mucosa and the discharge are likely to conceal the foreign body. Shrink the

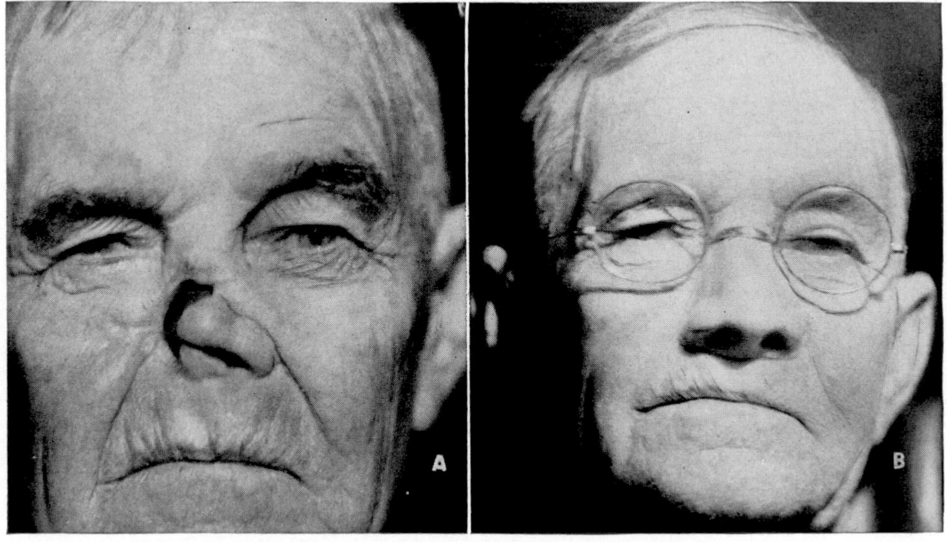

FIG. 447. A. Controlled epithelioma of the nose. B. Nose restored by prosthesis (courtesy of Dr. T. E. Schaeffer).

mucosa with cocaine and adrenalin and wipe away the discharge, then search for the foreign body. In very young children or youngsters hard to handle, it may be necessary to resort to a general anesthetic for examination and removal. A two and one-half per cent cocaine solution may be sprayed into the affected nasal chamber and the foreign body located and removed with an appropriately bent

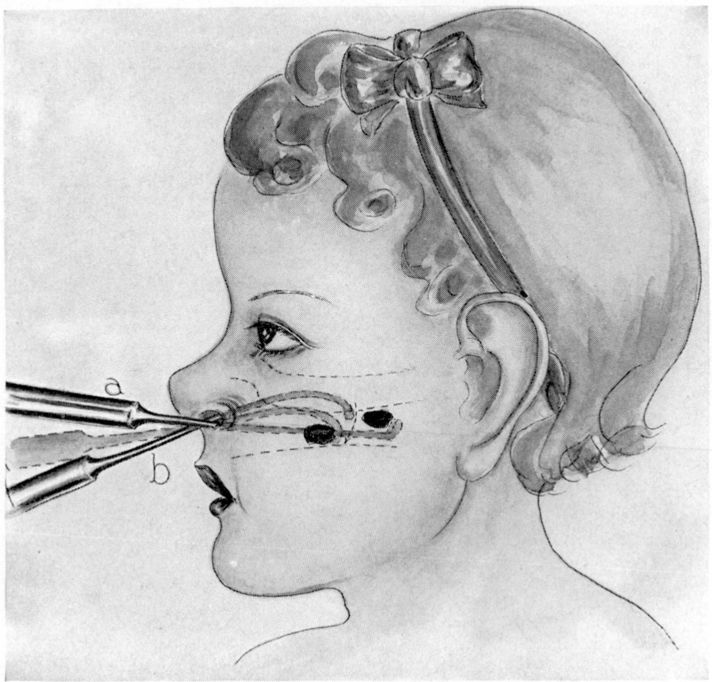

FIG. 448. a. Removing foreign body from nose by insinuating a blunt angulated instrument behind it and drawing it forward; foreign body being guided along roof of nasal chamber. b. Foreign body being propelled along floor of nasal chamber.

probe, or a forceps (Fig. 448). A suction apparatus may be employed to remove any remaining débris.

CHAPTER 17

SURGERY OF THE NECK AND CERVICAL ENDOCRINE GLANDS

INJURIES TO THE NECK

CUT THROAT

In cases of attempted suicide, the superficial structures alone are injured in about 50 per cent of cases. Occasionally the larger vessels in the neck are severed with a fatal outcome. The treatment here is obvious, aseptic repair of the divided tissues.

Deep Wounds in the Neck

These are divided by Hamilton Bailey into definite categories, depending upon the position of the injury inflicted, viz.: (Fig. 449).

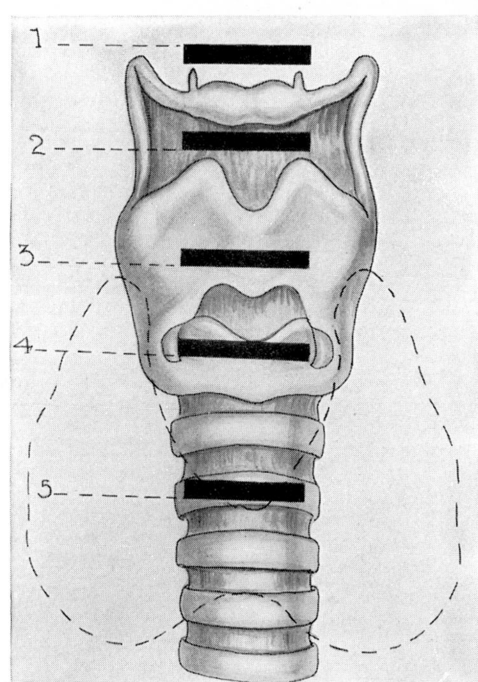

Fig. 449

WOUNDS ABOVE THE HYOID BONE

In this locality, the wound may often lead into the mouth and the epiglottis will in many cases be found injured. The principles of treatment are:

Step 1. Asepticize the wound.
Step 2. Repair the epiglottis with catgut sutures.

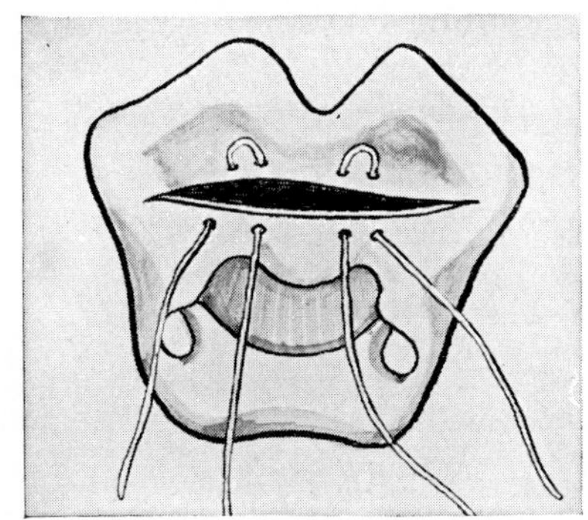

Fig. 450

Fig. 449. Position of the wound into the air-passages of 57 cases of suicidal "cut throat" with a deep wound. 1. Above hyoid (8). 2. Thyrohyoid membrane (17). 3. Thyroid cartilage. (18). 4. Cricoid (10). 5. Trachea (4). (After Hamilton Bailey.)

Fig. 450. Suturing an injured thyroid cartilage. (After Hamilton Bailey.)

Step 3. Trim the mucosa of the pharynx and repair the wound.
Step 4. If the submaxillary gland is much traumatized, remove it.
Step 5. Ligate spurting vessels.
Step 6. Mop out the entire wound cavity with tincture of iodine.
Step 7. Close the cutaneous wound.

WOUNDS OF THE THYROHYOID MEMBRANE

Step 1. Repair the epiglottis as above.

Step 2. Suture the thyrohyoid membrane and close any chance opening into the pharynx.

Step 3. **Laryngotomy** is indicated in most cases. Bailey lauds this procedure and prefers it to tracheotomy. In the presence of respiratory embarrassment laryngotomy (see p. 387) should be done before the wound is attended to.

WOUNDS OF THE THYROID CARTILAGE

Step 1. Perform laryngotomy as described on p. 387.

Step 2. Introduce mattress sutures of catgut as shown in the illustration (Fig. 450). Approximate the lips of the wound in the cartilage; do not tie the sutures too snugly because sutures pulled too snugly tend to cut out.

Wounds with loss of substance of the thyroid cartilage should be repaired by covering the defect with muscle—usually available from the prethyroid group of muscles.

WOUNDS ABOVE, BELOW OR THROUGH THE CRICOID CARTILAGE

Step 1. Expose the wounded structures thoroughly. Trim away crushed edges.

Step 2. Insert a laryngotomy tube.

Step 3. Approximate the tissues around it.

WOUNDS OF THE TRACHEA

Step 1. Good exposure here is essential.

Step 2. Bare the trachea by Digby's method which consists of making a tunnel with a pair of curved, pointed hemostats between the isthmus of the thyroid and the trachea. Divide the isthmus between two artery forceps, the hemostat behind acting as a protector of the trachea while the incision is being made. The trachea is now exposed.

Step 3. Insert an ample-sized tracheotomy tube into the opening in the trachea. Or, close the wound in the trachea and do a tracheotomy below the closed tracheal wound.

Step 4. Reunite the divided isthmus of the thyroid with catgut sutures.

Step 5. Insure hemostasis. Dress the wound.

Complications of "Cut Throat." (a) Bronchopneumonia, (b) cervical cellulitis (not frequent), and (c) oesophageal fistula.

WOUNDS OF THE VESSELS IN THE NECK

(See Chapter 21, p. 586)

FRACTURES OF THE LARYNX AND TRACHEA

(a) Simple fractures not interfering with breathing should be treated conservatively but the surgeon should always be prepared to interfere should an emergency arise.

(b) When respiratory embarrassment is present, do a tracheotomy at once.

RUPTURE OF THE TRACHEA WITH RETRACTION OF THE LOWER END

Search for the lower end of the windpipe, bring it to the surface, secure it there with sutures after a tube has been inserted. Transverse wounds of the trachea should be sutured.

FOREIGN BODIES IN THE PHARYNX AND ESOPHAGUS

If the foreign body has just been swallowed, introduce the index finger into the pharynx, sweep it to the back of the epiglottis. If you feel the foreign body, dislodge and extract it promptly.

If suffocation is imminent, do a tracheotomy promptly!

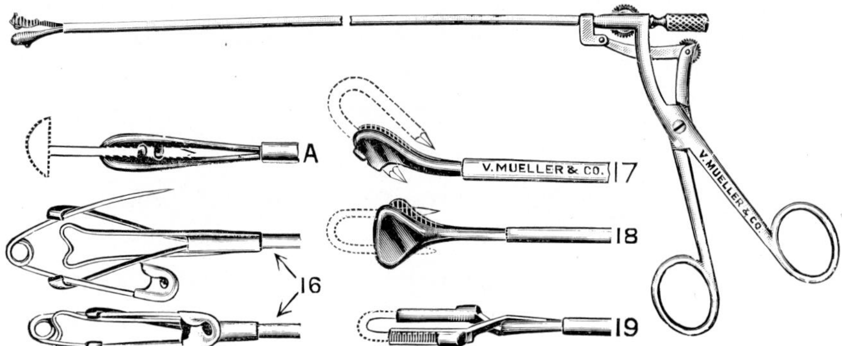

FIG. 451. Forceps for extracting foreign bodies from pharynx and esophagus.

Where no speed is indicated, explore the pharynx, hypopharynx and esophagus (sounds, x-ray, etc.). When located, remove the obstruction with a foreign body extractor (Fig. 451). When the foreign body is in the grasp of the instrument, proceed slowly, extricate methodically, without haste, lest serious injury to the esophagus and contiguous structures result.

Where esophagoscopy can be done it should be resorted to—it is the safest and best aid for exploration and extraction of foreign bodies.

BURNS AND SCARS

Scars caused by burns are always most disfiguring but seem to be doubly so when occurring on the neck where they frequently draw the mouth, chin and lips out of shape; they impede speaking, pull the chin downward and occasion different degrees of torticollis. Treatment of burns here requires great caution and care. If the burn covers a large area, a tent should be built over the patient and an electric lamp placed under it for heating purposes. Sterile vaseline and alboline are used to keep the surface soft and pliable. The tannic acid treatment is excellent (for which see p. 527).

As soon as possible, skin grafting should be resorted to (pinch grafts). On account of the movements of the neck, every effort should be made to keep the grafts in place with sea sponges.

Surgery of Scars

Scars which displace the chin downward demand surgical treatment in order to free the jaw. Often such operation, if carelessly performed, may lead to the formation of more scar tissue. Individual option and judgment must be exercised in each case. A number of plastic procedures may be necessary, and pedicled flaps from the skin of the breast or thorax may have to be resorted to. If a scar running from the chin to the neck contains a ridge of skin that is somewhat raised, make an incision along the length of the scar; fashion two leaves and

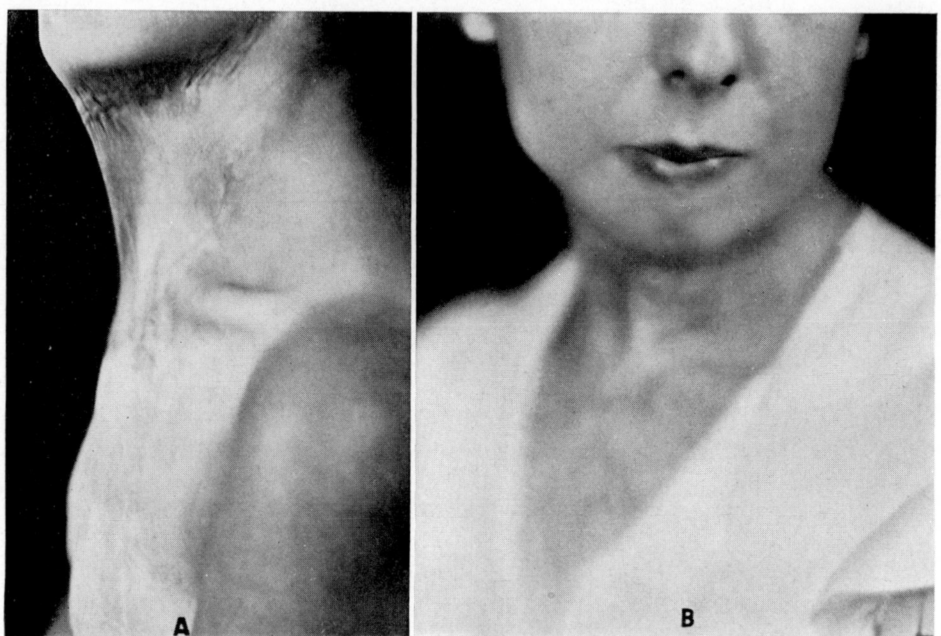

Fig. 452. A. Extensive scarring of neck and chest following burns. B. Same patient after multiple plastic operations.

incise these so as to form right angles to the original incision but at different points; separate flap one near the chin and the other farther down.

Figure 452A depicts a young woman who was desperately ill following a burn. The neck and submental region were a firm mass of scar tissue. Careful and painstaking plastic procedures enabled me to obtain the result shown in Fig. 452B.

INFECTIONS OF THE NECK

FURUNCLES AND CARBUNCLES OF THE NECK

Carbuncles should receive early attention. Poulticing and injections of antiseptics should be abandoned for more effective treatment thus diminishing the destructive process and bringing about quick relief. Ethyl chloride is recommended by Franke. It should be used properly to produce effective anesthesia and prevent the danger of gangrene. Occasionally block anesthesia is permissible.

Gas or ether anesthesia is usually employed. Operate quickly. L. Carp concludes that in large carbuncles of diabetic or non-diabetic origin, the treatment of choice is radical surgery. In preparing the skin before the operation, soap and alcohol are generally used in preference to iodine. Excision is the treatment of choice. (Figs. 453-454). The majority of furuncles are best treated by conservative measures (hot, saturated boric-acid applications and general sustaining

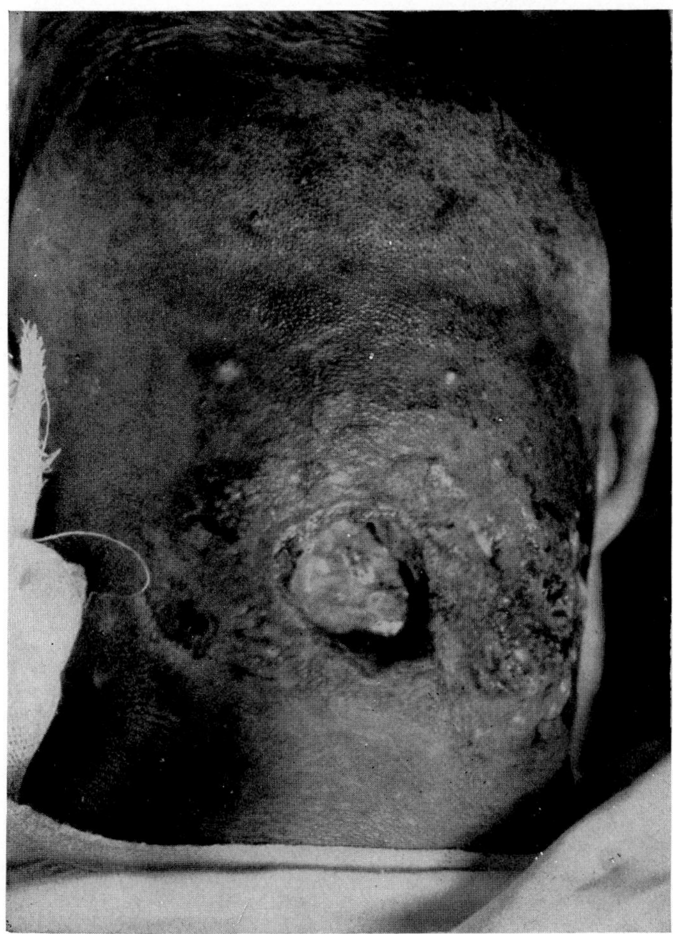

FIG. 453. Carbuncle of back of neck.

measures). When fluctuation presents, incise. Crucial incisions are often effective. (See also, x-ray treatment of, p. 197).

CELLULITIS AND LYMPHADENITIS

Infections in the upper neck are by no means rare; in school children enlarged lymph-nodes caused by colds or fevers are usually of no consequence. In some cases, however, periadenitis ensues, the nodes fuse together and an abscess may form; this should be guarded against by proper preventive measures. Iodine and other counterirritants are contra-indicated in acute cases but may prove useful in chronic conditions.

In deep infections where pus has accumulated in the structures of the neck, make a small, transverse incision in the deep fascia over the point where the abscess is suspected. "Hilton's method" is brought into use here. Insert an artery forceps or some similar blunt instrument into the wound and guide it toward the suppurating focus. When this is reached, open and withdraw the forceps thus enlarging the avenue which has been created through which pus may escape. Provide efficient drainage (cigarette or rubber drain).

A small, stab-incision is sufficient to afford egress to the accumulated pus even in cases of large pus collections of the uncomplicated type.

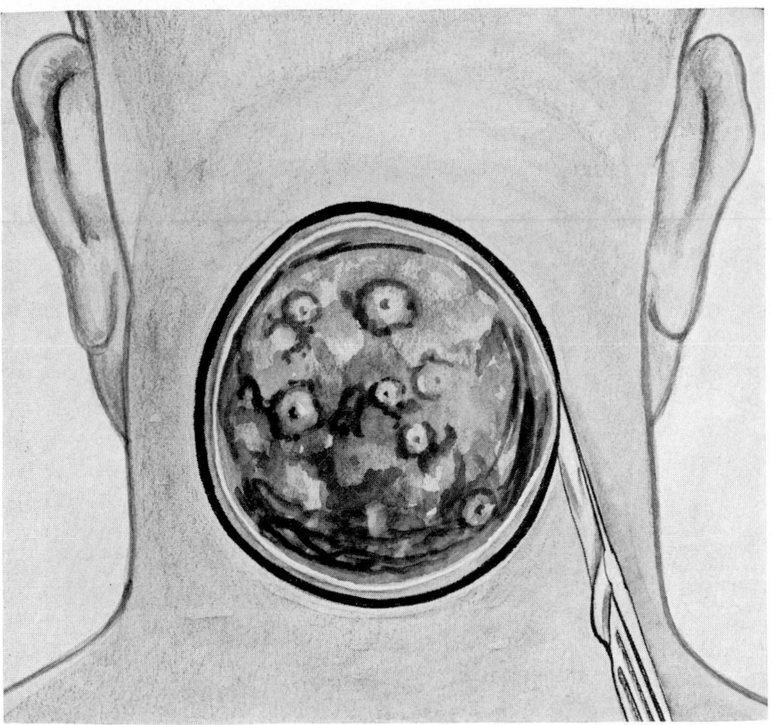

FIG. 454. Excision of carbuncle of the neck. (After Kirschner.)

The cellulitis generally found in adults usually has its origin in an abscessed tooth-root or osteitis. The tissues from the jaw down to the clavicle are swollen, the jaws cannot be opened and it is with difficulty that anesthesia is administered.

Make an incision along the anterior margin of the sternomastoid muscle, as soon as possible. The incision should be deep enough to lessen tension and circumvent the tendency toward edema of the glottis. Oftentimes there is little pus present; edema predominates.

LUDWIG'S ANGINA

The mortality in this condition is very high, death usually being caused by edema of the glottis. The regions under the jaw and inside the mouth are involved by a swelling. In every case of Ludwig's angina, have tracheotomy instruments and oxygen within close reach. The exact pathology of this condition is still somewhat obscure, although it is generally believed that it is essentially a virulent streptococcic cellulitis. The deep cervical fascia prevents its spread anteriorly; it tracks around the posterior free border of the mylohyoid muscle to the sublingual region, thus giving rise to the characteristic appearance of a phlegmonous swelling in the neck and floor of the mouth. If unrelieved, the pus burrows between the mylohyoid and middle constrictor of the pharyngeal muscles. "Herein lies the chief danger," says Hamilton Bailey, "for when the last situation is reached, edema of the glottis is imminent and often comes on with such dramatic suddenness that the patient is suffocated before laryngotomy can be performed.

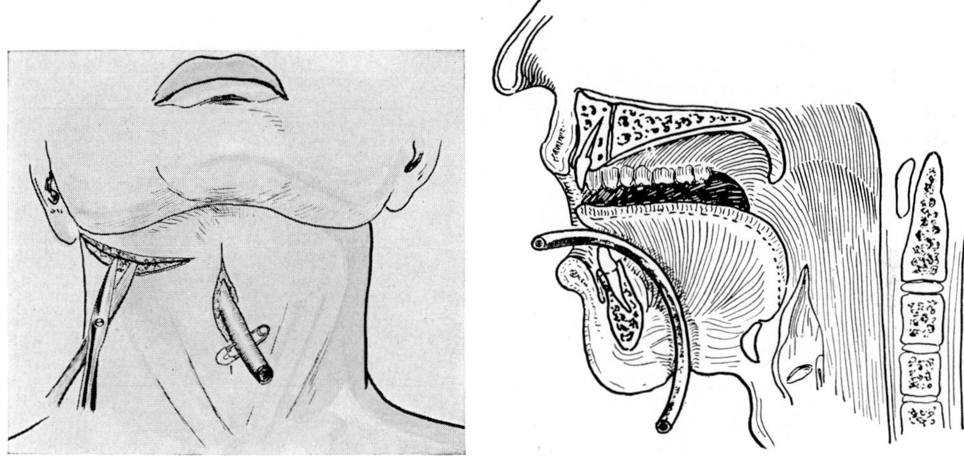

FIG. 455 FIG. 456

FIG. 455. Incision and drainage of the floor of the mouth in Ludwig's angina. Lateral submandibular incision, median incision between chin and hyoid bone.

FIG. 456. Drainage of the floor of the mouth in Ludwig's angina. A rubber tube traverses the affected area.

The very name angina tells of this danger for angina implies strangling." The treatment of this treacherous condition is drainage through the floor of the mouth.

Drainage of the Floor of the Mouth

Careful planning directed to relieving tension and evacuating pus should precede the surgical intervention. As stated, no time should be lost in performing the operation as the patient is in imminent danger of dying from sepsis or choking to death. In the majority of cases two incisions are adequate; however, if both sides of the neck are affected a third incision may be necessary.

Bailey speaks of decompression operation which is effected by an adequate incision which divides the mylohyoid muscle thus circumventing the pus and "tracking" it away from the vital area.

If the patient is very ill, anesthesia is unnecessary; however, procaine may be infiltrated through the skin; the deeper tissues require no anesthesia.

Step 1. Make a median incision between the chin and hyoid bone about 1 inch in length. Direct the scalpel through the median raphé of the neck into the gingivolingual sulcus back of the symphysis of the jaw.

Step 2. Introduce a curved Kelly hemostat into the wound and proceed through the floor of the mouth until the tip of the instrument is seen between the teeth. Grasp a fenestrated rubber tube with the hemostat and pull it from inside the mouth out through the neck-incision and secure both ends of it with safety pins (Figs. 455-456).

When combining the lateral submandibular and median incisions proceed as follows:

Step 1. Immediately under the angle of the jaw, make an antero-posterior incision 4 or 5 cm. in length, including only the skin and platysma (Figs. 445 and 457).

Step 2. Insert a curved Kelly hemostat into the wound, direct it across the sublingual space so that it enters the mucosa of the mouth near the tongue directly opposite the molar teeth. Grasp a fenestrated rubber tube with the hemostat and pull it from inside the mouth out through the neck incision, securing both ends of it with safety pins.

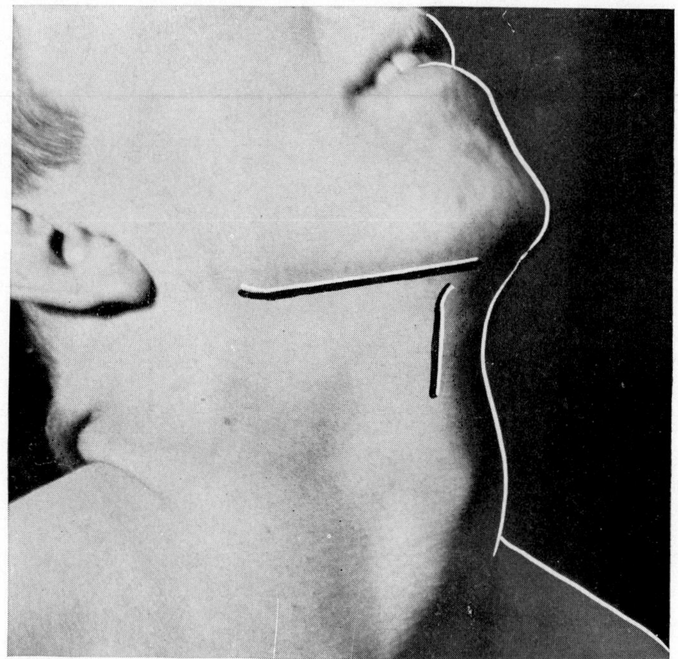

FIG. 457. Drainage of the floor of the mouth, combining lateral submandibular and median incision.

Make the median incision as previously described.

Make a second submandibular incision if the cellulitis involves the other side of the neck.

A. P. C. Ashhurst who recommends the above procedure, observes that relief of tension follows the above operation so quickly it may be discerned by watching the patient.

Apply dressings saturated with 2 per cent sodium citrate solution. Irrigate the tubes twice a day with boric acid solution. The wounds heal very satisfactorily.

Comment. Van Wagner and Costello advocate local block anesthesia of the cervical nerves by injecting novocaine solution behind the sternomastoid muscle (see cervical block under operations on the thyroid, page 446). Ethylene may be used, although Hamilton Bailey is prejudiced against gas in these cases having seen death occur in a case of Ludwig's angina at the hands of a competent surgeon who used gas (nitrous oxid) anesthesia.

PERI-ESOPHAGEAL SUPPURATION AND MEDIASTINITIS

These cases are treated by incision and drainage of the affected area. Begin at the anterior margin of the sternocleidomastoid muscle and advance cautiously down to the esophagus. Explore until the focus in the mediastinum is reached. In bilateral suppurations, make bilateral incisions. If the foreign body has not yet been removed, extract it and insert a stomach tube. Drain thoroughly and leave the wound completely open. Lower the head of the patient thus aiding drainage. A preliminary gastrostomy in such cases is often of great value.

DIAGNOSTIC OPERATIONS ON THE NECK

LARYNGOSCOPY

Indirect Laryngoscopy

This is a relatively simple method of examination of the larynx. It can be employed in all adults but in younger children it is often difficult, if not impossible.

Step 1. As a rule no anesthesia is required but in patients who have a sensitive pharynx, a spray of 4 per cent cocaine to the pharynx may be necessary. The laryngeal mirror, usually about one inch in diameter, is used. This is warmed by holding it for a few seconds in the flame of an alcohol lamp, to prevent the condensation of moisture on the mirror. The mirror should always be tested against the back of the examiner's hand, to be sure that it is not too hot.

Step 2. The tongue is then grasped with a linen cloth or gauze and pulled forward. Care must be taken that the tongue is not injured against the lower teeth. Holding the tongue with the left hand, introduce the mirror; avoid touching the base of the tongue else the patient may gag. The mirror is turned to the angle at which the light from a head-mirror is reflected into the larynx. It must be remembered that the mirror causes the anterior portion of the larynx and the posterior portion to be reversed in the image (Fig. 458, I, II, III and IV).

Direct Laryngoscopy

There are several methods of examining the larynx directly, including the use of the Jackson laryngoscope, the Hasslinger directoscope (Fig. 459) and the Lynch suspension apparatus. The theory of their use is the same, that is, to retract the epiglottis and other intervening structures so that the interior of the larynx is in the direct line of vision. Local or general anesthesia may be used.

Step 1. Employing local anesthesia, the pharynx is first sprayed with 4 per cent cocaine. Cotton pledgets dipped in 10 per cent cocaine are then applied to the base of the tongue, the epiglottis and the pyriform sinuses. This is done by means of a curved laryngeal applicator. The arytenoid cartilages and the interior of the larynx are then touched with the solution, using a mirror and a laryngeal applicator.

Step 2. The patient is placed on a table in the recumbent position. An assistant holds the patient with the shoulders on the table, the neck is flexed

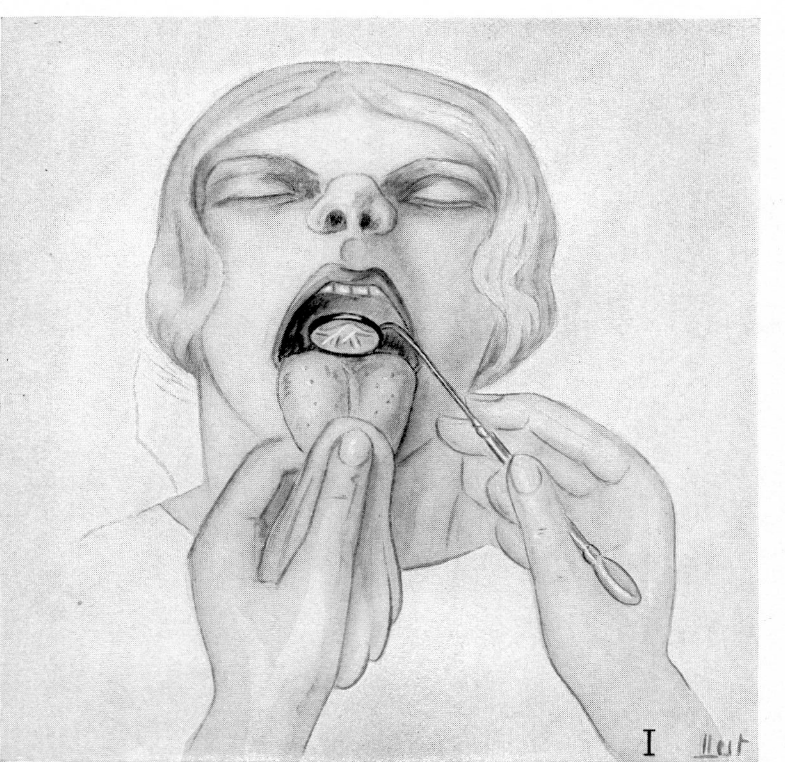

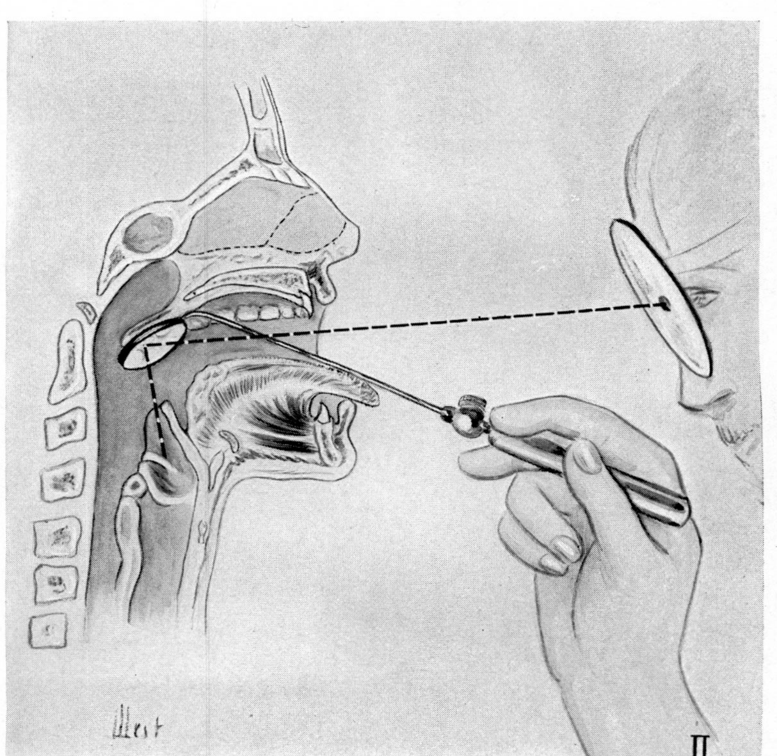

FIG. 458. Indirect laryngoscopy (indirect view). I. Method of introducing laryngeal mirror. II. Examination with laryngeal mirror. (Continued on next page.)

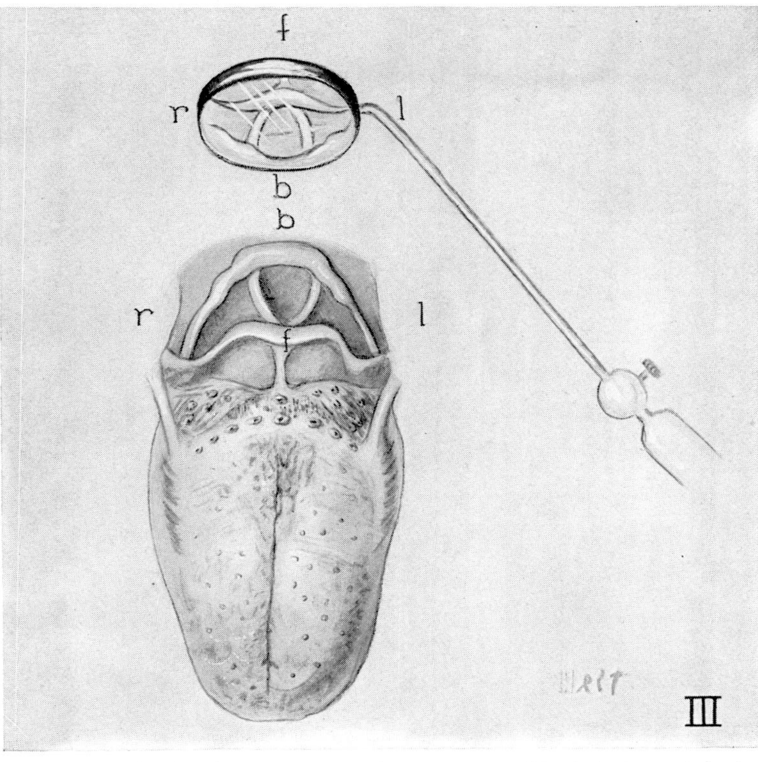
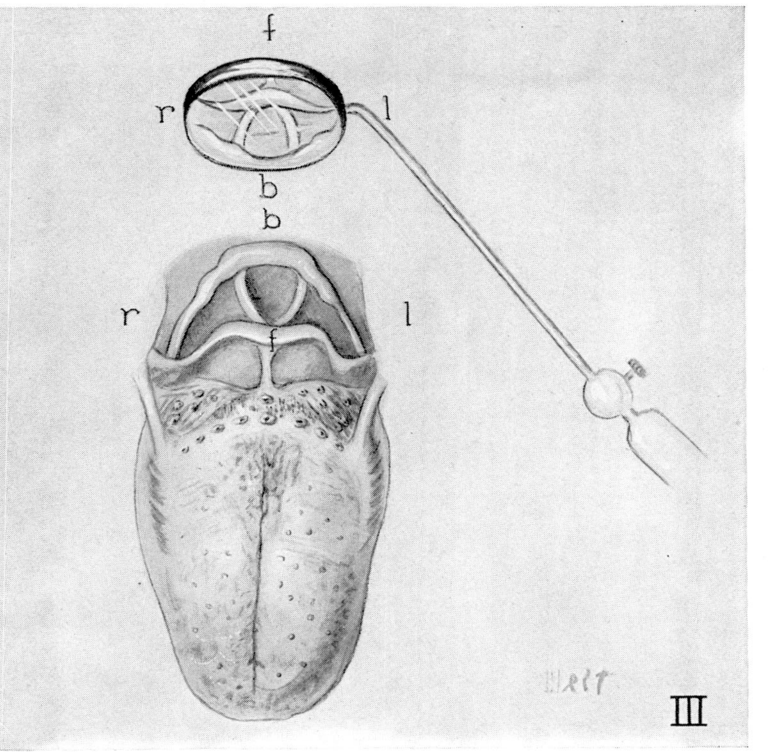

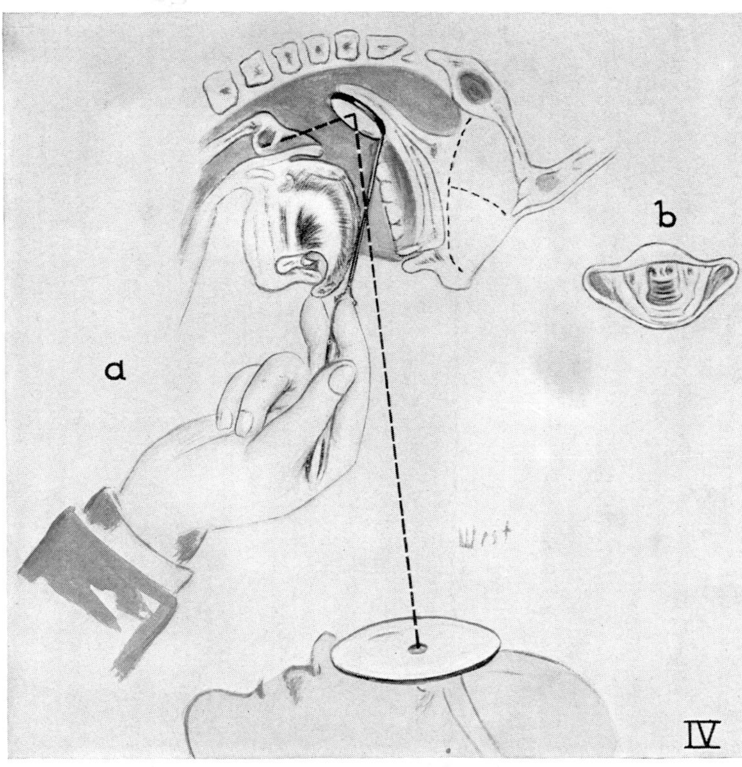

FIG. 458 (Continued.) Indirect laryngoscopy. III. Relations of the laryngoscopic image to actuality, r. right, l. left, f. front, b. back. IV. Killian's method of indirect laryngoscopy: a. note position of patient and examiner and placement of laryngoscope, b. image of posterior laryngeal wall and bifurcation of trachea obtained by Killian's method of superior tracheoscopy.

on the chest and the head extended on the neck. This will afford a more direct exposure of the larynx.

Step 3. The surgeon stands at the head of the table and the laryngeal spatula is held in the left hand. It is introduced along the dorsum of the tongue, the epiglottis coming into view. This is then picked up with the tip of the spatula. The laryngoscope is then introduced one or two inches further, the

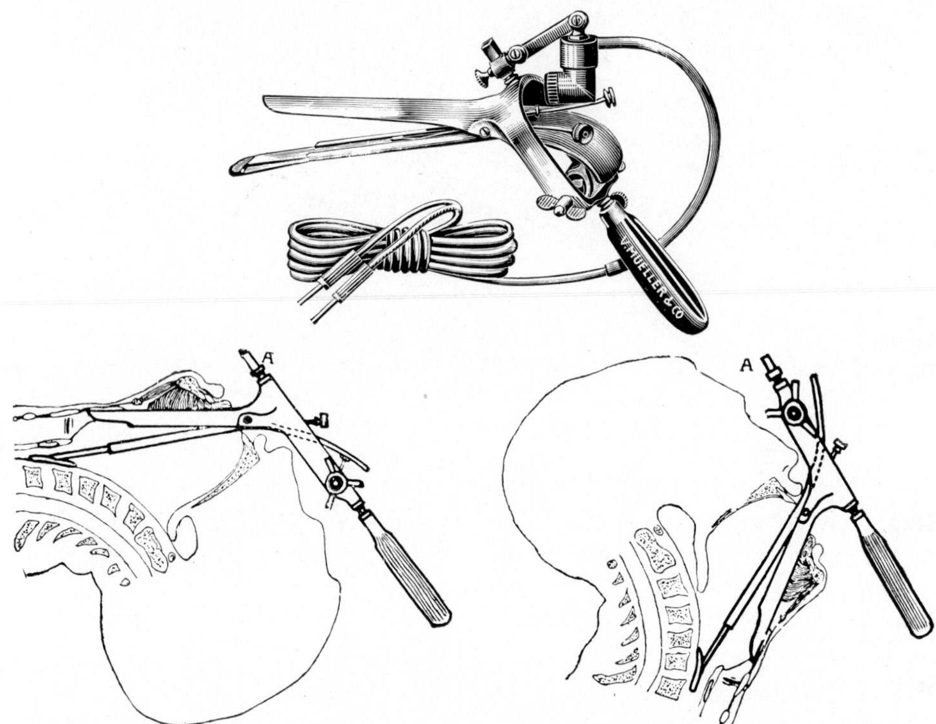

FIG. 459. Hasslinger's directoscope. This is a self-retaining adjustable speculum for examination and treatment of the larynx. The hypopharynx and the underlying vertebrae are used as the fixed point, from which counter pressure is used to advance the tongue and epiglottis forward, thus exposing the larynx. For introduction the instrument is closed and the pharyngeal blade is drawn back all the way. The operator advances the instrument along the patient's tongue, over the epiglottis until the posterior wall of the larynx is exposed, then with the thumb of the left hand, the advancing rod is pushed forward to its entire limit in order to bring the hypopharyngeal plate in proper position. Lower figures show the instrument in proper position with the patient in the upright and reclining positions.

whole pressure being directed in an upward direction. Avoid using the teeth as a fulcrum. The entire interior of the larynx may now be effectively exposed. If the anterior portion is not readily seen, gentle pressure on the thyroid cartilage from the outside will give a better view.

The Lynch suspension apparatus is a device that holds the spatula in position and allows the operator free use of both hands in performing intralaryngeal manipulations.

ESOPHAGOSCOPY

Von Mikulicz, in 1881, was the first to use straight esophagoscopic tubes.

Anatomic Notes. It must be recalled that the distance between the dental arcade and the cricoid cartilage in the adult is 15 cm.; the length of the esophagus is about 25 cm. The distance from the dental arcades to the cardiac orifice is about 40 cm.

Direct endoscopy of the esophagus is done with a straight esophagoscope (Fig. 460). Exploration may be done with the patient sitting or in the recumbent position. In many patients no anesthetic is necessary. On occasion, general anesthesia may have to be resorted to. After the tube has cleared the cricoid cartilage, it may be readily passed to the cardiac orifice of the gullet if no obstruction impedes its

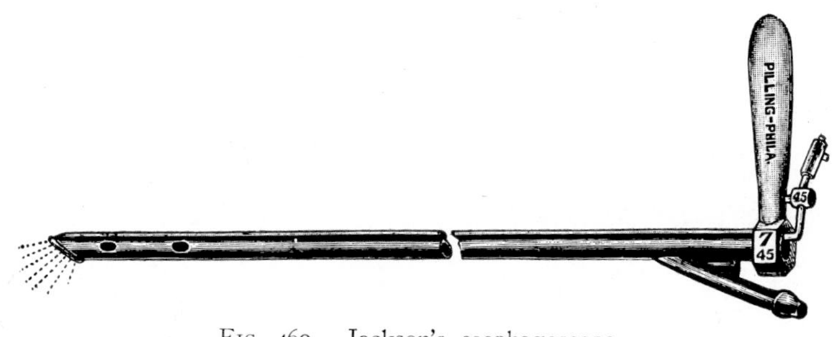

Fig. 460. Jackson's esophagoscope.

passage. Doyen remarked that endoscopy of the esophagus is within practical range of all surgeons and is wrongly made a specialty.

OPERATIONS ON THE NECK

INTERCRICOID LARYNGOTOMY

Step 1. Extend the head of the patient. Pick up a vertical fold of skin so that its center corresponds to the upper level of the cricoid cartilage. Local anesthesia (Fig. 461).

Step 2. Transfix the skin and make a transverse incision about one inch in length.

Step 3. Open the crico-thyroid membrane (Figs. 462 and 469) with a pair of pointed curved scissors, close to the upper border of the cricoid cartilage, thereby avoiding the small transverse artery.

Step 4. A laryngotomy tube, by preference Butlin's (Fig. 463), is inserted into the opening created, between the blades of the scissors.

Step 5. Check bleeding. Dress.

TRACHEOTOMY

Anatomic Considerations. In the adult the trachea is about 4½ inches long. Two and one half inches lie above the sternum and comprise about eight to ten rings. One should locate the following landmarks from above downward: the hyoid bone and its greater cornua, the thyroid cartilage and the cricoid cartilage. The tracheotomy triangle is formed by drawing a line transversely across the cricoid cartilage to the anterior borders of the sternocleidomastoid muscles. The thyroid isthmus covers the second, third and fourth tracheal rings. The pretracheal fascia is attached to the anterior surface of the cricoid cartilage forming the suspensory ligament of the isthmus. It covers the anterior surface of the trachea. The arteries are: the cricothyroid, running transversely across the cricothyroid space, a branch of the inferior thyroid, coursing behind the isthmus and occasionally a thyroidea ima (from the innominate) passing upward in front of the trachea. The veins are: branches of the superior thyroid veins passing to the upper border of the isthmus, the inferior thyroid veins descending from the lower border of the isthmus in front of the trachea to the left innominate; the left innominate vein which crosses the front of the trachea (obliquely) and may lie from one half to an inch above the suprasternal notch.

Tracheotomy, under certain conditions, is a very simple procedure. Again it may be difficult to accomplish (emergencies, alarming dyspnea, improper surroundings, poor assistance, etc.).

Types of Operation. High tracheotomy (above the isthmus of the thyroid gland).

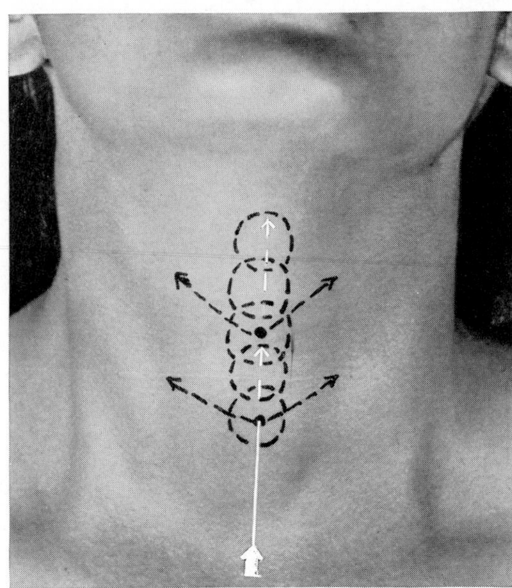

Fig. 461

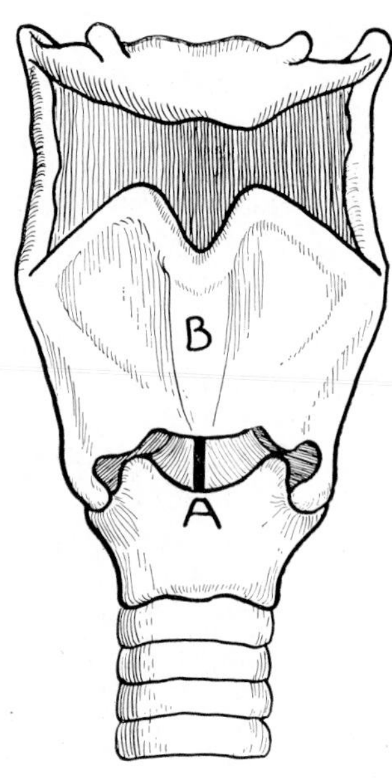

Fig. 462

Fig. 461. Laryngotomy. Infiltration anesthesia for laryngotomy. The circles represent the intracutaneous wheals created by the novocaine solution. The needle and white arrow point in the direction of the needle while making this infiltration. From these points down the tissues between the skin and trachea are infiltrated in the direction indicated by the arrow. The length of the first infiltration is about 3 inches, its highest point being a little below the upper margin of the thyroid cartilage. Hertzler pointed out that theoretically if the needle is passed too deeply there is danger of blocking the pneumogastric nerve. Such danger is negligible since this nerve lies deeply behind the superior thyroid nerve. After incision of the skin, the needle is passed through the cricoid membrane where the mucosa is infiltrated, care being taken not to perforate the mucosa. About 1 cc. of anesthetic is here deposited slowly. A similar deposit is made at the higher point. If the injection is properly performed, no reflexes are excited when the interior of the larynx is exposed. Should a sensitive area be touched, a pledget of cotton moistened with cocaine solution is pressed against it. It is to be hoped that "laryngologists will realize they have here a method that is superior to the hanging method."

Fig. 462. Intercricothyroid laryngotomy (diagrammatic). A. Cricoid cartilage. B. Thyroid cartilage. Between the two a vertical line indicates placements of incision.

Caution. In low tracheotomy the skin incision must be ample in order to avoid subcutaneous emphysema. In making the incision, keep close to the median line. Deviation to one side or the other may cause undesirable bleeding and culminate in an improper opening in the trachea. The trachea must be steadied while being opened. A dry field is essential. A blood clot or mucous plug in the trachea may prevent proper areation. Any tendency to dyspnea must be investigated and the causative factor eliminated.

Complications. 1. Aspiration of blood or mucus causing respiratory embarrassment (bronchopneumonia, tracheobronchitis, etc.).

2. Pressure necrosis from improperly placed tube.

3. Dislodgement of the tube with ensuing threatened suffocation. (Act promptly; remove the tube at once.)

High Tracheotomy

Position of the patient. Place the patient on his back with the shoulders raised on a pillow or sand bag and the head extended. Good illumination is essential.

Anesthesia may be local or general. Palpate the thyroid and cricoid cartilage.

Step 1. From a point below and in the middle of the thyroid cartilage, make an incision exactly in the midline, about 1½ inches in length (Fig. 464 A). The sterno-thyroid and the sterno-hyoid muscles are retracted laterally and the isthmus of the thyroid is pushed downward. Catch all bleeding vessels and ligate them (anterior jugulars). Expose the pretracheal fascia and incise it transversely at the level of the cricoid cartilage (Fig. 464 B). If the isthmus cannot readily be displaced it is best to divide it between two ligatures (Fig. 464 C). The upper three or four tracheal rings are thus exposed.

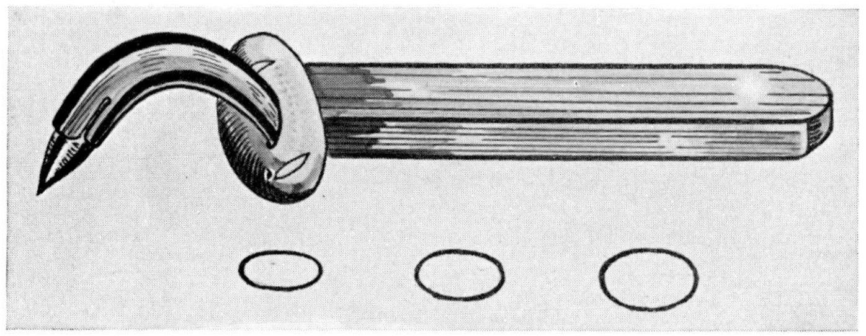

FIG. 463. Butlin's laryngotomy tube with a pilot.

Step 2. Steady the cricoid cartilage with a sharp hook which pulls the cartilage upward (Fig. 464 D). **Incise the trachea from below upward.** Care should be taken not to push the knife so far in as to injure the posterior wall of the trachea. Two or three tracheal rings are divided. The incision in the trachea is about ¾ of an inch in length. A pair of hemostats spreads the opening transversely. Introduce a tracheotomy tube (Fig. 465) or, suture the edges of the tracheal opening to the edges of the skin. One suture on each side suffices to keep the tracheal opening patent.

If a tube is used its size should suit the opening in the trachea (Fig. 466). After the tube is properly placed, it should be secured by a tape around the neck to prevent it slipping out.

Low Tracheotomy

Step 1. The incision in this operation begins near the cricoid cartilage and extends downward for about 2 inches.

Step 2. Divide the fascia and expose the trachea. Ligate and divide vessels as they appear. Vigil is essential to discover any abnormal vessels crossing the operative field. (Fig. 467 A.) If the isthmus of the thyroid interferes with exposure pull it out of the way (upward). A study of Fig. 467A shows why

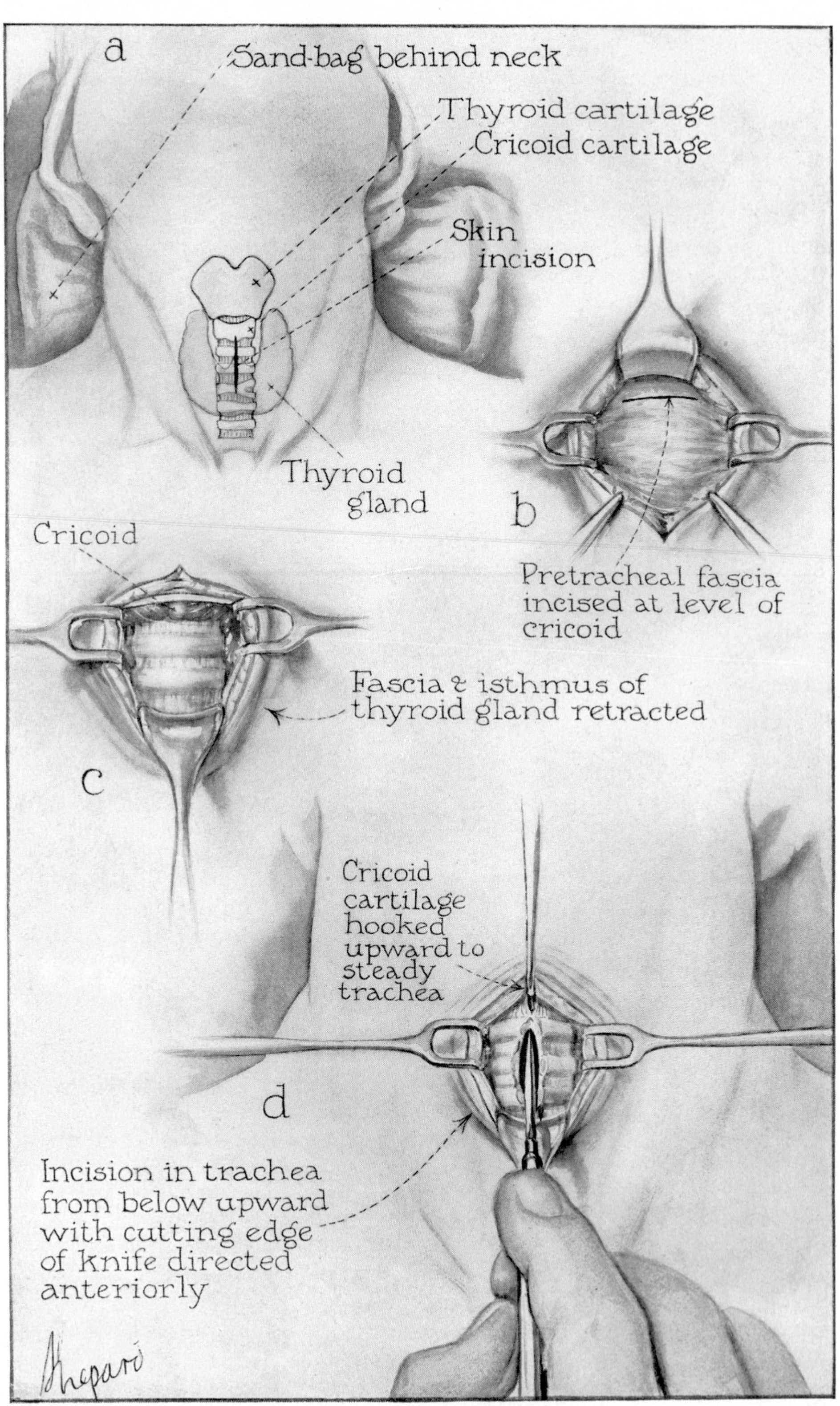

Fig. 464. High tracheotomy.

the low operation should not be used in children (vascular anomalies, deep position of the trachea, short necks, thymus gland).

The trachea is opened in the same manner as in the high operation. (Fig. 467 B.) Some object to high tracheotomy because of the possibility of laryngeal stenosis.

Comment. The inner tracheotomy tube should be frequently removed and cleaned. During the first few days after the operation the outer tube should never be removed except by the surgeon. The nurse or patient should never be permitted to remove the outer tube until the surgeon is satisfied that they are capable of replacing it.

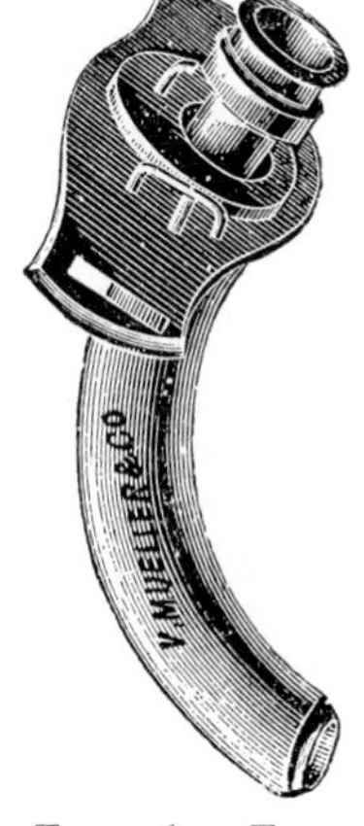

Fig. 465. Tracheotomy tube.

DIGBY'S TRACHEOTOMY TECHNIC

Step 1. (Fig. 468) Make an incision in the midline extending from the upper border of the cricoid cartilage and continued downward for about 1½ inches. Divide the cervical fascia longitudinally. Expose the cricoid cartilage.

Step 2. Make a transverse incision into the fascia attached to the lower border of the cricoid cartilage, thus exposing the beginning of the trachea (Fig. 469).

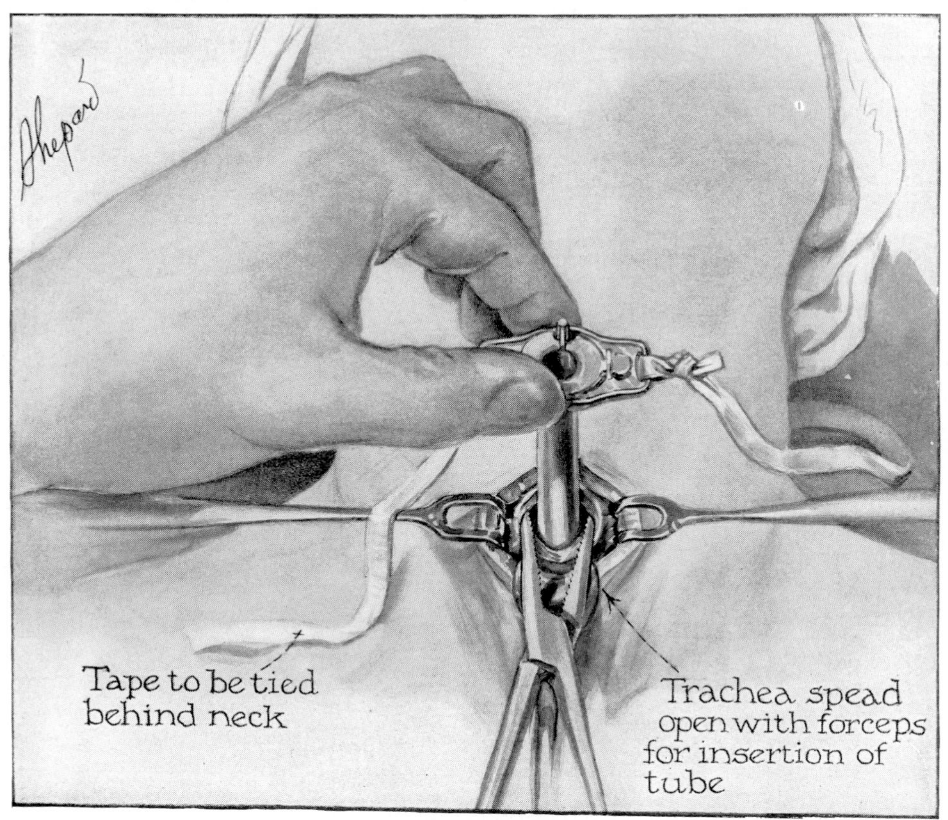

Fig. 466. Insertion of tracheotomy tube.

Step 3. Introduce the point of a closed artery forceps between the trachea and the isthmus of the thyroid gland. A to-and-fro motion of the slightly opened

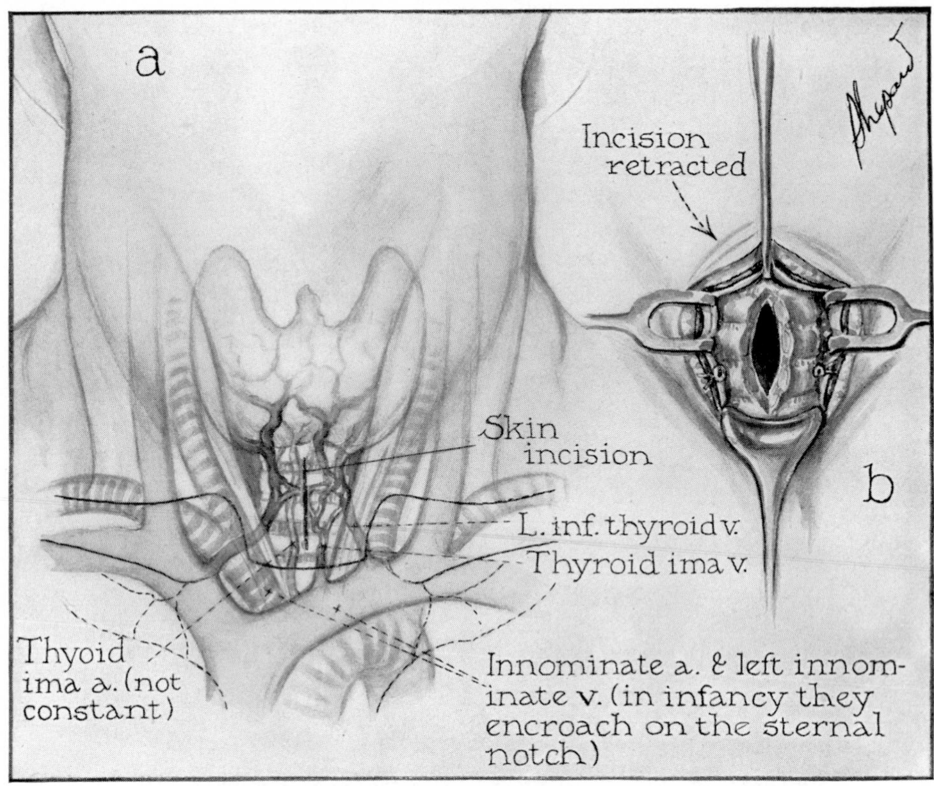

FIG. 467. Low tracheotomy.

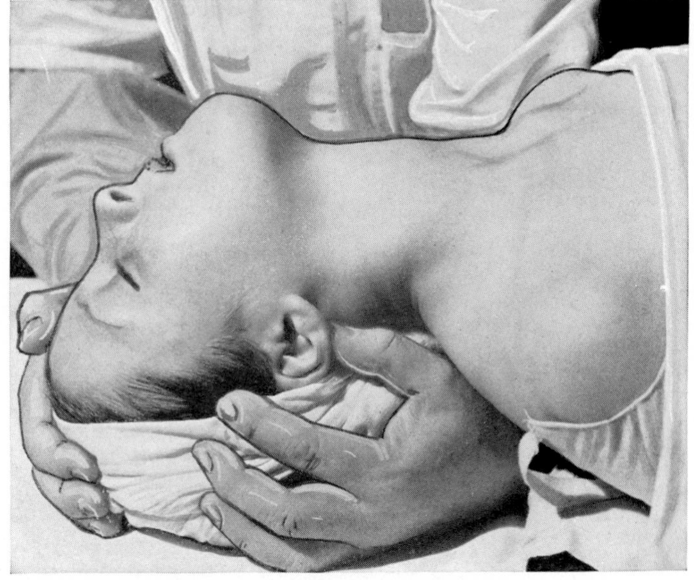

FIG. 468. Tracheotomy. The assistant standing on the patient's left, places his right hand on the forehead and his left on the occiput. He then fully extends the neck, and holds the head firmly in this position until the tracheotomy tube is safely placed. (After Hamilton Bailey.)

forceps will aid in its passage. The isthmic-tissue is raised and the hemostat is kept close to the midline. A second artery forceps is placed parallel to the first (Fig. 470).

Step 4. Divide the isthmus between the artery forceps and rotate these laterally to about 90 degrees; in so doing depress the handles of the forceps somewhat so as to raise the points of the hemostat, thus separating the tissues from the trachea; this is to be aided by a snip of the scalpel where necessary. The first four rings now lie clearly exposed.

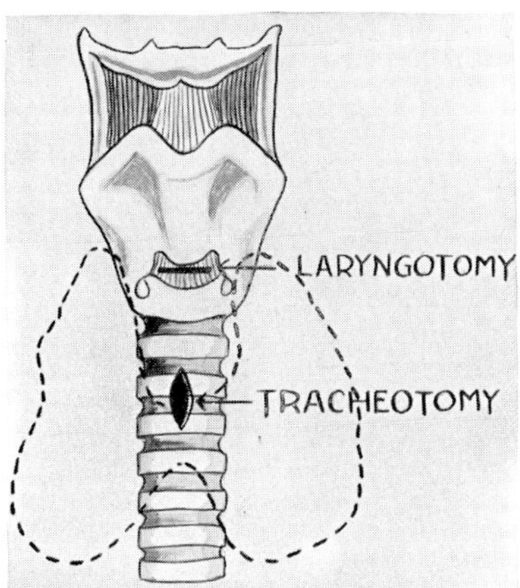

FIG. 469. Emergency openings of the trachea. (Hamilton Bailey.)

Step 5. Now make a vertical incision dividing the second, third and fourth tracheal rings. Pick up one edge of the wound in the trachea with a dissecting forceps, snip off one or two of the tracheal rings and repeat the procedure on the other side—an oval window thus results on the anterior surface of the windpipe. This is preferable to passing the tube through a tight vertical opening.

Step 6. Ligate the divided isthmus. Insert the tracheotomy tube as described above.

Step 7. Close the skin around the tube.

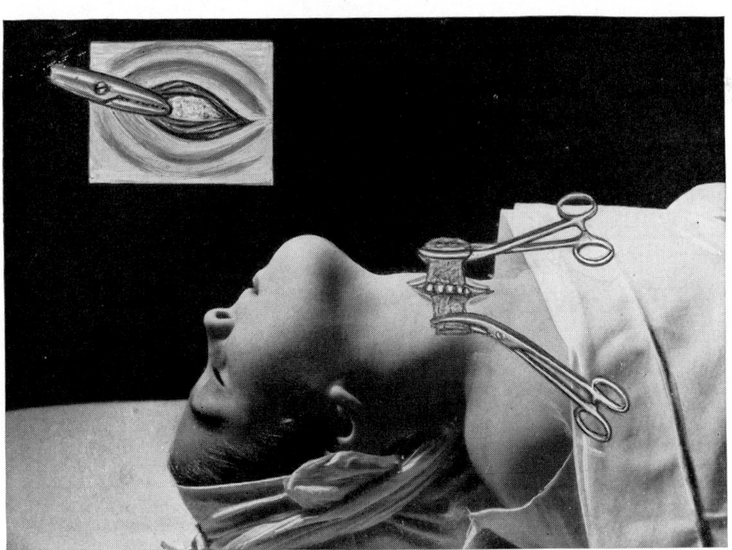

FIG. 470. The isthmus of the thyroid is divided between artery forceps and the trachea is exposed. The insert shows how an artery forceps tunnels the isthmus to separate it from the trachea. (Emergency Surgery, Hamilton Bailey, John Wright & Sons, 1936.)

ST. CLAIR THOMSON'S PROCEDURE—(TRANQUIL TRACHEOTOMY)

Sir St. Clair Thomson characterized his procedure in the following terms: "The calm with which this procedure takes place is in striking contrast with the agitated, hurried and often bloody and dangerous operation of former days."

The principal underlying the procedure is based on the elimination of the commotion which attends the first entry of air into the trachea. This is accomplished by the use of intratracheal infusion of cocaine which is accomplished as follows:

Step 1. Fill a hypodermic syringe with 20 drops of a 2½ per cent solution of cocaine for an adult; for a child, 5 drops of a 1 per cent solution.

Step 2. Lay bare the tracheal rings as described above. Grasp the syringe as you would a fountain pen, placing the forefinger about an inch down from the extremity of the needle. The middle, ring and little fingers rest on the patient's neck thus preventing the point of the needle from entering the lumen of the trachea for more than a quarter of an inch.

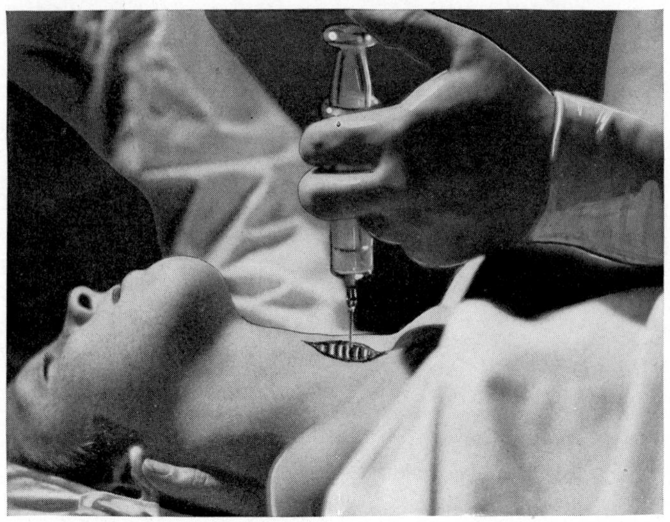

FIG. 471. Tranquil tracheotomy by injecting a solution of cocaine into the lumen of the trachea. (After Sir St. Clair Thomson.)

Step 3. Inject the cocaine solution into the lumen of the trachea (Fig. 471). Withdraw the needle briskly. Immediately upon the solution entering the trachea a slight cough is promptly produced which, however, does not cause much distress. If the condition is not urgent about ten minutes should elapse to allow the cocaine to take full effect. At the end of that period the incision can be made into the trachea and the tube inserted without spasm or cough.

Step 4. Complete the operation as outlined above.

TRACHEOTOMY IN DESPERATE CASES

Step 1. Extend the patient's head. Palpate the cricoid cartilage. Make the skin of the precricoid region tense. (Fig. 472.)

Step 2. Make a longitudinal incision exactly in the midline, about 3 inches in length.

Step 3. Lift up the larynx by placing a sharp hook under the cricoid cartilage which is steadied with the left hand.

Step 4. Direct the cutting edge of a narrow bladed knife toward the patient's chin and thrust the knife about half an inch below the cricoid cartilage, into the trachea. Extend the incision somewhat upward. Air will now rush into the opened trachea.

Step 5. Guide the point of an artery forceps along the blade of the knife into the opened windpipe. Spread the blades of the hemostat while the scalpel is withdrawn.

Step 6. Insert a tracheotomy tube. Release the sharp hook from under the cricoid cartilage.

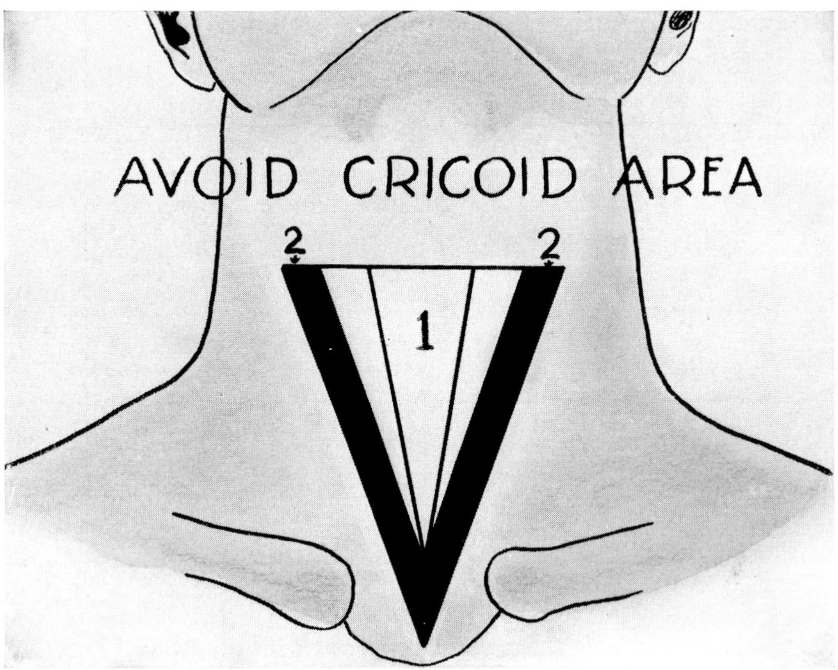

Fig. 472. Jackson's tracheotomy triangle: 1. safety zone, 2. danger zone.

Step 7. Close the wound. Dress.

Comment. In these urgent cases, waste no time in preparations. Procrastination often spells death. Act promptly! On occasion, the resourceful surgeon will have to depend upon a pocket knife and a tube. The desideratum is to get air to the suffocating patient as promptly as possible.

INTUBATION

(Tubage)

This operation was first recommended by Loiseau and Bouchet (France 1880). In England the procedure was championed by Sir W. Macewen and in America by O'Dwyer of New York.

Advantages of intubation.

1. No anesthetic is required.
2. No operation is performed.
3. Performance is rapid.

4. Breathing is continued through natural air passages.
5. Better results are obtained in children under five years of age.
6. Recovery is quicker.

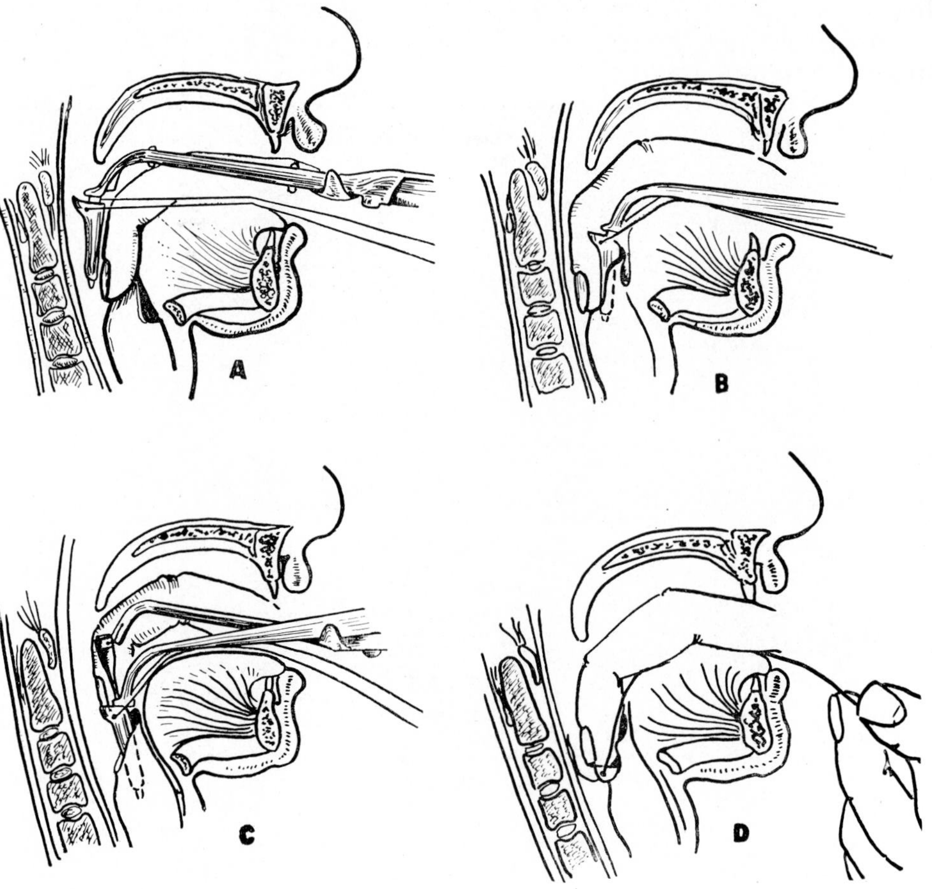

FIG. 473. Intubation. A. Elevate the epiglottis and draw the tongue forward with the finger directing the tube into the larynx; string in the tube. B. The tube is passed under finger. C. The tube is pressed into place with the finger and detached from the obturator. D. The tube is held in place by the finger.

Disadvantages.

1. Requires special training and instruments.
2. Must be performed quickly; respiration is embarrassed during introduction of the tube.
3. The tube may be coughed up or blocked; drainage is inefficient.
4. Complications are frequent (bronchopneumonia, ulceration, stenosis).
5. Exacting after treatment demands constant watchfulness.
6. Secondary tracheotomy is frequently necessary (about 30 per cent).
7. Tube difficult to keep in place.

The choice between tracheotomy and intubation depends upon the experience of the surgeon. Generally it may be stated that in selected cases with an experienced surgeon, the method is valuable.

In this procedure it is necessary that the surgeon's fingers be trained to recognize the epiglottis, the arytenoid cartilages and the laryngeal entrance since the hands place the tube almost entirely without sight.

Step 1. Fix the mouth open. Locate the entrance to the larynx with the left index finger which has been protected by bandages.

Step 2. Now place the left index finger on the posterior surface of the epiglottis to serve as a guide for the tube which is mounted on a special curved instrument and carried into the larynx where it remains in place without aid because of its length and shape (Fig. 473 A, B, C and D). The larger part of the tube rests below the cricoid cartilage and its funnel-shaped upper end on the arytenoepiglottidean folds.

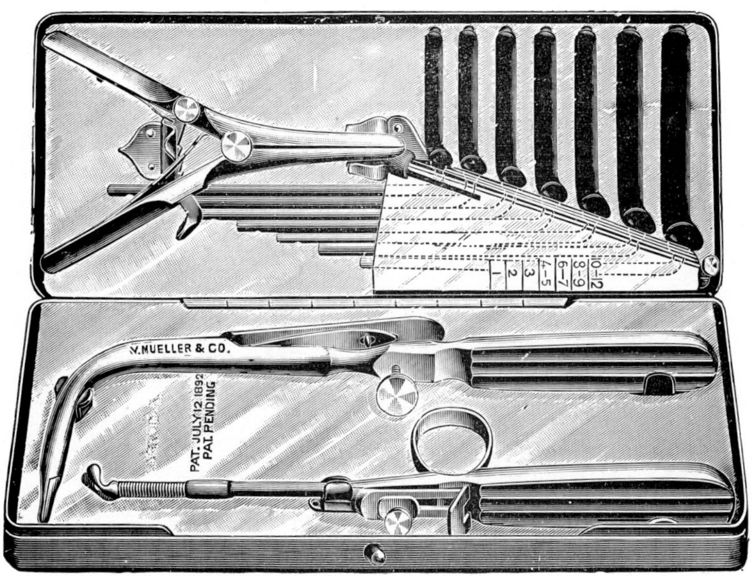

Fig. 474. Ermold-O'Dwyer's intubation set.

The instruments which are absolutely necessary are a mouth gag, an introducer and a laryngeal tube of proper dimensions. (Fig. 474.)

Comment. No anesthesia is employed. An assistant is necessary to help hold the patient and expedite the procedure. The patient is held between the knees of the assistant who sees that the body is kept in an upright position with the head on the assistant's left shoulder; the patient's hands are held firmly by the assistant. The surgeon takes his position on a stool facing the patient. The cannula is inserted alongside of the finger until it reaches the larynx (Fig. 473 A and B). At the first inspiration of the patient the cannula is inserted into the glottis and the carrier withdrawn (Fig. 473 C). The string which has been placed in the cannula need not be removed as it is helpful in removing the tube. In order to be sure the tube is properly placed, insert a finger after the tube has been placed in position; if the larynx can be palpated posteriorly, the tube is correctly placed. If not, the tube must be replaced. If the tube cannot be properly placed in three efforts, do a tracheotomy. It is usually left in about 4 days.

PHARYNGOTOMY

While the patient is lying on his back with his head extending over the operating table and a cushion under his shoulders, locate the hyoid bone and thyroid cartilage with the fingers (Fig. 475).

Step 1. Incise the skin transversely parallel to and directly under the hyoid bone (Fig. 476). An incision 2 inches long is adequate to expose the entrance of the larynx, but if there is a growth in the pharynx or upper larynx, the incision must be longer.

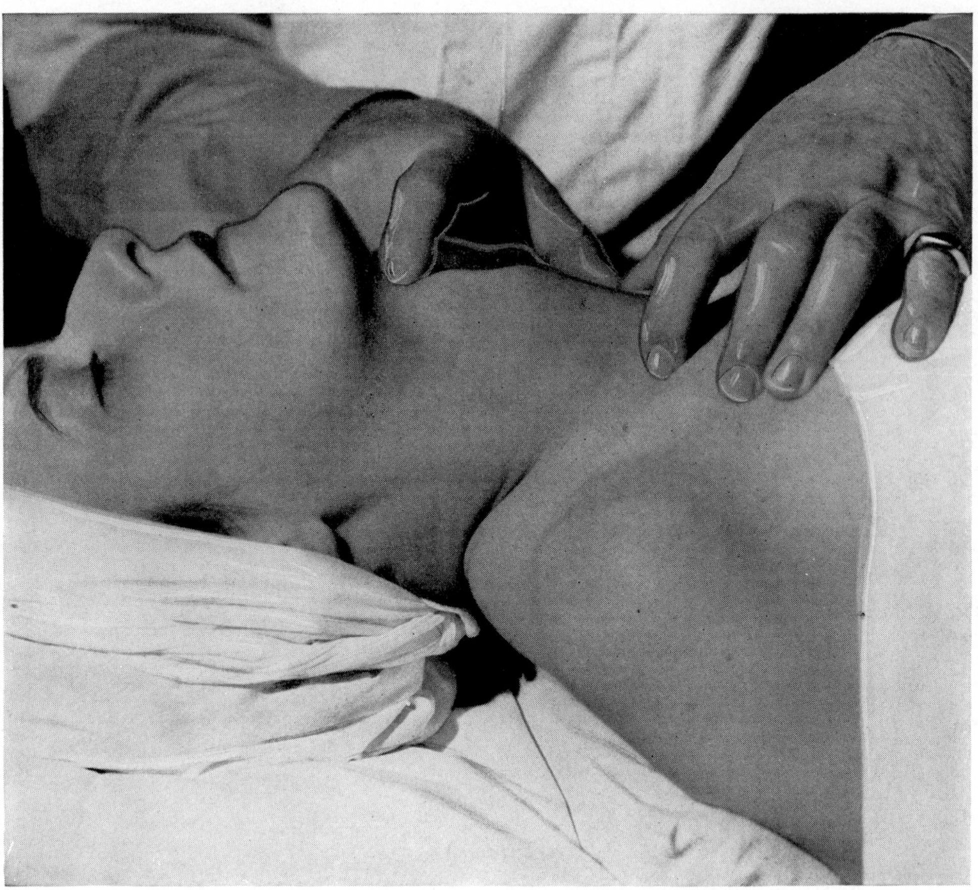

FIG. 475. Subhyoid pharyngotomy. Locating the thyrohyoid space.

Step 2. Incise the platysma myoides, omohyoid, sternohyoid and thyrohyoid muscles near the hyoid bone, permitting enough of their structures to remain so that they may be sutured (Figs. 477-478).

Step 3. With a cutting instrument directed backward and upward, incise the thyrohyoid membrane near the posterior surface of the hyoid, allowing enough of the membrane to remain for resuturing purposes. Check bleeding.

Step 4. While exercising care so that the epiglottis is not injured, grasp the mucosa with a forceps during expiration and incise it. In the upper margin of the incision, place two sutures of catgut to act as guides when the edges of the wound are being approximated. Place a suture in the epiglottis for the same purpose. Adequate exposure of the upper larynx or lower pharynx is now accomplished. In cases of malignancy of the upper larynx or if undue bleeding is expected, perform a preliminary tracheotomy. A foreign body or a tumor may now be removed, or the latter electrocoagulated.

Step 5. Reunite the incision in the mucous membrane with fine catgut sutures,

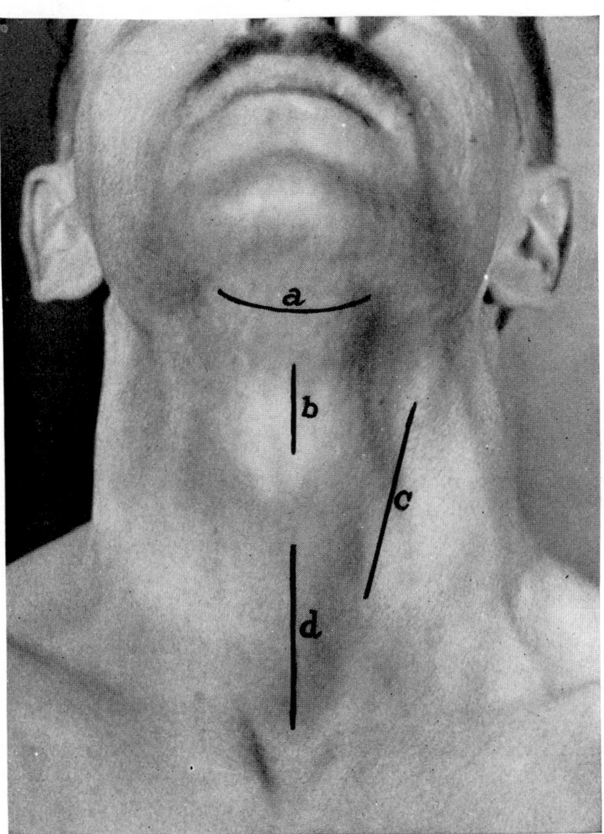

FIG. 476. Incisions used in some operations in the neck. a. Infrahyoid pharyngotomy. b. Cricothyreotomy. c. Lateral esophagotomy. d. Inferior tracheotomy.

uniting the thyrohyoid membrane, muscles and skin separately. Drain through gauze or oiled silk inserted down to the suture-line in the mucous membrane. If most of the pharynx has been dissected, fill the space with gauze and leave the incision partly open. In such cases a tracheotomy becomes imperative.

Transhyoid Pharyngotomy

Vallas advocates mesial division of the pharynx.

Step 1. Incise the skin, subcutaneous tissue and mylohyoid muscles in the midline from a point slightly above the hyoid to the notch of the thyroid.

Step 2. Completely expose a small piece of the hyoid bone in the middle and divide it by means of scissors or forceps.

Step 3. Create a space about 1½ inches wide by retracting the two portions of

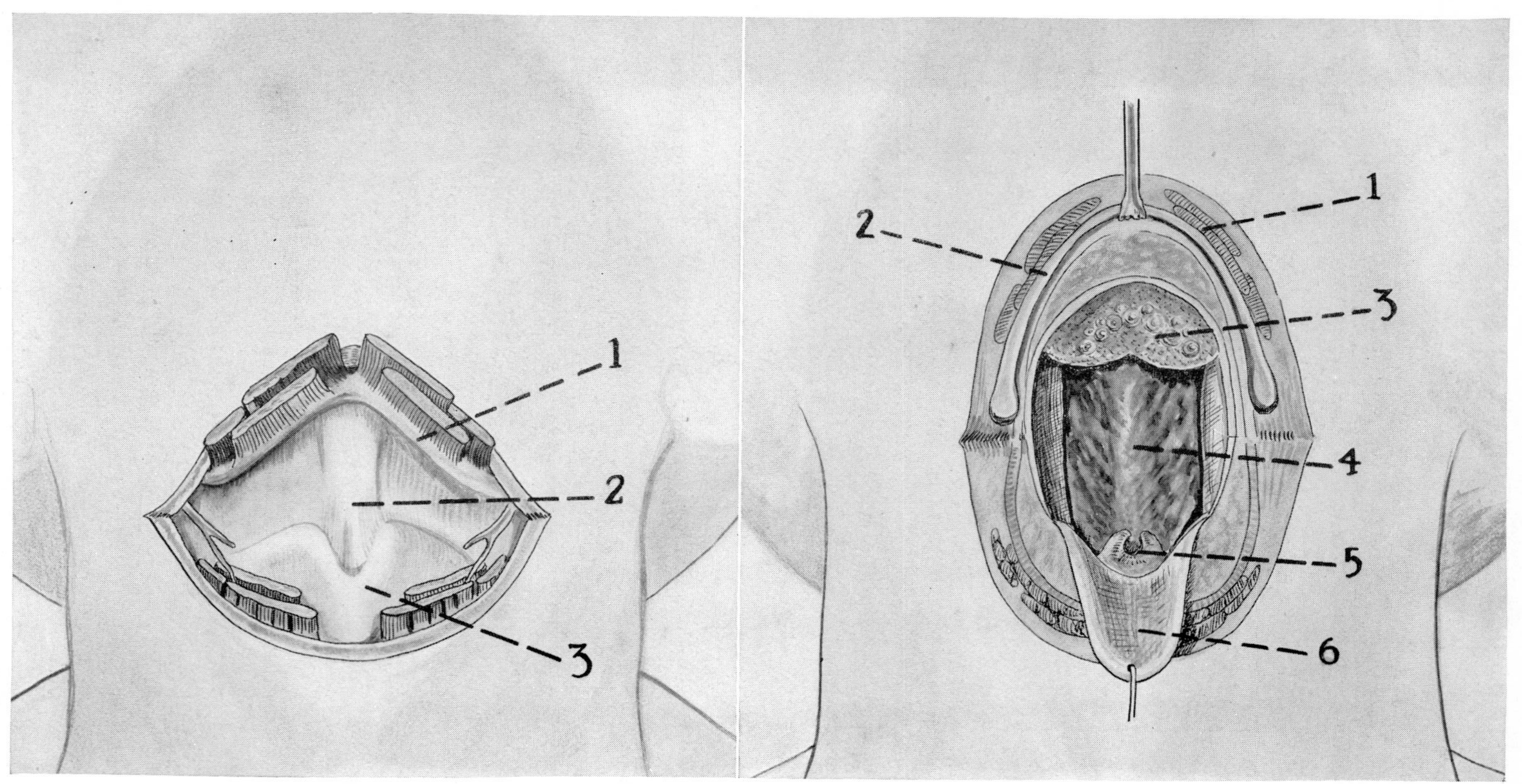

Fig. 477

Fig. 478

Fig. 477. Median subhyoid pharyngotomy: 1. hyoid bone, 2. thyrohyoid membrane, 3. larynx.

Fig. 478. Median subhyoid pharyngotomy: 1. subhyoid muscles, 2. hyoid bone, 3. base of tongue, 4. posterior wall of pharynx, 5. arytenoid cartilages, 6. epiglottis. (After Doyen.)

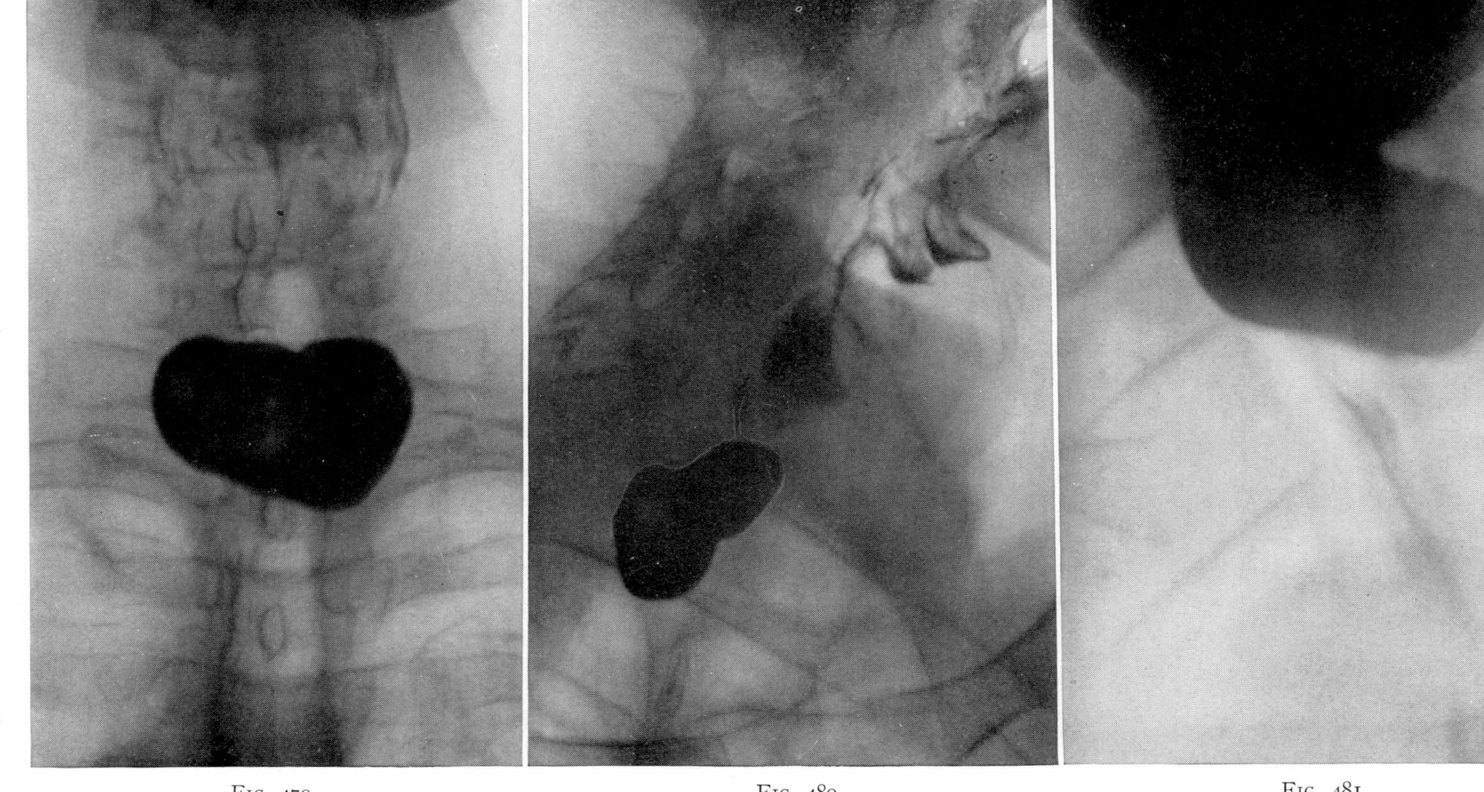

FIG. 479

FIG. 480

FIG. 481

FIG. 479. Diverticulum of the esophagus; front view.
FIG. 480. Diverticulum of the esophagus; lateral view.
FIG. 481. Diverticulum of esophagus; posterior view. (Author's Service, Cook County Hospital.)

the hyoid bone, thus obtaining exposure of the mucosa of the pharynx above and the thyrohyoid membrane below the bone.

Step 4. Incise the pharynx from above downward, being guided by a finger introduced into the pharynx through the mouth.

Step 5. Attend to the corrections which prompted the operation; provide appropriate drainage; suture the tissues in layers. The hyoid bone need not be sutured.

Suprahyoid Pharyngotomy

This operation is recommended by Ermitsch, Grünwald, Federoff and many others when tumors are present, particularly if at the base of the tongue and the epiglottis. No preliminary tracheotomy is required. The patient is placed on his back, his head falling backward over the end of the operating table; a cushion is placed under his shoulders.

Step 1. At a point a quarter of an inch above the hyoid bone make a transverse, concave incision upward including the skin and platysma.

Step 2. The submaxillary gland which now comes into view is drawn back. Protect the insertions of the digastric muscle. Separate the mylohyoids, geniohyoids and hyoglossi muscles by a transverse incision. The pharynx is incised carefully avoiding the epiglottis, and complete exposure of the pharynx, soft palate, tonsils, epiglottis and base of the tongue is accomplished. If it is necessary to operate on the base of the tongue, a sharp tractor is used to draw that organ into the wound.

EXTERNAL ESOPHAGOTOMY

This is indicated in cases of **foreign bodies** which cannot be attacked otherwise, also in treating strictures which are so situated that dilatation per os is impossible and in certain diverticula (Figs. 479-480-481). Where the indication is the removal of a foreign body, external esophagotomy should be undertaken within 24 hours after other modes of attack have failed. Do this operation where the up and down movement of the foreign body threatens to inflict serious injury or where bleeding forces the surgeon to prompt action. Periesophageal infections and symptoms of mediastinitis indicate immediate operation.

Infiltration, block or general anesthesia may be resorted to in approaching the esophagus in its cervical portion.

Strictures in the neck should be incised longitudinally so that healing takes place transversely thus widening the diameter of the esophagus. In strictures located below the upper thoracic opening the operation is performed for the purpose of permitting dilatation, also for dividing strictures located below the upper opening of the thorax through the esophagotomy opening. External and internal esophagotomy may be combined (see also Surgery of the Esophagus in Chapter on Surgery of the Chest).

Operation. This may be performed on either side of the neck but is usually done on the left side. Guard against injury to the recurrent laryngeal nerve (Fig. 482). If a foreign body is to be removed, its location determines the side to be operated upon.

Step 1. Make an incision along the front margin of the sternocleidomastoid muscle extending from the hyoid bone to the clavicle. The skin, platysma and superficial fascia are included in the incision.

Step 2. Draw back the sternocleidomastoid muscle laterally and the sternohyoid mesially. Incise the omohyoid muscle mesially to the carotid sheath, exposing the middle layer of deep cervical fascia covering the thyroid gland and permitting access to the esophagus (Figs. 482 and 483 A).

Step 3. Draw the thyroid gland, larynx and trachea to one side and the sternothyroid, sternocleidomastoid, sternohyoid muscles and large vessels to the other, exposing the inferior thyroid artery and the longus colli muscle in the background.

Step 4. Doubly ligate the inferior thyroid artery and divide it between ligatures, exposing the esophagus. Avoid injury to the recurrent laryngeal nerve between the esophagus and trachea; if necessary draw the nerve toward the middle with a hook.

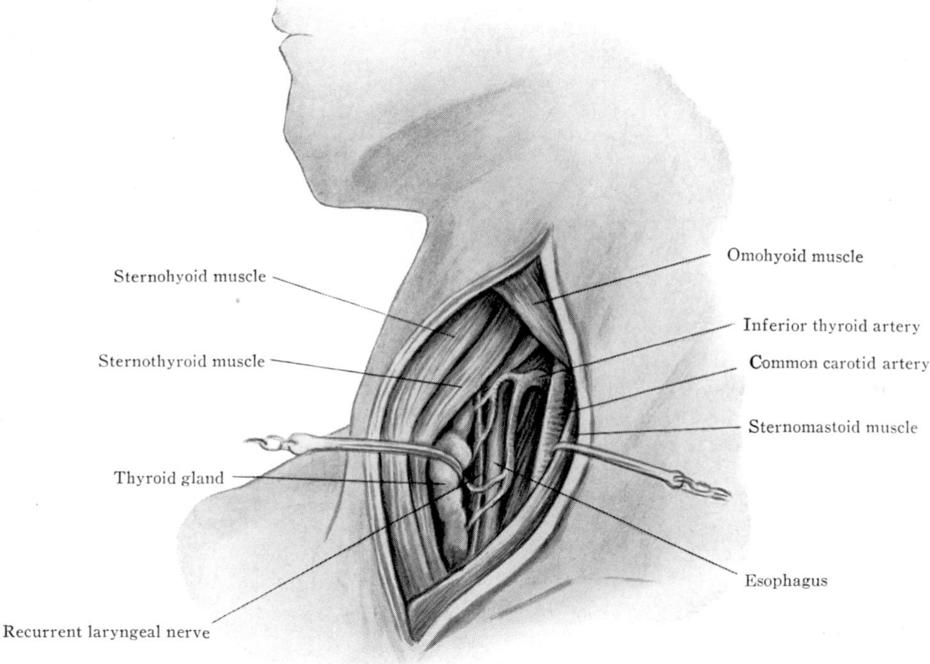

Fig. 482. Exposing the esophagus. (Davis' Applied Anatomy.)

Step 5. Incise the esophagus on its posterolateral aspect. The insertion of a bougie is very helpful. If a foreign body is to be removed, grasp and extract it carefully (Fig. 483 B).

Step 6. Introduce a stomach tube through the esophagotomy incision for feeding purposes. Place one cigarette drain in the esophagus below the tube and another in the direction of the mediastinum. Close the remainder of the wound in the esophagus in two layers. In some cases temporary gastrostomy may be indicated.

Leave the wound entirely open, changing the dressing frequently if symptoms of periesophageal inflammation are present. Remove the tube in about a week.

Apply a gentle compression dressing to the wound for a few days following the removal of the tube.

If during the manipulations little trauma has been inflicted on the esophageal wall, a double row of catgut sutures are used to close the wound. Suturing, however, is generally done under difficulties since only the more serious cases are treated by surgical means. Even though the incision in the esophagus is closed, thorough drainage must be provided for the external incision as well as toward

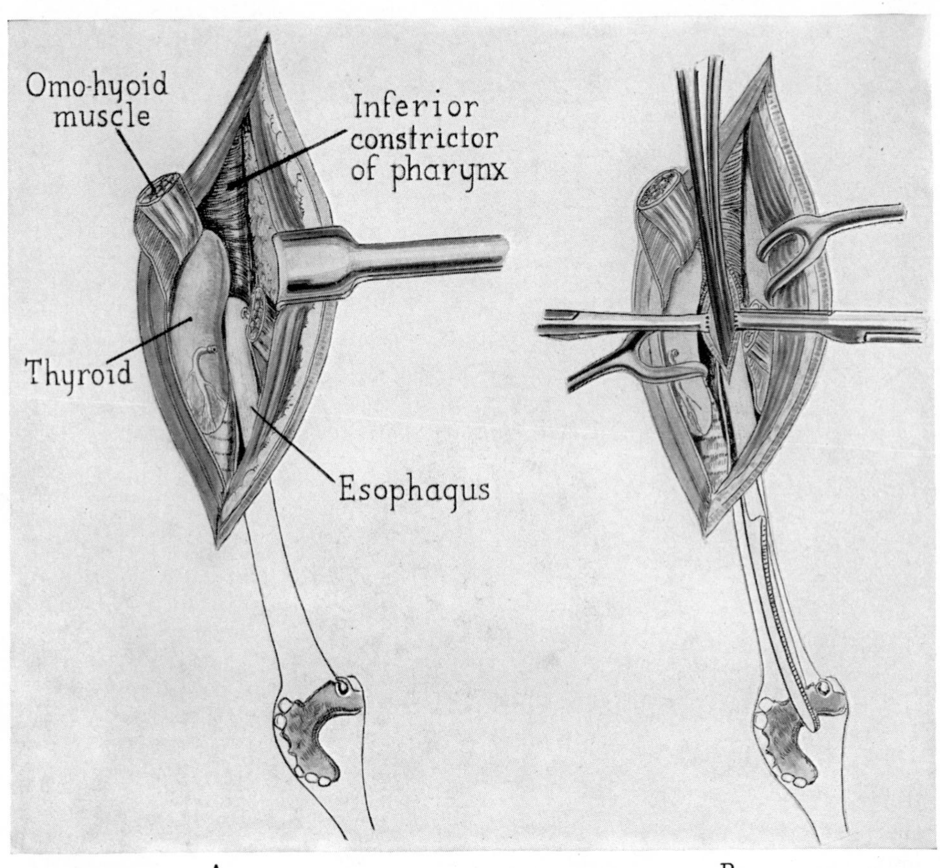

FIG. 483. External esophagotomy. A. Note the omohyoid muscle has been divided and the inferior constrictor of the pharynx exposed. The thyroid and the sternocleidomastoid muscles have been retracted to expose the esophagus. B. Removal of foreign body from the esophagus by external esophagotomy. Observe v. Graefe's instrument hooked beneath the dental plate pulling it upward (modified after Doyen).

the mediastinum. Hans counsels mesial incision of the esophagus following a median cutaneous incision in cases which can be sutured. He states that this is less difficult and the sutured closure less dangerous by reason of the trachea lying over it.

Dangers. Aspiration pneumonia, the result of anesthesia, swelling of the throat, the result of manipulations, and local inflammation and suppuration as well as mediastinitis may ensue following the operation. Metastatic abscesses or sepsis are possible sequels. Esophageal and mediastinal fistulae often close spontaneously but occasionally they call for surgical repair.

LARYNGECTOMY

Billroth performed the first laryngectomy for carcinoma of the larynx in 1873 (Fig. 484). Total extirpation of the larynx is usually called for when malignant disease is present to such an extent as to involve both lateral halves of the organ. Although in some technics it may be omitted it is more usual to perform a prior

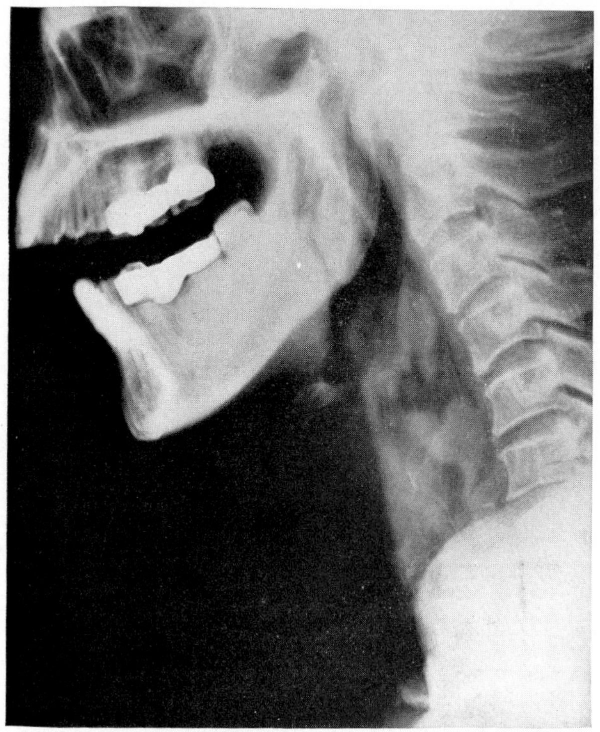

FIG. 484. Carcinoma of the larynx.

tracheotomy which may be done some days previous to or immediately preceding the main operation. The greatest danger in laryngectomy is not so much the immediate risk of the operation as aspiration pneumonia.

Median Thyrotomy or Laryngofissure

This procedure is indicated for diagnostic purposes, removal of foreign bodies or growths from the larynx or preparatory to some other operation; it is not a serious procedure. Complete exposure is obtained by dividing the anterior aspect of the larynx in the middle and separating it; the larynx is later sutured.

Hemilaryngectomy or Partial Laryngectomy

This procedure holds a median position between laryngofissure and total laryngectomy and may prove more dangerous than either. It is indicated in cases of chondritis accompanied by cartilage necrosis and malignancies which involve the subjacent cartilage. It consists of the removal of a portion of the larynx.

It may be performed under local (infiltration or block) anesthesia.

Total Laryngectomy

Step 1. Make an incision in the median line of the neck starting above the hyoid bone and extending to about an inch above the sternum (Fig. 485 a). The thyroid cartilage and tracheal rings are exposed (Fig. 485 b).

Step 2. Divide the isthmus of the thyroid gland in the midline and ligate the stumps (Fig. 485 c). The infrahyoid muscles are drawn back after being detached from the thyroid cartilage. Retract the sternohyoid and divide the sternothyroid muscles; retract the lobes of the thyroid gland from the larynx and trachea to the desired distance.

Step 3. Ligate the superior and inferior laryngeal arteries and branches as well as their related veins.

Step 4. A single median incision may suffice but it is generally advisable to make additional incisions above and below forming flaps which when drawn back facilitate dissection.

Step 5. Insert two strong silk sutures transversely through the anterolateral aspects of the trachea between the first and second rings of cartilage, then pass one end of each suture through the skin and clamp the loose ends in pairs.

Step 6. Incise the trachea above the sutures between the first tracheal ring and the cricoid cartilage, directing the instrument from the front to the back and from below upward, being careful not to injure the esophagus. The lower end of the trachea is dissected from the esophagus and drawn forward.

Step 7. Make a small transverse incision above the suprasternal notch. Make a tunnel by blunt dissection through the connecting tissue to the main incision.

Step 8. Bring the two pairs of sutures attached to the trachea through the transverse wound by means of an artery clamp, with the end of the trachea following. One suture of each pair is inserted through the adjoining skin on either side and tied to its partner; in like manner a suture is passed above and below. The trachea should be sutured as far down as possible.

Step 9. Insert a tracheotomy tube in the tied end of the trachea and continue anesthesia through it, thus protecting the lungs from aspiration (Fig. 485 d and e).

Step 10. Retract the margins of the wound and subjacent muscles; detach the muscles from the thyroid cartilage; the inferior constrictors to the posterolateral aspects of the larynx are cut; ligate the cricothyroid artery; sever the internal laryngeal nerves where they join the thyrohyoid membrane.

Step 11. If greater exposure is desired the thyrohyoid membrane is incised above the thyroid cartilage. The procedure from here on is determined by the individual involvements. Separation from below is generally preferred.

Step 12. Separate the tracheal stump and larynx from the esophagus by means of blunt dissection accomplished by the use of a forceps, blunt dissector, Mayo scissors and the fingers. This is an exacting part of the operation and should be done very carefully.

Step 13. Sever the inferior constrictors of the pharynx close to the thyroid cartilage. Detach the larynx from the esophagus at the arytenoid cartilages

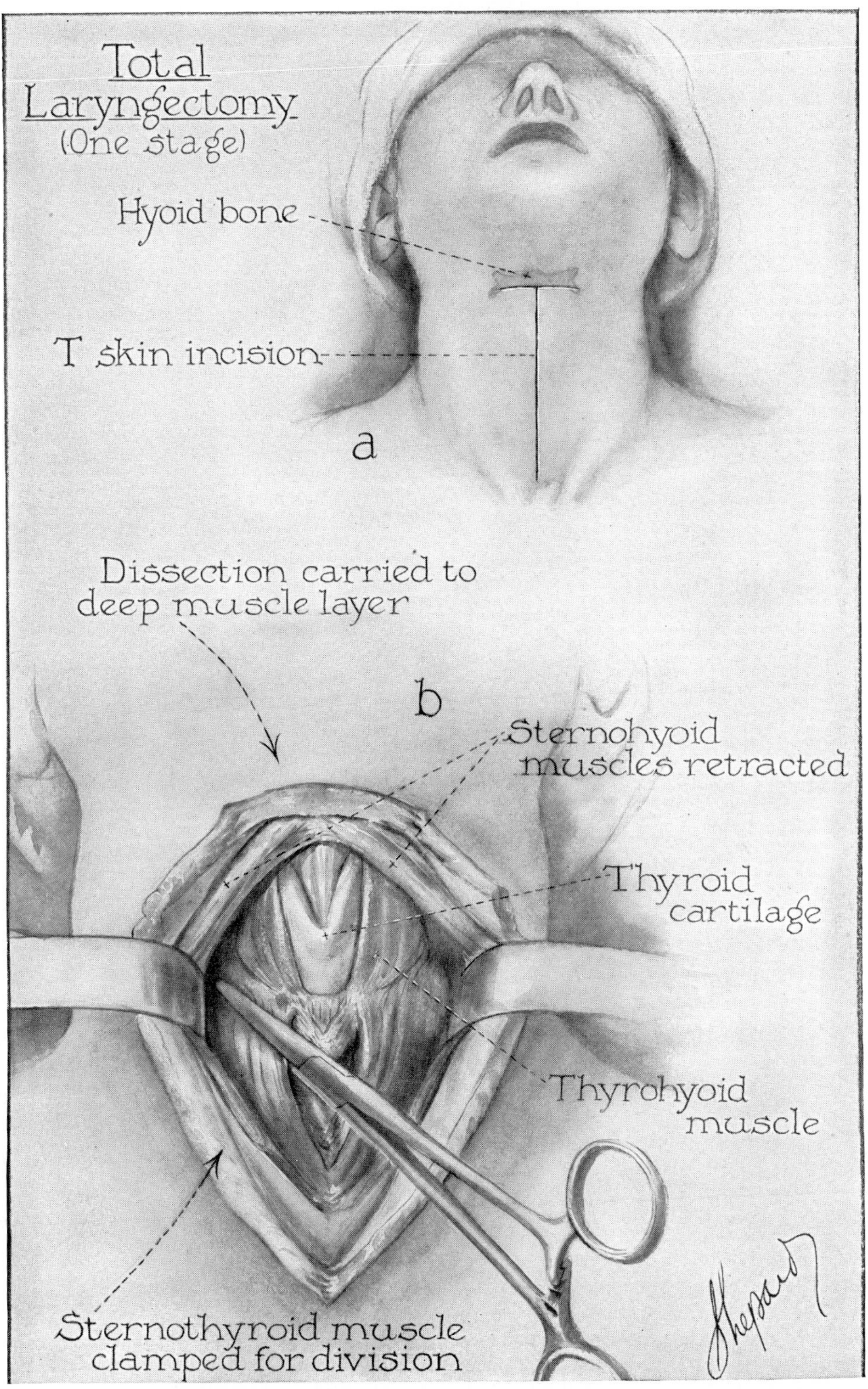

FIG. 485. Total laryngectomy in one step. a. T-skin incision. Note relation of the transverse line of the incision to the hyoid bone and extent of vertical line to the jugulum. b. The superficial tissues have been divided; skeletonization of the larynx has been begun by dissecting the superimposed structures. The illustration depicts the division of the sternothyroid and thyrohyoid muscles.

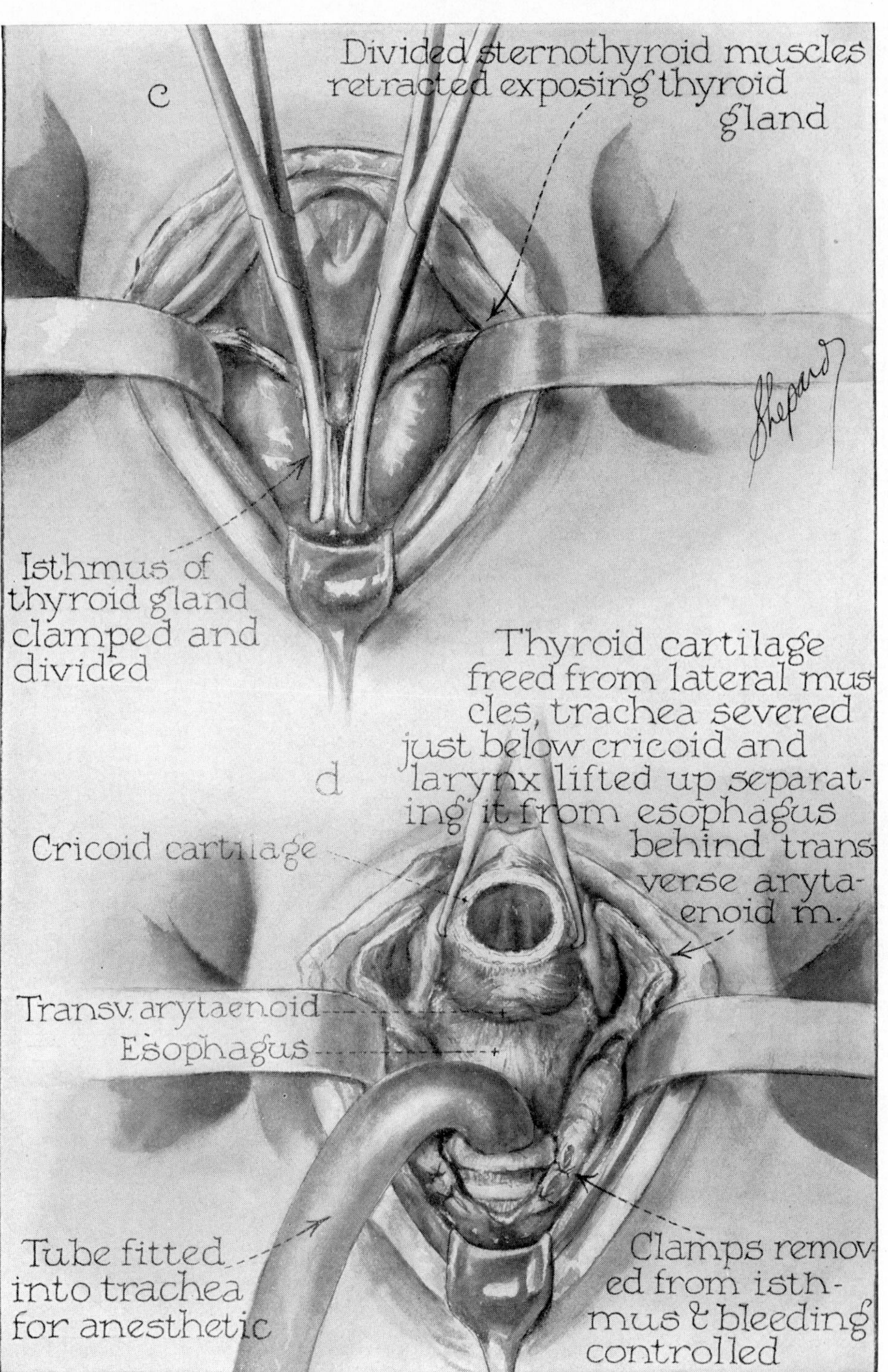

FIG. 485. Total laryngectomy in one step (continued). c. Strap muscles of the neck have been divided and retracted exposing the thyroid gland. Clamping and division of the isthmus of the thyroid. d. The thyroid cartilage has been freed from its muscular attachments. The trachea is severed just below the cricoid cartilage. The larynx is lifted up with hook and forceps and is separated from the esophagus and from the transverse arytenoid muscles in the back. A tube is fitted into the trachea for intratracheal insufflation anesthesia. e. The hypopharynx is opened between the hyoid bone and the attachment of the epiglottis. All arterial trunks have been ligated. The buccal cavity has been packed with iodoform gauze. A nasal tube is introduced for gavage (nasal feeding). Observe that during this step of the operation, the anesthetic is continued by intratracheal insufflation. f. The larynx has been severed from the

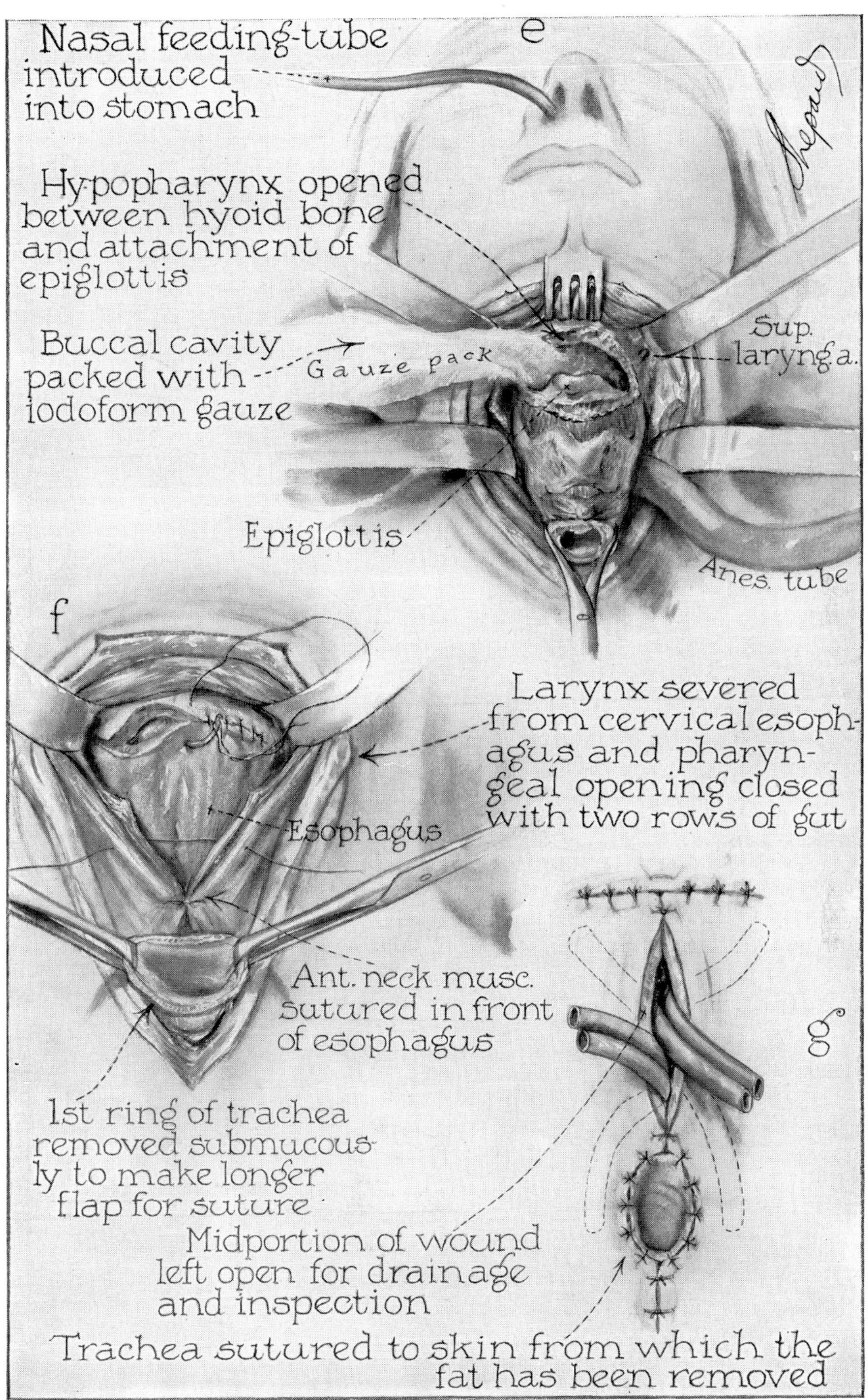

FIG. 485. Total laryngectomy in one step (continued). cervical esophagus. The opening in the pharynx is closed with two rows of interrupted catgut sutures. The strap muscles are reunited in front of the esophagus. The first ring of the trachea has been removed in a submucous manner to afford a longer flap for suture. g. Operation completed. Observe that the midportion of the wound was left open for drainage and dressings. Note the placement of the drainage tubes. The trachea has been sutured to the skin from which the fat has been removed.

(Fig. 485 f). Divide the pharyngeal mucosa transversely a half inch beyond the growth. Divide the thyroid membrane in front transversely.

Step 14. The epiglottis may be removed with the larynx which is dissected leaving the pharyngeal cavity open.

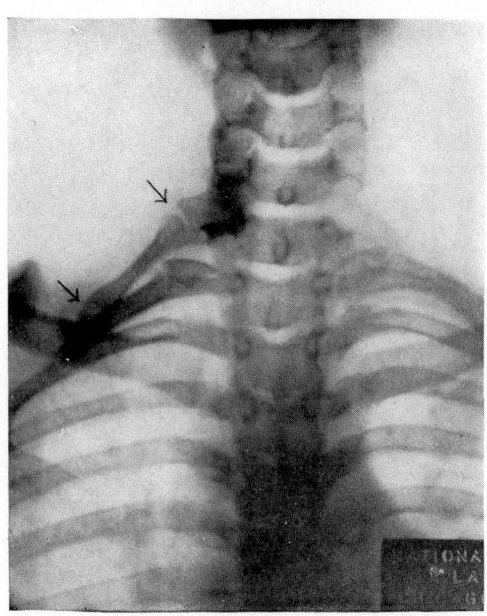

Fig. 486

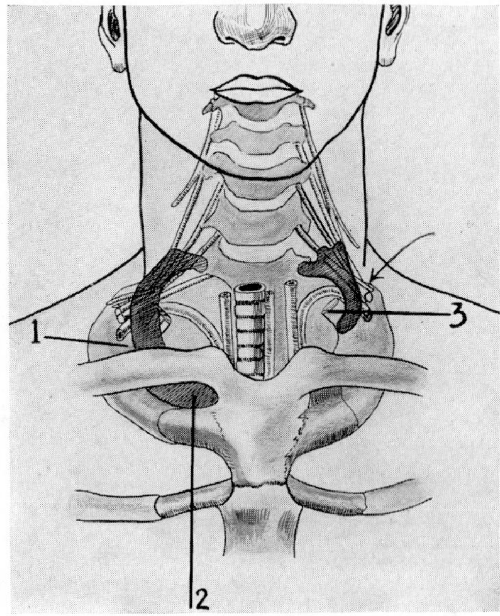

Fig. 487

Fig. 486. Cervical rib.

Fig. 487. Topography of cervical ribs: 1. first rib, 2. (shaded area) servical rib extending to the sternum, 3. scalenus anticus muscle. The arrow points to the direction of the pressure exerted upon the brachial plexus. The shaded area also represents the cervical rib (after Corning).

Step 15. Where it is possible to close the wound by suturing, the trachea is fastened to the lower part of the neck. Temporary drains are inserted (Fig. 485 g).

EXCISION OF CERVICAL RIB

Cervical ribs are unilateral or bilateral and are not of the same size. They are joined to the seventh cervical vertebra and in some instances terminate in the neck tissues; in other instances they are joined anteriorly to the first thoracic rib or sternum (Fig. 486). Ordinarily, there are no symptoms; however, in some cases the rib presses on the vessels or nerve-trunks passing over it (Fig. 487). If pressure symptoms do not respond to simple treatment, surgical intervention becomes necessary. Sometimes the connective tissue which extends beyond the rib is the source of trouble and must be excised.

Anterior Operation

Step 1. Approach:

(a) Make an incision beginning a finger's breadth over the clavicle and extending from the sternomastoid to the trapezius, or

(b) Make an oblique incision along the front edge of the trapezius muscle or slightly in front of it, or

(c) Make a vertical incision over the most prominent part of the swelling.

These incisions possess equal merit provided adequate exposure is obtained; it may be necessary, in some instances, to combine two incisions.

Step 2. Incise the platysma and superficial fascia; ligate the external jugular vein doubly and divide it between ligatures. Incise the deeper tissues so as to obtain exposure of the brachial plexus and large vessels. Carefully draw back the vessels and nerves lying over the cervical rib.

Step 3. Detach the rib from its tissues by means of blunt and sharp dissection; carefully avoid the pleura. Extraperiosteal excision of the rib is more difficult to perform than subperiosteal and seems to be somewhat superior. Expose a small middle part of the rib, divide it near the spine with a bone forceps, carefully cleaning away all sharp spicules adhering to the part left attached to the spine; divide the rib from its frontal attachment and remove it. Only the portion of the bone exerting pressure on the nerves and vessels need be excised, in cases where resection of the entire rib appears too difficult.

Step 4. Check bleeding. Effect closure of the wound by means of deep and superficial sutures.

Posterior Operation (Streissler's Method)

Step 1. Make an incision downward and parallel to the spine, beginning 2 cm. to the side of the spinous processes of the vertebrae and the width of a hand above the vertebra prominens and terminating the width of a hand below the vertebra prominens.

Step 2. Separate the trapezius, both rhomboids, serratus posticus and splenius; the complexus and semispinalis colli are also divided, thus obtaining exposure of the two lower cervical and two upper thoracic vertebrae, as well as the junction of the cervical rib and transverse process of the seventh cervical vertebra.

Step 3. Excise the transverse process exposing the neck of the rib, and divide it with a curved elevator, avoiding the nerve roots immediately in front of it.

Step 4. Grasp the rib with forceps and detach it as far as possible anteriorly by means of sharp and blunt dissection.

If removal of the rib proves too difficult on account of inadequate exposure, finish the operation through a front incision. The results, as a rule, are quite satisfactory.

Comment. Preserve, wherever possible, the posterior supraclavicular nerves; avoid the accessory nerve at the upper end of the wound. When mobilizing the sternomastoid muscle, pull it forward with the external jugular vein. When dividing the deep fascia, secure the transverse cervical vein as it passes over the posterior triangle where it merges with the external jugular vein. Free the posterior belly of the omohyoid muscle, displace it upward. Divide and ligate the transverse cervical artery where it crosses anterior to the brachial plexus. Be sure to identify the plexus at the lateral margin of the scalenus anterior muscle in front of the scalenus medius. In palpating the cervical rib through the scalenus medius, divide the muscles over the proximal portion of the rib, detaching them entirely from that structure. The rib is usually divided with its periosteum beyond the transverse process of the cervical vertebra. In clearing the rib forward and downward, free a layer corresponding to Sibson's fascia. Avoid injuring the pleura.

The front end of the cervical rib is generally attached to the first thoracic rib in the area of the scalene tubercle by bone or tissue fibers. To obtain exposure of this junction, carefully draw forward the lowest trunk of the brachial plexus and the subclavian artery. Divide the front junction and remove the rib.

In unusual instances where the rib reaches beyond the scalene tubercle, the rib may be excised at the level of the tubercle, since the front portion is harmless. In cases where pressure exists on the lower portion of the brachial plexus near the middle of the first thoracic rib, a similar procedure is followed. Expose the first rib; clear and remove the portion between the neck of the rib and scalene tubercle.

Control hemorrhage and apply a large pad of wool and a bandage to preclude a hematoma.

REMOVAL OF THE CERVICAL SYMPATHETIC

Anatomic and Practical Considerations. The cervical sympathetic is sometimes included in injuries of the neck; it is frequently compressed by a neoplasm, dilatation of an artery or an abscess. Motor fibers of the involuntary muscles of the orbit and eyelids, vasomotor fibers of the face, neck and head, dilator fibers of the pupil, accelerator fibers of the heart and secretory fibers of the salivary glands are furnished by the cervical sympathetic. Irritation of the cervical sympathetic results in the following conditions: wider opening of the palpebral fissure, exophthalmos, dilatation of the pupils, decreased perspiration, saliva and nasal secretion; the face and neck of the patient appears pale and cold. Its obliteration results in symptoms directly opposite those enumerated above.

Epilepsy, glaucoma and exophthalmic goiter have been indications for the removal of the cervical sympathetic. Jonnesco has been very successful in performing this operation in cases of exophthalmic goiter; he recommends it also in cases of hysteria, chorea and brain tumor. The cervical sympathetic is situated on the prevertebral fascia back of the carotid sheath and may be removed through an incision in front of the sternomastoid. Directly opposite the transverse processes of the second and third vertebrae appears the superior cervical ganglion whose branches extend upward near the external and internal carotid arteries, the ascending branch passing through its bony canal along the internal carotid artery in the base of the skull where the carotid and cavernous plexuses develop. The remaining tributaries form a communication with the cranial nerves, the pharyngeal nerves and the superficial cervical cardiac nerve. On the inferior thyroid artery opposite the sixth cervical vertebra appears the middle cervical ganglion; between the neck of the first rib and the transverse process of the seventh cervical vertebra is found the inferior ganglion.

The superior thoracic ganglia of the cervical sympathetic, which are four or five in number, emerge into the thoracic viscera, while the inferior, which are seven or eight in number, make up the splanchnic nerves and supply the abdominal viscera through the solar plexus. It should be remembered that the intercostal nerves originating from the spinal cord which correspond with the splanchnics which emerge from the ganglia and the ilio-hypogastric and ilio-inguinal nerves furnish the motor and sensory supply of the wall of the abdomen. Similarly, the same portions of the spinal cord furnish the abdominal viscera and their coverings of skin and muscle.

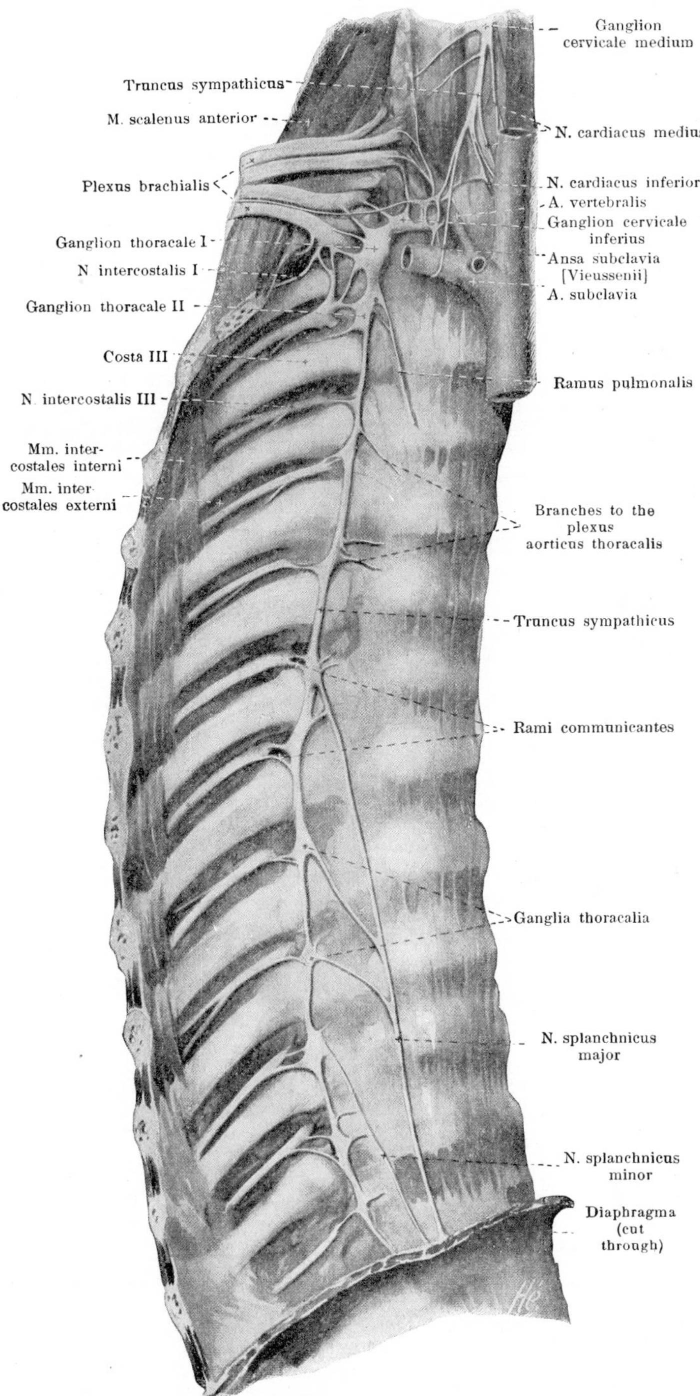

FIG. 488. Right sympathetic trunk in the thoracic cavity, viewed from the right and from in front. (The pleura and fascia endothoracica have been removed. Of the sympathicus only a few branches are drawn.)

The same pattern is followed by the nerves in the joints, the same nerve supplying the skin, joints and muscles, hence the sympathetic action of the joints under certain conditions. When a joint is inflamed in order to protect it, the skin becomes very sensitive, and the muscles stiffen making rest imperative. The abdominal muscles behave in the same way in case of inflamed viscera. (Fig. 488.)

Cervical Sympathectomy

Step 1. Make an incision beginning opposite the posterior margin of the mastoid process and continue it downward along the posterior border of the sternomastoid muscle to a point just below the clavicle. Divide the skin, superficial fascia and platysma. Ligate and divide the external jugular vein. Displace the sternomastoid muscle inward; expose by blunt dissection the common sheath of the exposed vessels (Fig. 520, page 444).

Step 2. Lift the unopened carotid sheath upward and retract it, thus exposing the cervical cord and superior and middle cervical ganglia. Isolate the trunk of the cervical sympathetic near the center of the incision and follow it up to the superior ganglion.

Step 3. Divide the communicating branches of the ganglion with scissors. Remove the ganglion with forceps.

Step 4. By making slight traction upon the distal end of the trunk, the cord is traced down to the middle ganglion; remove it in the same manner. Follow the main trunk of the sympathetic downward behind the clavicle to the inferior ganglion. Remove it. Exercise care not to injure the spinal accessory nerve and other important nerves and vessels in the vicinity.

Step 5. Unite with catgut sutures the separated muscles. Close the superficial wound.

Comment. Isolation and resection of the inferior ganglion is the most difficult step in the operation, as the ganglion lies deeply imbedded in a special pocket at the base of the neck or even in the thorax, behind the clavicle, against the neck and head of the first rib, between the scalenus anticus and longus colli muscles and just above the pleura. The trunk of the nerve should be used as a guide to the ganglion. It lies sometimes internal to, though rarely external to, the vertebral artery. The ganglion is adherent to the artery and enlaces it in a meshwork of its efferent and afferent fibers. To reach it, retract the scalenus anticus, the thyroid axis, and the vertebral artery and vein downward and outward; retract the sternomastoid muscle and the carotid sheath with its contents inward and forward. Divide the cellular and aponeurotic tissues covering the vessels and the ganglion. Isolate the ganglion from the vertebral artery externally and from the rib and spine internally. Isolate and divide the afferent and efferent fibers, and remove the ganglion.

Dangers.

1. Injury to the vertebral artery and vein.
2. Injury to the first intercostal artery or its cervical branch.
3. Injury to the subclavian artery, especially on the left side.
4. Injury to the pleura.
5. Morcellement may become necessary when the ganglion is friable.

6. Intimate union of the inferior cervical and first thoracic ganglia into one mass, from which a portion must be removed.
7. Injury to the retroclavicular venous plexus.

After the patient recovers from the operation performed on one side, the other side is operated on similarly.

TORTICOLLIS (WRY NECK; CAPUT OBSTIPUM)

There are several surgical methods to cope with this condition.

1. **Subcutaneous tenotomy** of the sternal and clavicular portions of the sternomastoid. (Fig. 489.) This operation is not much in vogue at

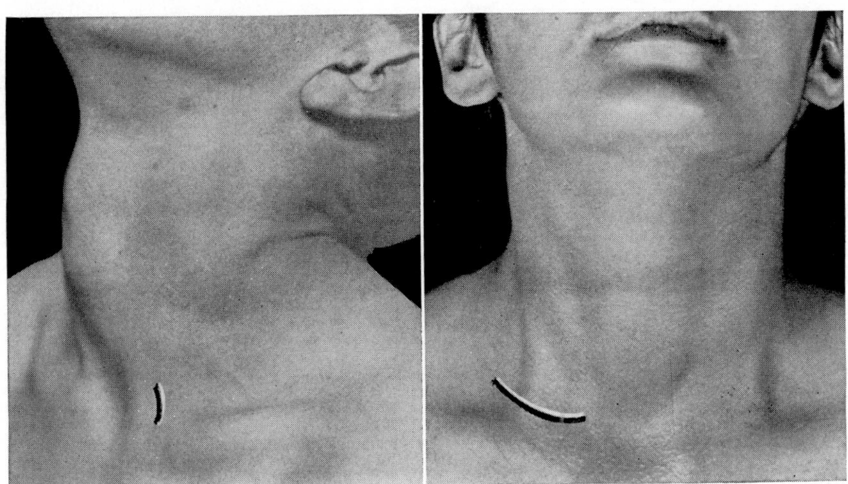

FIG. 489 FIG. 490

FIG. 489. Torticollis. Subcutaneous tenotomy of the sternal and clavicular portions of the sternomastoid.

FIG. 490. Line of incision in open tenotomy of the sternomastoid.

present; in its favor is the absence of scar, while against it appear the inadequacy of the procedure and its accompanying dangers.
2. **Open Operation.** This consists in dividing the constrictions and all fibrous bands which prevent rectification of the torticollis.
3. **Tendon Lengthening.**
4. **Mikulicz' procedure** which consists of excision of the degenerated sternomastoid.

In **spasmodic torticollis** the following methods may be used:

1. **Multiple myotomy** (Kocher).
2. **Finney's Operation** (see below).

Open Tenotomy of the Sternomastoid Muscle

Step 1. The tendon is divided ½ to ¾ inch above the clavicle; this is best accomplished by an oblique incision (Fig. 490). Begin the incision at the outer edge of the sternal attachment of the sternomastoid; the incision should be 1 to 2 inches in length and should extend upward and outward to the middle of the anterior margin of the clavicular portion of the muscle.

Step 2. Retract the wound thoroughly and expose both portions of the muscle.

Isolate and divide the attachments under visual guidance. The head of the patient should be rotated toward the sound side, thus putting all contracted structures on tension; these should be carefully divided.

Step 3. Attend to hemostasis. Close the wound. Dress.

Comment. Forcible overcorrection is advised by Lorenz before the patient comes out of the anesthesia. Retain the corrected or overcorrected position by an extension apparatus or by means of a proper dressing (plaster of Paris). Later resort to massage, etc.

Muscle Lengthening

This method is recommended by Thelwell Thomas. The object is to dispense with prolonged and tedious after treatment. No retentive apparatus is used.

Step 1. Make a transverse incision over the lower third of the sternomastoid. Expose the sternomastoid muscle and isolate its lower third. Compare for the degree of shortening on the affected side.

Step 2. Split the affected muscle longitudinally for a distance equal to a little more than half the amount of the shortening. Divide the anterior portion of the muscle transversely at the lower end of the vertical incision. At the upper end of the vertical incision divide the posterior portion of the muscle.

Step 3. Unite the ends of the muscle with chromicized catgut.

Step 4. Close the wound.

Comment. Besides lengthening the muscle, restraining bands should be thoroughly divided.

Mikulicz Operation—Myomectomy

In inveterate cases Mikulicz advised excision of the lower two-thirds of the sternomastoid, the upper one-third being preserved to avoid injury to the spinal accessory nerve.

Step 1. Expose and divide the sternal and clavicular portions of the muscle described above under open tenotomy.

Step 2. Grasp the divided ends of the muscle with forceps and pull these downward through the skin wound and while so doing, separate the muscle from its surroundings by thorough, blunt and sharp dissection. Avoid injuring the external jugular vein.

Step 3. When two-thirds of the muscle has been isolated, section and remove it.

Step 4. Attend to hemostasis. Divide all accessible cicatricial bands and close the wound. Dress. There is no need for postoperative orthopedic care.

Comment. Only one-third of the muscle is removed by Bruns. This operation should be reserved for severe or recurrent cases where all other methods have failed. The principle disadvantage of the operation is cosmetic disfiguration of the neck.

SPASMODIC TORTICOLLIS

John M. T. Finney and Walter Hughson made a study of thirty-two cases of spasmodic torticollis.[1] None were the common congenital and other acquired forms.

The disease derives its name from a sudden convulsive movement or spasm

[1] Annals of Surgery, 1925.

of one or more muscles or groups of muscles that move the head on the body. Not infrequently when one muscle or group of muscles—those primarily involved—are put out of commission by operation, the affection immediately manifests itself in an adjacent set of muscles, or may even involve the opposite side. This fact adds greatly to the uncertainty hitherto existing. Either for this reason or because incomplete operations have been performed, a comparatively large proportion of cases have required repeated operations before a cure has been effected.

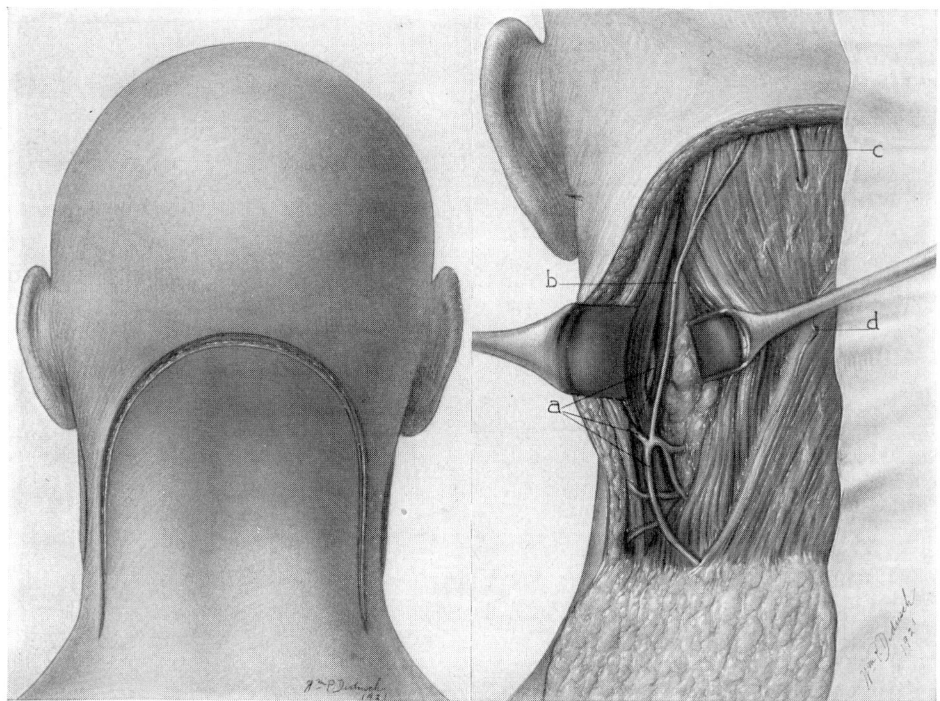

FIG. 491 FIG. 492

FIG. 491. Incision. Lower limit, level of angle of jaw; upper, 1½ cm. below occipital protuberance. (Courtesy of Dr. J. M. T. Finney.)

FIG. 492. a. Spinal accessory nerve; b. lesser occipital nerve; c. greater occipital nerve; d. third cervical nerve. View after skin and subcutaneous tissues have been turned back. (Courtesy of Dr. J. M. T. Finney.)

In a fairly large proportion of the cases maximum improvement was not attained for a considerable period—from six months to two or three years.

Finney Operation for Spasmodic Torticollis

Step 1. Make an incision along the posterior border of the sternomastoid muscle (Fig. 491), beginning at a point two finger-breadths below the level of the angle of the jaw and continuing upward along the edge of the muscle to a point about the level of the lobe of the ear, then curving over toward the midline to a point about two finger-breadths below the occipital protuberance, thence carried across the midline, following the same general direction as just described, in reverse order. When completed, the incision is in the form of an inverted "U."

Step 2. Reflect the flap of skin and subcutaneous tissue, taking care to identify and avoid the lesser occipital nerve which is quite superficial and lies along the posterior border of the sternomastoid muscle in its upper half. Having exposed and identified this nerve, follow it down to the point where it emerges from behind the posterior border of the sternomastoid muscle (Fig. 492).

Step 3. By retracting the sternomastoid muscle, the anterior divisions of the second, third and fourth cervical nerves now come into view together with the chain of deep cervical lymph nodes.

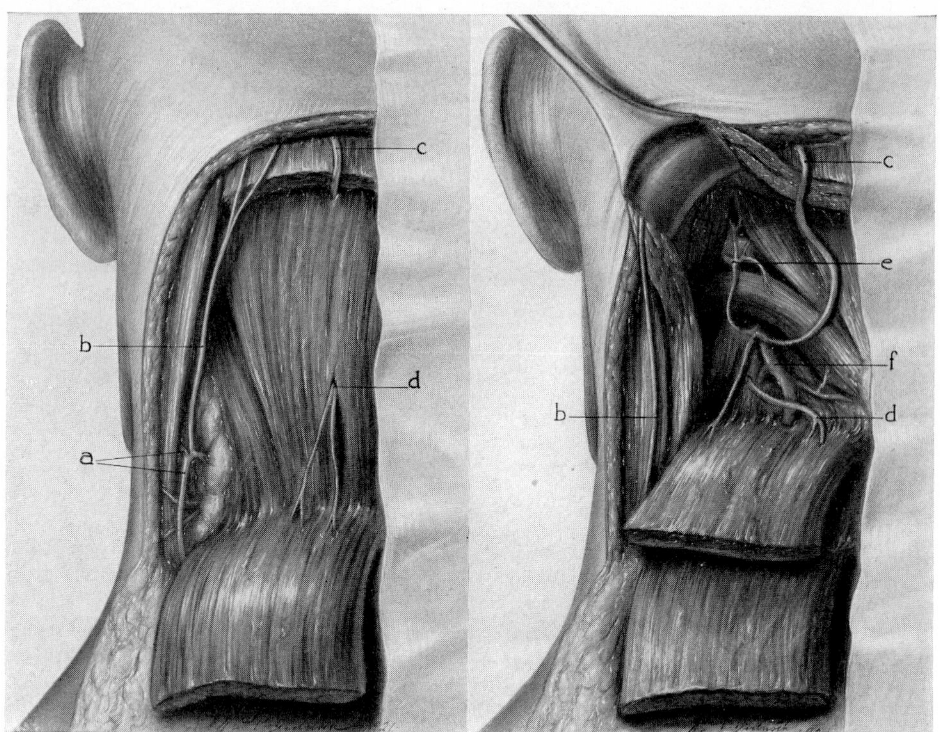

FIG. 493 FIG. 494

FIG. 493. a. Spinal accessory nerve; b. lesser occipital nerve; c. greater occipital nerve; d. third cervical nerve. Splenius and trapezius muscles have been divided and turned back.

FIG. 494. b. Lesser occipital nerve; c. greater occipital nerve; d. third cervical nerve; e. first occipital nerve; f. branch of venous plexus. All posterior muscles have been divided and turned back, exposing the suboccipital triangle. (Courtesy of Dr. J. M. T. Finney.)

Step 4. A little further in front of the nerve plexus, and consequently a little deeper in the wound, will be found the trunk of the spinal accessory nerve at the point where it emerges from the body of the muscle. The nerve having now been definitely identified (and here, as with all other nerve trunks involved, direct stimulation with a bipolar electrode makes the identification absolute) it can be resected at any point desired. No effort should be made to save the sensory branches of these nerves as, in Thomas' opinion, both efferent and afferent pathways should be interrupted.

Step 5. Search should next be made for the great occipital nerve where it emerges through the fibers of the splenius, about one cm. from the midline and just beneath the skin incision. Having identified this nerve, divide transversely at this point the trapezius and splenius muscles (Fig. 493), exposing the fibers of the complexus which is easily recognized.

Step 6. The fibers of this muscle are divided in turn through its whole thickness in the same planes as the skin incision, and it is then reflected backward in the same way, care being taken all the while to preserve the great occipital nerve which lies immediately below it. This exposes the two recti muscles (major and minor), and the superior and inferior oblique (Fig. 494), each of which can be distinguished by the direction of its fibers and their common point of origin.

Step 7. The trunk of the great occipital nerve should then be traced down to the point where it emerges from the vertebral foramen at the lower border of the inferior oblique muscle. At this point will be found its anastomosis with the suboccipital nerve running across the body of the muscle to the point where it is given off from the first cervical nerve in the suboccipital triangle. The great occipital nerve should be resected below the point of anastomosis with the suboccipital nerve.

Step 8. The suboccipital nerve can be traced out in the suboccipital triangle as it emerges between the vertebral artery lying deep in the triangle and the upper border of the inferior oblique muscle. Its branches to the recti muscles and the superior and inferior oblique muscles are given off here, and the main trunk of the nerve can be readily resected at this point. Care should be taken not to injure the vertebral artery which can be identified as it lies on the floor of the triangle.

Step 9. The splenius and complexus muscles should be reflected sufficiently to allow the exposure of the third cervical nerve where it emerges a fingerbreadth below the great occipital. At the level of the second and third cervical nerves is located a venous plexus of considerable size which may give rise to troublesome bleeding if care is not taken to avoid or control it, which, however, can be readily done. The third cervical nerve should be resected where it emerges from the vertebral foramen as it supplies fibers to the overlying muscles (splenius, trapezius and complexus).

Step 10. After the trunks of the upper three cervical nerves have been resected as described, the muscles may be replaced, layer by layer, and held in place by a few stitches, and the wound closed in the usual manner. In the earlier operations, portions of these muscles were excised, but subsequent experience has shown that with complete resection of the nerve-supply this rather mutilating procedure may be omitted. Formerly a drain, consisting of a small piece of protective, was always inserted at each corner of the incision, but with adequate hemostasis this is probably unnecessary.

At one time Finney applied a plaster of Paris bandage reinforced with wooden splints but this added greatly to the patient's discomfort and so was discontinued in favor of the ordinary gauze dressing and soft bandage, reinforced with light wooden coaptation-splints if desired. Notwithstanding the great extent of the wound, he has found the healing to be uniformly satisfactory and the resulting disability surprisingly slight.

The Spurling-Jelsma Technic in Spasmodic Torticollis

R. Glenn Spurling and Franklin Jelsma[1] point out:

While it is true that there are many reports in the literature commending the treatment of psychoanalysis and medical measures, such reports have been, on the whole, unconvincing.

There are cases in which the spasmodic contractures seem to be sharply limited to one sternocleidomastoid muscle or perhaps one sternocleidomastoid and one trapezius muscle. While cases of this sort are rare, yet they do occur, and a unilateral section of the spinal accessory nerve may effect a cure. Judging from the reports of some authors, it would seem that improvement is likely to be temporary because the spasmodic contractures soon develop on the opposite side or in the other muscles of the neck on the same side.

Spurling and Jelsma believe that all of the muscles of the neck are involved in severe cases; and nothing short of the radical intervention will suffice to relieve the symptoms. This attitude is the one held by the majority of surgeons who have written in recent years upon the treatment of this malady. The Keen operation forms the basis of treatment now generally employed. Finney and Hughson in 1925 described an operation which is a great improvement upon the original Keen procedure. It consists of sectioning the first three cervical nerves and the spinal accessory nerve bilaterally, also the division of most of the posterior neck muscles attached to the occipital bone. Their results in a series of thirty-two cases were highly satisfactory.

In 1924, McKenzie, from Cushing's clinic, reported the intradural section of the first, second and third cervical nerves and the spinal accessory nerve on one side for the relief of a severe case of spasmodic torticollis. In this report, a statement by Dr. Cushing indicated that as early as 1902 he had performed an intradural section of the first and second cervical nerves in the treatment of a case of this disease.

Coleman, in 1927, reported the first case in which the first four cervical posterior roots on both sides were sectioned intradurally. He resected the spinal accessory nerves in the neck at the secondary operation. The result in his case was highly satisfactory.

Since McKenzie's report appeared, neurosurgeons generally have adopted the intraspinal operation as the method of choice. The result seems more satisfactory than that by any other procedure heretofore employed.

The only variation in the technic of the intradural operation is that some authors advise cutting the spinal portion of the accessory nerve intradurally, while others prefer to section the nerve in the neck. Spurling and Jelsma believe that the operation can be performed safely by division of all the nerves, viz., the first three cervical anterior and posterior roots and the spinal portion of the accessory nerve intradurally. Thus, the entire procedure can be completed in one session through one operative incision. It is unnecessary to remove a part of the occipital bone as originally advised by McKenzie in order to section the accessory nerve. Inasmuch as

[1] South. Med. Jour., March, 1933.

we are concerned only with the spinal portion of the nerve, it can be divided easily through the dural incision at the level of the foramen magnum. It is unnecessary to section the cerebral portion of the accessory nerve, since it plays no part in the disease.

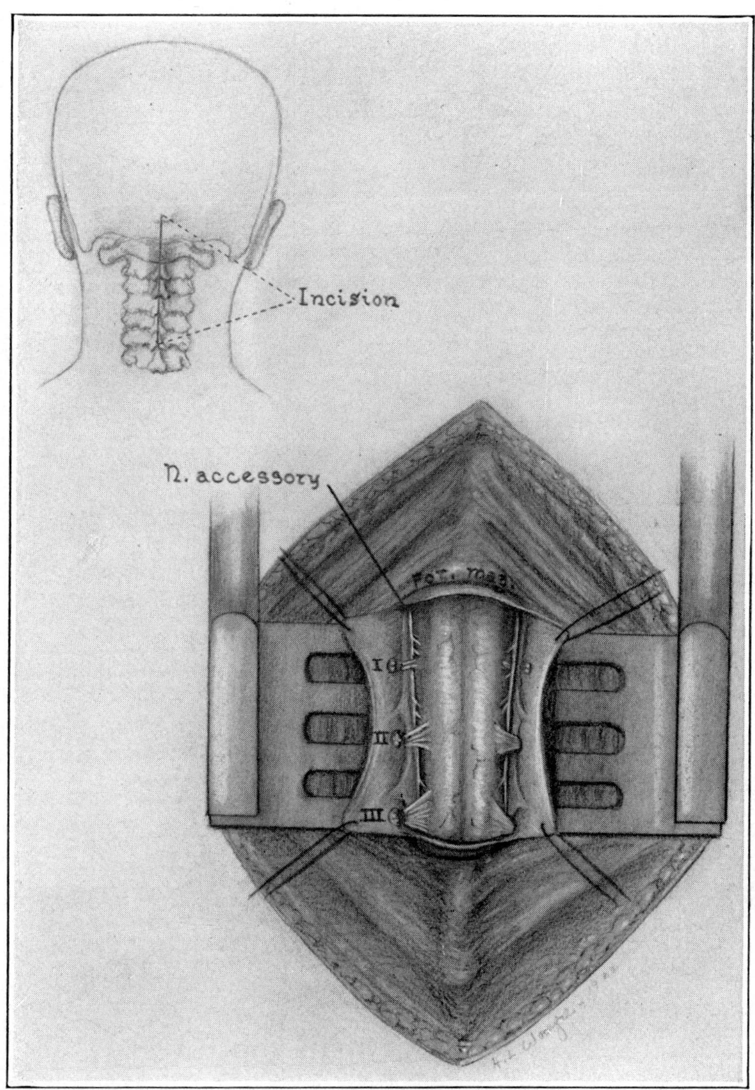

FIG. 495. Spurling-Jelsma operation. First, second and third posterior roots are shown on the left side. On the right side, the first posterior root is absent. The trunk of the spinal portion of the accessory nerve is shown bilaterally. Insert shows line of skin incision.

Step 1. Make a midline incision from the occipital protuberance to the spinous process of the fifth cervical vertebra. Free the muscles and periosteum from the spinous processes and the base of the occipital bone. Remove the laminae of the upper three cervical vertebrae.

Step 2. Open the dura mater in the midline over the first three cervical segments and extend the incision upward to the rim of the foramen magnum, being careful to avoid the cerebellar dural sinus.

Step 3. Identify and section the posterior and anterior roots of the first three cervical nerves. (Often the posterior root of the first cervical nerve is absent.) Identify the filaments of the spinal portions of the eleventh nerve between the posterior and anterior cervical roots. Where these filaments unite to form the spinal part of the accessory nerve, a small artery is seen. Apply silver clips to include the artery and nerve trunk before cutting the nerve (Fig. 495).

Step 4. Close the dura and neck muscles with layers of interrupted silk sutures. Immobilize the patient's head for the first two days with sandbags. After this the patient should turn his head from side to side, gradually strive to support it while sitting in bed and after two weeks start active motion of the neck muscles.

Spurling and Jelsma comment as follows:

"Convalescence in the two cases which we have treated by this method has been rapid and uneventful. Spasmodic contractures disappeared immediately following the operation. At first, the patient will complain of considerable difficulty in supporting the head. In both instances the patients have been able to walk around with little or no discomfort after four weeks. In the first patient, upon whom we operated eight months ago, the weakness and fatigue of the neck muscles have entirely disappeared, although he still recognizes the fact that movements of the head and neck are limited considerably.

"The choice of which radical operation should be used in the treatment of severe spasmodic torticollis seems to us to be one of individual preference, because both the Finney operation and the intradural operation seek to accomplish the same end. We believe that the intradural operation is by far the simpler procedure, provided the operator is accustomed to intraspinal operations. The mortality for either operation should be practically nil. It seems to us that there is more likelihood of missing important nerve roots by the Finney operation than by the intradural approach. There again, such a contingency would depend largely upon the skill and experience of the individual operator. When the Finney operation is employed, there is always the possibility of regeneration of the nerves after section outside the spinal cord. This possibility does not occur when the nerves are sectioned intradurally."

CYSTS AND TUMORS OF THE NECK

REMOVAL OF TUMORS OF THE NECK IN GENERAL

Removal of tumors of the neck requires mature surgical judgment and experience. It is beset with many pitfalls and dangers. Beginners and those of limited experience tred dangerous ground in undertaking removal of tumors of the neck.

"Block dissection" of the tumor and regional lymph nodes is the goal. In other words, an attempt is made to dissect out the neoplasm and its lymph apparatus en bloc (Fig. 497).

Dangers of the Operation.

1. **Hemorrhage.** Careful dissection and ligation of vessels as encountered will do much to minimize bleeding.
2. **Air Embolism.** We must remember that during inspiration the blood in the cervical veins is under negative pressure and that, under these circumstances, if a vein is injured, air may be sucked into the vessel and through it into the heart with fatal results. This may be obviated by painstaking technic and prompt action should the accident occur (salt solution; pressure).

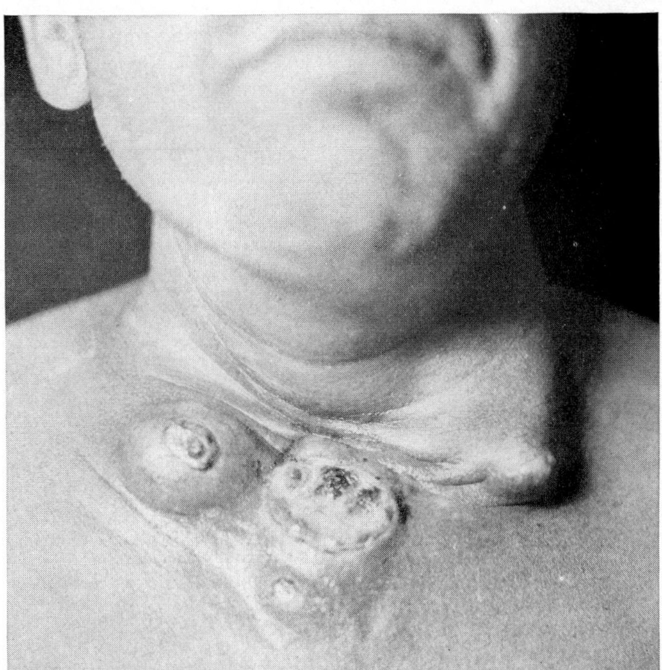

FIG. 496. Lymphosarcoma of glands of neck; metastases in the mediastinum. (From Author's Service of Cook County Hospital.)

Precautions.

1. Always work with ample exposure and good illumination.
2. Keep the **wound moist**; should the slightest "hissing" sound be heard, promptly press the finger against the tissue at a point nearer the heart than is the wounded vein. "Hissing" means air has found its way into the vessel, or injury to the pleura; ascertain which. Throw salt solution into the wound.

   The late John B. Murphy placed a small pack of gauze to which a thread was attached to keep it from being lost, under the sternal attachment of the sternomastoid muscle. The object was to exert pressure to keep the cervical veins full, thus making the veins visibly prominent and preventing the danger of negative pressure. This step is of great value.

   Leave inoperable cases alone. (Fig. 496.) (See also air-embolism.)
3. Use blunt dissection in preference to sharp division of the tissues.

4. **Stop! look! and touch!** before you divide any structure about which you are in doubt.
5. Insure hemostasis as you go along. Respect tissues; treat them kindly; don't tear.

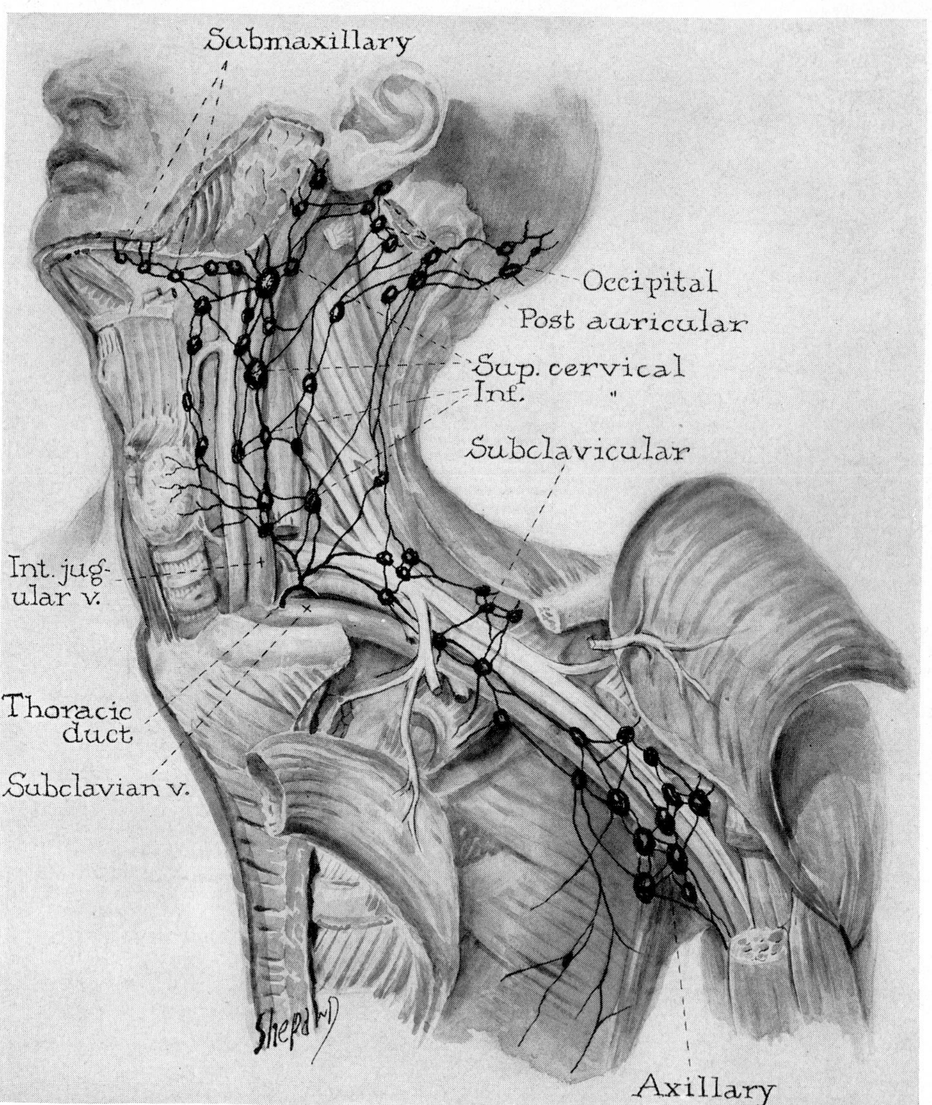

FIG. 497. Distribution of the lymphatics in the neck.

If, in spite of all precautions, air has been sucked into a vein, Binnie advises packing the wound in the neck loosely; do not apply forceps to the vein or forcibly compress the chest during the succeeding expirations; and do not lower the head and shoulders of the patient.

6. **Avoid injury to the thoracic duct.** When the duct has been injured a little clear fluid (chyle) is seen escaping. Usually such mishaps are not

fraught with danger. Lecéne points out that the discharge will continue for about three weeks. It usually yields to compression and proper gauze tamponade. During this period patients lose considerable weight.

7. **Avoid injury to important nerves**: the spinal accessory, vagus, phrenic, recurrent laryngeal or cervical sympathetic nerves.

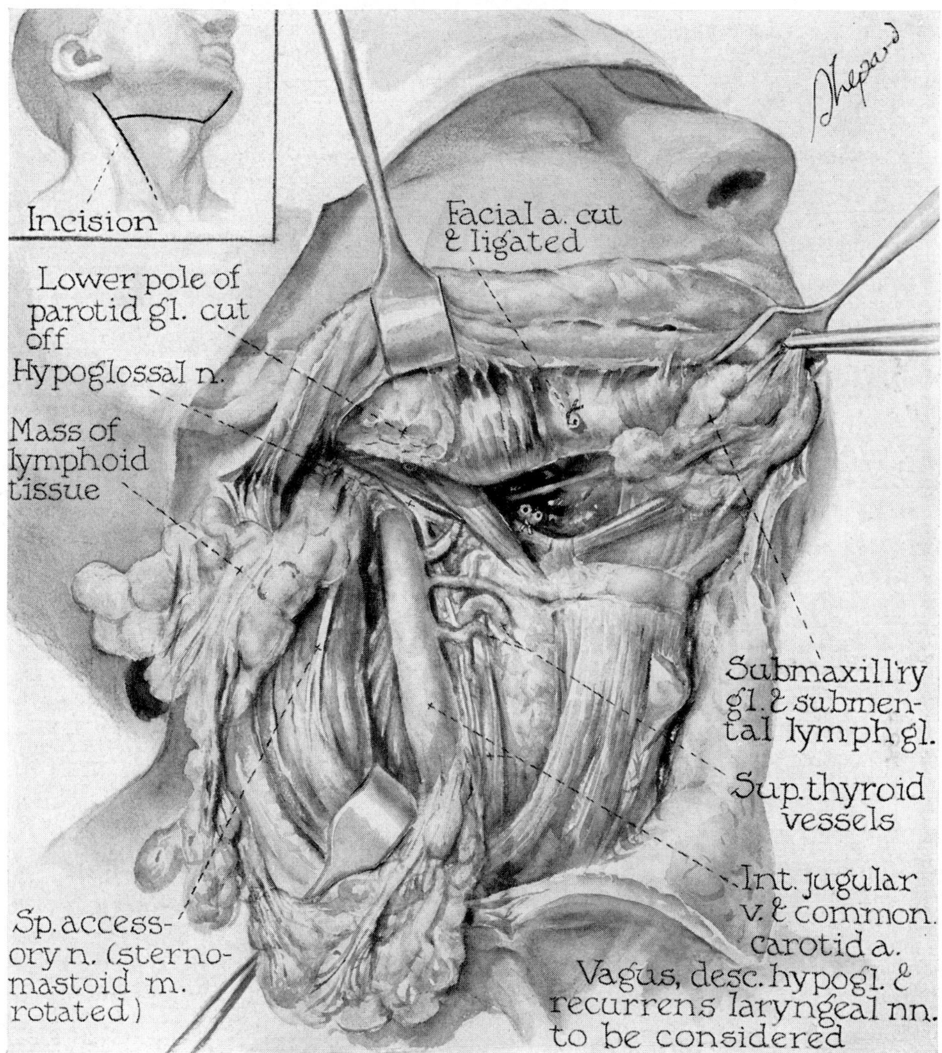

FIG. 498. Block dissection of the lymph nodes of the neck, submaxillary and submental regions.

Where the affected lymph nodes are few or not adherent, the operation is simple. Under such circumstances, make an incision over the tumor and shell it out by blunt dissection through the incision.

Step 1. Drape the scalp with a gauze or rubber cap to keep the hair out of the way. Support the patient's shoulders and turn his head to the opposite side.

Step 2. Make an oblique incision along the sternomastoid muscle beginning at the mastoid process and ending near the sternoclavicular articulation. Expose the external jugular vein and divide it between two ligatures (Fig. 498). Keep the field of operation constantly free from blood.

Step 3. Dissect the skin liberally from the subjacent tissues anterior and posterior to the incision and retract it. If necessary, make another incision beginning at the lower end of the oblique incision and continue it outward, parallel to and close to the clavicle. A variety of incisions have been recommended for block dissections in this region. The resourceful surgeon will plan the incision to meet the requirements of the case.

Lay bare the sternomastoid muscle and liberate it from its surroundings through its entire extent. Divide the deep cervical fascia at the upper border of the clavicle from the symphysis menti to the mastoid process and downward across the hyoid bone to the sternal portion of the sternomastoid muscle; ligate and divide the sternomastoid muscle.

When the internal jugular vein is to be ligated and divided, do so just above the clavicle. Look for the omohyoid muscle which has been exposed and find the internal jugular vein beneath it. Dissect the vein out of its sheath. Do not injure the internal carotid artery or vagus nerve.

Notice the point of exit of the superficial cervical nerves at the posterior edge of the muscle. These nerves are of considerable size and with careful dissection are readily identified. Identify the spinal accessory nerve as it emerges from behind the sternomastoid muscle. This nerve enters the muscle about two inches below the tip of the mastoid process, after passing over the prominent transverse process of the atlas. It is important to preserve this nerve in young individuals. Christian Fenger has shown that if the nerve is severed, drooping of the shoulder and scoliosis result.

Step 4. Dissect out the packet of fascia which enfolds the carotid artery, the internal jugular vein, and the vagus nerve. Once exposed, protection of these important structures from trauma is facilitated. Clear out the supraclavicular space. Ligate the transverse cervical artery here. Look out for the thoracic duct. If divided, no harm will result (see above). Respect the phrenic nerve and cupola of the pleura at the apex of the lung.

Step 5. Systematically remove the diseased lymph nodes. Begin the dissection near the lower end of the wound and by the side of the carotid packet. This is not difficult to accomplish. No blind work is permissible. If these important structures are not carefully exposed and protected at an early stage in the operation, thorough removal of the nodes will become a difficult and dangerous task.

Step 6. Repair the wound in the cervical fascia by suture. Attend to thorough hemostasis. Unite the platysma. In careless suturing of the fascia an ugly scar will result because of stretching of the skin. Drain at the lower angle of the wound.

Step 7. Close the skin wound with interrupted sutures or Michel clips. Apply a voluminous dressing.

Comment. If the operation is performed for tuberculous lymph-nodes some may be ruptured and permit caseous material to escape. In such case, wipe the escaped material away. It is good practice to scrape the remnants of the caseous material from the ruptured gland, subsequently mopping the part scraped with liquid carbolic acid.

In dissecting the nodes for malignant disease look for the external maxillary artery in the upper part of the dissection and identify it where it enters the groove in the submaxillary gland. Clamp and doubly ligate it. Remove the submaxillary gland with its nodes and ligate its duct close to the floor of the mouth. Include the submental nodes in the dissection. When working along the horizontal ramus of the mandible a number of facial veins will also call for division and ligature. Along the submental region great care should be exercised not to leave any nodes behind. Crile insists, and justly so, that complete block dissection of the neck in all cases of carcinoma of the tongue is of cardinal importance. To this must be added complete ablation of the fascial structures surrounding the lymph nodes and complete removal of the sternomastoid muscle. Block dissection is done with greater facility when the sternomastoid is removed together with the anterior jugular vein and lymph structures. In some cases removal of the primary growth with the cautery instead of the scalpel is of distinct value. In working in the submaxillary region, do not injure the hypoglossal nerve.

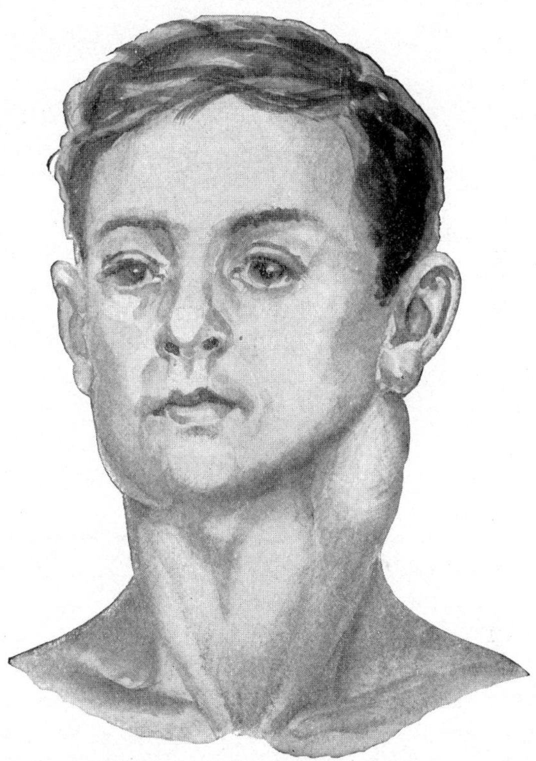

FIG. 499. Tuberculous lymphoma of the glands of the neck.

HODGKINS DISEASE; MALIGNANT LYMPHOMA; TUBERCULOUS CERVICAL ADENITIS

Much surgery has been done in this class of cases heretofore. At present the scalpel has yielded to x-ray, radium and heliotherapy with much more gratifying results than before; particularly is this true in tuberculous lymphadenitis, while Hodgkins disease is, it needs no emphasis, not amenable to surgical interference (Figs. 499 and 496, p. 423).

The surgeon of today rarely subjects cases of tuberculous lymphadenitis to operation without having first given the measures enumerated above a trial. If a block dissection should, for some reason, be decided upon, the technic of that operation will be found elsewhere in this chapter.

THYROGLOSSAL CYSTS AND SINUSES (FISTULAS)

These congenital conditions are usually found in one of three situations (Fig. 500):

1. Between the foramen cecum of the tongue and the hyoid bone (Fig. 501);
2. Between the hyoid and larynx;
3. Below the larynx overlying the trachea.

The second variety is the most common.. The tumefactions appear as cysts which approach the skin and rupture or are incised so that, as a rule, the surgeon has a sinus rather than a cyst to treat. Suppuration may complicate the condition.

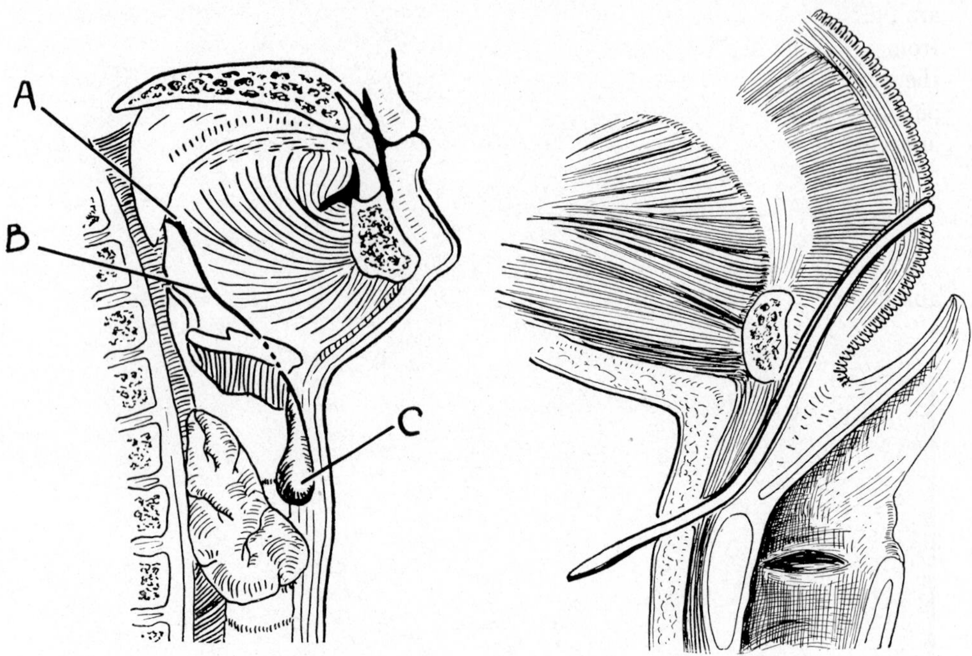

FIG. 500 FIG. 501

FIG. 500. Excision of thyroglossal cysts and sinuses (Sistrunk's technic). Lateral view of the remains of the thyroglossal structures: A. foramen cecum, B. thyroglossal duct, C. thyroglossal cyst, showing their embryologic connection with the pyramidal lobe of the thyroid gland.

FIG. 501. Median branchial fistula connected with the foramen cecum of the tongue.

Operation for Second Variety of Thyroglossal Sinus

Step 1. To point the way in exploring the sinus, inject it with a strong methyl blue or brilliant green solution.

Step 2. Circumincise the scar or sinus around a probe introduced into it.

Step 3. Identify the borders of the sternohyoid muscles; retract these. Grasp the sinus with an Allis forceps. Dissect it out by sharp instruments taking care not to sever its superficial part from the deep portion. Follow the course of the sinus which is usually inward, toward the lower edge of the hyoid bone.

Step 4. Cut off the sinus with the lower border of the hyoid bone. As a rule, this is not difficult because most of these operations are on the young when the hyoid is still cartilaginous. Only in so doing can one be sure that the very bottom of the sinus has been removed.

Step 5. Place a small drain at the bottom of the wound.

Median cysts below the larynx and about the sternal notch between the thyroid lobes are very rare. In attacking these, one may shell them out. A pedicle attaches them to the deeper structures (isthmus of thyroid); the pedicle is to be divided.

Cysts below the foramen cecum were referred to by Bland Sutton as "lingual dermoids." Occasionally they are small and are situated just under the foramen cecum producing a tumefaction in this region. Excision is difficult. If they assume considerable proportions, they push the tongue out of the mouth and are palpable between the mandible and the hyoid bone. They must be attacked from below through a midline incision or a curved incision running parallel with the mandible. The latter gives better exposure. Exercise care not to leave any portion of the cyst-wall behind. The attachments are usually to the hyoid bone and foramen cecum.

Excision of Thyroglossal Sinus
(Sistrunk's Technic)

Either local or general anesthesia may be used; general anesthesia is preferable due to the gagging which accompanies the insertion of the finger about the

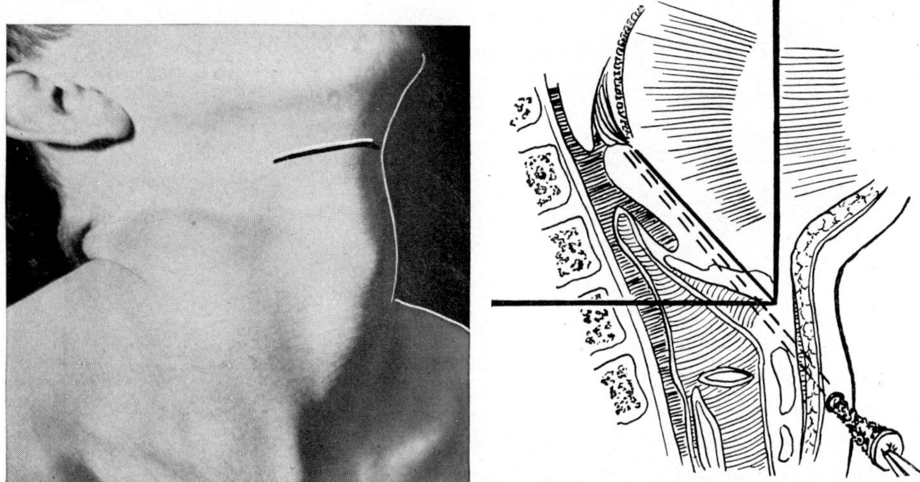

FIG. 502 FIG. 503

FIG. 502. Excision of thyroglossal cysts and sinuses (Sistrunk's technic). Line of incision.

FIG. 503. Ascertain the direction of the course of the thyroglossal duct by drawing imaginary lines, one longitudinal and the other perpendicular to the center of the hyoid bone. "Coring out" of the cyst and duct is done along the line represented by the 45 degree bisection of the right angle extending from the distal end of the cyst just below the center of the foramen cecum.

foramen cecum. If a sinus is present, it should be injected with a solution of methylene blue. Place a pillow under the shoulders and head of the patient. Extend the neck in the same way as for thyroidectomy.

Step 1. Make a transverse incision over the cyst about 1 or 1½ inches long, including the skin, subcutaneous tissues and platysma muscle (Figs. 502-503).

Step 2. Divide the raphé joining the sternohyoid muscles in the midline. The cyst is visible immediately under this raphé; dissect it free and in an upward direction toward the hyoid bone. In most instances the tract runs under the hyoid bone making it advisable to remove a small portion from the center of the bone with stout scissors.

Step 3. After introducing a mouth-gag, insert the left index finger into the mouth.

Draw the tongue forward by means of a suture. Direct the finger backward over the tongue thus locating the circumvallate papillae two rows of which form a "V" near the base. Immediately back of this point the foramen cecum appears. Insert the finger, pressing upward and forward and in this way shorten the distance between it and the hyoid bone. Be mindful of the thyroglossal duct. Core an area about 3 mm. in diameter from the muscles of the tongue with a knife or long-bladed scissors. Make no attempt to isolate the duct; its fragility renders such a step inadvisable.

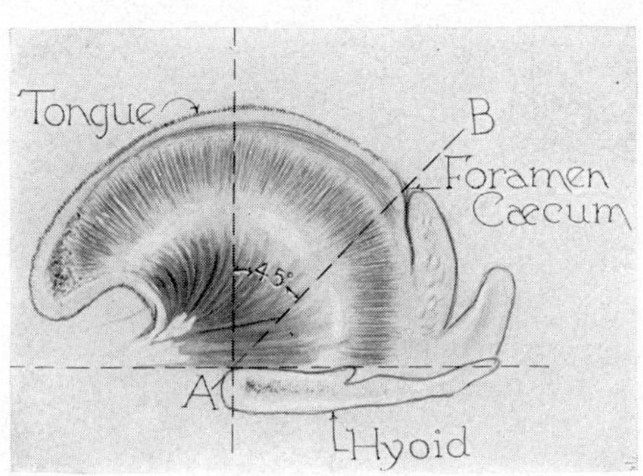

FIG. 504. Sistrunk's operation for the removal of thyroglossal tract. The illustration shows the suprahyoid portion of the thyroglossal tract by "coring out" the tissues along the lines indicated, A-B.

Step 4. With a finger about the foramen cecum acting as a guide, avoid entering the mucosa of the mouth. With a scissors or knife, cut off the cored-out muscles of the tongue when the foramen is reached.

Step 5. Repair the defect in the muscles with a few interrupted catgut sutures; avoid injuring the hypoglossal nerves by placing the sutures superficially.

Step 6. Introduce a small split rubber tube deeply into the muscles of the tongue allowing it to protrude over the hyoid bone. Repair the defect in the bone by approximating the edges with chromic catgut sutures including the periosteum and adjoining tissues. As a rule, two sutures are sufficient. Separate closure is unnecessary for the raphé wound. Close the skin with interrupted sutures of horsehair or any non-absorbable material. Permit the rubber drain to remain in place for four or five days.

Comment. The thyroglossal duct follows a direction in accordance with a line drawn at an angle of 45 degrees backward and downward in the direction of the foramen cecum through the intersection of lines drawn perpendicularly and horizontally toward the center of the hyoid bone (Fig. 504.) An important factor to observe in connection with this operation is the complete disregarding of the duct and the coring out of the tissues through which it passes. A guiding finger in the mouth prevents entering the mouth or pharynx.

Cervical Auricles: Branchial Cysts and Fistulae

The second, third, and fourth branchial clefts have their external orifices along the anterior margin of the sternomastoid muscle. The opening of the second, the one most commonly affected, is situated about the level of the angle of the mandible. It opens into the space in which the tonsil is lodged. If accompanied by a fistula, its dissection with closure of the pharyngeal opening is one of the most difficult things to accomplish. The reason for this is obvious when we recall that the sinus winds its way into the pharynx between the internal and external carotid arteries.

The third and fourth clefts enter the upper part of the larynx; the superior laryngeal nerve is seriously jeopardized if these are attacked.

The cysts of the second cleft are quite common and are distinguished with some difficulty from an enlarged lymph-node in the same situation. Their wall is thick. Their surgical removal does not differ from the operation for a tuberculous lymph-node or other localized tumor (Fig. 505).

Branchial sinuses opening externally are but slightly disfiguring. They require no interference. The scar resulting after their removal will be more conspicuous than the small skin depression in the neck. **"Accessory auricles"** are rare. They consist of tabs of skin and cartilage (termed cervical auricles) found in the neck or just in front of the ear. They are not particularly difficult to remove except when complicated with sinuses.

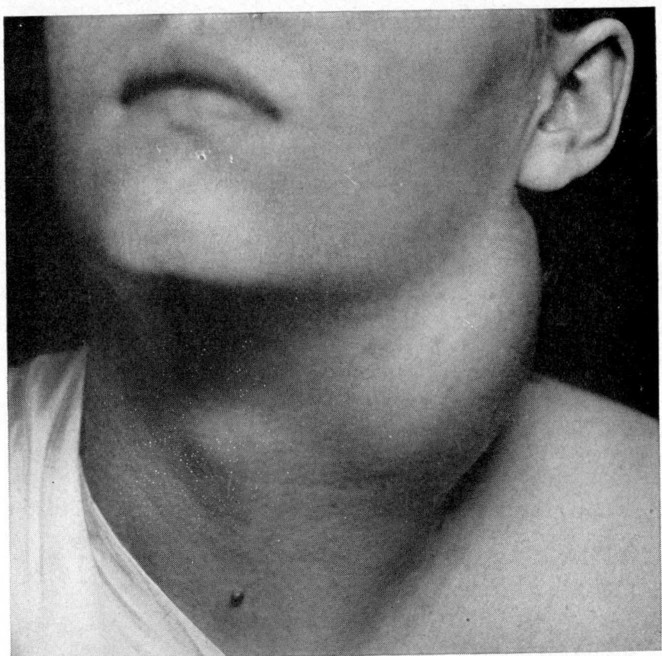

Fig. 505. Branchial cyst diagnosed as malignancy gland of the neck.

Olan R. Hyndman and George Light[1] comment as follows concerning the etiology of branchial cysts:

"1. Branchial cleft anomalies (cysts and fistulas) result from a failure of absorption of the included ectodermal and entodermal epithelium that is buried during the growth and fusion of the branchial arches in early embryonic life. This is most probably the sole explanation, the thymic stalk playing no rôle.

"2. Branchial cysts, in truth, are epidermoid cysts of the neck whose parent epithelium was buried during the development of the branchial apparatus. Their characters are more varied, of course, than those of the commoner epidermoid or inclusion cysts owing to the activity of the entodermal or ectodermal epithelium or both. Many of the submaxillary cysts and so-called granulae are of branchial origin.

[1] Archives of Surgery, September, 1929, Vol. 19.

"3. Branchial fistulas may be familial and hereditary, and they seem to be inherited through the mother only.

"4. More attention should be given to the possibility that a tumor in the neck is of branchial origin, especially in view of their frequent simulation of tuberculous glands and their occurrence in early youth. This is enjoined even more by the fact that results from treatment are in proportion to the completeness with which the epithelial wall is excised.

"5. An adequate and simple classification of the cysts would be (a) branchial cleft epidermoid cysts and (b) branchial cleft mucous cysts."

TUMOR OF THE CAROTID BODY

These tumors are of rare occurrence and are often referred to as paragangliomas or as pheochromoblastomas or chromaffinomas (Fig. 506). They are usu-

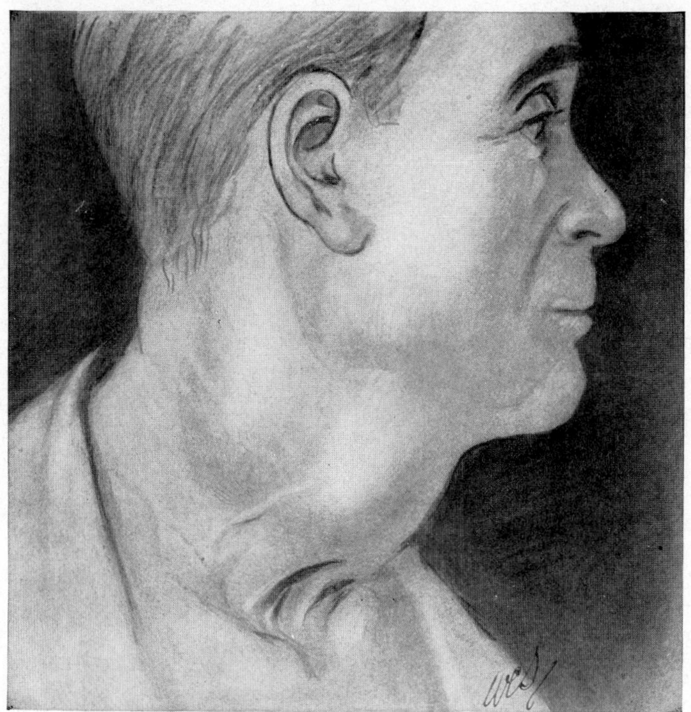

Fig. 506. Tumor of the carotid gland.

ally benign and are encountered in the parasympathetic system. While described as a slow-growing, benign neoplasm, recurrences after removal and metastases have been described in about 25 to 30 per cent of cases, the latter reproduce in the main the histologic structure of the carotid gland. These tumors may grow very slowly for many years and ultimately display malignant characteristics. The tumor originates at the bifurcation of the common carotid artery, in the carotid sheath, hence the pneumogastric, hypoglossal and sympathetic nerves are affected early. It tends to displace the pharyngeal wall inward; the opposite is true of lymph-nodes in the same locality. Carotid body tumors when of considerable size are so vascular that a bruit and expansive pulsation have caused them to be misdiagnosed as aneurysms.

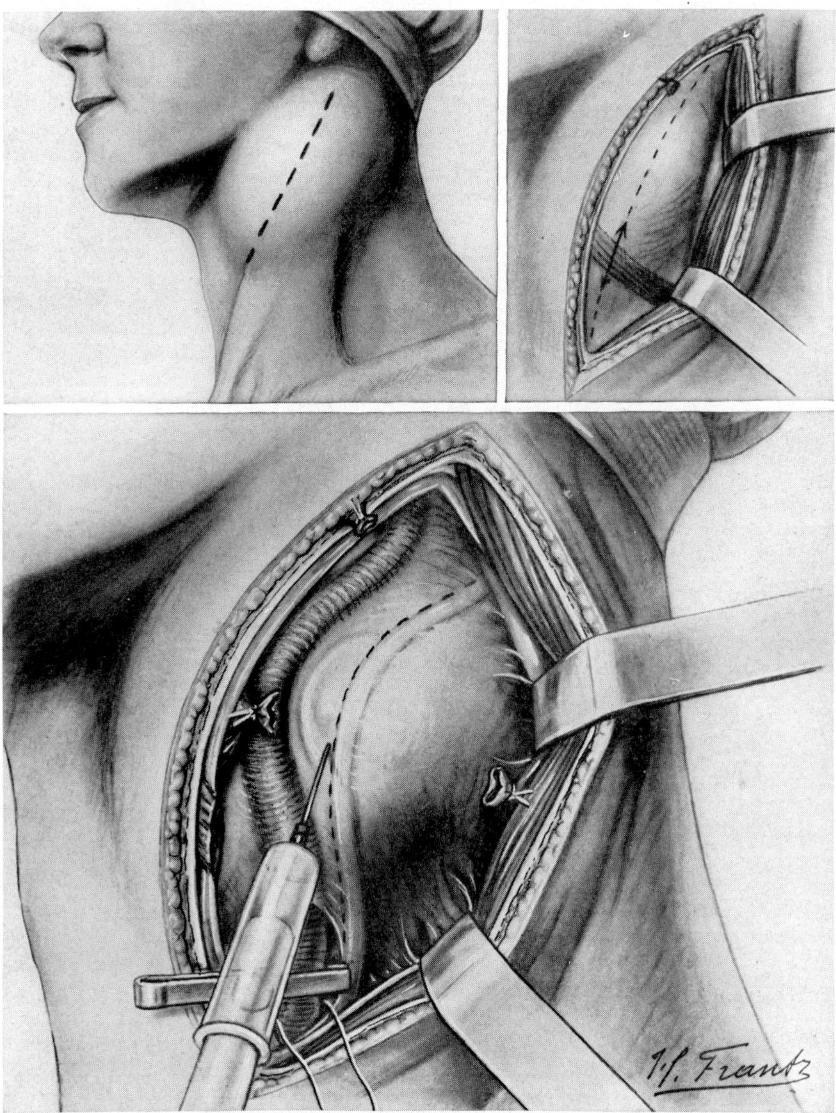

FIG. 507. Upper left insert shows the line of incision over a carotid tumor. Upper right insert depicts the sternomastoid muscle retracted; the omohyoid is seen to traverse the operative field toward the inferior angle. After incising the middle cervical aponeurosis, the omohyoid muscle and the vascular nervous bundle, which is shown ligated in the illustration, the internal jugular vein is retracted together with the sternocleidomastoid muscle. A rubber covered hemostatic clamp is shown compressing the common carotid artery. Observe that the pneumogastric nerve, which passes on the external surface of the tumor, is being injected with an anesthetic.

Step 1. Make an incision along the anterior border of the sternomastoid muscle.

Step 2. As soon as the tumor is exposed, endeavor to determine whether or not it is operable. Often such violent bleeding ensues that **ligation of the carotid** becomes imperative. In such an emergency, the common carotid artery is ligated first, then the external, and finally the internal, at the base of the skull. The ligation of the common carotid has, it should be remembered, a high mortality.

Step 3. Remove the tumor. Close the wound.

Dangers of the operation.

1. Immediate high operative mortality.
2. Effects of ligation on the common artery (softening of the brain, hemiplegia, etc.
3. Injury to the hypoglossal, pneumogastric and sympathetic nerves.

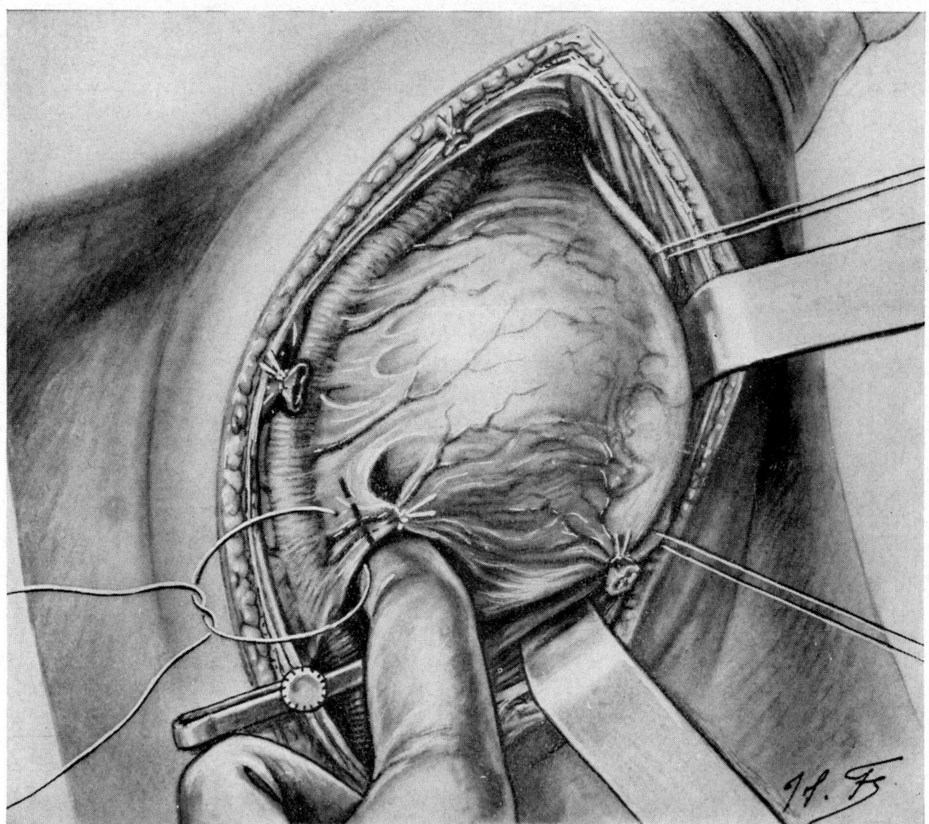

FIG. 508. The pneumogastric nerve is surrounded by a ligature and is displaced backwards. A ligature is placed on the carotid artery near its bifurcation.

Comment. In view of the comparative benignancy of these tumors radium may be tried if danger is sensed should an operation be undertaken. In one of my cases I was able to control bleeding by tamponade (the tumor was not large) after removal of most of the tumor. The patient was then subjected to radium treatment. The tumor diminished in size and at the present writing (3 years after the operation) the patient is at work (housemaid) and enjoys good health.

In the young, therefore, when the tumor is of limited size, radical extirpation should be attempted. In persons of advanced years with atheromatous vessels which would render ligation of the carotid hazardous, it is better to counsel against operation.

P. L. Mirizzi[1] has described a method of removal of a large carotid tumor, the steps of which are illustrated in the subjoined (Figs. 507-508-509).

OPERATIONS ON THE THYROID GLAND

Terminology. One is impressed with the confusion still existing in the denominations of surgical procedures dealing with operations on the thyroid gland. Excision, enucleation, resection, hemithyroidectomy, lobectomy, are terms used frequently and indiscriminately.

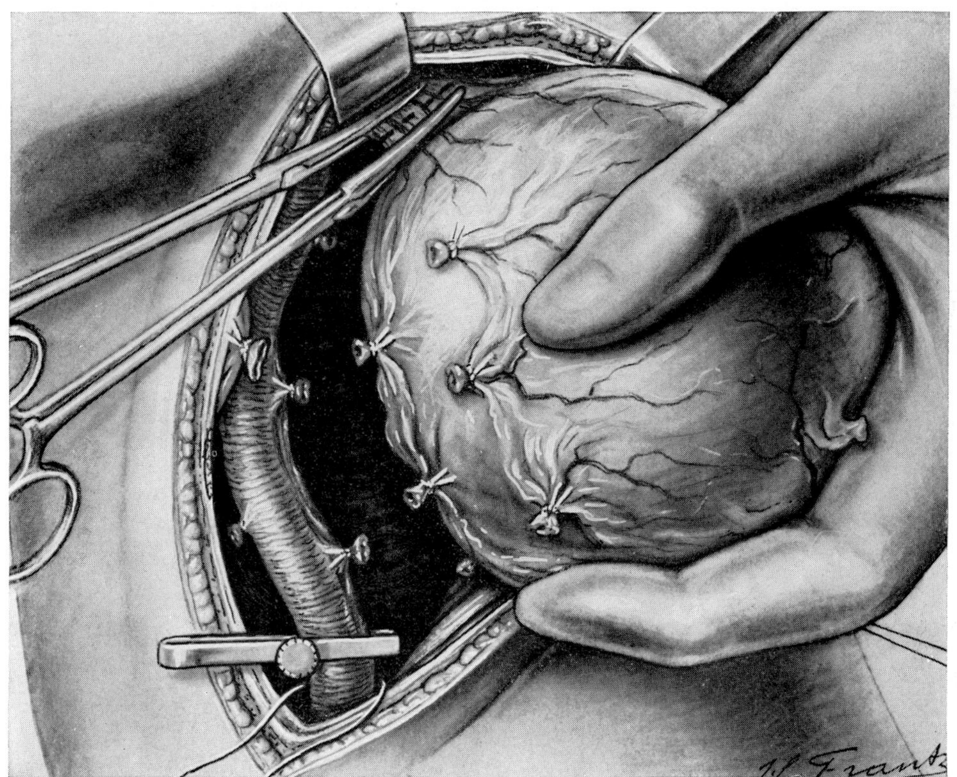

FIG. 509. The vessels supplying the tumor have been ligated and divided between two mosquito forceps. Isolation of the vessels is aided by putting the tumor on traction which exposes the vessels to better advantage (courtesy of Prof. P. L. Mirizzi).

1. Excision (Kocher) refers to a complete removal of one or both lobes. The method is applicable in malignancies of the thyroid only.

2. Resection (Mikulicz) indicates a partial extirpation of one or both lobes of the thyroid.

3. Enucleation (Socin, Billroth) means the removal by separation of one or more nodes or cysts from the thyroid substance.

4. Combined procedures of enucleation and resection are often done. In the majority of cases melon (cuneiform) or marginal resections are performed.

Anatomic Considerations. (Figs. 510-511.) The thyroid gland consists of two lateral lobes and an isthmus. Each lateral lobe is conical in shape with the base directed downward. The superficial surface is slightly convex. It is covered by the

[1] La Presse Medicale, Cordoba, Argentine, No. 92, du 16 Novembre, 1935.

sternohyoid, sternothyroid and the anterior belly of the omohyoid muscles. It is also overlapped by the anterior border of the sternocleidomastoid muscle. Its deep surface is concave and rests upon the lower part of the thyroid cartilage, the side of

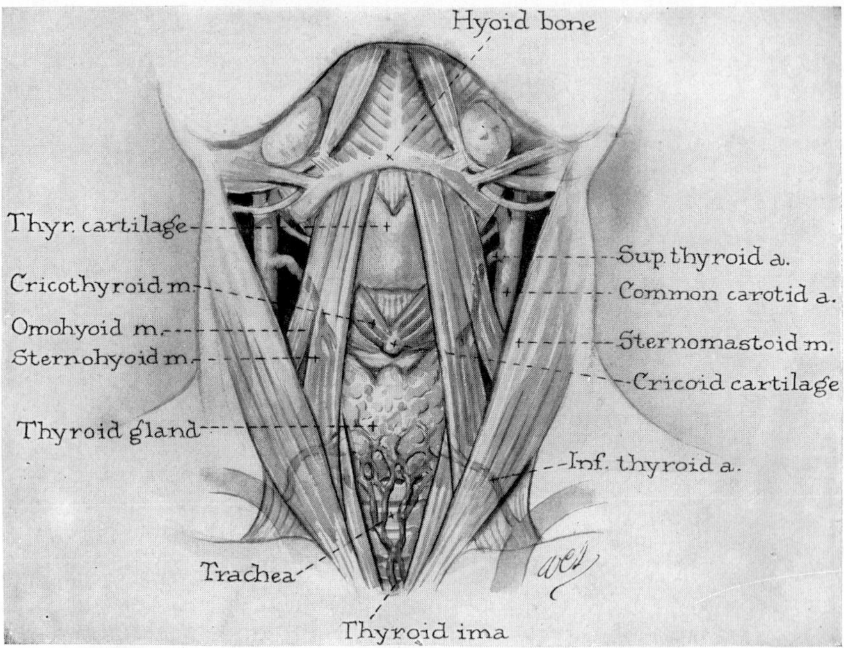

FIG. 510. Anatomy of the anterior thyroid region.

the cricoid cartilage and the sides of the upper five or six rings of the trachea. Its posterior border is rounded and rests upon the pharynx, the esophagus and the prevertebral layer of the deep cervical fascia. If enlarged the lateral lobe may overlie the carotid sheath.

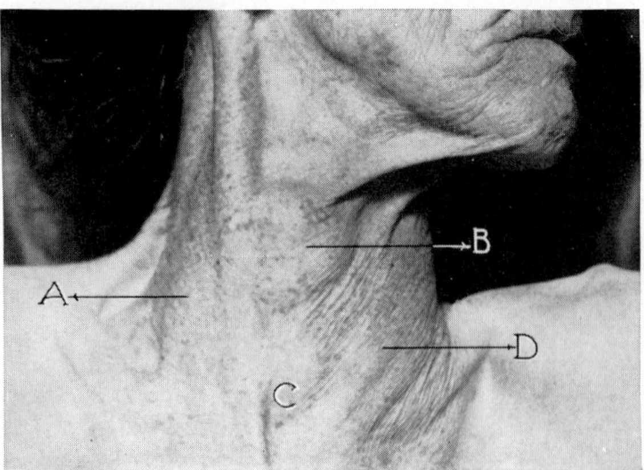

FIG. 511. Surface markings of thyroid gland: A. right lobe, B. pyramidal lobe, C. isthmus, D. left lobe.

The apex of the gland lies upon the inferior constrictor of the pharynx. The isthmus connects the anterior borders of the lateral lobes; it is inconstant, in both size and position and covers the anterior surface of the second, third and fourth rings of the trachea. The pyramidal lobe, if present, runs upward toward the body of the hyoid bone to which it is attached by a fibro-muscular band.

Rather frequently the lower border of the lobes of the thyroid extend to the superior margin of the sternum. Occasionally they may dip past the clavicle into the superior mediastinum. We then speak of an intrathoracic goiter.

The capsules of the thyroid. For the beginner particularly, these are rather confusing anatomic entities. After dividing the prethyroid muscles a connective tissue layer of variable thickness is encountered. It is a component of the deep cervical fascia. It is known as the external capsule of the thyroid, or prethyroid membrane. (Kocher.) Reverdin called it the "envelope aponeurotique." The best descriptive term, however, adopted by many surgeons is that of the surgical capsule. This capsule is derived from the pretracheal fascia. It is composed of loose connective tissue and is easily detachable. It surrounds the thyroid in all directions and is attached to the trachea and the cricoid cartilage. This membranous structure is of great importance because the parathyroid glands are situated posteriorly on its inner surface. The thyroid gland itself is surrounded by the glandular capsule, often referred to as the capsula interna or capsula propria. It is a peritoneum-like structure through which the large veins are seen coursing on the surface of the thyroid gland. There are three cleavage spaces which are of great importance in operations on the thyroid.

(a) The **sternomastoid space** (deQuervain) between the **sternocleidomastoid muscle** and the prethyroid muscles,

(b) The **musculo-capsular space** between the prethyroid muscles and the surgical capsule, and the

(c) **Intercapsular** or **surgical space,** located between the glandular capsule and the surgical capsule. This is the most important of the three cleavage spaces. It is composed of loose connective tissue and contains numerous arteries and veins. It surrounds the thyroid gland entirely, extending from one side of the trachea and esophagus to the other side. It is only at the postero-internal surface of the thyroid that they come into more intimate contact. Normally, the relations between the glandular capsule and surgical capsule are very loose. Numerous vessels course here from and out of the thyroid. The surgical space plays an important rôle in operations on the thyroid. The carotid sheath is entirely independent of the spaces described. The inferior thyroid artery passes behind the carotid sheath but does not penetrate it.

Blood Supply. The thyroid gland receives its blood supply from the following sources: superior thyroid, middle thyroid and inferior thyroid. The superior thyroid veins, one or two on each side, leave the upper pole of the thyroid body and ascend to join the internal jugular or common facial vein. A middle thyroid vein in the average case issues from each lateral lobe of the thyroid, crosses the common carotid artery, and enters the internal jugular. This vein is extremely variable in position; moreover, it may be absent or may be represented by several veins. The inferior thyroid veins are of large size; they are formed by branches from the isthmus and lateral lobes of the thyroid. Their course is variable, but in general they descend along the trachea to the innominate trunks. At times they form a plexus on the front of the trachea below the isthmus of the thyroid. All these veins anastomose freely.

The **recurrent (inferior)** laryngeal nerves play an important rôle in operations on the thyroid gland. They are closely related to the lower posterior medial surfaces, (danger zones of Crotti) of the respective thyroid lobes. They course from below upward, lying in the groove between the trachea and esophagus. They pass under the lower border of the inferior constrictor of the pharynx, and enter the larynx behind the articulations of the inferior cornua of the thyroid cartilage with the cricoid. The nerve usually passes behind the inferior thyroid artery. This, however, is not constant; its course varies.

Nerve Supply. The nerves of the thyroid accompany and surround the blood vessels. They are derived from the superior ganglion of the sympathetic and from the superior and inferior laryngeal branches of the pneumogastric.

The Parathyroids. (Fig. 512.) These bodies which are referred to by Kohn as "epithelial bodies" have their origin in the branchial clefts. They appear as masses of closely connected epithelial cells on either side of the third and fourth branchial clefts. They are generally considered to be four in number although counting them is

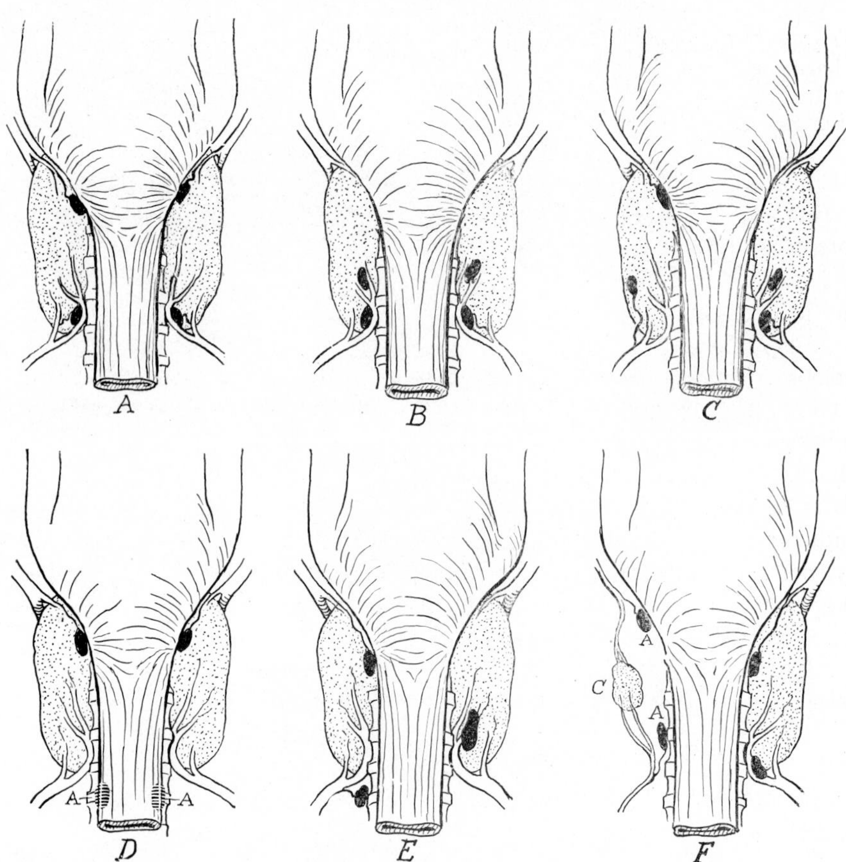

FIG. 512. Diagrams showing the different positions occupied, in different cases, by the parathyroid glands (after McCullum). *A*. Organs of the neck as seen from behind. Four parathyroids—represented as four black oval bodies—are seen in the positions which they commonly occupy. *B*. The two upper parathyroid glands lie close to the lower pair, which are in their usual position. *C*. The left upper and right lower glands are in their most typical position. The right upper gland lies in the region of the inferior thyroid artery; the left lower gland, supplied by a long arterial branch, is imbedded in the posterior surface of the thyroid near its outer margin. *D*. The two upper parathyroid glands are in the common position. The two lower glands AA lie on the anterior surface of the trachea. *E*. On the left side there are two parathyroid glands while on the right only one large gland is to be found. *F*. On the right side the condition of the parts (B) is practically normal; on the left side, however, the thyroid lobe (C) is almost completely atrophied, but the parathyroids (AA) are found about in their usual positions.

difficult because of their small size, inconstant position and resemblance to the surrounding structures. These bodies are enveloped in a capsule made up of thin fibers, have a reticular stroma and are furnished with a generous blood-supply.

These glands generally appear in pairs consisting of a superior (external) and an inferior (internal) body. As a rule, the superior is found close to the thyroid on the middle third of its back surface almost level with the lower margin of the cricoid cartilage. It appears posteriorly and external to the terminal tributaries of the inferior thyroid artery and recurrent laryngeal nerve. The inferior is generally found on the posterior part of the lower third of the thyroid, hence often appearing in front of the recurrent laryngeal nerve and inferior thyroid artery near the thyroid gland at the entrance of the lower arterial branches. It is also found at the inferior pole of the thyroid or immediately under it. Small masses of parathyroid cells have often been found below the thyroid, within the thymus and even within the thyroid (Getzowa).

The parathyroid glands are located external to the thyroid and are separated from it by the external capsule, although one or more may be found under the capsule but are hardly ever found imbedded in the gland itself. Their size averages about 6 to 4 by 2 mm. (Berkeley); however, it varies from 3 mm. to 15 mm. They are round, oval or reniform and generally flat. They have an unusual yellowish brown color.

Preoperative Medication

Emil Goetsch[1] discusses the correct and incorrect use of iodine particularly in preoperative medication and summarizes his observations as follows:

"Iodine has an important relationship to the normal function of the thyroid gland in which it is constantly present and is stored as a normal constituent.

"Simple colloid goiter, the inactive type of parenchymatous goiter, commonly develops whenever there is a deficient intake or a faulty metabolism of iodine in the body. Simple colloid or endemic goiter may be prevented by the prophylactic administration of minute amounts of iodine. Iodine, in small amounts, together with small amounts of thyroid extract is advised in the treatment of simple goiter. This is the only type of goiter in which the therapeutic administration of iodine is indicated. The prolonged administration of iodine to the simple colloid goiter may, however, occasionally stimulate the gland with the consequent production of hyperthyroidism. A correct diagnosis as to the type of goiter is therefore of the greatest importance in order to institute correct therapy.

"A nontoxic goiter may be activated and the symptoms of a toxic goiter may be exacerbated by the indiscriminate administration of iodine.

"The administration of iodine during pregnancy is indicated only in case inactivity of the thyroid gland is present. The physiologically overactive thyroid gland in pregnancy may be stimulated to further activity resulting in a state of true clinical hyperthyroidism.

"The administration of iodine does not prevent the growth and development of true adenoma and has no place in the medical treatment of this condition. Nontoxic adenoma is commonly activated by indiscriminate treatment with iodine and the symptoms of toxic adenoma are exacerbated by its use. The preoperative intensive preparation of the majority of patients with toxic adenoma does not produce improvement comparable to that seen in the case of exophthalmic goiter. The acutely toxic adenomatous goiter particularly when the metabolic rate is high, is often favorably influenced by the use of iodine, whereas those cases of adenoma with lesser degrees of hyperthyroidism may show relatively little improvement. An appreciable number in this group may be made acutely worse.

"The hyperplastic thyroid gland has an extraordinary affinity for iodine which causes the hyperplasia to revert to the colloid or resting state. Accordingly, when iodine is intensively administered to the patient with Graves' disease, previously untreated with iodine, a marked clinical remission in the course of the disease is produced. Operation should be and can be safely performed during this

[1] Amer. Jour. Surgery, 1934.

period of remission. The mortality of resection operations done during the period of remission has been reduced almost to nil, and stage operations are rarely necessary. If thyroid resection is not done at this favorable time of remission, the patient often relapses into a state of clinical exacerbation in the course of one to two or even three months. A condition of uncontrollable hyperthyroidism may thus result. Similarly, exacerbation may follow upon the administration of iodine even in small doses, over a prolonged period.

"The hyperplastic thyroid gland in the phase of reactivation following a previous period of treatment with iodine becomes relatively insensitive or refractive to the further administration of iodine. The preoperative treatment wth iodine

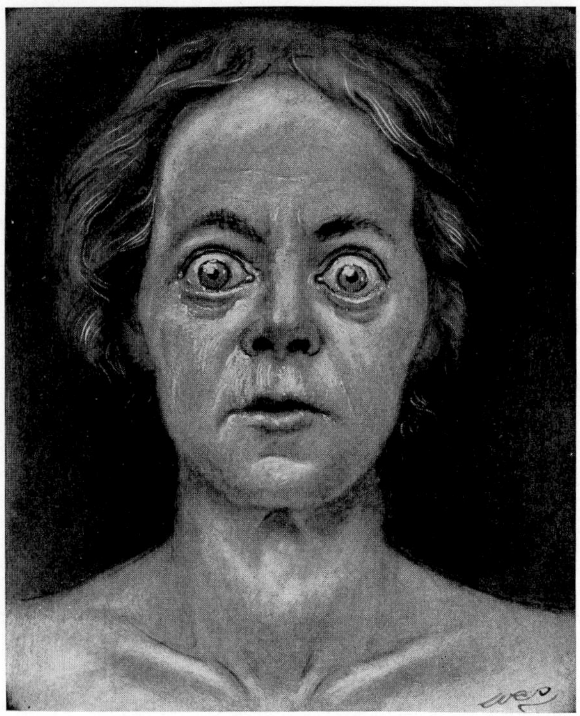

FIG. 513. Pronounced Graves' disease.

does not protect the iodized patient with toxic adenoma or Graves' disease in any way comparable to the protection afforded the patient not previously so treated. The patient suffering with an acute exacerbation following prolonged use of iodine may be a dangerous operative risk whether iodine is given preoperatively or not. It is particularly in these circumstances that recourse must be had to multiple operations such as preliminary ligation and single lobectomies to eliminate the increased risk involved in a primary double lobectomy.

"Iodine has little effect in controlling postoperative hyperthyroidism. There is no evidence that the postoperative administration of iodine reduces the incidence of recurrent hyperthyroidism. The spontaneous hyperthyroid crisis occurring occasionally in the course of severe Graves' disease may be effectively controlled by large doses of iodine given either orally or intravenously. When the crisis occurs as a result of the incorrect use of iodine, the further administration of iodine, even in large amounts, is ineffectual and a fatal outcome may ensue."

THYROIDECTOMY

"A uniform technic does not exist. Every surgeon puts into his work the seal of his own individuality; consequently, divergence of details will always be found; fundamental differences, however, do not exist any longer." (André Crotti.) (Figs. 513-514-515-516-517.)

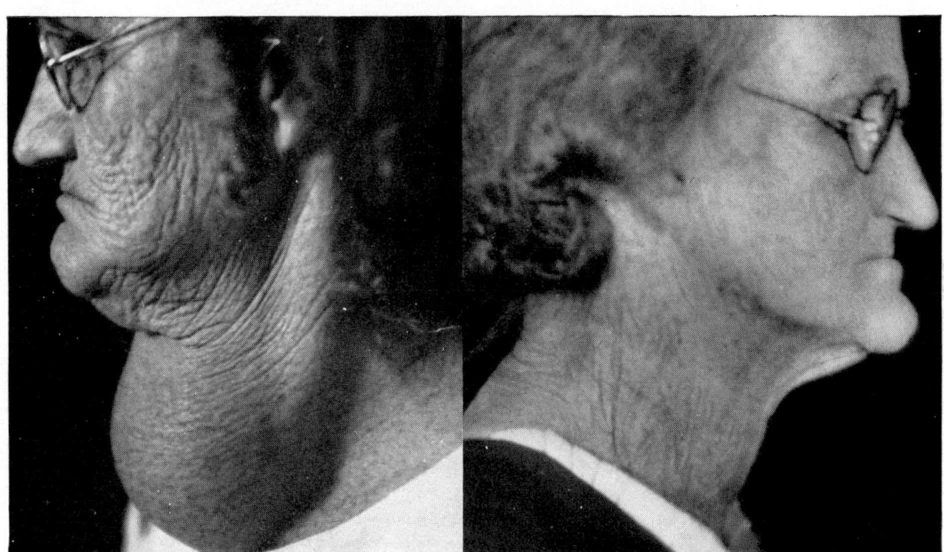

FIG. 514 FIG. 515

FIG. 514. Simple adenoma of the thyroid causing tracheal obstruction.
FIG. 515. Same patient after operation. (Author's Service, Cook County Hospital.)

Preanesthetic Medication

One-half to one hour before the operation, administer subcutaneously ¼ gr. of morphine and 1/120 gr. of atropine sulphate.

Local Anesthesia

In selected cases properly executed, local anesthesia is excellent. The advantages of local anesthesia are many. Among these may be mentioned: (a) the deleterious effects of the inhaled anesthetic on the lungs, kidneys and liver are avoided; (b) the recurrent laryngeal nerves are safeguarded; (c) the increased excitement, and consequently added strain, incident to taking and coming out of the anesthetic is avoided; (d) a more leisurely preparation of the field of operation and freedom from worry about the anesthetic during the operation is provided.

Many surgeons prefer this method to others (Kocher, DeQuervain, Socin, Rehn, Jaboulay, Crile). Numerous factors are to be considered in the successful execution of local anesthesia, viz., (a) proper selection of the patient; (b) a thorough knowledge of the surgical anatomy of the parts concerned in the operation; (c) the personality of the surgeon and his ability to quiet the patient (think of the unstable nervous mechanism of the thyrotoxic patient). We follow the teachings of Crile and "steal" the thyroid from the patient before whom opera-

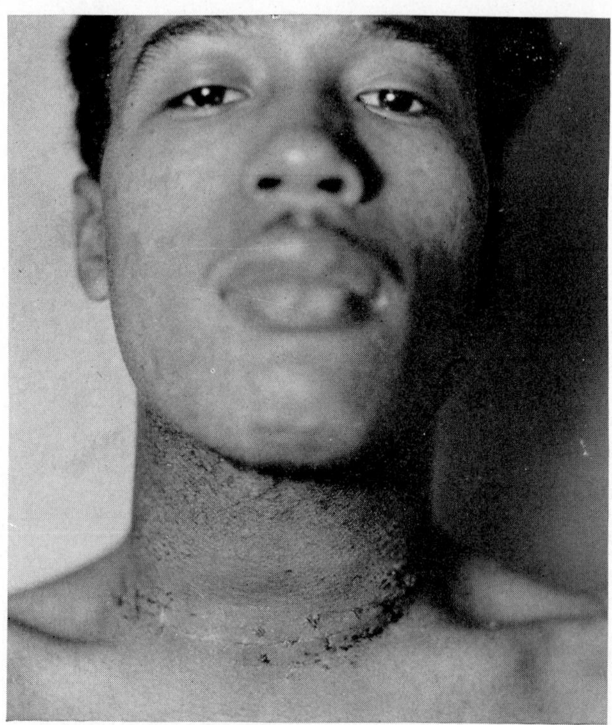

FIG. 516. Patient, from whom thyroid (shown in succeeding illustration) was removed; one week after operation.

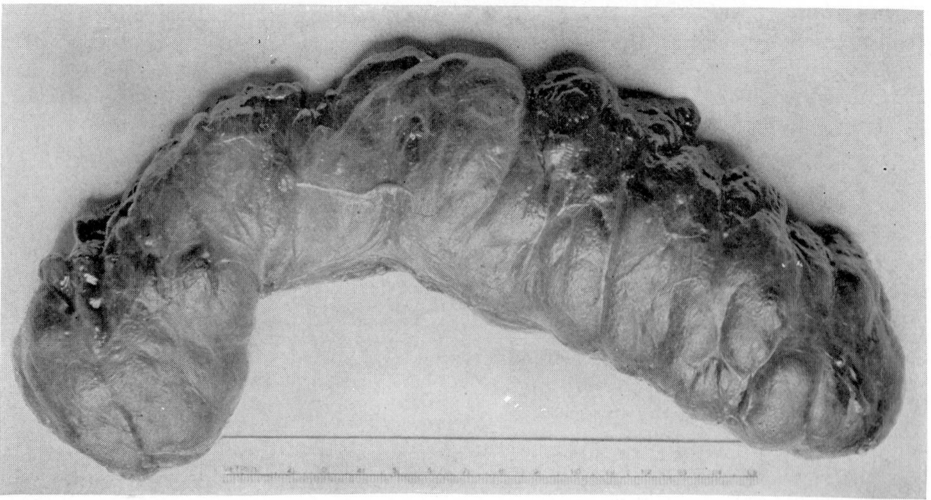

FIG. 517. Enormous thyroid fusing both lobes and isthmus into a sausage-shaped mass removed *en bloc*. (Author's Service, Cook County Hospital.)

tion is never discussed and who is unaware of the date set for the ordeal. Each day for a few days prior to the operation, give the patient a hypodermic injection of sterile water; a little later take him to the operating room where a pretext at anesthesia is made by allowing the patient to inspire a few whiffs of nitrous oxide-oxygen.

I have experimented with other drugs recommended but always returned to novocaine in ½ per cent solution. About 5 ounces can be used with safety, provided the solution is made up fresh and is thoroughly aseptic. Some surgeons add adrenalin to the novocaine solution. Let it be recalled that many thyrotoxic patients are supersensitive to adrenalin (**Goetsch test**). Yet, from a practical point of view, the amount of adrenalin used is so small that its deleterious effects are negligible. Its advantage is that it delays absorption of the novocaine and hence

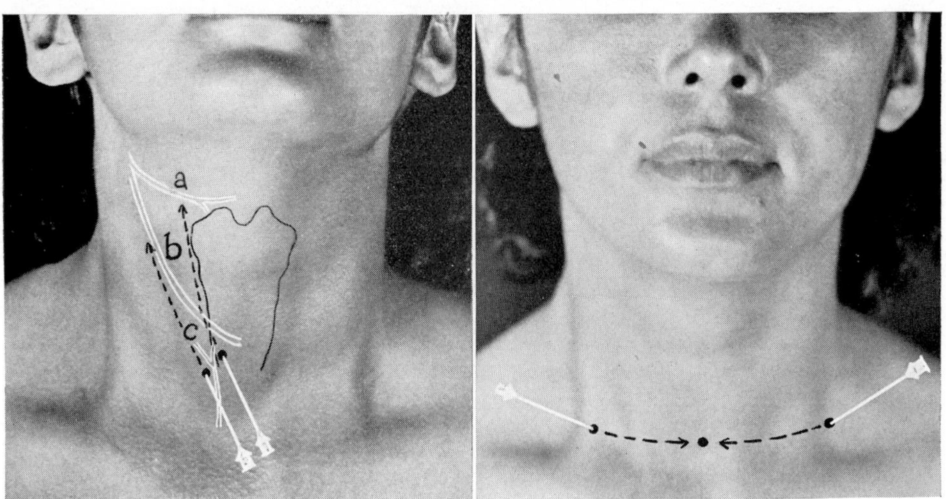

Fig. 518 Fig. 519

Fig. 518. Blocking of the superior laryngeal nerve: a. internal laryngeal branch, b. external laryngeal branch, c. recurrent laryngeal nerve. This nerve does not require infiltration.
Fig. 519. Local anesthesia in thyroidectomy. Line of infiltration in making Kocher's incision in thyroidectomy.

prolongs the time of anesthesia. We add four drops of 1:1000 adrenalin solution to every 100 cc. (3 oz.) of solution. Never exceed 1 Gm. (15 gr.) of novocaine crystals in the course of the operation. This amount of novocaine is present in 200 cc. (about 6 oz.) of the ½ per cent solution.

Precaution: Avoid entering a vein with the injecting needle. After the introduction of the needle into the tissues, draw the piston of the syringe a little back and note if blood is aspirated into the glass barrel of the syringe; if none appears, inject the anesthetic solution.

SUPERFICIAL NERVE BLOCKING

This consists of blocking the cutaneous nerve trunks at their exit at a point corresponding to about the middle of the anterior border of the sternomastoid muscle (Figs. 518-519-520-521).

Ten to twenty cc. of ½ to 1 per cent solution of novocaine are injected on both sides at the point shown in the illustration. (Fig. 519.) Here the cutaneous colli, the supra-clavicular and great auricular nerves emerge. The skin and subcutaneous tissues become completely anesthetized but the deeper structures remain unaffected.

Raise a wheal first and successively infiltrate the tissues along the line indicated.

Pass the needle vertically through the skin and fascia at the point illustrated; when a sense of release is felt after the point of the needle has penetrated the fascia and the surgeon has assured himself that he did not enter a vein (by withdrawing the piston of the syringe as outlined previously) the injection is made.

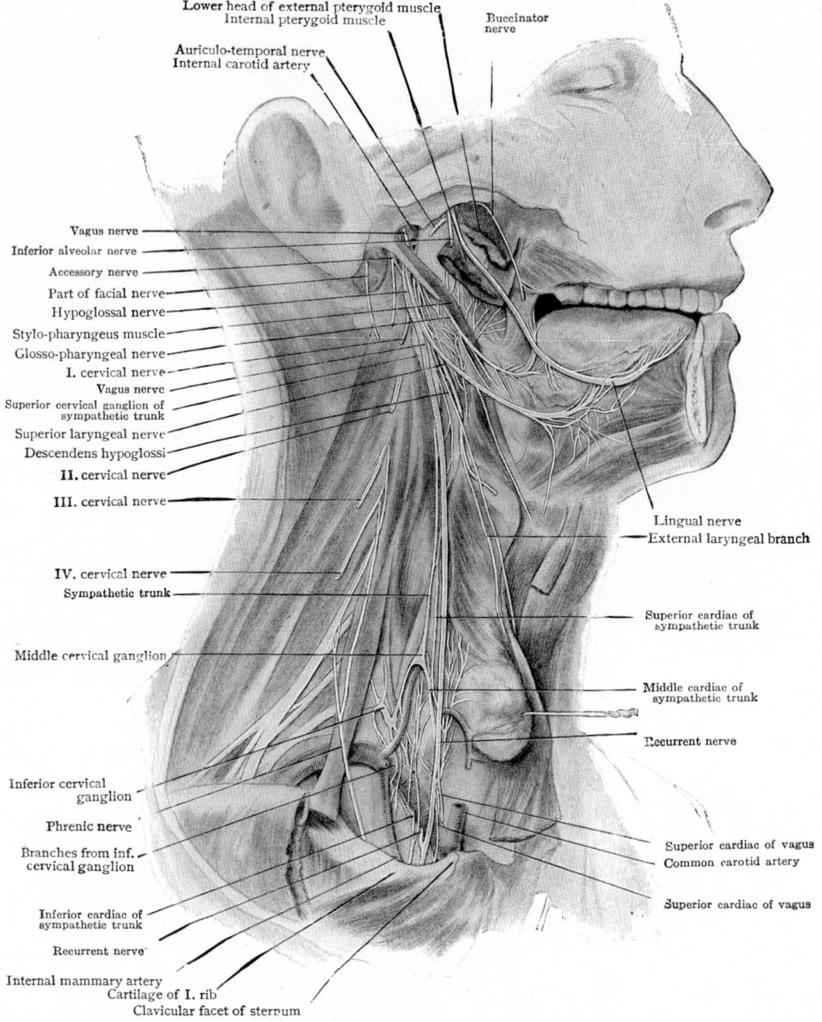

FIG. 520. Deep dissection of right side of head and neck, showing lingual, glosso pharyngeal, vagus and hypoglossal nerves and sympathetic trunk (Piersol).

Do not permit the needle to advance further lest deeper structures be jeopardized. It is for that reason that some surgeons limit the injection to bilateral subcutaneous infiltration in a line along the posterior border of the sternomastoid muscle. This reaches the nerves as they emerge through the fascia, is a simpler procedure, and is preferred by many.

The next step is to inject the subcutaneous and subfascial area of the skin incision (Figs. 522-523-524-525-526).

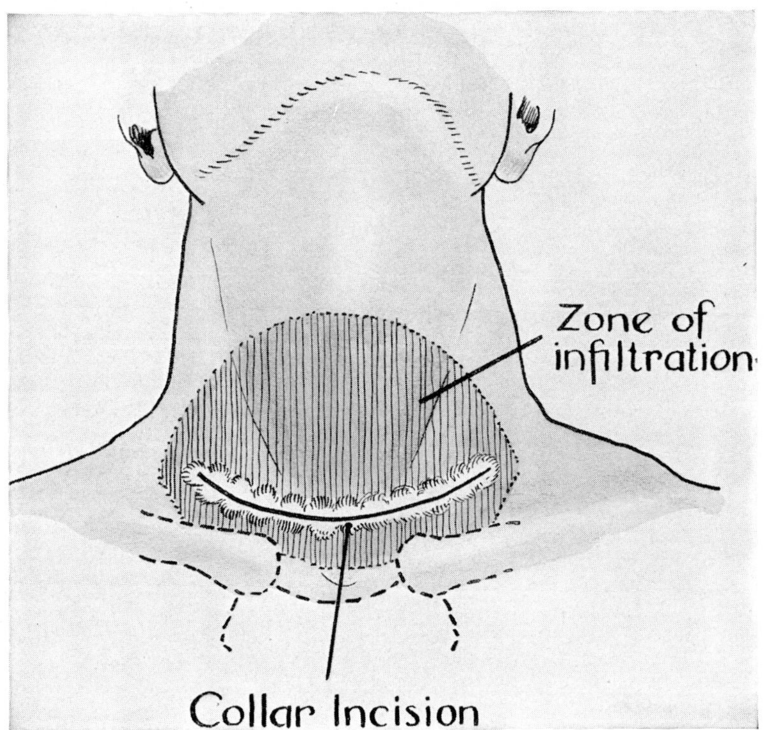

FIG. 521. Infiltration anesthesia in thyroidectomy.

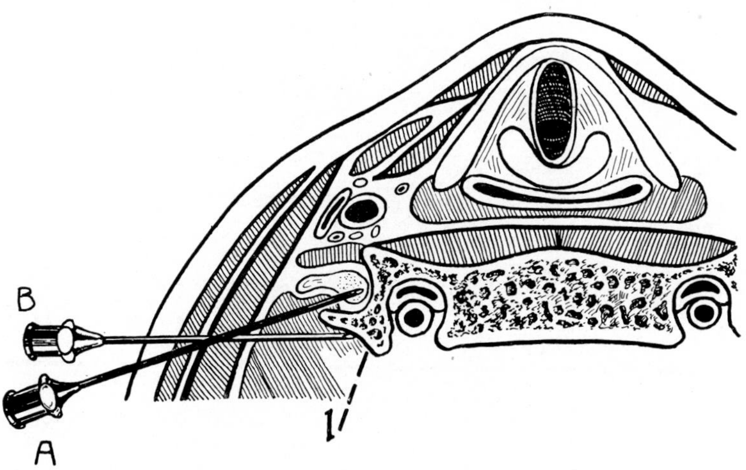

FIG. 522. Nerve blocking in thyroidectomy. Injection of cervical sympathetic nerves. 1. Transverse process of third cervical vertebra; A. needle passed on the posterior aspect of the third cervical vertebra; B. same needle withdrawn and placed about 1 cm. in front where it impinges the nerve supply sought.

Comment. Bilateral injection of the nerve plexus produces the most complete anesthesia, but is attended by the risk of bilateral blocking of the pneumogastric, sympathetic and phrenic nerves. Fatalities have been reported as the result of such accidents.

BLOCKING THE CERVICAL PLEXUS

This consists of injecting the points of junction of the second, third and fourth roots of the cervical nerves at their points of exit from the intervertebral foramina in front of the transverse processes (Figs. 527-528).

Haertel and Geyer's Paravertebral Nerve Block. Braun's modification of this method is as follows:

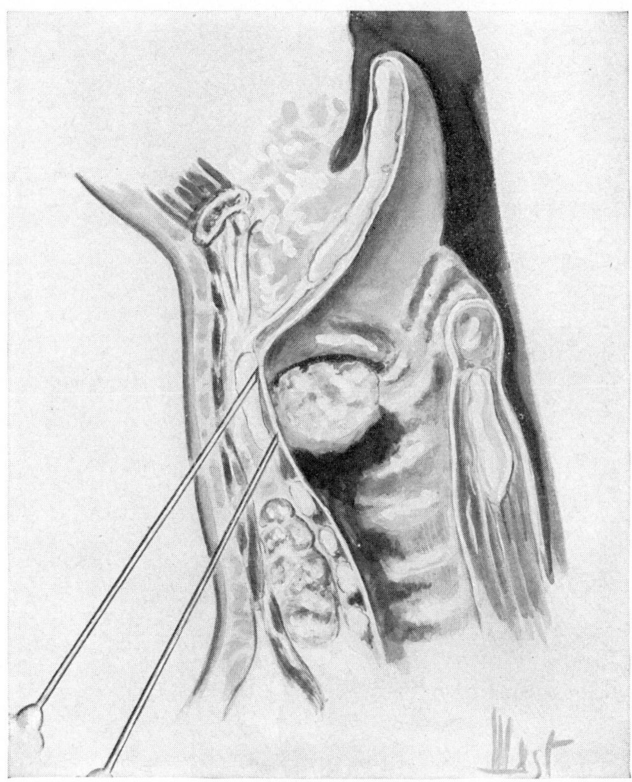

FIG. 523. Schematic diagram of a cross section of a larynx. The needles are pressed obliquely through the soft parts and through the cricothyroid membrane and the thyroid cartilage. Between these structures and the laryngeal mucous membrane the anesthetic fluid is deposited. The beveled edge of the needle should lie upon the deep surface of the mucous membrane. (After Hertzler.)

Draw a line extending from the anterior border of the mastoid process to the clavicle. This crosses Chassaignac's tubercle. Mark the point of junction of the first 1/3 with the second 1/3 of this line. Practically, this point corresponds to the level of the upper border of the thyroid cartilage. It is at this point that the needle is introduced and passed forward until the transverse process of the third cervical vertebra is felt. Withdraw the needle slightly and reintroduce it about 1 cm. or more in front of the transverse process (Fig. 529). Make sure that no vessel has been entered. Deposit 10 cc. of ½ per cent solution of novocaine. Withdraw the needle again for a short distance and inject the same amount of novocaine in front of the transverse process of the fourth cervical vertebra. DeQuervain admonishes the exercise of the greatest possible care to avoid inadvertently injecting the vertebral artery or vein which when entered may be followed by serious consequences or even death. If properly performed, complete anesthesia of both superficial and deep tissues result in about ten min-

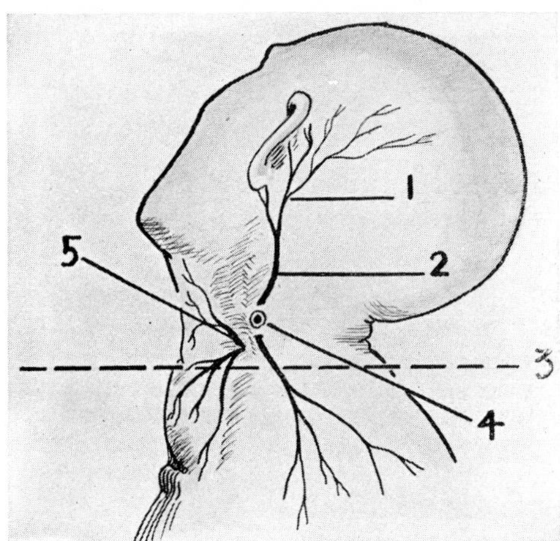

FIG. 524

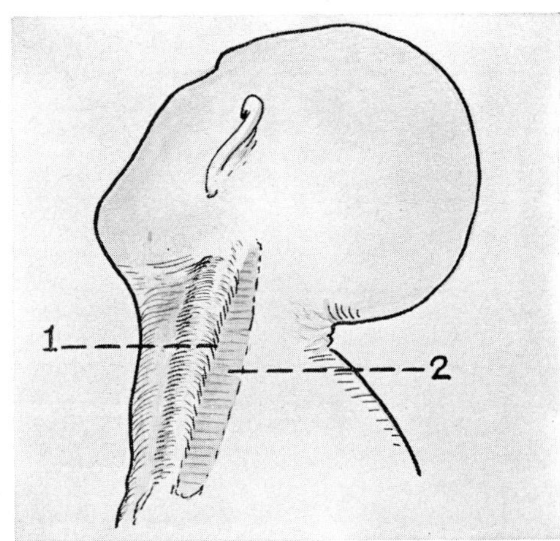

FIG. 525

FIG. 524. Diagram of cutaneous nerves, showing location of point for subfascial injection: 1. lesser occipital, 2. great auricular, 3. midpoint between mastoid and clavicular attachments of sternomastoid muscle, 4. point of insertion of needle, 5. cutaneous colli.

FIG. 525. Diagram of deep subcutaneous infiltration, along posterior border of sternocleidomastoid: 1. posterior border of sternomastoid, 2. zone of deep subcutaneous infiltration.

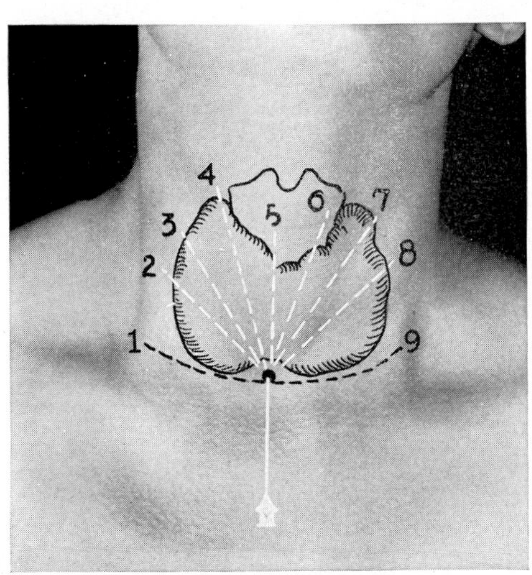

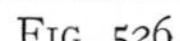

FIG. 526

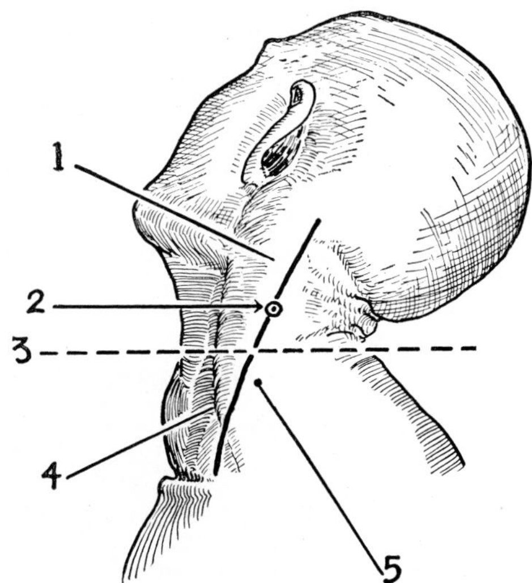

FIG. 527

FIG. 526. Infiltration anesthesia in thyroidectomy (modified from Hertzler). From the primary line of infiltration, the needle is passed between the platysma and the more deeply lying muscles. At 2 and 3 and 7 and 8 the anterior cervical and the supraclavicular nerves are blocked. At 4 and 5 and 6 the paratracheal structures are infiltrated. Line 1 to 9 represents infiltration of line of incision (Kocher).

FIG. 527. Location of point for insertion of needle in cervical plexus block: 1. sternomastoid muscle, 2. point for insertion of needle at junction of upper with middle third of line, 3. midline, 4. external jugular vein, 5. Chassaignac's (carotid) tubercle.

utes. Only one side should be blocked! Anesthesia on the other side is brought about by peripheral blocking.

INJECTION OF THE PARATHYROID SPACES

This is also not free from hazards and should be carried out with extreme caution.

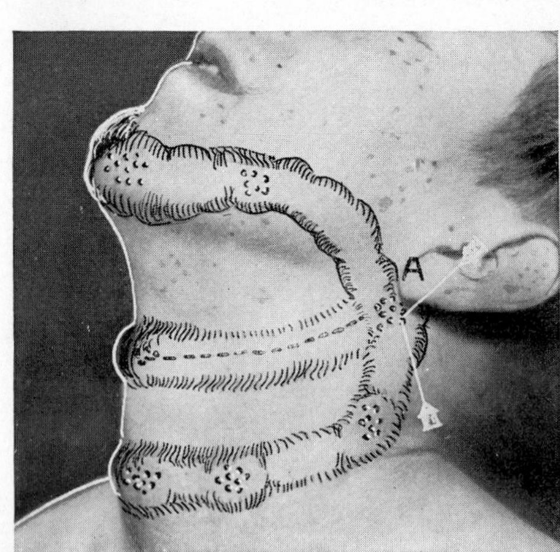

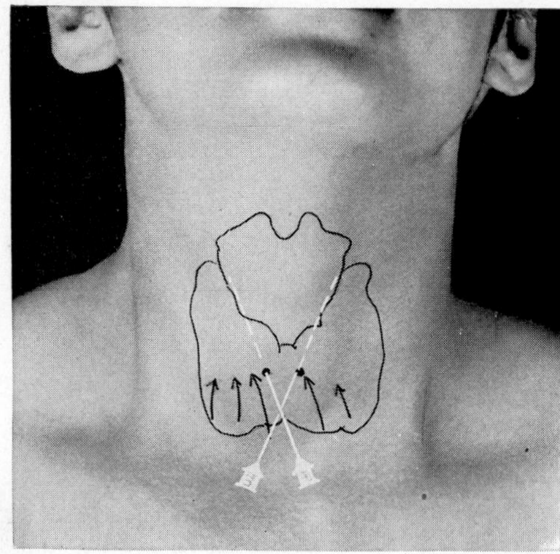

FIG. 528 FIG. 529

FIG. 528. Anesthesia for block dissection of the neck: A. point of entry of needles for blocking the cervical plexus.

FIG. 529. Paraglandular infiltration in thyroidectomy. A needle is passed between the gland and the overlying muscle. According to Hertzler (Local Anesthesia, Mosby, 5th edition) the soft parts over which the needle is passed should be depressed; its point may be made to reach the space between the trachea and superior lobe of the gland. A like maneuver makes it possible to infiltrate the entire paraglandular tissue.

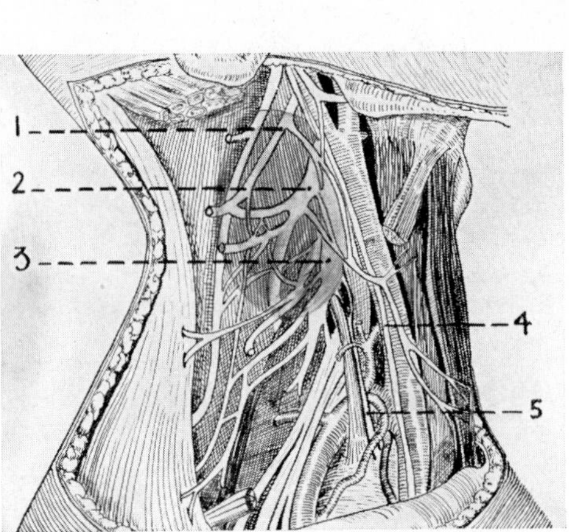

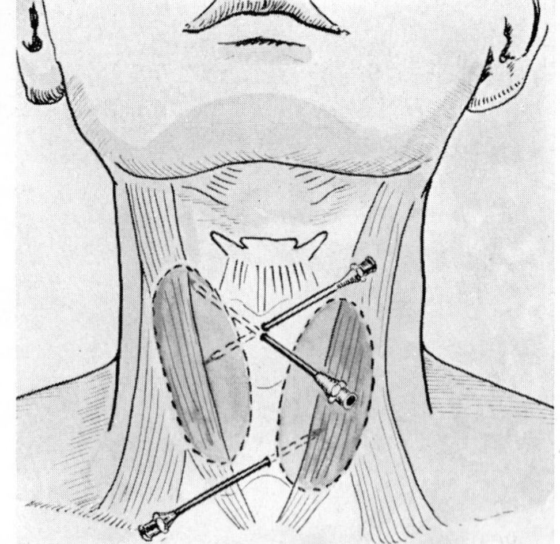

FIG. 530 FIG. 531

FIG. 530. Paravertebral injection (after Schultze). 1. Second cervical root. 2. Third cervical root. 3. Fourth cervical root. 4. Pneumogastric nerve. 5. Phrenic nerve.

FIG. 531. Injections of the parathyroid spaces.

In this procedure after the site for the collar incision has been determined and after the tissues have been dissected the parathyroid spaces are infiltrated as shown in Figs. 530-531. No solution is injected into the thyroid itself because it is not sensitive. Some degree of sensitivity is encountered at the upper and lower poles. Painstaking injection is paramount here. Crotti injects some novocaine-adrenalin solution into the surgical capsule of the thyroid before the goiter is luxated since this maneuver is very painful. This holds equally true for the regions about the trachea and esophagus and posterior surface of the thyroid, always keeping in mind the "danger zone." The isthmus is anesthetized by injecting the solution above, below and behind it.

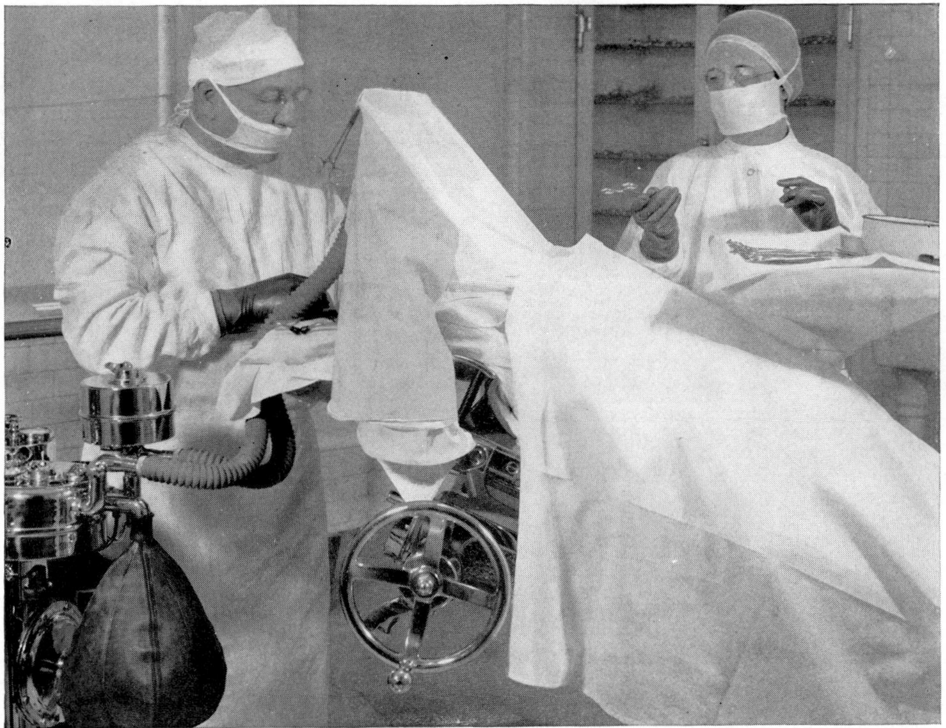

FIG. 532. Thyroidectomy. Arrangement of patient for removal of the thyroid. Observe bridge attachment on operating table which elevates the neck bringing the operative area nearer to the surgeon.

Operation

Do not begin to operate immediately after injection of the anesthetic is made but allow about ten minutes to elapse. Keep within the limits of the infiltrated area where regional infiltration has been resorted to.

Position of the Patient. Adjust the patient on the operating table in such a manner that there is a downward incline from head to foot. This lessens congestion in the field of operation. Elevate the shoulders on a sandbag. Extend the head; this renders the operative field prominent. Separate the face of the patient from the neck by a proper wire screen appropriately draped. (Fig. 532.)

Step 1. (Fig. 533a.) Make a low collar incision (Kocher) slightly curved, its concavity directed upward. It should be 1 or 2 cm. above the manubrium sterni. It varies in length with the size of the goiter. Let the incision correspond to a natural crease of the skin. If you want to avoid ugly scars, dissect the lower skin flap free so that it can be reunited without tension.

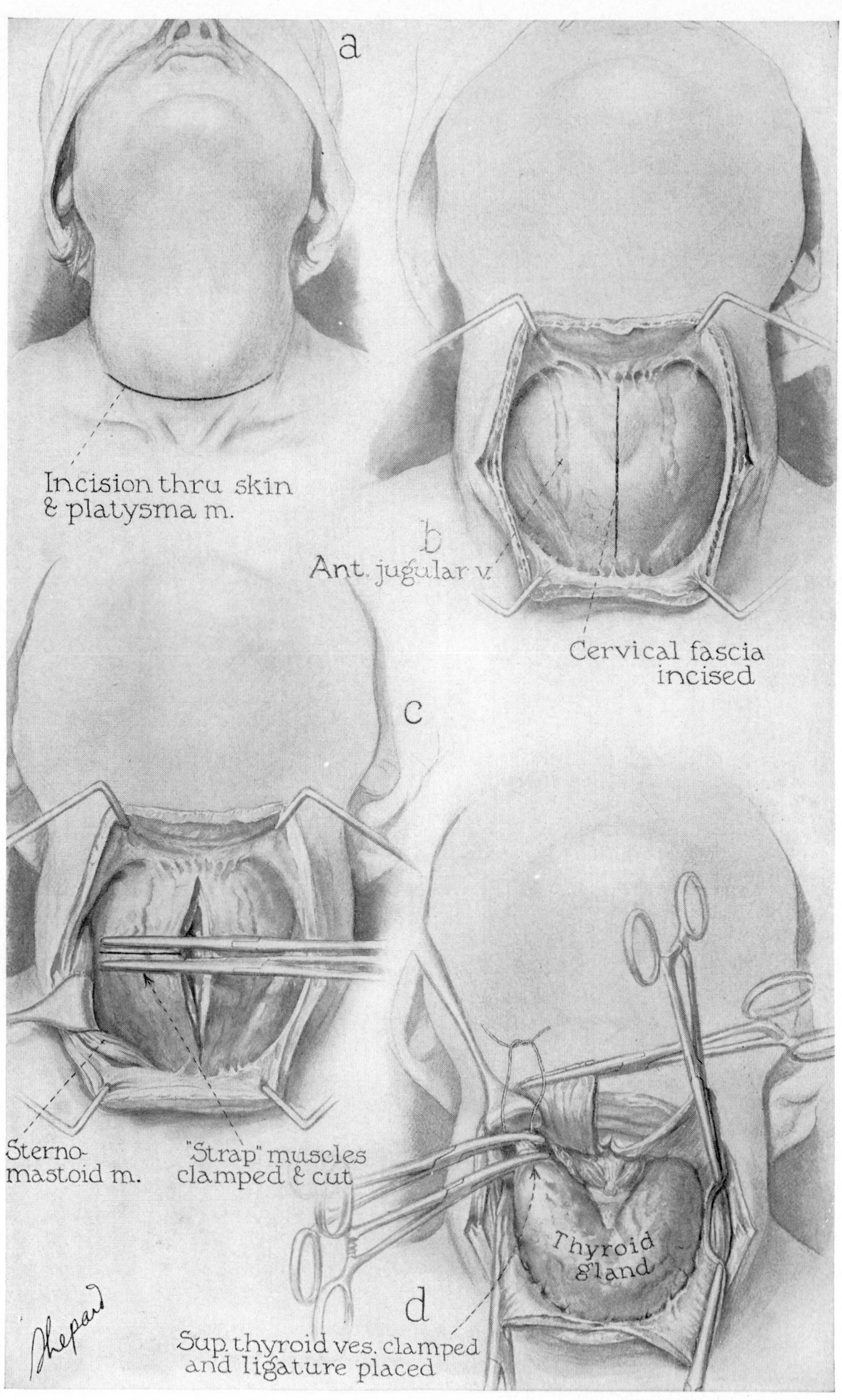

FIG. 533. a. Position of the patient's head. Incision (Kocher's) through skin and platysma. b. Longitudinal division of the cervical fascia. Ligation of the middle and oblique jugular veins. c. Division of the prethyroid ("strap") muscles between clamps. d. Exposure of the superior thyroid pole and vascular pedicle. Ligation of superior thyroid vessels. e. Superior pole freed. Surgical capsule opened and retracted. Glandular capsule clamped at various points, thus outlining the degree of contemplated resection of thyroid tissue. Resection of right lobe begun. f. Diagram showing relative amount of gland tissue removed. Also, protection of recurrent laryngeal nerve and parathyroid bodies afforded by careful operating in

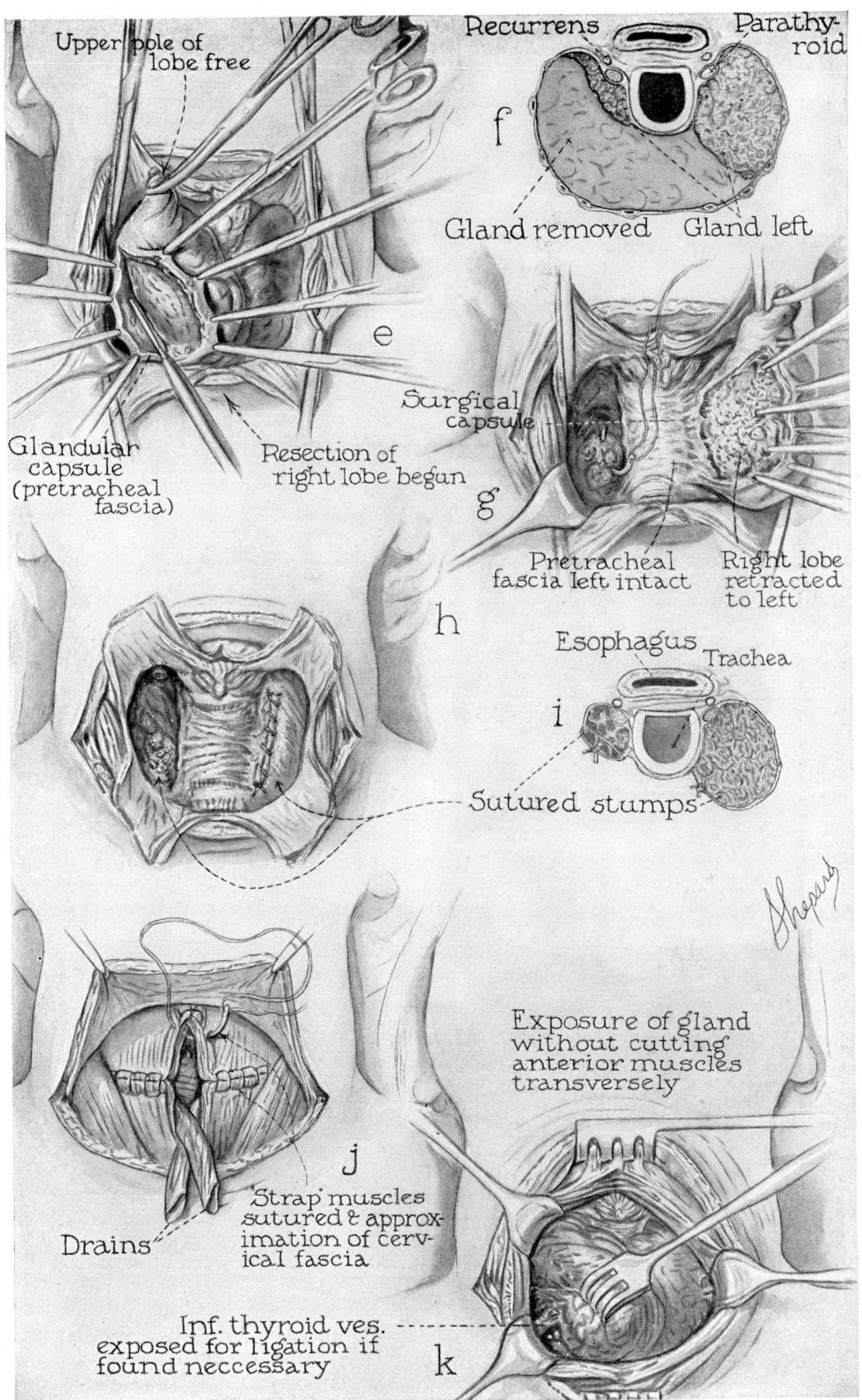

FIG. 533 (continued). the "danger zone" of Crotti. g. Pretracheal fascia left intact. Needle picking up the stump of the thyroid which may be attached to the posterior surface of a prethyroid muscle. (See text.) Right lobe of thyroid retracted outward and resection begun from within outward. h.-i. Sutured stumps and their relation to contiguous structures. j. Suturing of "strap" muscles and cervical fascia. Drains. k. Exposure of thyroid gland without dividing prethyroid muscles, which are forcibly retracted outward. Inferior thyroid vessels exposed for ligation, if found necessary.

Step 2. (Fig. 533b.) Divide and retract the subcutaneous tissues and platysma. Dissect the upper flap as high as the thyroid cartilage, the lower flap as low as the jugulum. Grasp and ligate small vessels as they present themselves. Divide the median and oblique jugular veins and, if necessary, treat the external jugular veins similarly. Drape and retract the flaps.

Step 3. Incise the cervical fascia vertically in the midline from the thyroid cartilage to the episternal notch, dividing the prethyroid muscles longitudinally. Introduce a finger under the muscles and separate them as far as possible in every direction from the subjacent structures. In so doing, direct the dissecting finger against the posterior surface of the muscles. This is for the purpose of avoiding injury to the veins in this situation. We are now in the musculo-capsular space.

Step 4. If the gland to be resected is of moderate size, and no operative difficulties are expected at this stage, the prethyroid muscles are simply separated with the fingers through the longitudinal incision made and are then amply retracted. In most instances this suffices. However, if the surgeon is not very experienced and sufficient space is desirable, it is safest to divide the muscles transversely (Fig. 533c). While it is better to do this step through a longitudinal opening, it is best in most cases to play safe. The muscles are divided at their upper end. The branches of the ansa hypoglossi, which supply the prethyroid muscles, enter the muscles in the lower part of the neck, so that if the nerve supply is to be preserved, the division of the muscles should be as high as possible. Another reason for dividing the muscles high is that after they are united again, the scar lies at a higher level than the scar in the skin. The omohyoid and sternocleidomastoid muscles are incised only when absolutely necessary.

Step 5. The surgical capsule having been divided, the glandular capsule is now in view. It is essential to orient one's self in the proper line of cleavage. The operation must now be continued in the surgical space. If this precaution is not observed, bungling instead of good surgery will result. Separate the lobe to be resected from its connections with the surgical capsule by blunt dissection with the finger. Retract the surgical capsule thoroughly but not too far posteriorly (parathyroid bodies). Respect the "danger zone" (region of the lower pole; parathyroids and recurrent laryngeal nerve). The middle thyroid veins are often encountered now. These must be doubly ligated and divided. Inadvertent tearing of these veins will flood the operative field with blood and will disturb the inexperienced considerably.

Step 6. Delivery of the thyroid lobe. Gently lift the lobe forward with two fingers introduced into the surgical space. Delivery with instruments may injure the large veins under the glandular capsule and cause undesirable bleeding. When by reason of inflammation or preoperative irradiations there are adhesions between the two capsules, luxation of the lobe will be correspondingly difficult. Forcible delivery may result in alarming hemorrhage. Under such conditions it is safer to resect the gland in situ.

Step 7. Free the upper pole from the surrounding structures. Guard the carotid sheath in so doing. Doubly ligate and divide the superior thyroid pedicle carrying the vessels. (Fig. 533d.) For safety, place another ligature above the first. Leave the ends of the ligatures long for the time being. Separate the superior pole from its attachments to the larynx. Work your way downward toward the (Fig. 533e) inferior pole. Occasionally difficulties are encountered if the upper pole extends high up into the neck or encroaches upon the larynx and esophagus. It must then be carefully and thoroughly resected. Remember it is safer to include in the ligature of the superior thyroid vessels a small knob of thyroid tissue than take a chance of the artery slipping out of the ligature.

Step 8. Ligation of the inferior thyroid artery. This is accomplished at a point internal to the carotid sheath. In so doing displace the thyroid lobe inward and upward and the carotid sheath outward. The inferior thyroid artery will usually be found about the junction of the middle with the lower third of the lateral lobe. Only the anterior branch of the artery is ligated and divided. The posterior branch is left undisturbed for nutrition of the remaining thyroid tissue (Fig. 533k).

Step 9. Map out the degree of resection to be accomplished. (Fig. 533f.) The procedure is a transglandular one and is accomplished from above downward. Apply hemostats to the glandular capsule all along the line of proposed resection. Divide the glandular capsule and resect the lobe until the region of the isthmus is reached. Only a thin layer of thyroid tissue is left along the posterior border of the resected gland. This is to be particularly observed in the "danger zone" (recurrent laryngeal, parathyroid). (Fig. 533h, i.) If a thyroidea ima is present it is ligated. Great care is to be exercised not to disturb the connective tissue covering the larynx and trachea (pretracheal fascia) lest the sensory fibers coursing here be included in ligatures and subjected to undue irritation (Fig. 533g).

Step 10. Resect the isthmus. Introduce a curved artery forceps between the isthmus and the trachea from below upward and separate these structures. The isthmus may now be divided between two clamps. In dividing the isthmus and lower lobe in this situation, bleeding from the superior communicating veins may be encountered. Clamp and ligate these vessels.

Step 11. If both lobes are to be resected the procedure is to be repeated on the opposite side. Resection may proceed from within outward or vice versa. (Fig. 533g.)

Step 12. If a pyramidal lobe be present dissect it out from below upward. Remove it thoroughly. If not, compensatory hypertrophy may ensue and cause a conspicuous bulge in the neck.

Step 13. Survey the field of operation. Hemostasis must be perfect. Redrape. Oozing is usually controlled by hot compresses.

Step 14. Examine the superior mediastinum for the possible presence of an enlarged thymus. If found, remove it (see Thymectomy).

Step 15. Resuture the prethyroid muscles and the cervical fascia (Fig. 533j).

Step 16. In thyrotoxic goiters drain for a day or two with a Penrose drain. Otherwise drainage is unnecessary.

Step 17. Reunite the platysma. If not resutured, spreading of the scar may result by reason of traction of this muscle on the edges of the skin incision.

Before proceeding to close the wound in the neck, flexion of the head will often reveal the presence of bleeding. Again, hemostasis must be perfect. Place the head in the normal position.

If the operation has been performed under local anesthesia, ask the patient to cough or speak. This will disclose whether or not the recurrent nerve has been injured or whether an insecure ligature is present. If the gland surfaces have not been approximated the posterior surface of the strap muscles may be sutured directly to the thyroid tissue.

Step 18. Close the skin with metal clips, Pagenstecher linen or horsehair. A subcuticular suture may also be used.

Intraglandular Enucleation

This consists of the enucleation of one or more nodes or cysts from the thyroid substance (Fig. 534):

Step 1. The extent of the skin incision depends upon the extent of the tumor to be enucleated. Primary ligation of principal vessels is unnecessary.

Step 2. Blunt dissection of the tumor is accomplished with the finger or with the Kocher dissector (Fig. 535) in a cleavage line between the tumor and thyroid tissue.

Step 3. The vessels are ligated as encountered.

Step 4. If a cyst is inadvertently opened during enucleation, grasp the edges of its sac with artery forceps and dissect it out thoroughly.

Step 5. Obliterate the spaces resulting from enucleated masses with interrupted catgut sutures.

Be sure of hemostasis. A hematoma in an incompletely obliterated space may give rise to compression of the trachea and become a source of danger. Should the bleeding become threatening during the enucleation or, by reason of existing adhesions, the enucleation become difficult, proceed at once to resection of the respective lobe.

If, instead of a finger, a cutting instrument is used to remove the intraglandular tumor, intraglandular or intracapsular excision is spoken of.

Resection-Enucleation

If the adenoma is large, or there are multiple adenomas, resection-enucleation is better than simple enucleation. Very large adenomas which occupy the greater part of one lobe are best treated by hemithyroidectomy.

Resection-enucleation is performed as follows:

Step 1. Expose the diseased thyroid.

Step 2. The adenoma to be removed together with about one-quarter to one-half inch of gland tissue surrounding it is outlined with artery forceps and removed (Fig. 536).

Step 3. Fold the remaining thyroid tissue on itself as shown in Fig. 537 and suture it as depicted. Insure hemostasis. Drain for a day or two, if deemed necessary.

Resection

This may be either **frontal (transglandular)** or **cuneiform** (melon resection). The former is shown in Figs. 538-539. It may be performed on one or both lobes of the thyroid. The raw surfaces may be anchored to the strap muscles.

CUNEIFORM RESECTION (ZOEGE VON MANTEUFFEL) 1898

Step 1. Ligate the blood vessels at their proper site.

Step 2. Dislocate the goiter. Ligate the thyroidea ima.

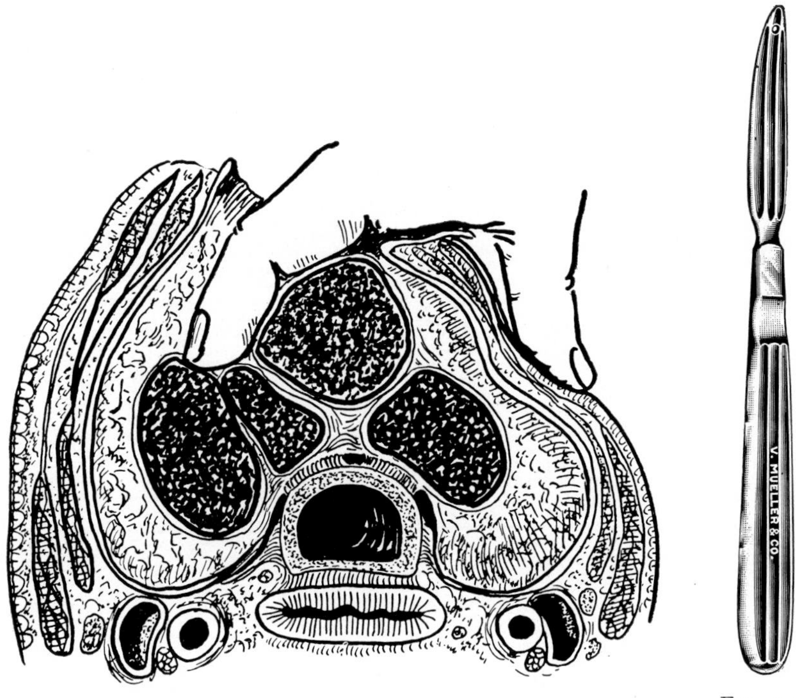

Fig. 534 Fig. 535

Fig. 534. Intraglandular enucleation of cystic goiter.
Fig. 535. Kocher's dissector, for use in goiter and bone work.

Step 3. Resect a wedge-shaped piece of thyroid from the respective lobe or lobes and the isthmus, if indicated. Wedge-shaped portions are removed not un-

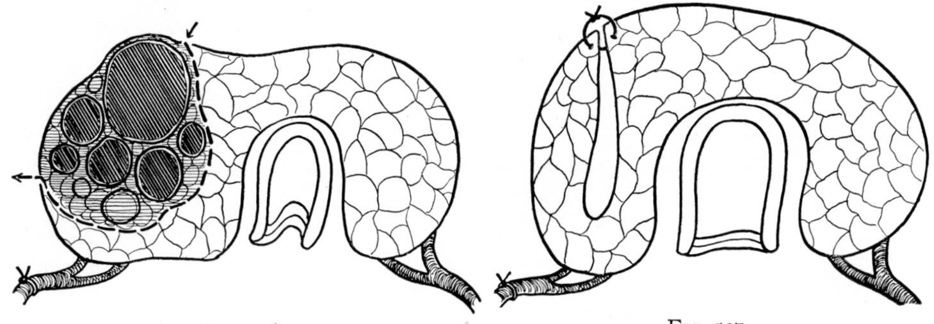

Fig. 536 Fig. 537

Fig. 536. Unilateral resection—enucleation.
Fig. 537. Thyroid tissue folded on itself and sutured.

like slicing a segment out of a watermelon (Figs. 540-541). The "danger zones" must, of course, be scrupulously avoided.

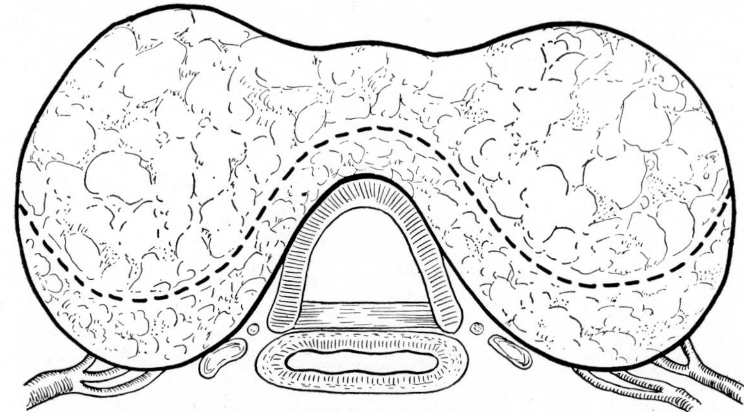

FIG. 538. Transglandular (frontal) resection; outline of line of excision. (After Crotti.)

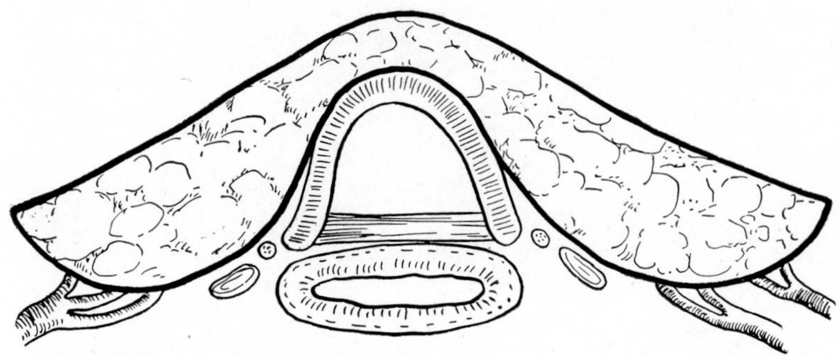

FIG. 539. Transglandular (frontal) resection; the raw surface may be anchored to the strap muscles.

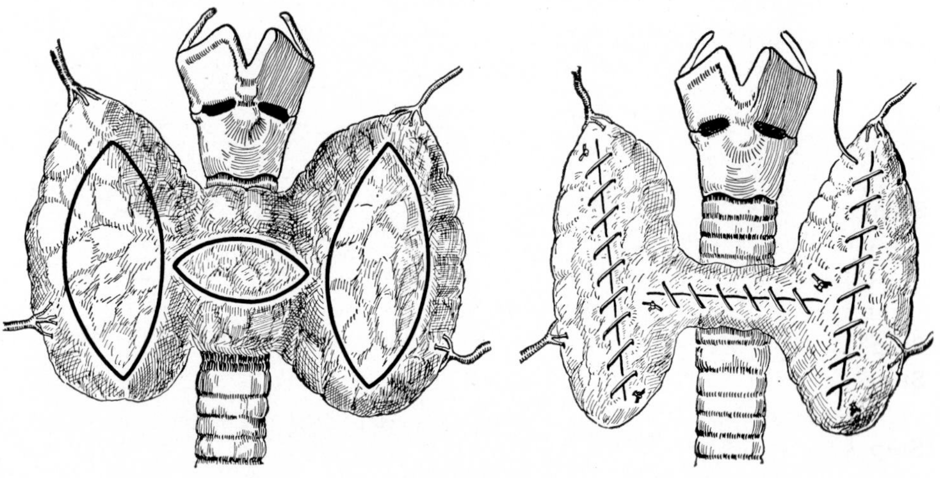

FIG. 540 FIG. 541

FIGS. 540-541. Cuneiform resection of the thyroid. Lines of excision and of subsequent suture. (After Crotti.)

Step 4. Reunite the remaining portions of the gland with interrupted catgut sutures (Fig. 541).

Step 5. Insure absolute hemostasis. Reunite the superimposed structures as above.

Intrathoracic (Substernal) Goiter

Thorough anatomic knowledge and considerable technical experience are essential in attacking substernal goiter (Fig. 542).

Step 1. Incision and exposure as before.

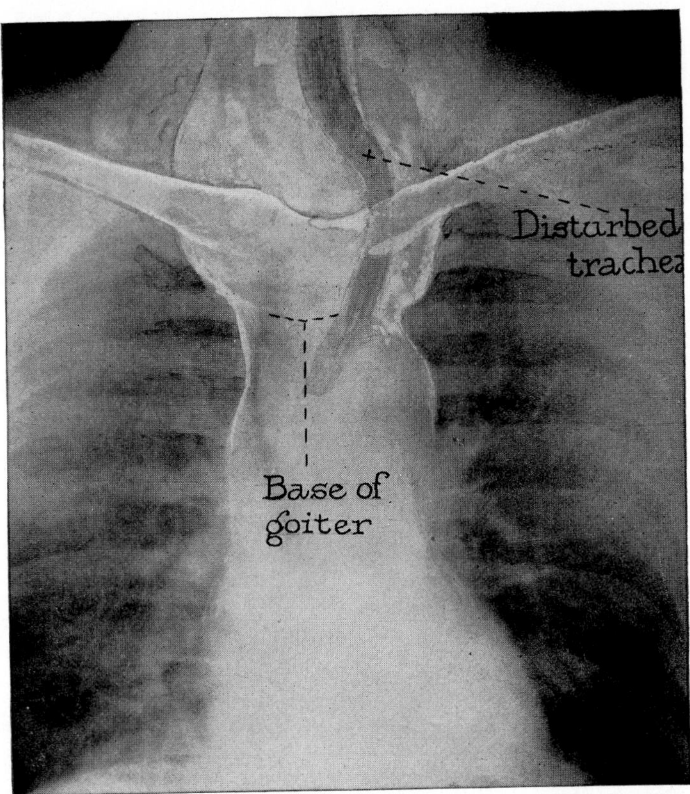

FIG. 542. Displacement of the trachea as a result of substernal goiter.

Step 2. Divide the muscles freely, particularly on the side where the intrathoracic goiter is located or "in cases of extreme gravity," says Joll, "there can be no serious objection to division of part or the whole of the sternomastoid muscle."

Step 3. Free the cervical portion of the goiter as thoroughly as possible.

Step 4. Ligate divided vessels as you go along. Perfect hemostasis is of utmost importance.

Step 5. Separate the substernal portion of the goiter and deliver it using the cervical portion of the thyroid as a tractor. The critical time of the operation is when the thyroid passes the upper opening of the thorax. Alarming hemorrhage and dyspnea may now ensue. The former may be due to injury of one or other of the large veins (internal jugular, innominate, subclavian); the latter the result of flattening of the trachea from compression, at the moment of delivery.

Step 6. In such case, replace the thyroid and allow the patient to breathe again. Do this a number of times until the goiter is successfully delivered.

Sometimes when the usual methods of delivery of the thyroid fail, recourse to resection of the manubrium sterni as advised by T. P. Dunhill (1922) may be the only avenue of approach. This, of course, is to be looked upon as a last resort and is performed as follows:

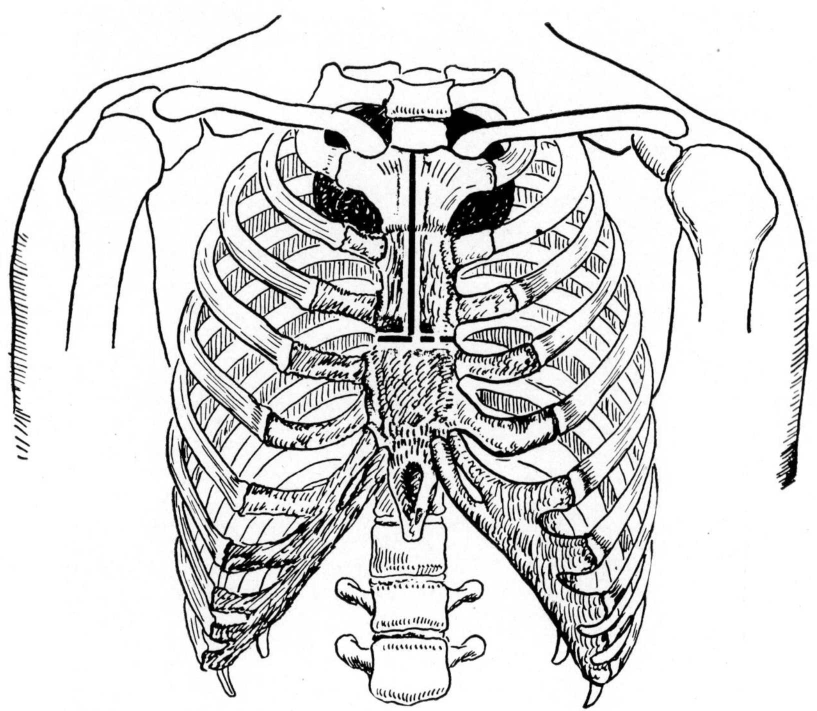

FIG. 543. Dunhill's method of dividing sternum to permit removal of impacted intrathoracic and malignant goiters.

Step 7. The sternum is divided in the median line (Fig. 543) down to or even beyond the junction of the manubrium with the gladiolus.

Step 8. A transverse incision joins the longitudinal thus creating a trap door.

Step 9. Reflect part of the clavicle and the required number of costal cartilages.

Step 10. Control bleeding in the cut surface of the sternum with Horsley's wax or muscle fragments.

Step 11. After removal of the thyroid the divided sternum and ribs are reunited with catgut sutures.

Step 12. The operation is completed in the usual manner.

Comment. Polycystic retrosternal goiter may be handled as illustrated in Figs. 544-545.

Operation for Malignancies of the Thyroid

The operation may be performed uni- or bilaterally.

Step 1. Make a collar incision a little higher than usual. After dividing the platysma, direct the cutting instrument toward the sternomastoid freeing its insertion over the sternum or resecting it if it is attached to the goiter.

Step 2. Divide the prethyroid muscles above and below, leaving them in contact with the goiter.

Step 3. Doubly ligate the superior thyroid vessels on the upper pole and divide them between ligatures.

Step 4. Raise the growth up; ascertain the location of the inferior thyroid artery; ignore the parathyroids and recurrent nerve if hopelessly fused with the growth.

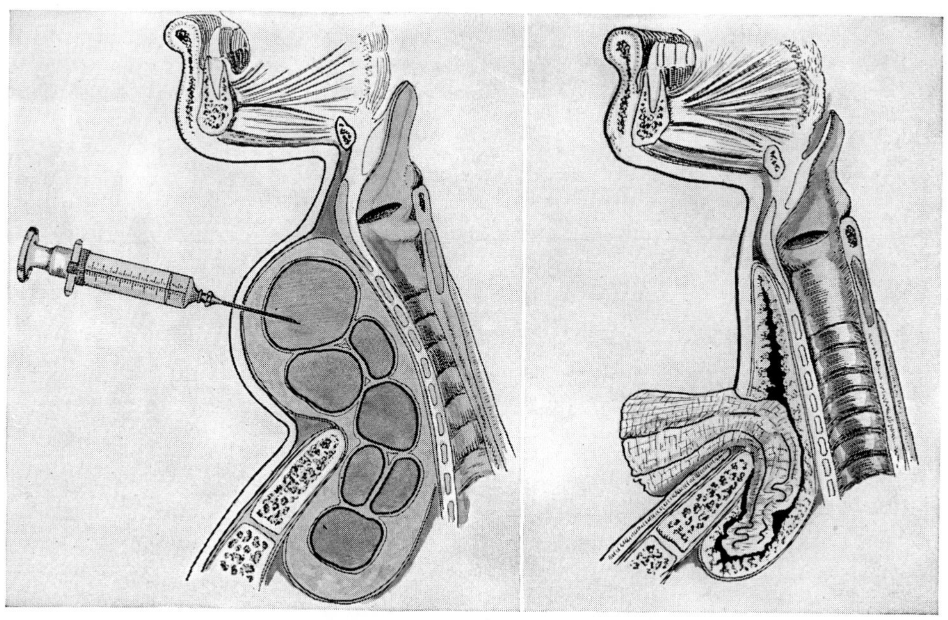

FIG. 544 FIG. 545

FIG. 544. Evacuation of cysts in retrosternal goiter.
FIG. 545. Tamponing of cavity following evacuation of polycystic retrosternal goiter.

Step 5. If the internal jugular vein is attached to the growth, resect it, after ligating it; this, to preclude air embolism. If in patients under forty years of age, the carotid is adherent to the growth, resect it; in older patients detach it carefully.

Step 6. Elevate the lower pole of the gland; doubly ligate the inferior thyroid vessels and divide them between the ligatures. Free the goiter toward the middle; separate it from the trachea and resect it. Ligate the antero-internal branch of the superior thyroid artery before the isthmus is dissected.

Comment. Where the tumor involves both lobes, the procedure requires careful study as to whether partial or complete removal of the thyroid should be done. In some instances the superior thyroid artery cannot be

reached at first; this necessitates approaching the tumor either through the isthmus or by detaching first the lower pole. The growth appears much more mobile before the operation than during it. A tumor fixed in the upper aperture of the thorax should not be interfered with. In fixation caused by neoplastic infiltration, the surgeon should hesitate before undertaking an operation. In some types of thyroid tumor where the growth is enclosed in the upper opening of the thorax chances of a successful operation may be very good, provided the tumor is not fixed.

It is sometimes difficult to distinguish between a malignant goiter and thyroiditis.

Stenosis of the trachea is treated in the same way as in non-malignant goiter; however, tracheotomy is performed more often for malignant goiter than for the innocent variety.

The after treatment in this type of case consists generally of radiation, arsenic and morphia in case of recurrence.

Injections of Boiling Water

In this procedure (Wyeth's operation) the blood and albuminoids of the tissues are coagulated by injections of hot water kept at the boiling point by using a Bunsen burner; the injections are made with a needle and syringe. The temperature of the water should range from 190° to 212° F.

Step 1. Prepare the skin as usual. Anesthetize the patient. Determine beforehand the temperature of the water to be injected into the growth as well as the amount and speed with which it is to be injected.

Step 2. When treating arterial and venous angiomas insert the needle deeply into the growth, injecting 30 to 60 minims of water at one location; withdraw the needle from ½ to 1 inch and repeat the injection. Continue this procedure until the entire tumor is made firm. Exercise care in using the needle so that the surrounding parts do not slough. Do not inject more than two ounces of water at one sitting.

Step 3. Dress and keep the parts quiet. If necessary, repeat the injection after 7 or 10 days.

Comment. Based on his thorough researches and careful scrutiny De Quervain concludes his observations as follows:[1]

The best immediate and lasting results are obtained in malignancies of the thyroid by early radical operation (calculated to protect the air passages), supplemented by radium.

Cases best yielding to treatment as shown by all statistics are those of the proliferating type of struma of Langhans (proliferating adenoma), papilloma and hemangio-endothelioma. The worst results are obtained in cases of sarcoma.

Irradiations supplementing incompletely operated cases prolong life and require further development of technic with reference to higher dosage.

Better results are obtained when patients are referred to the surgeon early in the disease at a time when there is a suspicion of malignancy. Some improvement may result from radiation-methods.

[1] Bull. Schweiz. ver. f. Krebs Forsch. No. 4, 1934.

Removal of benign goiters and efforts directed toward the systematic eradication of endemic goiters constitute prophylactic measures.

Electrosurgical Thyroidectomy

Advantages:

1. The radio knife is time-saving.
2. Hemostasis is better; fewer forceps are used.
3. In bad-risk cases the reduction in time and the facilitating of the operation are contributing factors in lowering mortality.
4. More thyroid tissue can be removed with less danger to the recurrent laryngeal nerves and the parathyroid glands than with the scalpel.
5. Less catgut is used, resulting in improved wound healing.
6. The radio knife is superior to either the scalpel or the cautery in the treatment of malignancy of the thyroid.
7. It is of particular value in resecting the hyperplastic or exophthalmic type of goiter.

Disadvantages:

1. The radio knife is not satisfactory for skin incision.
2. Occasional skin burns have resulted from coagulation too near the surface of the skin.
3. All important vessels must be ligated.
4. There is a tendency to postoperative hemorrhage.

Full cooperation of the nursing staff is necessary when the surgeon is using the radio knife. It would facilitate matters greatly in the operating room if a unit were available which could be manipulated entirely by the surgeon; there is need for much improvement on the present apparatus.

The technic may be summarized as follows:*

Step 1. The usual transverse incision is made either with a scalpel or a fine, purely cutting current, and the bleeders clamped and coagulated, avoiding damage to the skin margin. The scalpel gives a nicer scar.

Step 2. The usual exposure is made by dissecting the skin-platysma flaps downward and upward.

Step 3. The cervical fascia is incised in the midline, freed from the capsule by blunt dissection, and retracted laterally along with the sternohyoid muscles.

Step 4. The gland is gently mobilized with a finger and clamps are placed on the superior and inferior thyroid arteries.

Step 5. The gland is attacked in its superiolateral aspect with the combined coagulating and cutting current instead of with the scalpel and hemostats. The current is a valuable adjutant in cutting across the thyroid tissue, by controlling bleeding and lessening the toxic substances liberated into the blood and lymph streams.

Step 6. An occasional bleeding vessel will require clamping, but usually not more than four or five are needed on each lobe, and these, with the exception of the superior thyroid artery, are sealed by clamp coagulation. So small

* A. S. Jackson, Annals of Surgery, June, 1931. Martin B. Tinker, S.G., O Iii, 2. A. 1931; Kelly & Ward, Electrosurgery, 1932.

is the amount of current necessary, that these vessels are sealed with but little destruction of tissue.

Step 7. The wound is closed in the usual manner.

PROTECTION OF THE RECURRENT LARYNGEAL NERVE

The points at which the nerve may be most easily injured are (a) where it crosses the inferior thyroid artery and where it penetrates under the crico-pharyngeal muscle; (b) at the upper or lower pole. De Quervain says: "No surgeon has succeeded in avoiding these perils completely . . . The proposals made for safeguarding the nerve are diametrically opposed to one another. Payr, Hildebrand, Stierlin, Enderlen, and others deliberately expose the nerve. This anatomical dissection presupposes previous dislodgment of the goiter—a manipu-

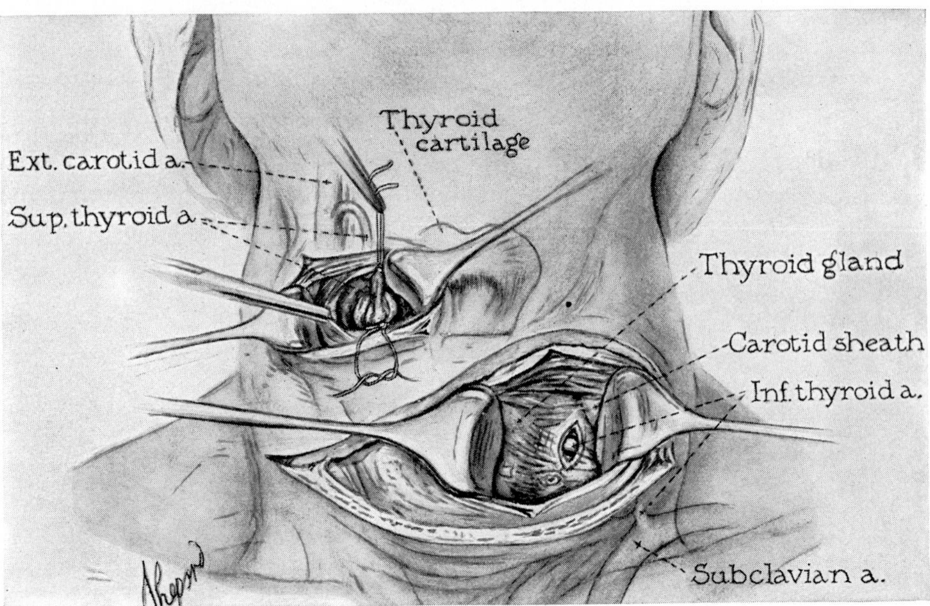

FIG. 546. Ligation of thyroid vessels, superior and inferior thyroid artery. Small collar incision. Carotid sheath retracted outward, thyroid lobe inward. Fascia overlying artery has been incised (see text). Incision of skin, platysma and deep cervical fascia along inner border of sternocleidomastoid muscle. Artery located in region of Chassaignac's tubercle. Another ligature placed around upper pole of the thyroid gland.

lation which the most expert cannot perform without the risk of injuring the nerve by dragging on it. This anatomical dissection is, therefore, no absolute guarantee of immunity—although it saves the nerve from injury by forceps, or from being included in a ligature, or from an inadvertent cut with scissors. Personally, we think that the remedy is worse than the disease, because the nerve is exceedingly sensitive, and practical experience supports this view. It is hardly necessary to mention the risk to the parathyroids involved in such a dissection of the retrothyroid region."

LIGATION OF THE THYROID ARTERIES

Ligation of the Superior Thyroid Artery

Step 1. Make an incision about 1 inch in length along the inner border of the sternocleidomastoid muscle below the point where the hyoid bone crosses that muscle. Divide the platysma. Divide the deep cervical fascia vertically. Retract the sternocleidomastoid muscle laterally and the omohyoid muscle toward the midline. Palpate for pulsations and identify the vessel (Fig. 546). If there are difficulties encountered expose the superior pole of the thyroid. Ligate the artery with a blunt ligature carrier or with the author's olive-pointed needle (Fig. 547).

Step 2. Avoid injury to the vessel. Apply a second ligature around the upper pole of the thyroid gland. An additional ligature or two at the upper pole is effective in preventing return circulation through one of the anastomosing branches, as well as cutting off the superior thyroid lymphatics and sympathetic nerve fibers.

Step 3. Close the wound.

Ligation of the Inferior Thyroid Artery

This vessel is usually ligated between the carotid sheath and the sympathetic trunk externally and the thyroid gland and the recurrent laryngeal nerve medially.

Step 1. Make a small collar incision dividing the skin, fascia and platysma. Retract the sternocleidomastoid outward.

Step 2. Incise vertically the fascia covering the sternohyoid muscle. Expose the carotid sheath. Ligate and divide any veins crossing the field. Displace the carotid artery laterally and the thyroid medially.

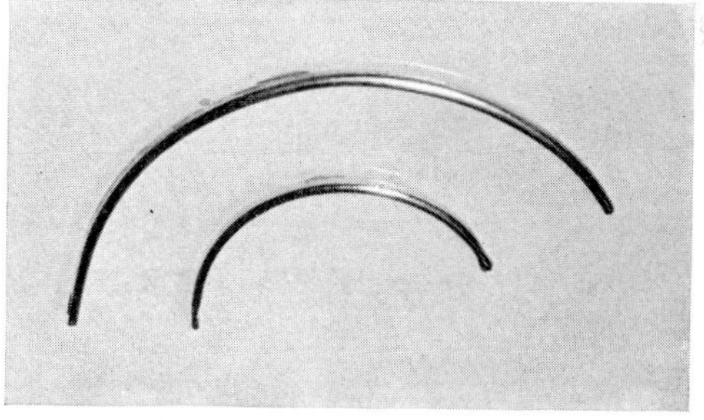

Fig. 547. Author's olive-pointed needles for ligating poles in thyroidectomy or in ligation of individual thyroid vessels.

Step 3. Locate the carotid tubercle (Chassaignac's) on the transverse process of the sixth cervical vertebra. The inferior thyroid artery can be palpated immediately below this and to the inner side of the thyroid. Free the artery. Ligate it doubly. Occasionally, anomalies are encountered (direction, number of arteries).

Step 4. Close the wound.

Comment: Should the condition of the patient become alarming during a thyroid operation do not continue to operate. Leave hemostats on the vessels, pack the wound with gauze, apply a retentive dressing to the neck and return the patient to bed promptly. To persist in operating on a patient who is apparently succumbing on the table is foolhardiness. The operation may be continued, if deemed advisable, a few days later. Many a calamity may be averted by adopting this rule.

Ligation of vessels first, prevents entrance of gland secretions into the general circulation. Particularly is this of value in dealing with carcinoma of the thyroid. Another reason for such ligating is that as the operation proceeds the weight of a multitude of hemostats tugs at the trachea and thus often embarrasses respiration.

In exposing the large veins think of the possibility of air embolism. To avoid this divide the veins promptly after first doubly ligating them.

Practice ligations of the external carotid on the cadaver; it will fortify your confidence in doing thyroid surgery.

Avoid injuring the trachea during the separation of the thyroid from it. If the trachea is opened inadvertently, repair it at once. A thin layer of thyroid tissue left on the trachea insures against its accidental opening. A collapsed trachea must be combated promptly with tracheotomy.

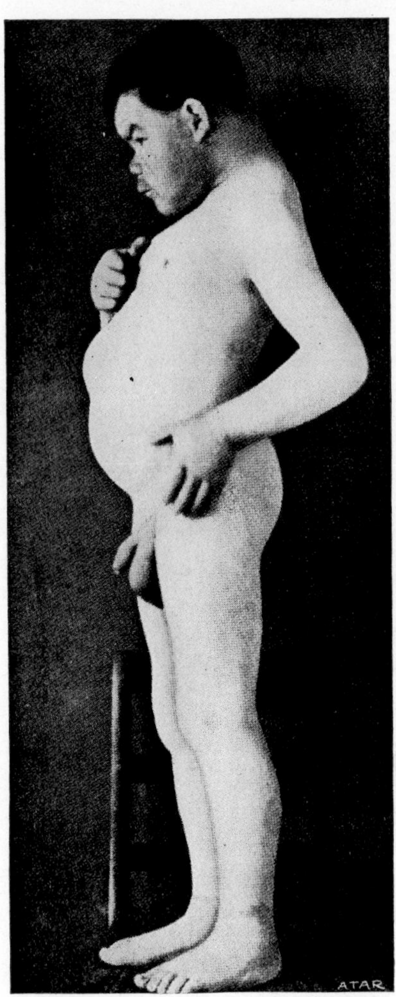

FIG. 548. Postoperative cachexia strumipriva after removal of thyroid. Patient aged 26. (Courtesy of Prof. de Quervain.)

If hoarseness develops on the day following thyroidectomy, do not conclude that there is an injury to the recurrent laryngeal nerve. Postoperative edema is usually responsible for hoarseness. With the recession of the edema, the patient's voice will return.

It is better not to remove the isthmus completely, unless it causes definite symptoms of compression of the trachea. Have a competent laryngologist ascertain the condition of the vocal cords prior to thyroidectomy. This is good insurance to your reputation and the patient's welfare. Unilateral or bilateral operation? The consensus of opinion is in favor of the latter. How much thyroid should be removed? That depends upon the case. Too little is just as bad as too much (hypothyroidism, myxedema, etc., Fig. 548).

In hyperthyroidism only an amount of thyroid tissue sufficient to carry on normal function should be left behind.

It is safer to resect from the inside outward (less danger of injuring the parathyroids).

Asepsis in thyroid operations is of vital importance. Do not be alarmed by a transitory rise in temperature following thyroidectomy. It is a common occurrence. In preparing thyrotoxic patients for thyroidectomy do not use iodine on the skin.

Complications Arising During Thyroidectomy

Dyspnea. If threatening, ascertain its cause promptly; in desperate cases tracheotomize at once.

Hemorrhage from the Superior Thyroid Artery. I have learned to leave a rather small button of superior pole tissue embraced by the ligature and place another ligature above it instead of depending upon the latter alone for security.

Commenting on this precaution De Quervain says: "Slipping of this artery should never occur if the precaution is taken of preserving a small tip of the upper pole."

Hemorrhage from the Inferior Thyroid Artery. Displace the carotid artery outward, press the lobe of the thyroid against the trachea and, simultaneously pulling it upward, locate the bleeding vessel and ligate it. Be cool! If a surgeon loses his head at this point, he will lose his patient. Pack the bleeding area for about five or ten minutes—look for the vessel again—you will find it!

Hemorrhage from the Middle Thyroid Veins. This should also be treated by compression and ligature. If the bleeding comes from the capsular veins or from those of the upper or lower pole, quick dislodgment of the respective lobe will tend to arrest the bleeding; greater opportunity is thus offered the surgeon to search for the bleeding point and control it. If the field of operation is suddenly flooded with blood, pack promptly and properly; wait a few minutes and proceed as suggested above.

Injury to the Esophagus. While rare, I have injured the esophagus once in extirpating a large goiter which embraced the retrotracheal space for a considerable distance. Fortunately, the opening was small and in the upper part of the esophagus. The patient was fed through a tube for a fortnight and the fistulous tract closed spontaneously.

Perithyroiditis Causing Adhesions. These often render the operation difficult and usually result from previously given x-ray or radium treatments or antecedent operations on the thyroid. Radium and x-ray-therapy obliterates the cleavage planes, and only meticulous and painstaking work will circumvent the constantly lurking dangers in these cases.

Should drainage be instituted after thyroidectomy? I always drain every toxic goiter. I never drain goiters of the non-toxic variety provided the operation has proceeded smoothly with no operative complications and one is reasonably sure of thorough hemostasis.

Tracheal Collapse and Conditions Which Simulate It. According to Cecil A. Joll[1] the term tracheal collapse is used to describe certain rare cases of acute respiratory distress occurring during or immediately after thyroidectomy. The theories advanced to explain its production are: (1) that the walls of the trachea are softened by the long-continued pressure of the goiter and, the latter being removed, there is not sufficient rigidity remaining in the tracheal wall which is therefore sucked in at each inspiratory movement and acts as an obstructive valve; (2) that although there is no actual softening of the wall of the trachea (a point emphasized by Berry), the peculiar physical characters of the cartilage-ringed walls of the trachea render it liable to collapse after removal of the tissues which surround its walls and, to some extent, hold them apart.

The difficulty Joll finds in accepting either of these explanations as invariably applicable is that he has met with three cases in which sudden respiratory distress occurred during thyroidectomy, the whole length of the cervical trachea being under direct observation, yet no trace of collapse of its walls or of any serious kink or stenosis was visible. The passage of a large intratracheal tube from above temporarily overcame the respiratory difficulty, but as soon as the tube was removed the dyspnea recurred. In each case tracheotomy cured the condition. It is difficult to resist the conclusion that some of the cases designated

[1] Diseases of the Thyroid. Wm. Heinemann, London, 1932.

tracheal collapse may be due to laryngeal spasm. It has been suggested that sudden onset of dyspnea during thyroid operations is due to bilateral injuries to the recurrent nerves; but in the cases to which Joll referred, the fact that the tracheotomy tube was removed within a week and that no subsequent trace of laryngeal paralysis could be found makes this explanation untenable.

Air Embolism in Thyroidectomy was first seen by Donald Guthrie* in 1907, while he was an assistant at the Mayo Clinic. A. Kocher was present and assured Guthrie that no ill effects would ensue. Kocher was right. Guthrie points out that arterial air embolism which may occur in any thoracic operation, beginning with pleural paracenthesis, is far more dangerous than the venous type, because it can lead to embolism to the brain or coronary arteries. He considers "pleural epilepsy" not as a pleural reflex, but as a consequence of arterial embolism. The entrance of larger amounts of air into the veins leads to exitus. In the seventeenth century, horses and cattle were killed by blowing air into their veins. The first case in the literature of a fatal air embolism in man was reported in 1818. In abortions and confinements, air embolism can lead to death, especially in placenta praevia. Postmortem examinations in these cases show foamy blood in a dilated right ventricle and in the large veins. Death occurs only if the amount of air reaches a certain maximum. Death is caused by mechanical and biologic changes. Anemia of the center of the fourth ventricle through primary cessation of breathing leads to death. Timely artificial respiration may sustain life. If after the heart has continued to function for a certain length of time, and breathing has stopped a second time, death will result. Small amounts of air compressed into the circulation cause shortness of breath and lower blood pressure; injection of large amounts can also result in heart palpitation. Patients having hyperthyroidism, with resultant cardiac changes, are in greater peril if an air embolus occurs than are patients with other diseases. Because of the typical hissing noise, followed by "bruit de soufflement" of the French, a whirring, splashing sound which can be heard even at a distance of 1 or 2 meters from the operating table, diagnosis is not difficult. Sometimes vision is impaired; in some instances one may even see gas bubbles in the retinal vessels. Guthrie has seen, since 1932, four air emboli in goiter cases, three being secondary operations, one of which was fatal. In one case, the patient developed a postoperative paralysis on one leg without losing sensibility. The best method of prophylaxis consists of curtailing the collection of too many clamps in the thyroid bed before ligation. In shock, resort to artificial respiration supplemented by the administration of salt solution because heart-paralysis precedes paralysis of respiration; intracardiac injection of adrenalin should be used.

Denk reported one fatal and two mild air embolisms in 378 goiter cases during the last four years and believes they can be prevented by ligation of the veins before separating them and that air embolism may occur even after closure of the wound. It is recognized by the cessation of breathing. The suggestion of Claremont to draw out the foamy blood may perhaps succeed by introduction of a urethral catheter into the right ventricle through the cubital vein. A research worker demonstrated the possibility of reaching the right ventricle by a catheter introduced into the cubital vein on his own person. Von Eiselsberg believes that with accurate hemostasis, air embolus, of which he has seen a great number as a student, has become much more rare. He has observed, during a secondary lami-

* Guthrie, Donald: Wiener klinische Wochenschrift, Vienna, 50:1667 (Dec. 10) 1937.

nectomy, a fatal air embolus, into the coronary artery as a result of a congenital communication of both ventricles in a case of a war injury. Finsterer (1914) observed an air embolism in a sixty year old woman, in two separate instances. At first, during the development of a retrosternal struma, a hissing noise was heard for a minute or two from which the patient recovered quickly. That same afternoon she vomited, became cyanotic and unconscious. The chest was opened, and the heart incised. Artificial respiration brought relief after several minutes. Since that time, Finsterer operates goiters in Trendelenburg's position, which he considers the best preventive. Sternberg saw embolism twice. The vein was immediately compressed with the finger. Ranzi calls attention to the fact that most of the emboli are not fatal. He saw an exitus only once. Since the air enters in consequence of negative pressure the patient should immediately have the head lowered and the field of operation covered with moist gauze. In severe goiter cases the positive pressure apparatus should be ready, because positive pressure prevents entrance of air into the veins, while Schnitzler emphasizes that the lowering of the head diminishes the danger, but does not prevent it, especially in tracheal stenosis. Albert in all his lectures advises removal of blood from the heart by suction. Werkgartner examined the records of the Institute of Forensic Medicine since 1919 and found fifty cases of death from air embolism, more than half of these followed operation. Next in frequency to this, are abortions and puncture wounds. Several times emboli occurred in operations for injuries, four times in goiters, once in an operation for lymphoma. At postmortem the point of entrance is hard to find. One would have to fill the pericardium with salt solution, puncture the right ventricle and, if necessary, press out the blood from the pulmonary veins. Radical procedures should be used, because these cases invariably terminate fatally when less radical measures are employed.

COMPLICATIONS FOLLOWING THYROIDECTOMY

Hyperthyroidism

Comment: My experiences coincide with the subjoined conclusions of Donald Guthrie who emphasizes that:

Severe postoperative hyperthyroidism may be largely prevented by the proper preoperative treatment. It is important to consider each patient with hyperthyroidism as a separate problem and not to apply set rules or standardized methods of preparation. The cooperation of an experienced internist is invaluable in this work.

It is important to appreciate the disturbed psychic state of the patient and to understand how proper forms of suggestion will be of benefit. It is equally important to appreciate the deleterious effects of fear upon bodily physiology and to understand how easily disturbed mental states will aggravate toxic symptoms.

Anoci-association and general anesthesia are both important safeguards against the development of severe postoperative hyperthyroid reactions.

Safe thyroid surgery demands the services of a skilled anesthetist and of a well-trained goiter team.

The condition of a large group of former hyperthyroid patients, not weeks or months, but years after operation, should be the gauge by which a method of preparing and operating upon these patients should be judged.

No set rules can be applied to suit all cases. Every patient is a separate problem.

Crotti uses, with success, diasporal, a colloidal iodine preparation, pre- and postoperatively in hyperthyroid states and to frustrate postoperative thyrotoxic crises. Cole uses sodium iodide, intravenously, for the same purpose.

MORTALITY FOLLOWING THYROIDECTOMY

Emil Goetsch,[1] analyzing 3,610 operations on 3,321 patients performed between 1920 and 1934, found that there were forty-two fatalities: operative mortality, 1.16 per cent; patient mortality, 1.26 per cent. Of these fatalities, seventeen (40 per cent) were due to postoperative crisis with secondary cardiac failure and seven (17 per cent) to primary cardiac failure unassociated with severe postoperative crisis. Five were due to pneumonia, five to embolism, and one to tetany which could have been obviated. The remaining seven fatalities were mostly accidental, of the type which do not now occur with refinement in technic.

TRANSPLANTATION OF THYROID TISSUE

Historical Notes. To Schiff is given credit for first transplanting the thyroid in animals; Kocher receives credit for the first attempt in man in a case of cachexia strumipriva in 1883. In both cases, the functional results were only temporary. Bircher and others met with the same results when attempting transplantation of the thyroid for myxedema. v. Eiselsberg and Christiani seem to have met with the first success with this operation both as regards life and function of the transplanted thyroid tissue. Unusual results have been reported by Payr in both animal and human experiments. A large piece of thyroid tissue from a mother was transplanted into the spleen of her child, who was a victim of congenital myxedema, with very favorable results.

Serge Voronoff* describes his results followed up twenty years after grafting thyroid tissue in cases of myxedema.

Kocher met with a certain degree of success by transplanting thyroid tissue into the medulla of the tibia. He employed the following procedure.

Step 1. Form an osteoperiosteal flap in the diaphysis of the tibia. Make a pocket near the epiphyseal line where the blood supply is adequate, and in the medulla.

Step 2. Introduce into the opening a silver ball about 1 cm. in diameter and close the bone and skin flap over it.

Step 3. A few days later reopen the incision after granulation has taken place, remove the ball, irrigate the wound with normal saline solution and place the implant, which is of the same size as the ball, in the blood-free pocket. Use normal or hyperplastic thyroid tissue from which the capsule has been dissected.

ANCILLARY THYROID OPERATIONS

The Surgical Relief of Progressive Exophthalmos

NAFFZIGER OPERATION

While, after thyroidectomy, exophthalmos usually recedes, in certain individuals the exophthalmos not only does not recede but becomes progressively

[1] Criteria of Operability for Goiter, Minnesota Medicine, Oct., 1935.
* Bull. Soc. Path. Comp. No. 492. Oct. 1937.

pronounced. If not relieved, the symptoms (lacrimation, epiphora, corneal ulcerations and ophthalmitis) may become so marked that only enucleation or death relieves the patient from a pitiable existence. The disease is one of mechanical origin, viz., the result of a pronounced swelling of the extra-ocular muscles (often to 10 times their normal size). H. C. Naffziger devised an ingenious operation for the relief of this condition which is indicated in progressive exophthalmos following thyroidectomy and which has yielded him and others gratifying results.

The rationale of the operation is a decompression of the orbit and the optic foramen to afford adequate space for the increased orbital content and constricted optic nerve brought about by reflecting bilateral frontal flaps, elevating the dura of the frontal lobe, unroofing the orbit and removing the upper portion of the optic foramen, wide exposure of the orbital fascia and the ring of Zinn (Fig. 549).

Before operating, x-ray studies are to be made to show (a) the height and extent of the frontal sinuses; (b) the projection of the frontal and ethmoid sinuses into the orbital plate and (c) views of the optic foramen showing the immediate relationship of the sphenoid sinus to it. These roentgenologic studies will point the way to avoid opening into spaces and sinuses during the operation.

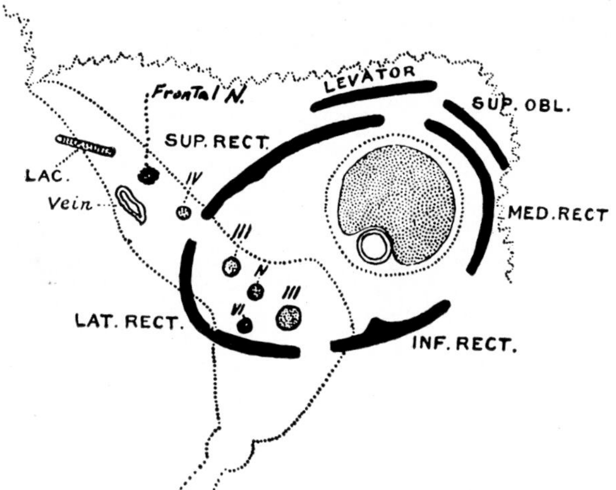

FIG. 549. Scheme to show the position of the annulus of Zinn and its relation to the structures in the apex of the orbit (after S. Whitnall).

Anesthesia. Avertin 85 mgm. per kgm. of body weight and 0.5 per cent procaine hydrochloride for local anesthesia.

Step 1. Expose the frontal bone by a transverse incision from the temporal fossa on one side, across the frontoparietal region, immediately behind the hair line, to the temporal fossa on the other side. (Fig. 550.) Dissect the scalp from the pericranium and reflect it forward thus exposing the frontal bone on both sides down to the frontal sinus. Bilateral frontal flaps are fashioned, the hinge of each being the temporal muscle. A small ridge of bone is left in the midline for the purpose of stabilizing these flaps when replaced.

Step 2. Separate the dura from the floor of the anterior fossa. Carry this stripping of the dura back to the sphenoid ridge and the base of the anterior clinoid process. Mesially, it is continued almost to the cribriform plate. The roof of the orbit is then opened (Fig. 551). Carefully separate the orbital fascia.

Step 3. Remove the roof of the orbit with rongeur forceps. Carry the opening in the bone forward, anteriorly, to the frontal sinus and laterally to a point where the orbital roof merges into the lateral wall of the skull and posteriorly to the sphenoidal ridge. Leave only a thin line of bone attached to the small sinus which is to be found in the dural reflection. Remove the roof of the optic foramen and its superolateral margin (Fig. 552). X-rays of the optic foramen will show its relation to the sphenoidal sinus. The orbital contents will bulge into the opening as it is enlarged.

Step 4. Open the orbital fascia. Avoid the frontal branches of the fifth nerve, working by blunt dissection. Expose the levator superioris and superior rectus muscles. Avoid the nerve supply, which enters from below.

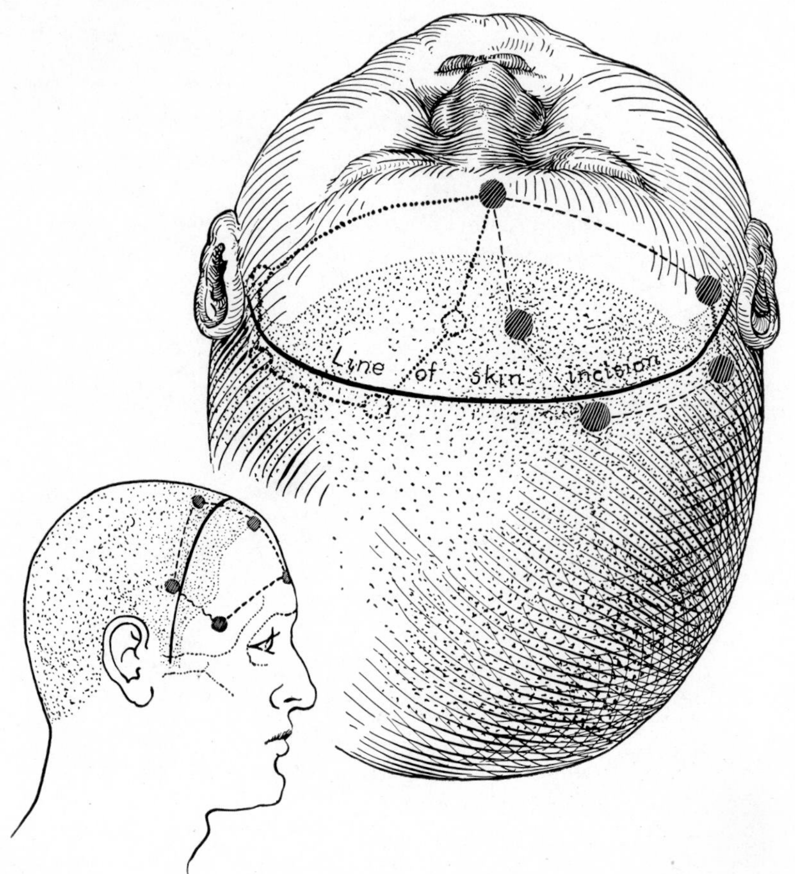

FIG. 550. Incision used. The solid black line indicates the coronal incision; the dotted lines, the two osteoplastic flaps. (Courtesy of Dr. Howard C. Naffziger.)

Step 5. Expose the internal and external recti similarly. The muscles are usually enormously enlarged (Fig. 553). In some patients, Naffziger carried the dissection down to expose the capsule of Tenon and the optic nerve as it enters the globe. Ordinarily this is unnecessary, the orbital fascia being open in all directions. The zonule of Zinn surrounding the orbital fissure and the optic foramen may be slit, usually at the outer margin of the superior rectus muscle.

Step 6. Hemostasis. Allow the dura to come down and rest directly on the orbital content. Carry out a similar procedure on the opposite side. Replace the bone flaps and fasten them together across the ridge of bone in the midline. Replace and suture the scalp in position. Suture the galea and skin separately. Fill the openings in the bone with bone dust. Protect the cornea carefully.

OPERATIONS ON THE PARATHYROID GLANDS

"Hyperparathyroidism[1] is a distinct disease-entity associated with a definite train of symptoms and a characteristic disturbance of calcium and phosphorus metabolism. It is constantly associated with a demonstrable adenoma usually of

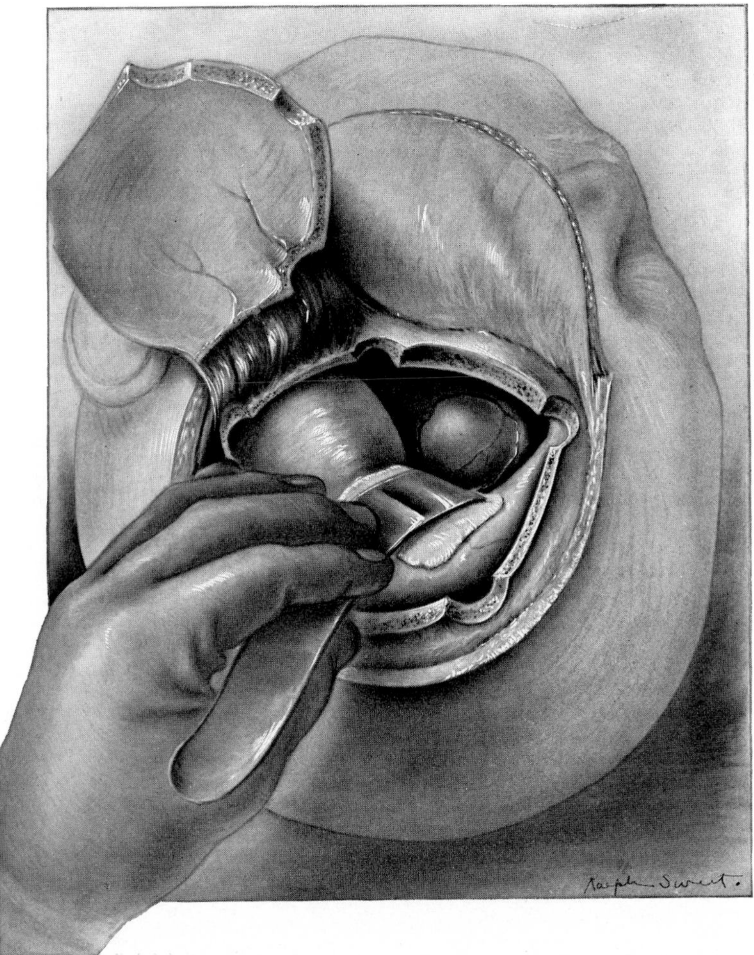

FIG. 551. Intracranial approach to the orbit. Part of the orbital plate is removed, exposing the fascia of the orbit. (Courtesy of Dr. Howard C. Naffziger.)

gross size of one or more parathyroid bodies. Following the total or subtotal resection of the tumor the calcium and phosphorous metabolism returns to normal, usually after a more or less prolonged period of tetany.

"The beneficial effects said to follow the removal of one or more normal parathyroids in certain cases of arthritis or in Paget's disease are, to say the least, viewed with skepticism. . . .

"The removal of normal parathyroid bodies or interference with their blood

[1] Churchill, E. D., and O. Cope, Surg. Gynec. and Obst., 58:255, 1934.

supply when operating with a definite diagnosis of hyperparathyroidism is absolutely contra-indicated.

"Subtotal resection of a parathyroid tumor is advisable when normal glands have been removed or damaged at a previous operation. Subtotal resection may also prove to be the operation of election in a very sick patient to lessen the

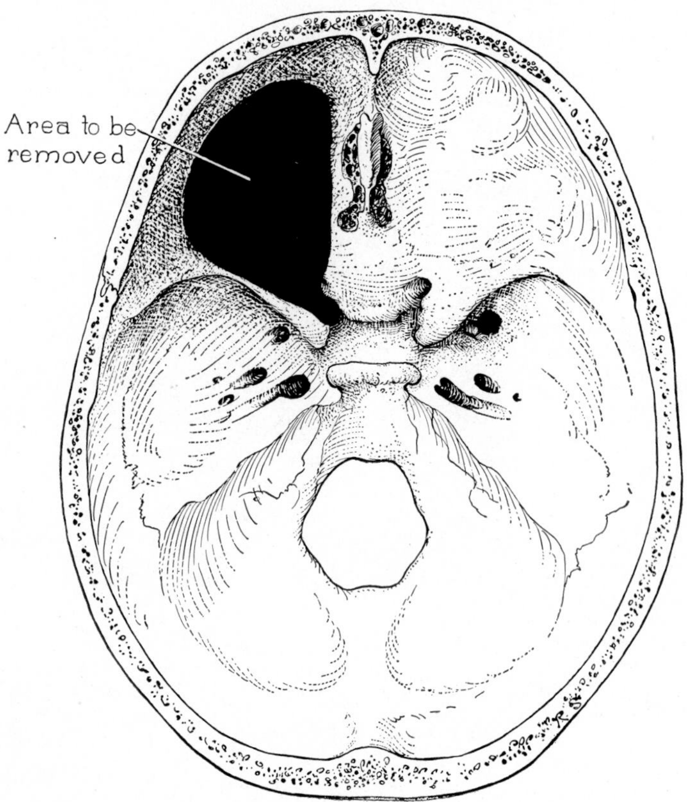

FIG. 552. Naffziger operation. The base of the skull showing the area of bone removed from the orbital plate and from the optic canal. (Courtesy Dr. Howard C. Naffziger.)

dangers of severe tetany. It has been done in one such case. The fate of the residual tissue being unknown at the present time, complete resection is the operation of choice.

Felix Mandl pioneered, in 1926, in parathyroidectomy as a means of cure in von Recklinghausen's disease. Others verified Mandl's findings.*

PARATHYROIDECTOMY

Removal of a parathyroid tumor is sometimes called for in cases of generalized osteitis fibrosa. Parathyroids are seldom palpable; therefore, free excision is essential.

Step 1. Make a wide collar incision as for thyroidectomy. Divide the depressor muscles transversely.

Step 2. Expose the whole thyroid gland thoroughly. Incise the thyroid sheath over each lobe.

* M. Chifoliau and A. Amdire, Jour. Chir. 38, Nov. 1931.

Step 3. After ligating and dividing the middle thyroid vein, rotate the corresponding lobe mesially and complete the separation of the thyroid fascia from the capsule covering the posterior surface of the lobe. The existing tumor of the superior or inferior parathyroid body is now exposed. The tumor may be found on either side of the trachea or in the superior mediastinum.

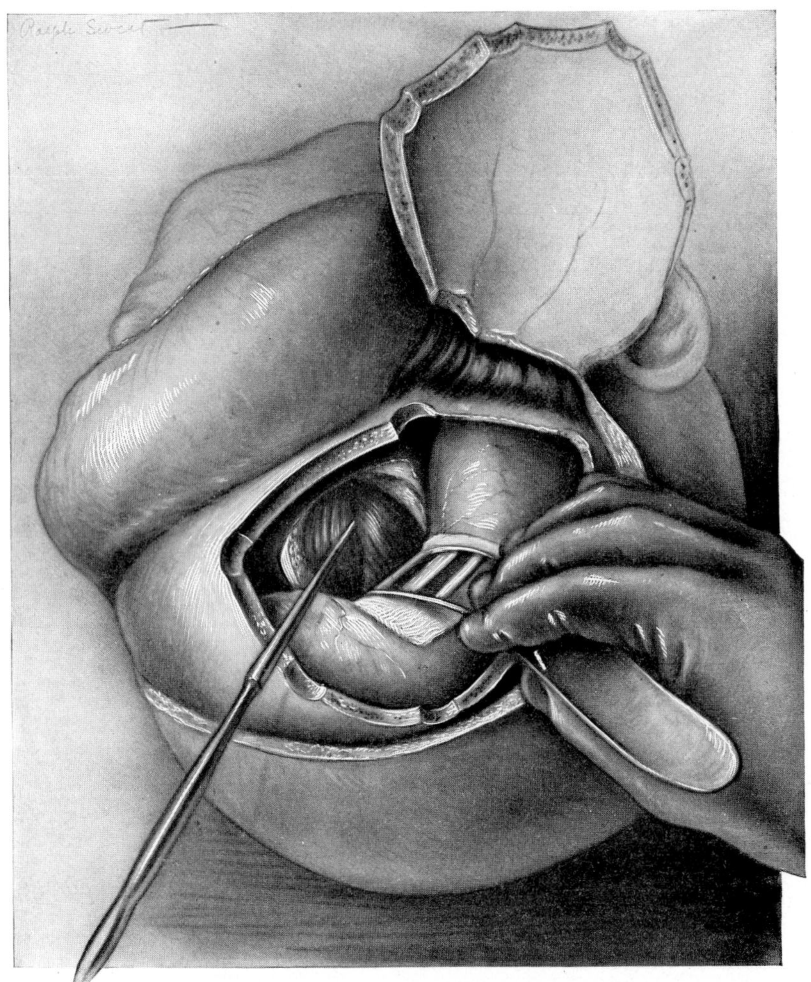

FIG. 553. Naffziger operation. Enlarged levator superioris and superior oblique muscles. (Courtesy Dr. Howard C. Naffziger.)

Step 4. Remove the tumor. This is usually not difficult. Walton calls attention to the fact that when the parathyroid tumor cannot be found in any of these situations it is probable that it involves one or other of the inferior parathyroid glands which may lie behind the thyroid sheath. It is necessary, therefore, in such instances to incise the thyroid sheath on one or both sides immediately above the level of the inferior thyroid artery and to search for the tumor alongside the esophagus, or within the thorax, where it may have passed down behind the esophagus to rest upon the bodies of the upper thoracic vertebrae.

Churchill's and Cope's Operation for Parathyroid Tumors Associated with Hyperparathyroidism

It is best to locate a small parathyroid adenoma in the first surgical exploration of the neck. Strict attention should be paid to hemostasis, as the staining of the tissue with blood makes it difficult to identify the parathyroid tissue. Doubly ligate even the smallest vessels before sectioning. It is imperative that all tissues be carefully handled by sharp dissection, as a hematoma may quickly develop

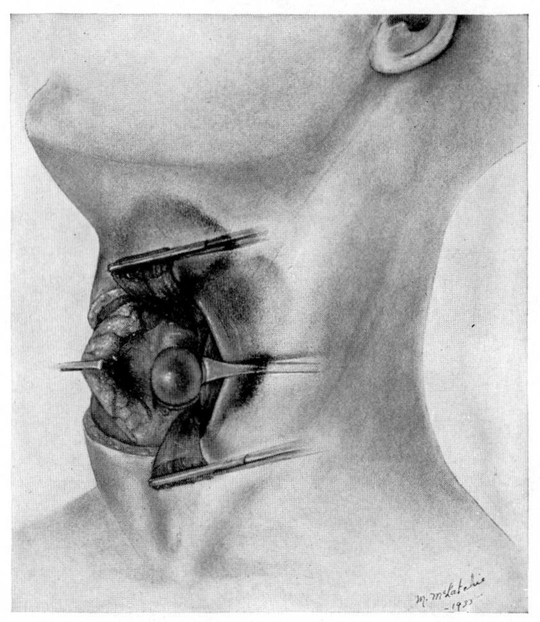

FIG. 554

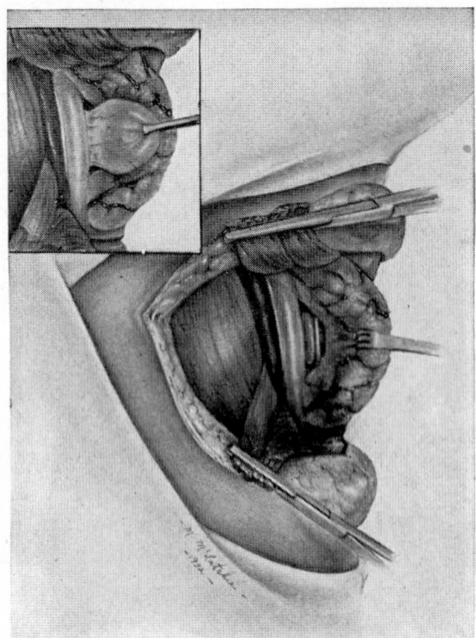

FIG. 555

FIG. 554. Parathyroid tumors associated with hyperparathyroidism. A parathyroid tumor exposed by elevating lobe of thyroid. The inferior thyroid artery formed a sling which may have prevented this tumor from descending into the posterior mediastinum, as it lay on the deep cervical fascia. Only the upper third of the tumor is shown in the cut.

FIG. 555. Parathyroid tumor situated between trachea and esophagus posterior to the recurrent nerve. Insert shows the tumor when delivered. (Courtesy of Drs. Edward D. Churchill and Oliver Cope and Surgery, Gynecology and Obstetrics.)

following an injury to the parathyroid body. A parathyroid with a hemorrhage in its tissue resembles a ripe currant. If this is present there is danger of postoperative tetany.

Do not cut into the thyroid gland, as the resultant hemorrhage will obscure the operative field. Use traction stitches of fine silk instead of double hooks to retract the thyroid. After hyperparathyroidism has been established proceed as follows:

Step 1. Try to locate the tumor by means of an x-ray. Take films to outline the trachea and penetrate the superior mediastinum. Look for a calcified capsule or displaced trachea. Use a swallow of thick barium to outline the esophagus in both anterior and lateral views. A filling defect or displacement of the esophagus may indicate the position of the tumor.

Step 2. After anesthetizing the patient, preferably with ether, make a wide collar incision; section the pretracheal muscles and dissect the middle cervical fascia from the surface of the thyroid. Look for any indications of tumor behind the thyroid.

Step 3. Identify the carotid sheaths and cut the lateral thyroid veins between ligatures. Palpate the posterolateral aspects of the thyroid and examine them directly. Continue the dissection downward on one side until the recurrent laryngeal nerve is identified and the region of the terminal divisions of the inferior thyroid artery exposed. Repeat this on the opposite side.

Step 4. Expose the trachea and esophagus and carry dissection upward to the larynx and downward into the superior mediastinum (Figs 554-555). Sever the branches of the inferior thyroid artery individually as they enter the capsule of the thyroid, making sure the blood supply of any normal parathyroid body is left intact (Fig. 556).

Step 5. Insert the finger back of the sternal notch deep to the middle cervical fascia; explore the anterior mediastinum. Insert the finger into the posterior mediastinum behind the trachea and esophagus. At the same time introduce a finger of the other hand into the posterior mediastinum on the other side. Palpate the structures of the mediastinum between the two fingers. If a substernal tumor is identified, deliver it into the operating-field with gentle traction. **Do not remove normal parathyroid bodies if no tumor is found.**

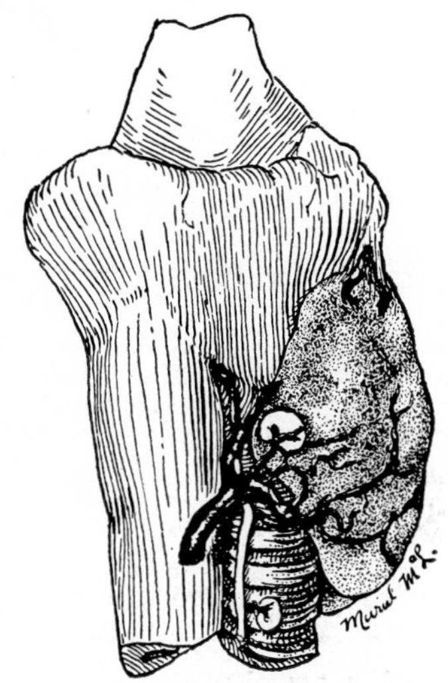

FIG. 556. Parathyroid tumors associated with hyperparathyroidism. Sketch from actual autopsy dissection (by R. R. Linton). The inferior thyroid artery may be divided at a point between the artery to the parathyroid and the capsule of the thyroid gland. This technic has been useful in complete thyroidectomy. A second parathyroid body is shown on the lateral aspect of the trachea. (Courtesy of Drs. Edward D. Churchill and Oliver Cope, and Surgery, Gynecology and Obstetrics.)

If no tumor is found after complete dissection of the neck and palpation of the mediastinal structures, recheck the diagnosis during convalescence. At the conclusion of an unsuccessful operation remove a small button of bone from the sternum if that has not already been done. If the diagnosis is confirmed, explore the mediastinum under direct vision by section of the sternum. Under positive pressure-anesthesia make a midline incision downward from the sternal notch sweeping to the right at the level of the third costal cartilage. Insert a finger into the mediastinum and direct it upward behind the sternum pushing the great vessels backward to avoid injury. Split the sternum with a Lebsche sternum knife and retract the two halves bringing the anterior mediastinum into view (Figs. 557-558-559-560).

In a final attempt to locate a tumor undertake block dissection of the neck above the larynx.

SECONDARY OPERATION

Churchill follows the principles of Clute for secondary operations on the parathyroid (Fig. 561).

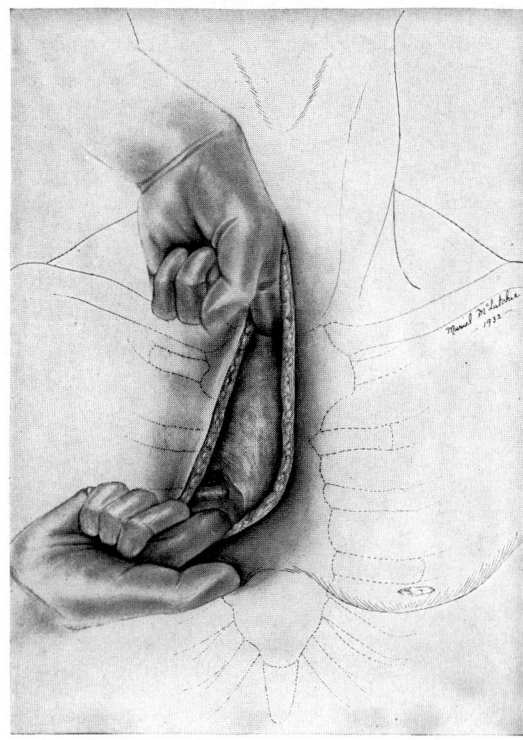

FIG. 557. Parathyroid tumors associated with hyperparathyroidism. First step in anterior mediastinotomy (after Sauerbruch). (Courtesy of Drs. Edward D. Churchill and Oliver Cope and Surgery, Gynecology and Obstetrics.)

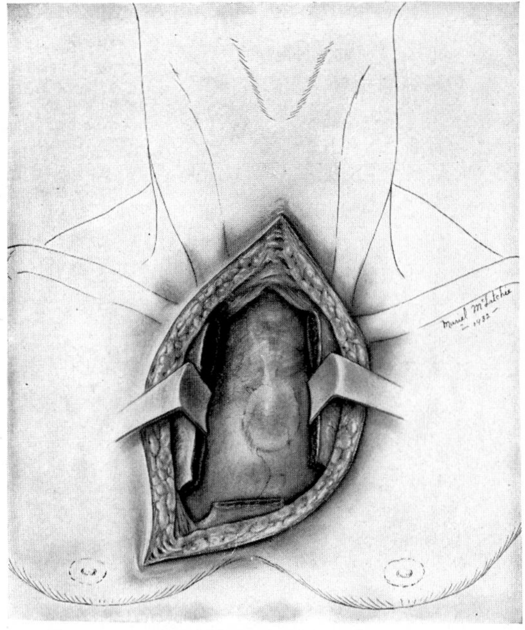

FIG. 558. Parathyroid tumor exposed by retraction of the two halves of the sternum. The vascular pedicle extended downward from the neck, the tumor lying below the left innominate vein. (Courtesy of Drs. Edward D. Churchill and Oliver Cope and Surgery, Gynecology and Obstetrics.)

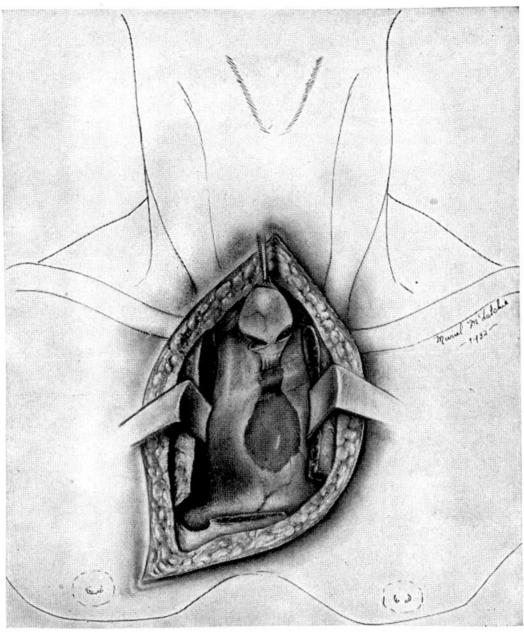

Fig. 559. Subtotal resection of the tumor because of the fact that at least two normal parathyroids had been previously removed. (Courtesy of Drs. Edward D. Churchill and Oliver Cope and Surgery, Gynecology and Obstetrics.)

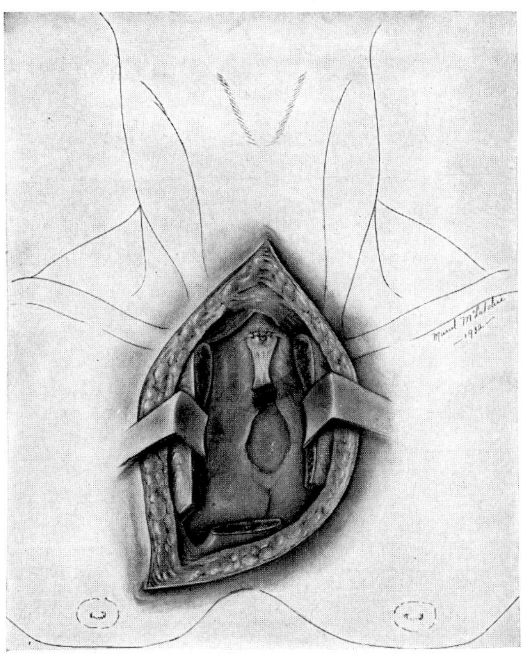

Fig. 560. Fixation of residual tumor tissue in the sternal notch with vascular pedicle intact. (Courtesy of Drs. Edward D. Churchill and Oliver Cope and Surgery, Gynecology and Obstetrics.)

Step 1. Section the pretracheal muscles; enter the deep areas of the neck on both sides through the carotid sheaths.

Step 2. Identify and retract the great vessels and the vagus nerves laterally; find the trunks of the cervical sympathetics marking the deep cervical fascia. Isolate the recurrent nerves as low as possible and trace these upward toward the larynx. Identify the thoracic duct.

Step 3. Explore the scar-tissue around the thyroid only after the exploration has been carried "far afield." Normal parathyroids or their vascular pedicles may be injured here, but a tumor would likely have been identified by the first surgeon.

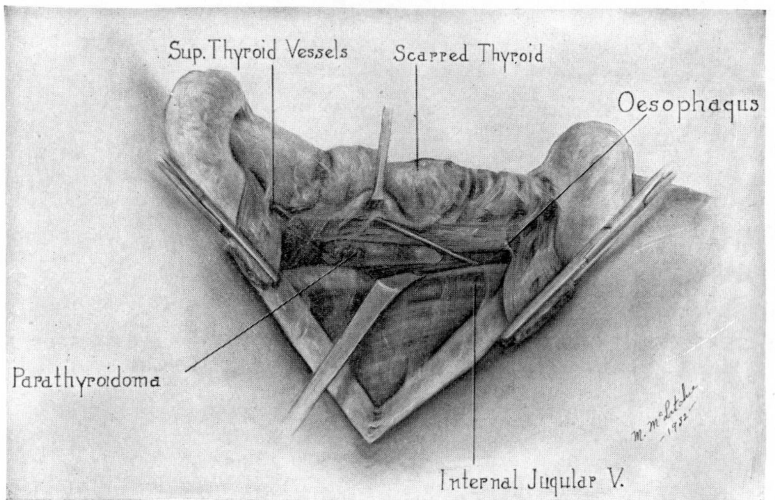

FIG. 561. Parathyroid tumors associated with hyperparathyroidism. Parathyroid lying behind the esophagus discovered at secondary operation. (Courtesy of Drs. Edward D. Churchill and Oliver Cope and Surgery, Gynecology and Obstetrics.)

SUBTOTAL PARATHYROIDECTOMY

This operation is indicated where damage has been done to normal glands or their blood supply. The capsule is resutured to form a compact body and its location clearly marked. In the case of mediastinal tumors, transfer the residual tissue, with its vascular pedicle intact, to the neck. The cases operated on showed marked tetany even with subtotal resection.

In some advanced cases accompanied by extensive decalcification of the bones, subtotal resection is indicated even if the normal parathyroids are intact. Severe tetany sometimes follows the removal of a large adenoma even when a limited dissection made damage to other parathyroids impossible. Death has been known to follow from uncontrollable metabolic disturbance caused by total resection of a tumor.

Comment. In speaking of the results of the operation, Churchill and Cope state: "The immediate result in the cases from which a parathyroid tumor has been removed either completely or by subtotal resection, has been a correction of the disturbance in calcium and phosphorus metabolism. In fact, postoperative studies showing the return to normal constitute the final step in establishing the diagnosis and efficacy of the treatment. They are notably lacking in the reported cases of Paget's disease and arthritis. Following removal of the tumor in true hyperparathyroidism the serum-calcium values fall with dramatic rapidity. Symptoms and signs of tetany may appear even with a serum-calcium above the normal level when hypercalcemia has been present for a long time. The tetany is controlled by high calcium diet, administration of calcium gluconate, irradiated ergosterol and parathormone.

Improvement in many of the symptoms of hyperparathyroidism may be expected within a few days. In several instances the patient has only been made conscious of certain long standing but ill defined symptoms such as loss of energy, constipation or fatigue by their abrupt cessation following operation. These symptoms are then recognized in retrospect as manifestations of the disease. The muscle and joint pains as well as bony tenderness are promptly relieved. The replacement of calcium in the bones takes a longer time and many months may elapse before any change becomes apparent by x-ray. The bone tumors being osteoclastomata, may be expected to disappear, but the bone cysts formed by fibrous replacement of bone substance persist.

"How far the kidney damage may be repaired is not known. In certain cases some improvement in renal function has been observed. The only fatality in the 11 cases here presented occurred following the removal of a ureteral stone several weeks after the resection of a parathyroid adenoma."

PARATHYROID TRANSPLANTATION

In discussing Transplantation of Living Grafts of Thyroid and Parathyroid Glands Harvey B. Stone[1] concludes:

"In dogs, certain endocrine tissues may be transplanted successfully from one individual to another. Factors of success in such transplants include the choice of a proper site for the graft, proper size and form of the graft, and biochemical adaptation of the graft to the host. The axilla and groin are proper sites. The grafts should be tiny fragments or tissue cultures. The grafts should be grown in culture in a medium containing the blood fluids of the host to adapt it before implantation.

"In human beings, ten cases have been submitted to grafting treatments, using the methods developed by experiments on dogs. Five of these were grafts of thyroid tissue and five were grafts of parathyroid tissue. Of these ten cases, only two are of sufficiently long standing to permit an opinion as to the success of the experiment—both of them being parathyroid tetany cases. In both of them we believe we are justified in assuming that the grafts were successful."

Tissues chosen to receive this implant should have a generous blood and lymph supply; the subcutaneous tissues, properitoneal tissue, omentum, spleen and bone marrow have all been recommended.

Step 1. Select a parathyroid in a location free from blood in a patient who is undergoing a goiter operation but is otherwise healthy. The surgeon should make sure that the patient will suffer no ill effects from parting with a parathyroid. The removed parathyroid is placed in Locke's solution and kept at body temperature until implantation takes place; implantation immediately upon removal is to be preferred.

Step 2. Anesthetize the patient and form a properitoneal pocket free from blood

[1] Annals of Surgery, October, 1934.

under the rectus abdominis muscle. Local anesthesia is best avoided as it may interfere with the transplant.

Step 3. Split the parathyroid without taking it out of the solution or incise it so that there are two raw surfaces; the procedure varies according to the size of the organ. Place the implant in the pocket made for it with as little han-

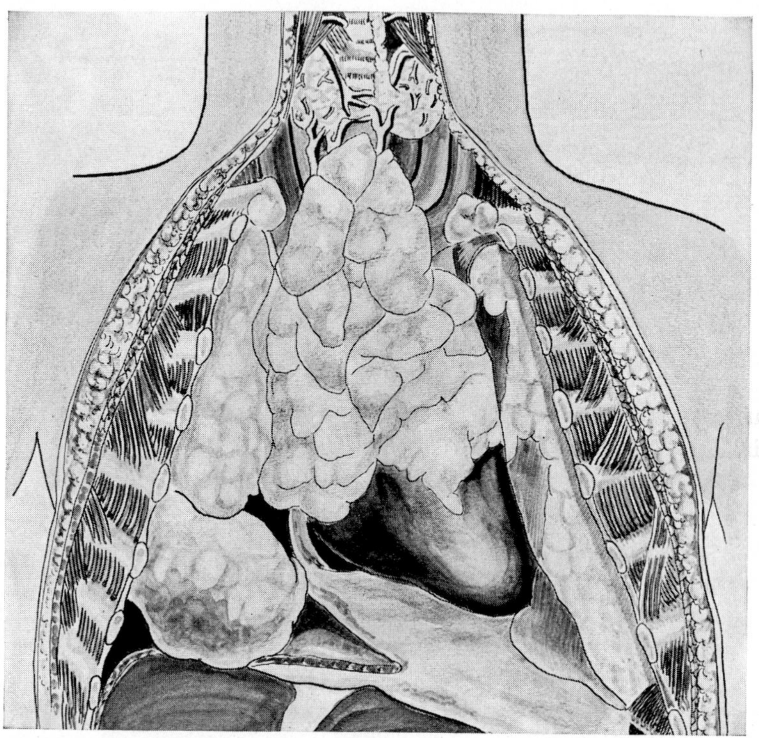

FIG. 562. Thymus of newborn baby (natural size). Note that the thymus fills almost the entire mediastinum and extends upward as far as the thyroid gland. The figure illustrates very well what is called the "cervical" and the "intrathoracic" portions of the thymus. Note, too, the vessels extending from the thyroid to the thymus (after Crotti).

dling and exposure to the air as possible. Check bleeding and close the incision without drainage.

Frugoni and Binde reported a case (Il Policlinico, Sezione Pratica, 44, 1937) in which a graft from a simian gland persisted for eight years in a patient twenty-one years of age. The operation was performed by Serge Voronoff.

OPERATIONS ON THE THYMUS

THYMECTOMY

Anatomic Considerations. To all appearances, the thymus seems to be associated with the nourishment of the unborn child and infant (Fig. 562). It increases in size in proportion to the rest of the body until the child is about two years old. After that it grows larger in some parts, diminishes in other parts, adipose formations appear followed by degeneration of the gland. Before degeneration takes place, it is firm and pink in color; later it is similar in appearance to adipose and areolar tissue and is very easily torn.

The thymus is enveloped in a capsule of fibers from which branches project among the lobules. It is found behind the upper part of the sternum and when it reaches its greatest size it projects for a short distance into the neck and extends down to about the fourth costal cartilage and in unusual cases as far as the diaphragm. The thickest part of the thymus rests on the pericardium, emerging from here into two flat lobes which become thinner and more divergent as they descend. The left lobe overlaps the right and is separated by a tissue of fibers. The left lobe is generally the larger of the two. Irregularities of the fibrous septa sometimes result in the fusion of the two lobes so that a third one appears between them.

The thymus is in touch with most of the aortic arch while the innominate veins and superior vena cava form a furrow on its posterior surface. It extends into the

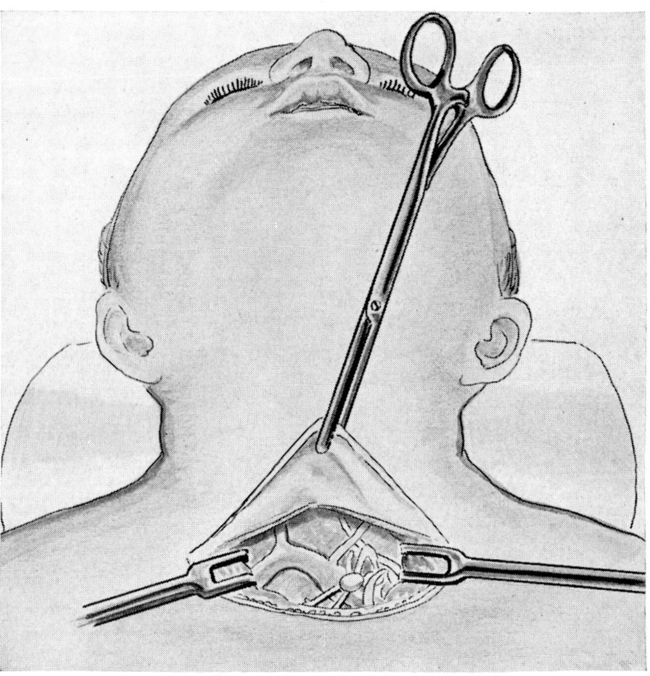

FIG. 563. Thymectomy. Transverse incision over manubrium. The superficial fascia of the neck is shown divided. The veins overlying this fascia are ligated.

space between the pericardium and pleura on either side. Before atrophy takes place, the thymus resembles a thick crescent. The suspensory ligaments connect the thymus capsule to the thyroid. The internal mammary vessels follow their course in front of it. Authorities differ widely concerning the weight of this body at birth; 3 gm., 5 gm. and 13.75 gm. being given as average figures. It is heaviest at puberty after which it becomes thinner and softer being replaced by fat and areolar tissue but rarely disappears completely although after 20 years of age it is not easily discerned as a rule. The internal mammary, thyroid and pericardial arteries furnish the blood supply for the thymus through capillaries at the junction of the medulla and cortex. The veins join together forming larger trunks, the left innominate being the most important. There are many large lymphatics which empty into the nodes behind the sternum and form a plexus around the lobes.

Anesthesia. Crotti admonishes that "in children, especially in the newborn, the dyspnea may be so intense that anesthesia, no matter what form, may only increase the dyspnea, consequently in such conditions the operation may have to be performed under local anesthesia or with no anesthesia at all as in the newborn for instance. . . . In small children chloroform seems to be preferable to ether."

The patient's position is the same as in classical thyroidectomy.

Step 1. Make a transverse incision above the manubrium of the sternum. Retract the lips of the wound. Divide the cervical fascia in the median line (Fig. 563).

Step. 2. Separate the prethyroid-muscles in the midline. Retract them laterally. Look for the upper limit of the thymus, which will ascend and descend during the respiratory excursions.

Step 3. Deliver the thymus into the wound by gentle traction on its upper pole. Attend to hemostasis during delivery (Fig. 564).

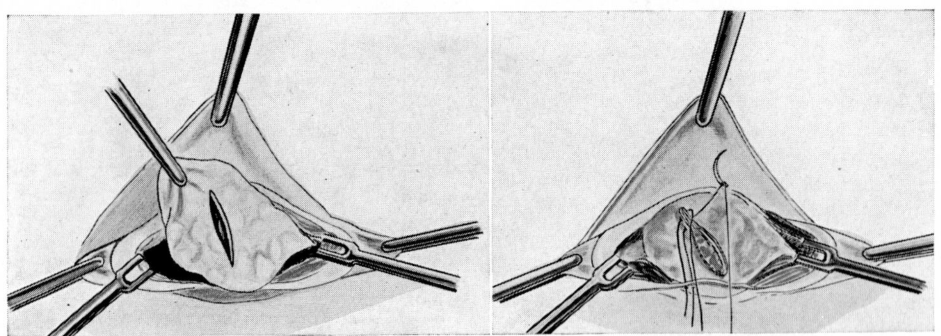

Fig. 564 Fig. 565

Fig. 564. Thymectomy. The capsule of the thymus is grasped with a pair of forceps, pulled upward, forward, and incised.

Fig. 565. Thymectomy. The thymus has been removed. The capsule of the thymus is sutured to the fascia and sternum.

Step 4. Crotti counsels extracapsular resection of the thymus, stating that "usually the thymus is easily loosened from the surrounding structures. Whenever, however, there is some perithyroiditis and consequently there is some difficulty in getting the thymus up, it is better then to perform an intracapsular thymectomy." Under such circumstances the capsule of the thymus is opened, permitting the parenchyma of the gland to protrude during the respiratory excursions (expiration). Shell out the gland digitally with care (Fig. 565).

Step 5. Ligate the base of the thymus snugly. Ablate it sufficiently above the ligated base to avoid slipping of the ligature. In an emergency (hemorrhage) tight packing should be resorted to.

Step 6. Attend to hemostasis. Reunite the prethyroid muscles. Suture the platysma. Close the skin. Dress.

TUMORS OF THE THYMUS

This surgery is of a very different type.

Lilienthal says: "Greater progress would be made if it were possible to perform more exploratory operations for suspected tumors in this region before such proportions have been reached that a transpleural operation with its added dangers has become necessary. Also, there would be less embarrassment from the greatly dilated veins which are present later on in the disease. The method of approach when the tumor does not extend too far beyond the borders of the sternum is by Milton's operation (Chap. 29) or one of its modifications. The thymic arteries are small in size and should not add greatly to the dangers, but means for differential pressure must be ready with an anesthetist skilled in their use in case one or both pleurae are wounded. When it is obvious that we are dealing with an inoperable condition some relief may be secured by the decompression afforded by a longitudinal division of the sternum and its posterior periosteum. Large mediastinal tumors spreading laterally need not of necessity cause distress by pressure upon the trachea as do those confined to the mediastinum itself."

CHAPTER 18

PRINCIPLES OF PLASTIC SURGERY AND SKIN GRAFTING

Historical Notes. The Hindus practiced skin grafting and plastic surgery two thousand years ago. A customary form of punishment was cutting off the nose; men belonging to the tile-maker's caste consequently became skilled in grafting on noses formed from the skin of the gluteal region. It is doubtful if similar operations could be done so successfully today, since there is no record of the exact technic employed by these operators. It was believed at that time that the graft atrophied or grew healthy in accordance with the state of health of the original donor.

There is very little recorded concerning the progress of this art during the middle ages. Toward the end of the eighteenth century Indian methods of grafting were introduced into Europe. At about this time Tagliacozza, a famous Bologna surgeon, is given credit for some very fine work in rhinoplasty.

RECONSTRUCTIVE AND AESTHETIC PLASTIC SURGERY

Plastic surgery designates that branch of general surgery which deals particularly with repair and reconstruction in connection with defects and malformations, whether these may be congenital or acquired; it includes not only the improvement of appearance but, so far as possible, the restoration of function. Plastic reconstructive work may, and generally does, consist in building up local defects with tissue obtained from the immediate vicinity or even from a considerable distance from the defect; but it also often includes removal of the localized redundant tissues and remodeling what is left so as to produce a normal or approximately normal appearance. This type of plastic reconstructive work and all operations which are undertaken principally for the removal of unsightly disfigurements may in a general sense be described as **aesthetic plastic surgery**; but many of these operations have not merely an aesthetic but also an economic and therapeutic value. (See Surgery of the Breast, etc.) Aesthetic plastic work, at present, is to a great extent confined to the facial and other exposed regions, but in the case of women, it may include the breasts, abdomen and other parts which have become unsightly and burdensome. General plastic work not only includes the aesthetic type but also work on bones, joints, tendons, etc., so as to eliminate pain and restore function. This type of plastic work may be called for in any region of the body following the healing of traumatisms or to remedy such congenital defects as webbed fingers, deformed feet or the like. The plastic work may require manipulation of bone, muscle, fascia, fat and skin, either in situ or transposed from a distance. By the term "take" we mean that the entire graft has healed in its new position. By a "partial take" we mean that the tissue transplanted has only partially healed.

The surgeon who undertakes plastic work should, therefore, be thoroughly familiar with the behavior of such tissues under all conditions and very particularly with their mode of healing when traumatized. He should also be conversant with the possibilities of **tissue-transplantation** and the use of **free** and **pedicled flaps** and **grafts.** By a "**flap**" is meant a segment of tissue detached from its natural bed for the greater part of its extent. The part by which it is left attached to its original surroundings (pedicle) carries blood vessels, thus supplying nourishment to the detached part of the flap. The detached part may be applied to a raw, granulating surface and, if this latter is well vascularized, the flap will, as a general rule, soon become itself vascularized and when this occurs, the flap may be entirely detached from its nutrient base. A "graft" may be entirely detached from its surroundings and connections and transferred to the place for which it is intended, where in due time it may become vascularized and live incorporated in its new surroundings. Bone, cartilage, skin and perhaps other tissues may be freely grafted or transplanted and under certain conditions will permanently live in the new site; other tissues and even parts of internal organs can be transplanted, become vascularized and live for a greater or lesser time in their new environment (Alexis Carrel). The free ends of the same or different tendons may be sutured together and will in time become integrate.

It will be seen that the operations of plastic surgery are manifold and the knowledge of technic demanded from the plastic surgeon is extensive if he covers all the fields embraced in this type of surgical work. Many procedures, such for instance as arthroplasty, are undertaken by the general surgeon as a part of his general work.

TWO MAIN PRINCIPLES OF PLASTIC REPAIR

1. The proper preparation or vivification of the surface or site of the plastic work;

2. Complete absence of tension when and after flaps or grafts are applied. These principles are perhaps more applicable to superficial than to deep plastic work and in this chapter, we will confine our attention principally to superficial plastic work.

The first of the main principles just referred to must of necessity presuppose some general conditions in regard to the patient; he should be free from all active disease such as syphilis, tuberculosis or suppurative disease of any kind: he should not be aged or feeble and his general health should be good. In the case where a plastic operation is being performed to remedy defects due to traumatism, such as a burn, the healing process should be complete and the patient in good general condition. All scar tissues must be completely removed from the superficies and all bleeding arrested before a flap or graft is applied to it.

METHODS OF PLASTIC REPAIR

When a superficial defect has to be repaired by a plastic operation which includes a skin covering, the following methods may be employed: (a) **Skin grafting**; (b) The French Method (gliding the edges together and suturing). This method was originally devised by Celsus. In such cases of tension, the skin may be mobilized to a great extent by undercutting; in this manner large areas of skin may be shifted without impairing the vitality of the transplant. (c) The Indian Method, which consists of using pedunculated flaps from tissue in the immediate neighborhood with more or less torsion of the pedicle. (d) The Italian or Tagliacotian Method: the use of pedunculated flaps from distant parts, as for instance when a nasal defect is to be repaired by a flap of tissue from the arm. While the method is inconvenient for the patient requiring immobilization of the arm for a long period, the procedure assures nourishment of the flap. (e) The Gillies Tubed-Pedicle Flap: In treating soldiers who had been wounded during the World War, it often happened that no local flaps were available to fill in defects where something more than epithelial covering was needed and it became necessary to obtain flaps from a distance; thus Gillies tubed-pedicle flap was

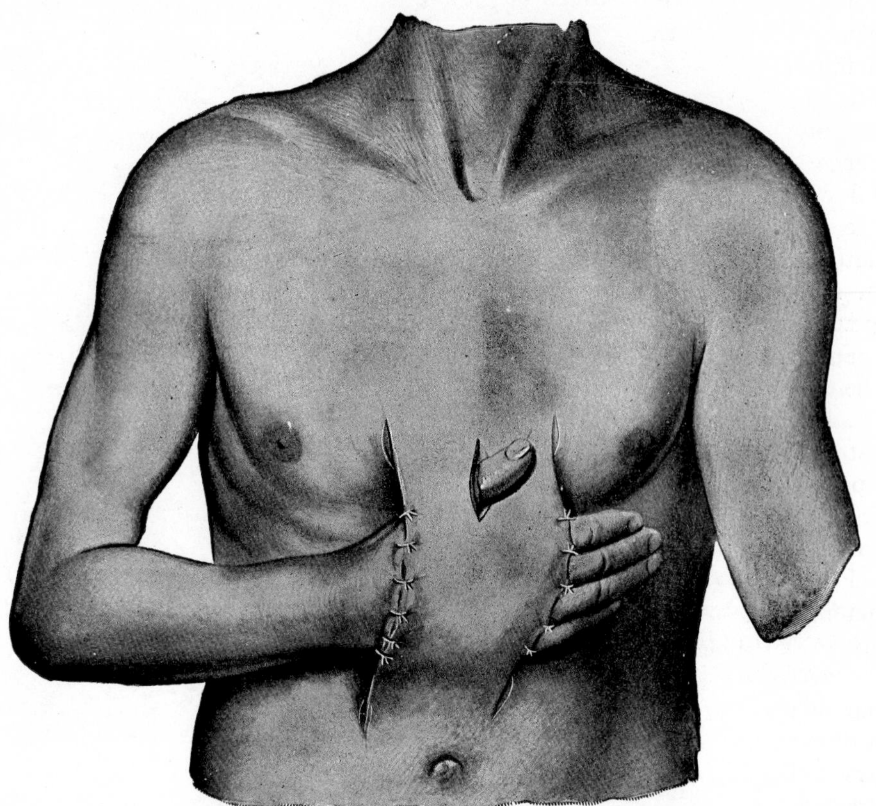

FIG. 566. Plastic surgery. Making a new dorsum and palm of the hand through a bridge flap taken from the abdominal wall.

developed. It is an excellent way to transfer whole skin together with the necessary amount of subcutaneous tissue from one part of the body to another. The wall of the abdomen usually furnishes this flap. The accompanying illustrations describe better than words the method of procedure (Fig. 566). The flap may be used for repairing various defects.

Flaps

Flaps for plastic work are usually thick and include the subcutaneous tissue which contains the blood vessels supplying the skin, so that vitality is not impaired. The deep fascia is not, as a rule, included in the flap. In some cases, as in certain kinds of rhinoplasties a flap may be cut containing bone and periosteum.

It is not within the province of this chapter to describe the many types of defects for which flaps may be employed nor the manner in which they may be utilized. Each type of defect will have to be handled according to its own particular circumstances and the judgment of the surgeon. There are, however, certain generalities which apply to flaps of all kinds. When a flap is obtained from the vicinity of a defect it may be glided into its new position and fixed there by sutures. In the case, for instance, of an external wound left following amputation of the breast, when the edges cannot be approximated, a flap may be obtained from the axillary or shoulder region and slid into the defect (sliding flaps). There is more danger of necrosis when such a flap is transplanted.

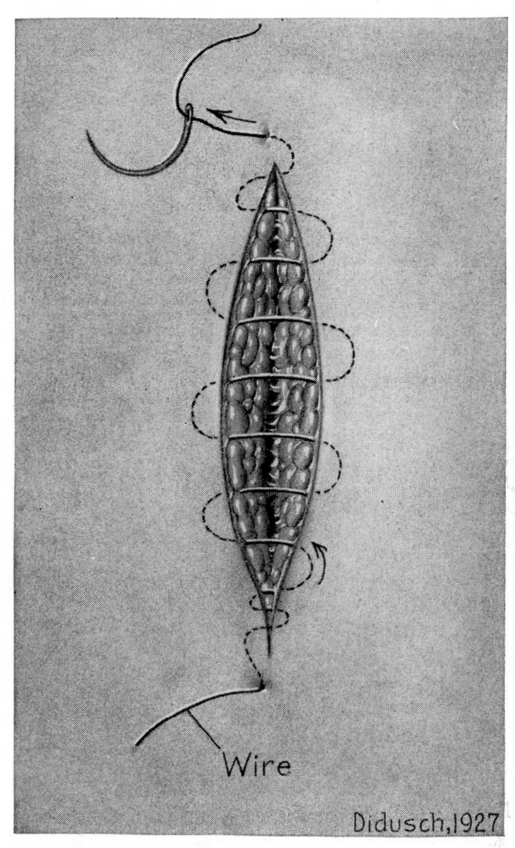

Fig. 567. Illustrating the Halsted subcuticular suture. This suture was first used by Dr. W. S. Halsted in closing hernia wounds, and when properly inserted in closing a straight incision gives the minimum skin scar. A small curved needle is used, and this penetrates the epithelial layer of the skin only at its point of entrance at one end of the wound and of emergence at the other. The skin edges are brought together by drawing the suture snug after taking short lateral bites on each side through the deeper layers of the corium. Although any suture material may be used, silver wire is the most satisfactory, as it has enough rigidity to splint the coapted edges. Care must be taken not to kink the wire while making the closure and also the wire must be freely loosened as the stitch is being placed so that it will slide through the skin after the suture is completed; otherwise it may be difficult to remove and may even break off and remain in the skin. The wire is usually removed after ten days. (Davis and Traut in Lewis' Practice of Surgery.)

Davis and Traut have ably illustrated and described the various types of flaps used in modern plastic work. A study of the illustrations and legends (Figs. 567-587 incl.) will do more to elucidate the factors under consideration than any amount of text.

According to circumstances, a flap in plastic work may be used in different ways. There is the reversed flap in which the cuticle is directed inward, the outer surface being later covered by a skin graft. This may be indicated in repairing defects in the cheek or other regions having a mucous lining. In the superimposed flap, the first reversed flap is itself covered by a second flap with its cuticle outward, or the first reversed flap may be folded on itself. A granulating flap is a double pedicled one in which the superficial tissues are dissected up but the extremities left intact. The isolated part forms a kind of bridge, the undersurface of which is prevented from uniting to its surroundings by some protective material and then allowed to granulate for from ten to fourteen days. Experience has shown that the vitality of such a flap in its new position is more assured after the pedicles have been divided if the deeper parts are granulated. Moreover, such a flap can be cut much longer in proportion to its width than a free flap without fear of sloughing; the length may be three times the breadth.

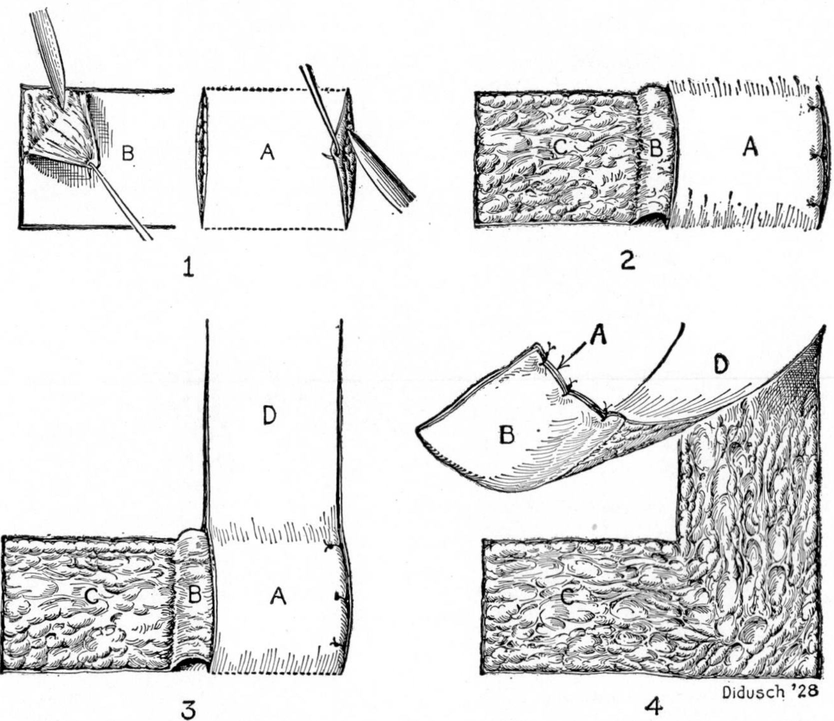

FIG. 568. Illustrating a method of lining the desired portion of a flap by the use of a lateral flap adjacent to the lower pedicle (Lauenstein).

1. The dotted lines and incisions in A mark out what will evenutally be the lower end of the pedunculated flap which is to be lined. This area is completely undercut. B indicates the lateral flap which is raised with its pedicle adjacent to A and which will be turned over and drawn under A to line it. A long lateral flap whose pedicle is at a greater distance from A and in which delayed transfer has been used might be more sure of success in certain situations.

2. Shows the lateral flap B drawn under the undercut area A and sutured so that the raw surface of B is in close contact with the raw surface of A.

3. After healing is complete between A and B, the length of the future shank D is outlined with incisions and may be undercut, leaving it attached at each end, and either be replaced for delayed transfer or tubed. The pedicle of B is then divided and the raw margins of B and A on that side are sutured. The desired portion of the flap is now lined and consists of a double thickness of subcutaneous tissue with whole-thickness skin on both sides. After gradual division of the lower pedicle of A, this lined area can be shifted into any position to which the length of its pedicle will carry it.

4. Shows the lined portion of the flap after division of the lower pedicle has been completed. After the lined portion has been grown into its new position, the pedicle is either divided close and the shank returned to its bed, or the shank may be utilized. The defects left by the removal of the flap should be grafted with skin. This suggestion may be very advantageous in various ways. (Davis and Traut in Lewis' Practice of Surgery.)

When a flap has been used for filling up a defect or other plastic procedure, it will, of course, be necessary to fit and trim it so as to leave no projections over the contiguous tissues. When its exact figuration has been accomplished, it should be sutured in place. The suturing of a plastic flap in place is a most important procedure. Silkworm gut or fine linen is commonly used, every effort being made to obtain good apposition between the edges of the flap and those of the prepared bed. Catgut may be used for buried sutures if they are necessary, or for the union of mucous surfaces. Fine horse-hair is employed where the situation calls for the avoidance of stitch marks.

The management of tension is a delicate matter; there should be enough but not too much; the condition of the sutured edges should be constantly inspected and any dragging stitches removed. Usually after suturing there is always some swelling of the flap and of the tissues surrounding it; a stitch, therefore, that may when put in appear slack, will soon tighten up; too much tension may occur with the appearance of a zone of inflammation which, if not corrected in time, may be followed by sloughing.

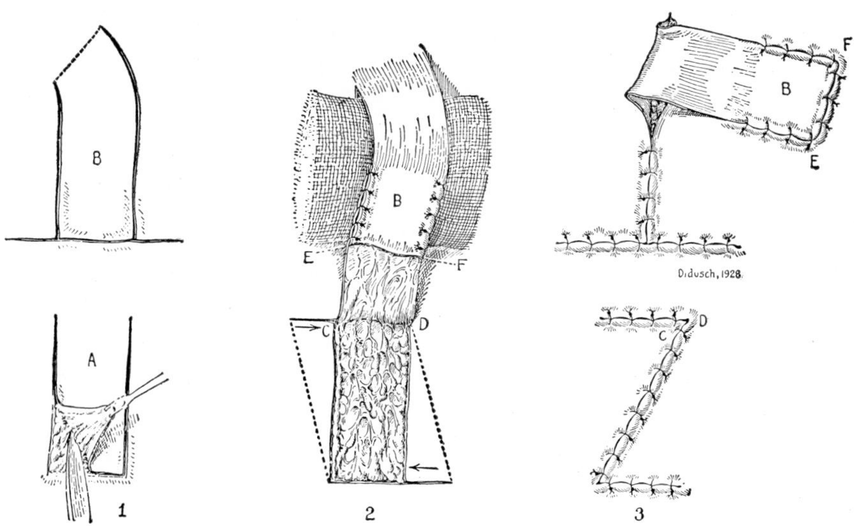

FIG. 569. Illustrating a method of forming a double-faced flap by utilizing portions of two pedunculated flaps.

1. A and B show the outlines of the two flaps of the same width and of the required length, both having their pedicles above.

2. Shows the flap A raised and turned upward and its lower third placed under the lower third of flap B and sutured raw surface to raw surface. Note the roll of gauze to prevent kinking of the pedicle of flap A. Also note the outline of the lateral triangular flaps which will be advanced to close the defect made by raising flap A.

3. After healing has taken place the double-faced portion is separated from flap A, and on the pedicle of flap B is shifted where necessary. Note the closure of the defect left by raising the flaps. This procedure may be used very advantageously in certain situations and has been utilized in making compound flaps, for instance, when including a portion of the clavicle in the section to be lined. (Davis and Traut in Lewis' Practice of Surgery.)

Different modes have been devised for the closure or filling of deformity gaps of varying shapes. Triangular-shaped gaps, if small, may have the edges brought into apposition by simple undermining of the subcutaneous tissues and suturing the skin edges together. When such gaps are of a larger size, an incision is made continuous with one side of the triangle; the subcutaneous tissues beneath the edge of this incision and of the side of the triangle next to it are undermined by dissection; the loosened-up skin may then be sutured over the defect. If necessary, the original incision may be continued on both sides continuous with one side of the triangular gap and the same procedure followed on each side. Quadrilateral and elliptical gaps may be dealt with in a similar manner by undermining the subcutaneous tissues around them.

The most satisfactory method of suturing skin edges in plastic work is the single on-end or vertical mattress suture as it prevents overlapping of the edges. This suture may also be used for coapting mucous membranes. A continuous mattress suture may also be employed.

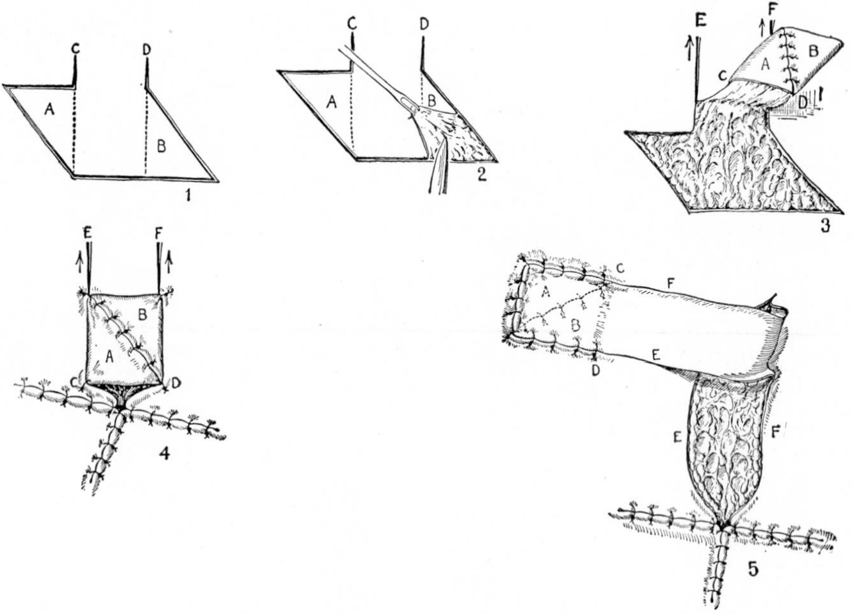

FIG. 570. Illustrating a method of lining a portion of a pedunculated flap by infolding two lateral triangular sections (after Cole).

1. The dotted lines indicate the width of the flap to be lined. The incisions show the shape of the flap to be raised. The triangles A and B are to be turned under for lining.

2. The flap being raised.

3. The flap raised and the triangles A and B folded backward and sutured, thus lining the selected portion of the flap. Note the diagonal suture line.

4. The lined portion is laid back against the underlying tissues and kept stretched by sutures. The defect from which the flap came should be closed by sutures if possible, but where this cannot be done skin grafting is required.

5. After healing is complete, the pedicle of the flap is gradually lengthened and the lined portion of the flap is shifted wherever desired. The shank of the pedicle is returned to its original position after it is finally separated from the lined portion. This is a more complicated method than we usually employ, but is illustrated to show the idea, which may be modified to suit conditions. (Davis and Traut in Lewis' Practice of Surgery.)

In the French method of cutting flaps for plastic work the skin edges, both of the flap and its bed, are undermined and the subcutaneous tissue pads removed. This enables the surgeon to bring the skin edges into better apposition and to avoid undue tension. Another method is to incise the edge of the flap on the slant so as to produce a bevel edge. This appears to give a larger area of epithelial surface for union, while the thin edge having the character of an epithelial graft tends to fuse with the opposite skin and to produce a rapidly fading scar. If this method be employed, it seems best to use a semi-subcutaneous mattress suture with a few interrupted edge-to-edge sutures. Tension sutures may be inserted occasionally along the united edges, care being taken to prevent cutting by tying them over strips of rubber.

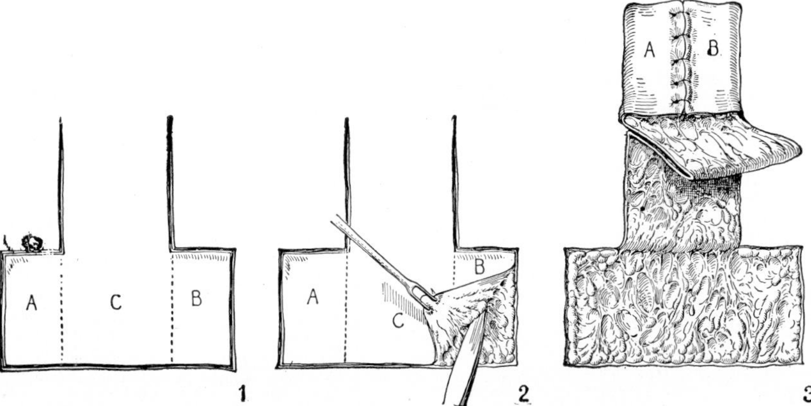

FIG. 571. Illustrating a method of lining the lower portion of a pedunculated flap by infolding two lateral rectangular sections (after Cole).

1. Shows the outline of the flap cut in the shape of a T. The dotted lines indicate the width of the portion C to be lined. The sections A and B are each one-half the width of the flap itself.

2. The entire flap is then undercut and raised.

3. The sections A and B are turned inward and the margins are sutured thus lining the section C. It is advisable for healing to be complete before attempting to shift the flap thus lined to its new location. The unused portion of the pedicle should be returned to its bed, and the rest of the defect left by raising the flap should be skin grafted. (Davis and Traut in Lewis' Practice of Surgery.)

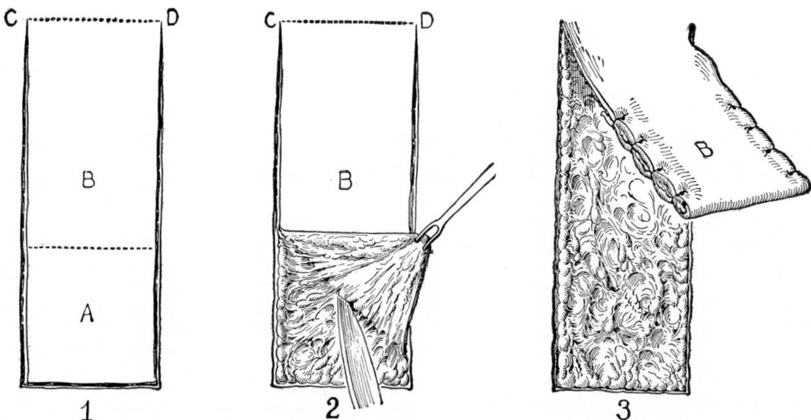

Suggestive methods for forming double-faced or lined flaps, in other words, flaps with skin on both sides. Many modifications may be made in carrying out the procedures, depending on the situation of the defect and the tissues available.

FIG. 572. Illustrating a method of lining a flap by folding it on itself.

1. Note the outline of the flap. The section A is the portion to be turned under to line a similar sized section of B. The dotted line CD indicates the extent of the undercut.

2. The flap being raised.

3. The section A has been folded under B and sutured so that raw surface is to raw surface. When healing is complete, the flap may be shifted as far as its primary pedicle will allow, or the pedicle may be gradually lengthened to give greater distance. Should the flap be on the arm, it may be carried to the face or elsewhere by the Italian method. The area from which the flap was raised may be snugged by sutures and skin grafted. (Davis and Traut in Lewis' Practice of Surgery.)

ANCHORING OF FLAPS

Some surgeons doing plastic work have found it advantageous to approximate divided edges without suturing them together. This is accomplished in different ways. Strips of muslin to which hooks have been sewn may be glued

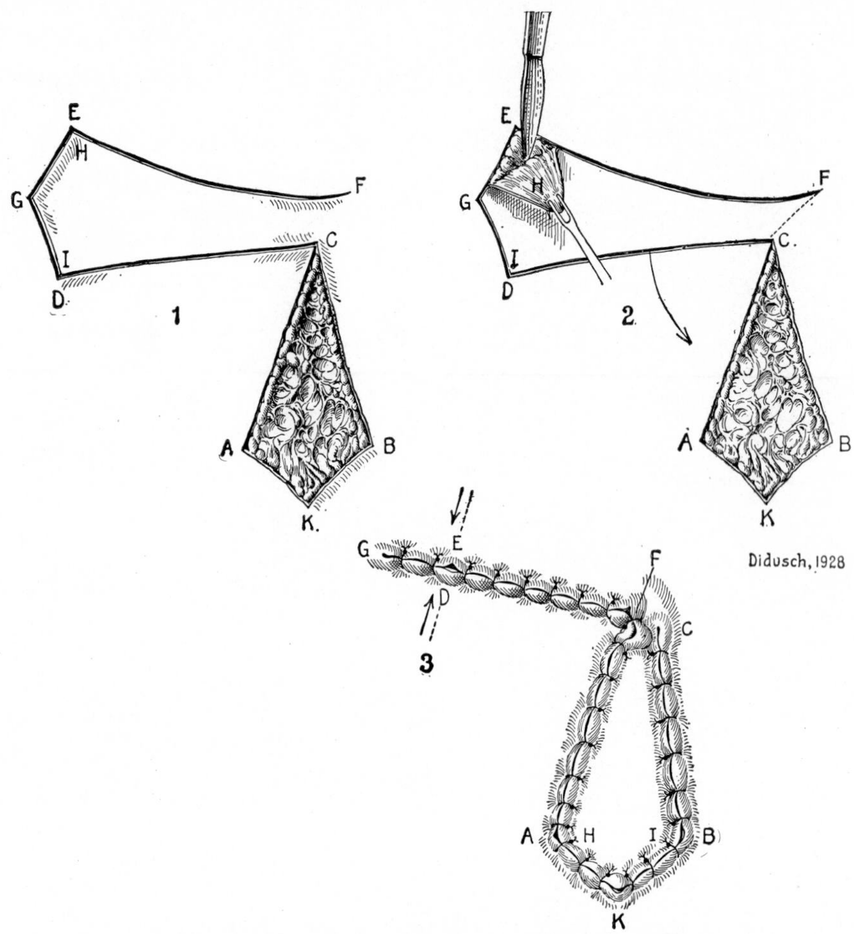

FIG. 573. Illustrating the closure of a defect with a pedunculated flap having a very narrow pedicle.

1. The defect with the outline of the measured flap. It will be noted that the pedicle is very narrow and the flap is long. A pedicle as narrow as this must carry an artery to nourish the flap, otherwise necrosis would surely take place, at least in part, even though delayed transfer was resorted to.

2. The flap being raised. Note the direction of the twist of the pedicle. Before inserting the flap the tissues adjacent to point C were undercut.

3. The flap sutured into the defect. The area from which it was raised was closed by sutures. Note the position of the points F and C as compared with that in 2. (Davis and Traut in Lewis' Practice of Surgery.)

to the shaved and cleaned skin-surfaces and the edges of the gap approximated by lacing up the hooks. Huessner's glue is one of the many similar preparations used for keeping the strips in place. It is composed of resin, 25 Gm.; alcohol (90%) 25 cc.; Venetian turpentine, 0.5 cc.; benzene 5.0 cc. There are various other non-suture methods such as the use of metal clips (Michel).

One thing to be borne in mind in connection with plastic work is that infinite patience both on the part of the operator and patient is called for. There must be no hurry and numerous operations may be required before a satisfactory result is obtained.

After-Care

Where there are no infective complications, the part should be immobilized and soft, non-irritant, dressings applied with even pressure. If the dressings are tight, the blood supply may be interfered with and a slough result.

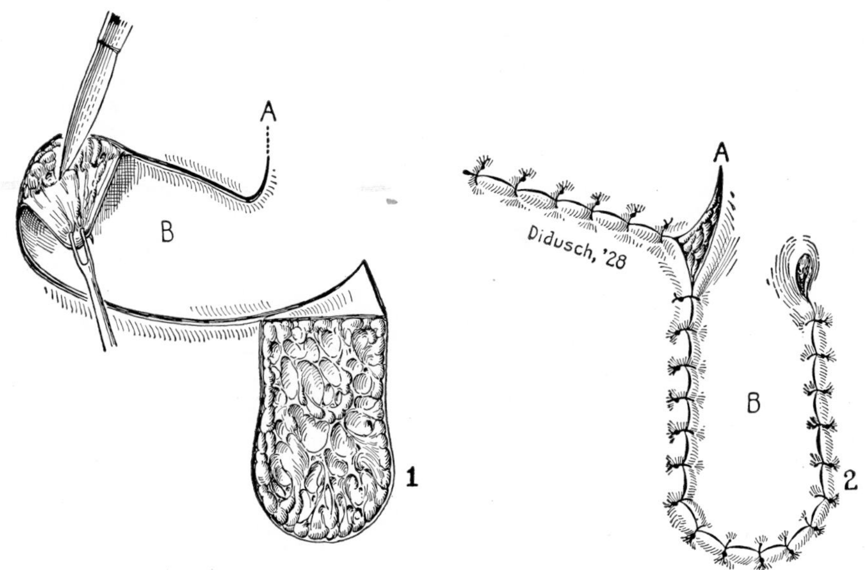

FIG. 574. Illustrating the closing of a defect with a single pedunculated flap from adjacent tissue with twisting of the pedicle by the Indian method.

1. The defect with the measured flap outlined. Note the triangle of skin between the pedicle of the flap and the upper end of the defect. In this instance it is advisable to remove this area in order to make a better closure.

2. The flap turned down with a partial twist of the pedicle and sutured into position. Note the closure of the area from which the flap was raised. When closure cannot be made, it is advisable to skin graft the defect. The pouting point caused by the twist of the pedicle can be removed later should it be objectionable. (Davis and Traut in Lewis' Practice of Surgery.)

Massage, or passive movement, is of great value both before and after operation. Before operation, scars may be made movable and the circulation in the region improved. Following operation, massage helps in restoring lost function; areas that have been grafted may be loosened up a bit and the color and circulation in the grafts improved. But massage should not be commenced until at least three weeks following operation.

In speaking of the Treatment of Superficial Granulating Wounds, John E. Cannaday[1] points out that Sir Walter Scott tells of the old belief among the Highland clansmen that a wound heals better if the first dressing is not changed for a long time and that the dried blood in the dressing was beneficial and promoted healing. Chutro, of Buenos Aires, in dealing with war wounded in Paris

[1] Am. Jour. Surg., Vol. XXV, No. 2, 1934.

during the World War, strongly stressed the great value of infrequent dressings and non-interference with wounds during the process of healing. He did not dis-

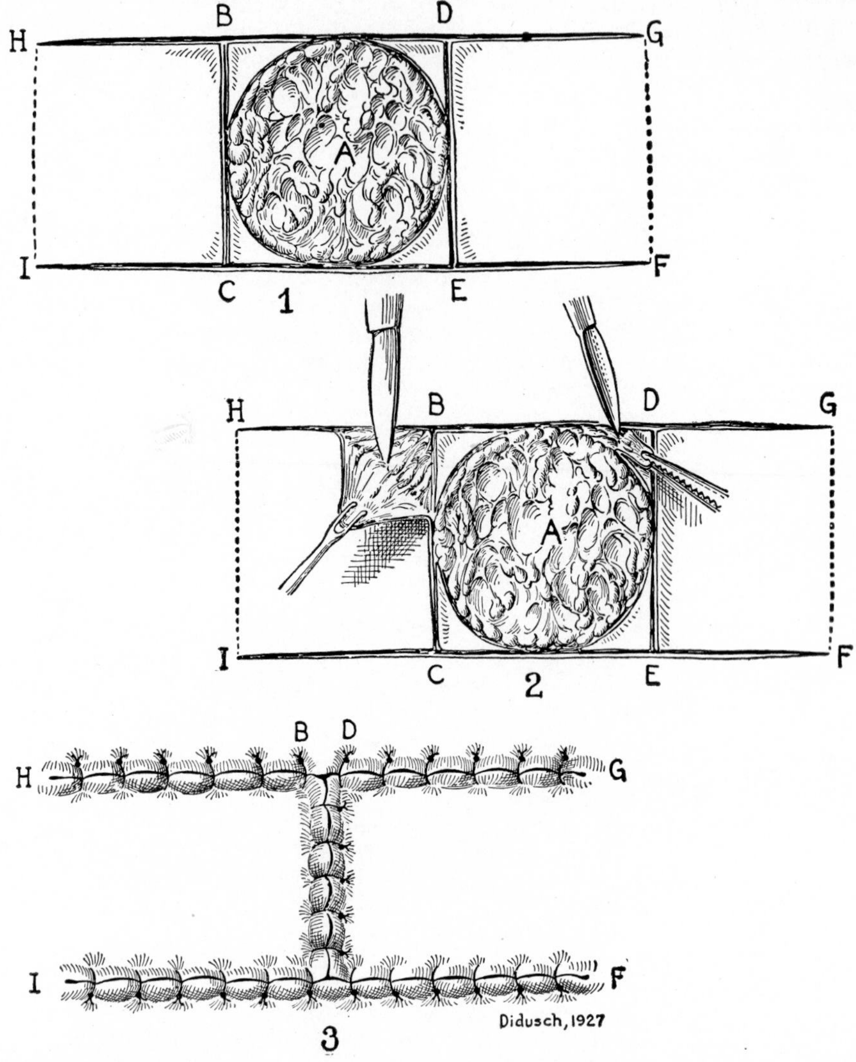

FIG. 575. Illustrating a method of closing a circular-shaped defect by the removal of four triangles of skin, thus changing the defect from a circle into a square. Lateral square flaps are undercut and advanced, and the closure is in the shape of an H (Szymanowski).

1. Shows the circular defect with the triangles outlined and the incisions made to form the lateral flaps.

2. Shows the removal of the triangles converting the circle into a square. Also the raising of the lateral flaps.

3. The lateral flaps have been advanced to meet each other and have been sutured. Szymanowski based the closure of all of these circular defects on Burow's method of excising triangles of tissue, combined with other well known procedures used for closing an ellipse, a triangle and a square. In other words, he used combinations of different procedures. In plastic surgery combinations must be frequently made in order to meet situations which unexpectedly arise. For this reason, it is essential for the operator to have mastered the methods of closing defects of various shapes. (Davis and Traut in Lewis' Practice of Surgery.)

turb the dressing for from two to three weeks or longer. Orr popularized a somewhat similar method. He packs the wound with vaseline gauze, applies a plaster cast over this and not infrequently does not disturb the dressing for a full month, the odor often being the indication for a change of dressing.

Wounds of the face that have not been dressed, apparently heal in a much more kindly and prompt manner than those that are covered with dressings. As far as the wound's healing is concerned, dressings are, as a rule, of no value

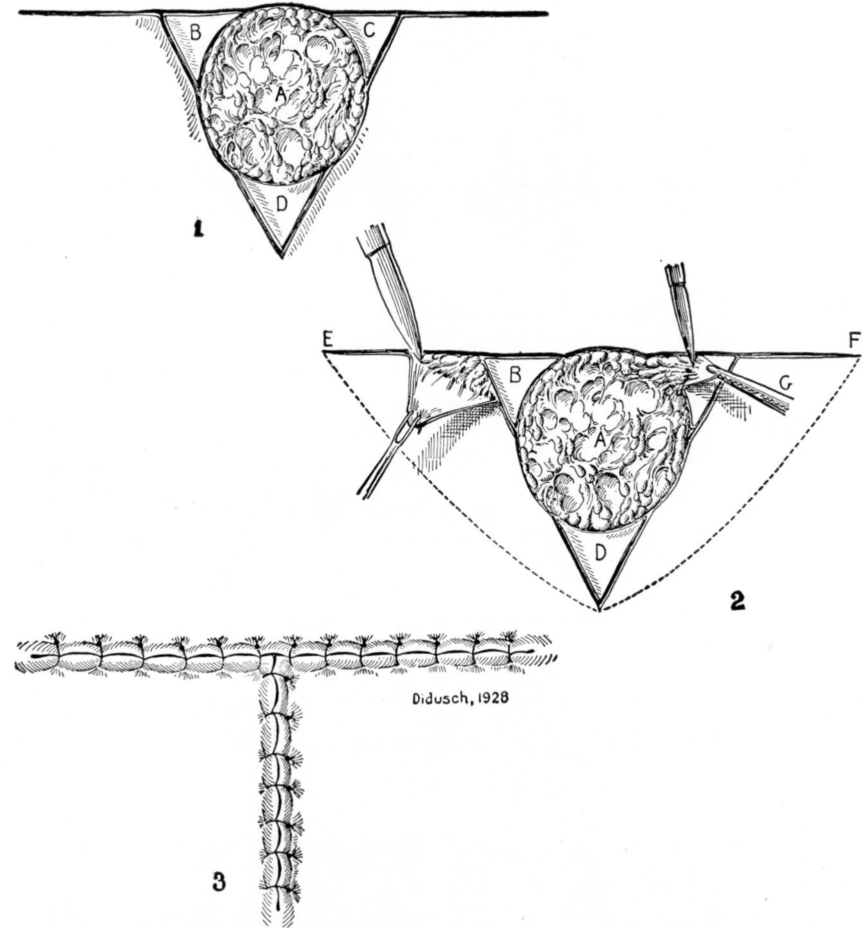

Fig. 576. Illustrating a method of closing a circular defect by the removal of three triangles of skin, thus changing the defect from a circle to a triangle. Lateral triangular flaps are formed and the closure is in the shape of a T (Szymanowski).

1. Shows the defect and the incisions outlining the three triangles, B, C, D, which are all to be removed. The incisions, E and F, on each side are continuous with the base of the large triangle and form the shorter side of the lateral flaps after they are undercut and raised.

2. Shows the process of removing the triangles of skin and raising the flaps which are undercut as far as the dotted lines.

3. Result obtained by sliding the flaps together and suturing the margins. (Davis and Traut in Lewis' Practice of Surgery.)

whatever. In some cases, they may protect tender, unhealed areas from contact with clothing. On a raw surface frequent application and subsequent removal of dressings or the more or less constant traumatism brought about by their presence, does a very great deal of harm: first, by keeping the skin edges in a moist, macerated and water-logged condition; second, by tearing away the epithelial new

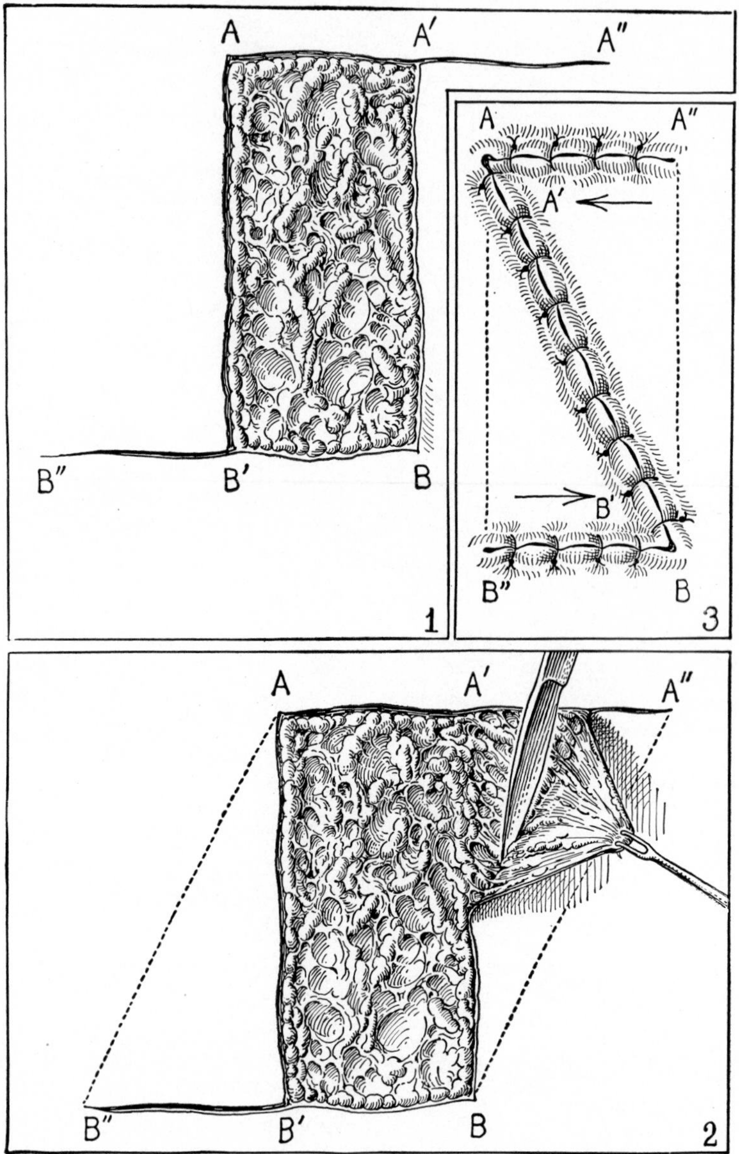

FIG. 577. Illustrating a method of closing either a large or a small rectangular defect by means of triangular flaps raised from opposite sides of the defect and advanced to meet each other.

1. Shows flaps formed by two incisions carried outward from diagonal corners of the shorter ends of the rectangle. Each of these incisions should equal in length the shorter side of the rectangle.

2. Shows the raising of a flap. The dotted lines indicate the size of each flap when completed.

3. Shows the flaps shifted inward and sutured, the final closure being in the shape of a reversed Z. This is an old procedure and a useful one. (Davis and Traut in Lewis' Practice of Surgery.)

growth thrown out for repair. Granulation tissue constituting the ulcer base becomes infiltrated with fibrous scar tissue, circulation suffers and the processes of repair are put to disadvantage.

Cannaday treats certain types of wounds, particularly those of a superficial nature, showing a tendency to delay in healing, by exposure to open air and sunlight; and, if the latter was not available, to the various types of electric light.

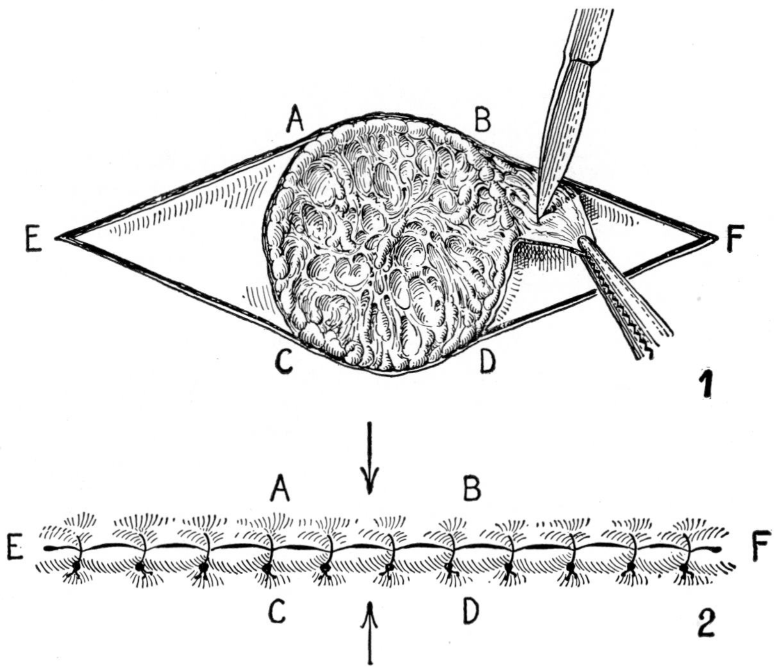

FIG. 578. Illustrating the simplest method of closing a circular defect which is too large to be drawn together by a purse-string suture. Two triangles of skin are removed and the defect is thus changed from a circle into an ellipse. The closure is in a line (after Szymanowski).

1. Shows the defect and the outline of the triangles of skin on each side which are to be excised.

2. The line closure made possible by the removal of the triangles. It may be necessary to undercut the margins considerably before the edges can be approximated if the defect is large or if the tissues are not freely movable. (Davis and Traut in Lewis' Practice of Surgery.)

He points out that the contact of dressings of the usual type with any granulating surface causes a free outpouring of serum, the so-called foreign-body reaction. This reaction is most strikingly seen in the response caused by a drain; the profuse discharge provoked usually disappears for the most part soon after the removal of the offending body.

Mouse-proof mesh and adhesive plaster is used to construct a screen or framework to be applied about the wound. The screen-wire is cut to the requisite size necessary to make an adequate shield over the wound. The edges are bound with strips of adhesive plaster and shaped so as to fit about the wound. (Fig. 588.) In many instances raw areas thus treated will heal in contradistinction to others that have been assiduously dressed day after day without apparent diminution in the size of the wound. If the wound is deep, as a rule, this form of treatment is supplemented by the application of heat, as by sunshine or lamp, which promotes healing by improvement of circulation as well as by the drying of the skin.

The position of the part involved often plays an important part in the healing process. If the wound is deep this form of treatment is not begun until the granulations are nearly flush with the surface. If the wound is superficial, such

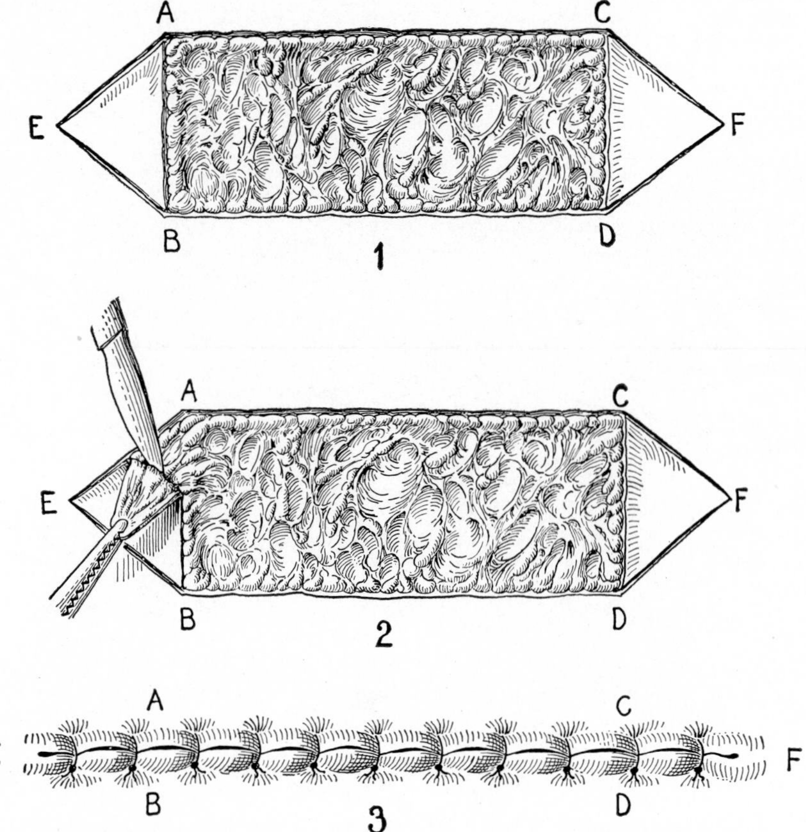

FIG. 579. Illustrating a method of closing a rectangular shaped defect by undercutting the margins, removing a triangle of tissue from each end and closing with sutures (v. Ammon).
1. Shows the defect with the two triangles of tissue to be removed marked out by incisions.
2. Shows the removal of the triangles on each end.
3. Shows the approximation of the edges and the closure in a straight line. This method can be used for closing larger defects than it would be possible to do with simple undercutting and suturing. (Davis and Traut in Lewis' Practice of Surgery.)

as that produced by removal of skin grafts for use elsewhere, the treatment can well be begun at once.

Skin Grafting

Skin grafting consists in completely removing a portion of skin or epithelium from one part of the body and transferring it to another part to correct a defect. It differs from plastic surgery in that the transplant used in plastic work is furnished with a pedicle through which it is nourished while uniting with the surrounding structures.

Skin grafting is often called "transplantation." The term "implantation" signifies the use of dead organic or inorganic substances. The word "graft" should be used in describing transplantation procedures while the word "flap" should be used in connection with plastic surgery.

Epidermal grafts are made up of epithelium alone in either large or small pieces; dermo-epidermal grafts consist of epidermis and a part of the true derm; total cutaneous or whole-thickness grafts are made up of the whole thickness of the skin and in some instances including the subcutaneous connective tissue.

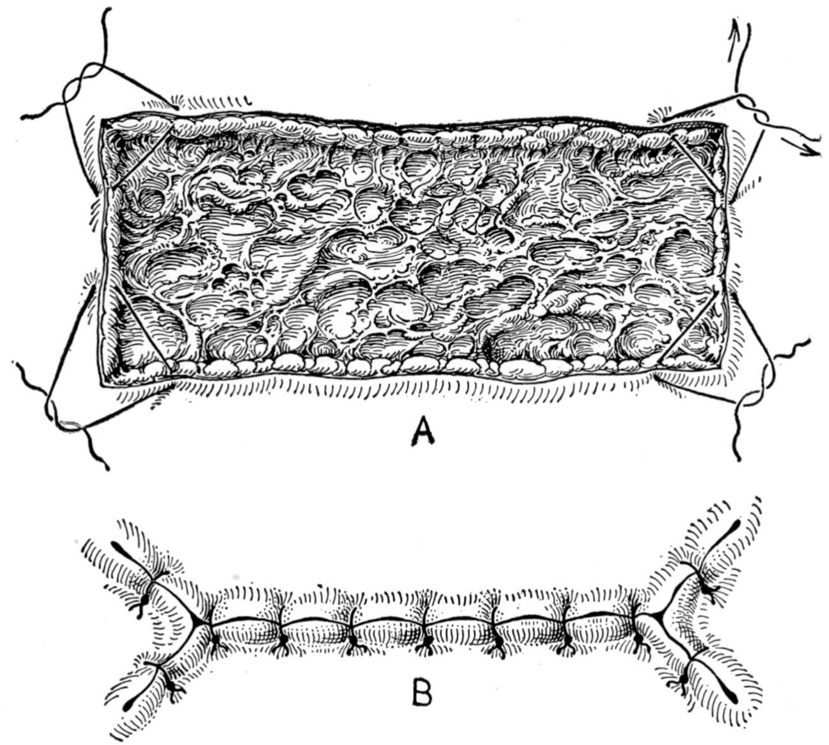

FIG. 580. Illustrating a method of closing a comparatively small rectangular defect by undercutting the margins and approximating the edges with sutures.
A. Shows the defect with the sutures which are first placed in the four corners.
B. After these are tied, the other sutures are inserted in such a way as to entirely close the defect in the shape of a double Y. This is a useful procedure and can often be advantageously employed. (Davis and Traut in Lewis' Practice of Surgery.)

Vegetable grafting although appearing somewhat similar to skin grafting is really quite different. Vegetable grafts grow more as parasites while skin grafts become a part of the tissue into which they are transplanted.

Autodermic grafts are those obtained from the patient himself. Those obtained from another individual are called hetero-, homo-, or isodermic; zoodermic is the term applied to grafts taken from animals.

If **zoodermic grafts** were successful, they would be classed as the favorite method. However, results are rather uncertain following this procedure. Reclus classes it as a "laboratory experiment." Colrat contends they are absorbed and that even though they appear to be successful at first, granulations are sure to appear later. Nevertheless many cases have been reported where the procedure was followed by gratifying results.

Out of 165 transplantations obtained from frogs, chickens, guinea pigs and rabbits, Cousin had 15 successes; out of 122 human grafts he reports successful results in 115 cases.

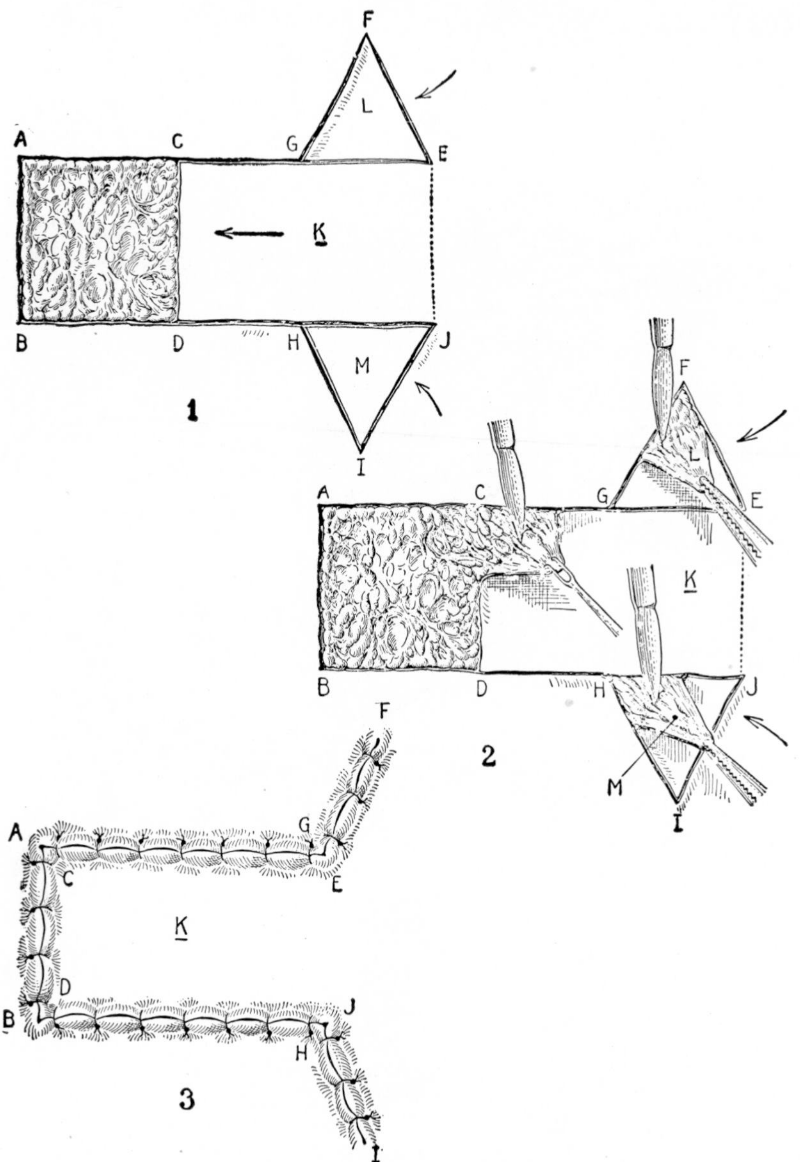

FIG. 581. Illustrates a procedure for closing a square defect by means of advancing a lateral flap and at the same time removing two triangles of tissue to facilitate the advancement, according to Burow's method.

1. Shows the defect and the outline of the flap, also the position of the triangles.
2. Shows the flap being raised and the triangles being excised.
3. Shows the closure. This is a more complicated method but is often useful in relaxing the shank of the flap. (Davis and Traut in Lewis' Practice of Surgery.)

There is a wide variation in the results obtained by the different surgeons in their experiments—some laud it highly; others condemn it.

Medieval history records an instance concerning the transplanting of a graft from an animal to man which is quite remarkable. During the seventeenth cen-

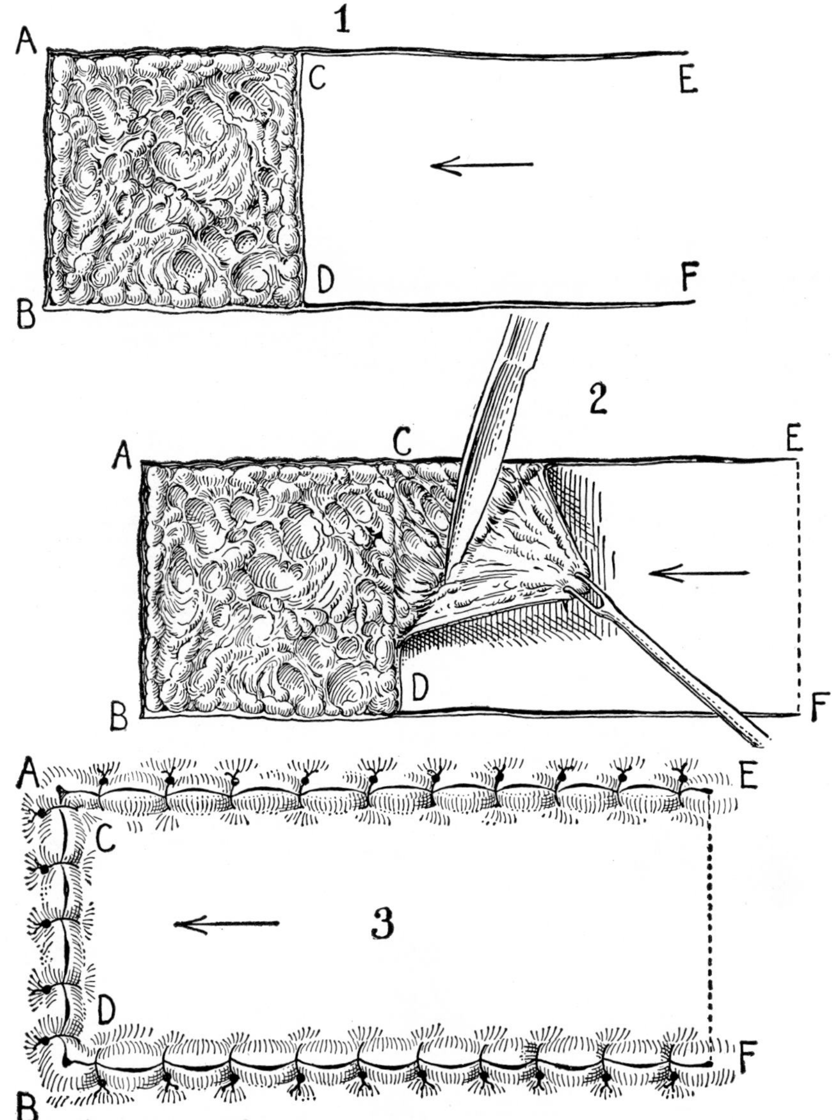

FIG. 582. Illustrates a simple method of closing a square defect by the use of a lateral flap which is advanced and sutured. This is typical of the French method and there are many modifications used, depending on the condition of the surrounding skin and on the situation of the lesion.

1. The defect with the flap outlined.
2. The flap partially raised. The dotted line indicates the outer limit of the flap.
3. The flap advanced in the direction of the arrow and sutured. (Davis and Traut in Lewis' Practice of Surgery.)

tury a surgeon placed a skin-periosteum-bone graft from a dog in a defect in the scalp and skull of a human; after it had grown in place, he was forced to remove it, under threat of excommunciation from the Church.

Skin from the frog furnishes perhaps the most successful zoograft. The skin from any portion of the frog's body may be used although that from the abdomen is usually employed. In 1884, Allen performed operations using this kind of graft; Baratoux and Dubousquet-Laborderie employed the method a few years later.

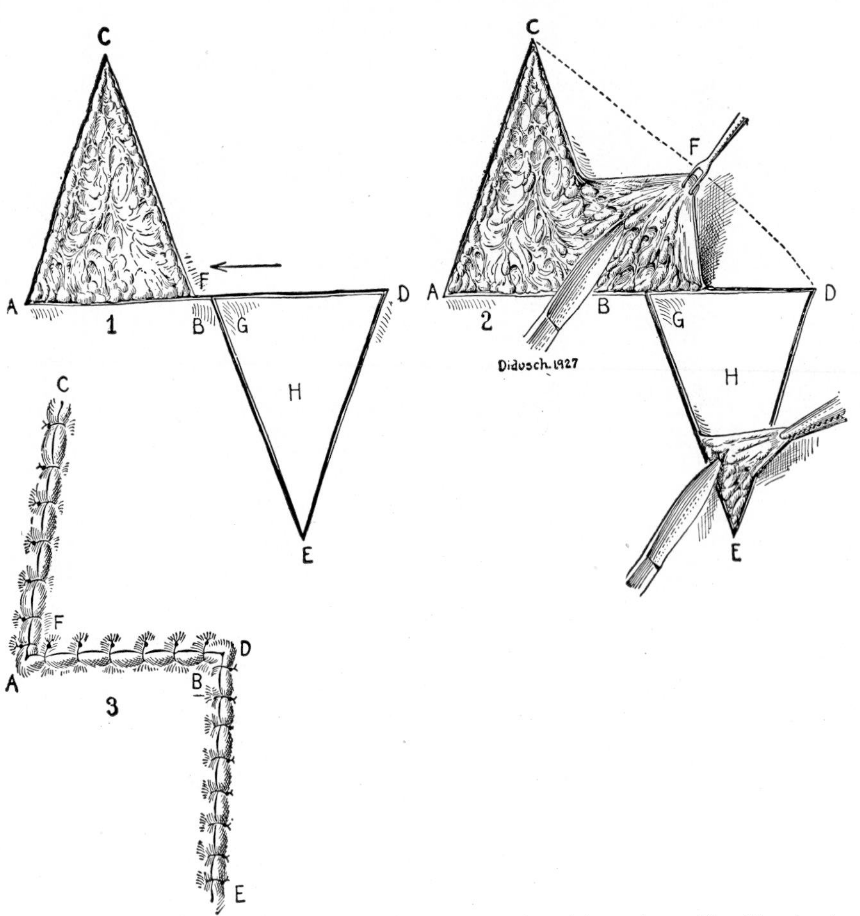

FIG. 583. Illustrating a method of closing a triangular defect of considerable size by the removal of a triangle of skin equal in size to the original defect. A triangular flap is then formed adjacent to the lesion and is advanced to fill it (after Burow).

1. Shows the defect and the outline of the triangle of skin, H, which is to be removed.

2. Note the formation of the triangular flap FCD. Also the removal of the triangle of skin H.

3. The point F of the flap FCD is advanced and sutured to the point A and the point B to the point D. This is rather an extensive procedure which is utilized only in situations in which for one reason or another other simpler methods cannot be used. However, the excision of triangles of tissues in the necessary situations, as first suggested by Burow, is most effective in aiding the closure of defects of various shapes found in everyday work and we frequently use the procedure. (Davis and Traut in Lewis' Practice of Surgery.)

The frog is prepared as follows: after scrubbing it is immersed as far as the neck for five minutes in a solution of corrosive sublimate or permitted to swim in a boric acid solution for some time.

Grafts may be wrapped in waterproof tissue with moist gauze and preserved for several hours.

The new skin becomes translucent and pink, appearing as a film through which the red surface beneath can be discerned. The pigmentation disappears in a few days but the new skin still seems to be slightly darker than the surrounding skin.

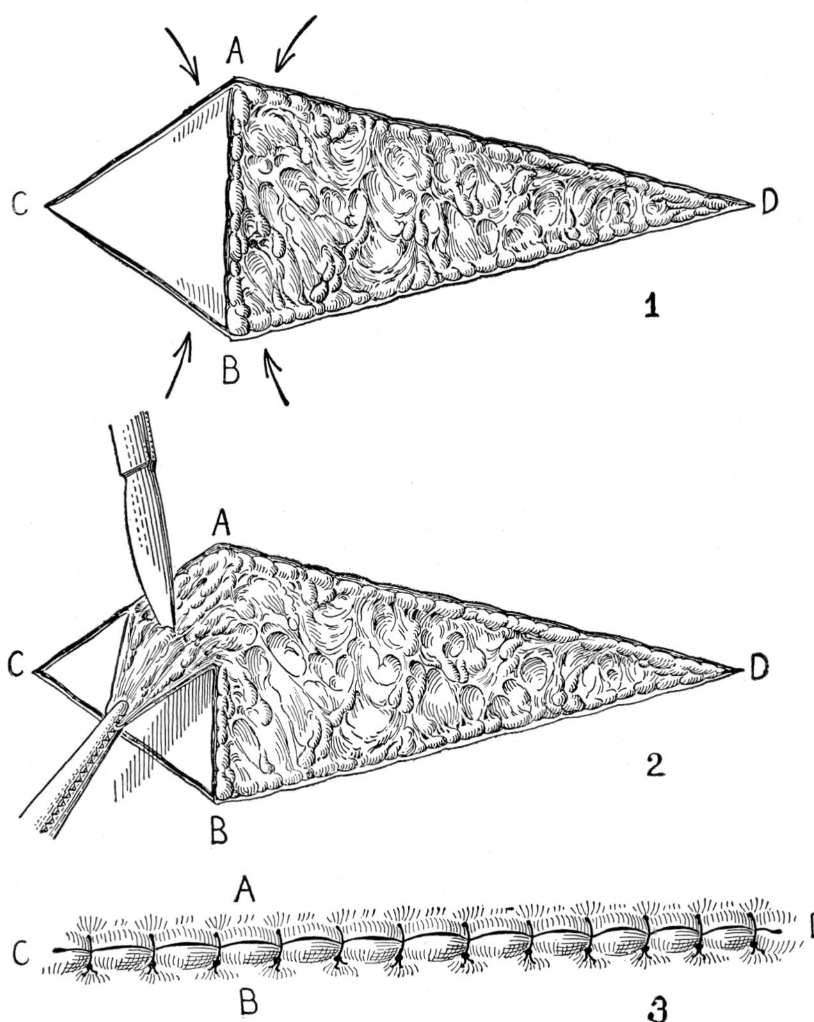

FIG. 584. Illustrating the closure of a larger triangular defect by the removal of a triangle of skin at the base of the triangular defect, undercutting the margins and approximating the edges with sutures (v. Ammon).

1. The defect with the outline of the triangle of skin which is to be removed.
2. Removal of the triangle of skin, which changes the shape of the defect from a triangle into a kite shape. The margins are undercut.
3. Shows the edges closed in a straight line. (Davis and Traut in Lewis' Practice of Surgery.)

Frog's skin must be given careful attention for at least three months, for although it makes a soft, pliable covering, it has a tendency to ulcerate and vanish.

A certain degree of success was attained by Redard by using the skin from the undersurface of a chicken's wing.

An ulcer was successfully grafted with pieces of cock's wattle by Altamirano.

Miles of Edinburgh grafted successfully the skin of a greyhound while Van Meter of Colorado employed the cuticle from a Mexican hairless puppy. The skin of a young pig was satisfactorily used by Raven and Hübscher.

Miles also used the skin of rabbits and kittens, after shaving the abdomen or flanks of the animals, he removed the skin in strips ranging from 1 to 6 inches long and from one-half to one inch wide. The edges of the grafts were placed

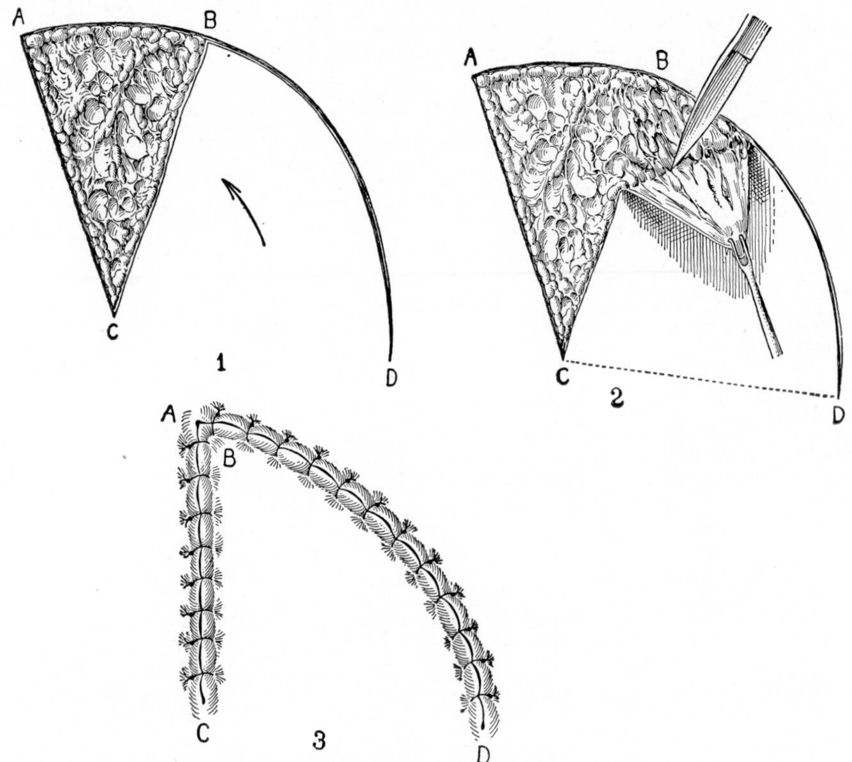

Fig. 585. Illustrating a method of closing a triangular defect of considerable size by the use of a unilateral flap which is advanced over the defect and sutured (after Jasche).
1. Shows the defect with the outline of the flap made by the curved incision BD.
2. Shows the flap being raised. Note the width of the pedicle CD.
3. The closure after sliding the flap over the defect. Smaller bilateral flaps can be used to accomplish the same purpose. (Davis and Traut in Lewis' Practice of Surgery.)

together and pressed down firmly being held in place by a dressing for forty-eight to seventy-two hours, after which it was carefully removed. If pustules have formed they should be opened. Granulations growing through the new skin which would seem to injure or destroy it should be removed with a sharp spoon. Out of 10 cases Miles reports 4 successes; only 2 were complete failures.

Based upon the idea that the testicle possesses a greater degree of cellular activity than other parts of the body, E. Aievoli used thin pieces of the testes of rabbits for grafting purposes with good results.

The lining membrane of an egg has been used advantageously for grafting purposes in the case of extensive burns, injuries to the tympanum, conjunctiva or pterygium.

Venable has reported excellent results using thin layers of skin from the shaved thigh of a young pig. Usually the skin is taken above the bristle layer; should a few bristles appear they are of no consequence, since the follicles in the graft soon atrophy. He reports 85 to 100 per cent of takes as against 30 to 75 per cent with other heterografts.

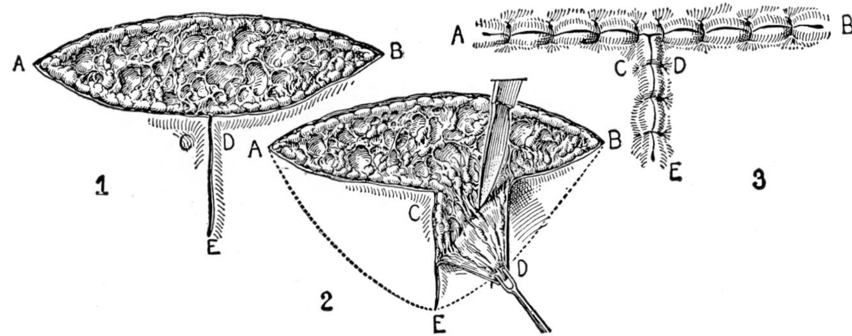

FIG. 586 I. Illustrating a method of closing an elliptical-shaped defect by the formation of two triangular flaps from the same side which are advanced and sutured (Lisfranc).

1. The defect. Note the vertical incision made from the central portion of the defect margin on the selected side.
2. Shows the formation and extent of the flaps which extend outward to the dotted line.
3. The closure in the shape of a flattened T. The principle of this procedure will be found helpful in many instances.

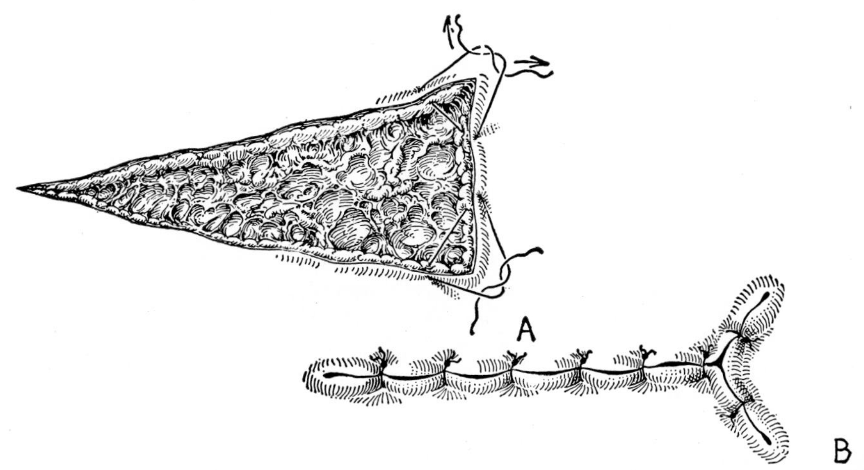

FIG. 586 II. Illustrates the simplest method of closing a small triangular defect by undercutting the margins and approximating the edges with sutures.

A. The defect, with the sutures which are first placed across the corners of the base of the triangle.

B. The closure in the shape of an elongated Y. (Davis and Traut in Lewis' Practice of Surgery.)

Transmission of Disease

Diseases of different varieties may be transmitted in skin grafting from one person to another. Syphilis, tuberculosis, small pox and even cancer are said to have been transmitted in this manner.

General Condition of the Patient

It is not necessary for the patient to be in an extremely vigorous state of health before a skin graft is applied but he should be free from toxicity.

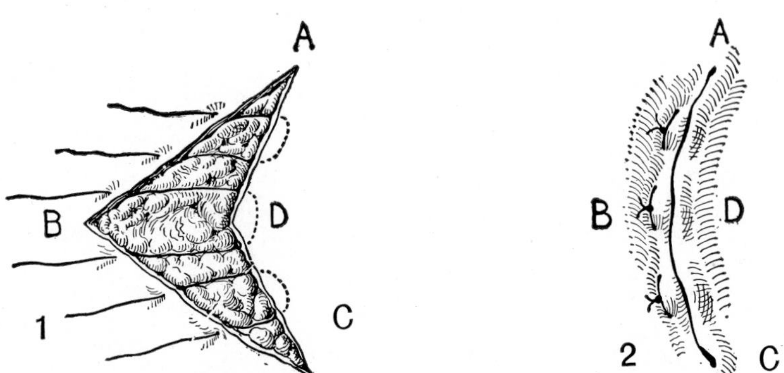

Fig. 587 I. Illustrating a method of closing an angled wound. 1. Note the modified mattress type of sutures which penetrates the full thickness of the skin on the side to which the tissue is to be drawn and loops through the deeper portion of the corium on the other side without penetrating the epithelial layer. 2. Sutures drawn snug and tied. This is a helpful type of stitch and can be used to advantage in many situations.

Where the patient has been suffering from erysipelas, grafts should not be undertaken until the disease has disappeared at least six weeks, for the streptococci

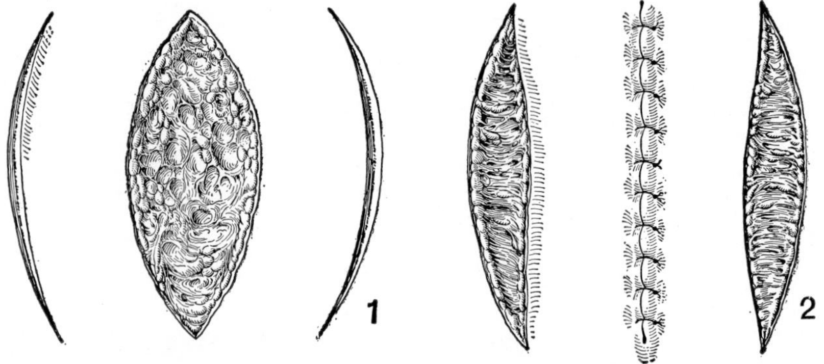

Fig. 587 II. Illustrating a method of closing an elliptical-shaped defect by means of bilateral relaxation incisions and approximation of the edges with sutures (Celsus).

1. Shows the defect with the bilateral curved relaxation incisions. When the defect is not too wide, the relaxation incisions will allow closure without extensive undercutting. In wider defects, the tissues must be undercut between the defect and the incisions in order to approximate the edges.

2. Shows the relaxation incisions gaping widely and the defect closed. These lateral defects may be allowed to heal by granulation or may be immediately skin grafted. A unilateral relaxation incision is sometimes sufficient. This is one of the oldest procedures in plastic surgery and the principle is very useful in everyday work. (Davis and Traut in Lewis' Practice of Surgery.)

are likely to cause dissolution of the grafts before or even after adhesions have taken place.

Successful grafts have been made in the presence of nephritis and diabetes although they exert an unfavorable influence.

Surgeons do not agree as to whether grafts can be satisfactorily implanted in the presence of syphilis. A great deal depends on the stage of the disease and whether the area to receive the graft is syphilitic. A skin graft should not be placed over a syphilitic ulcer. There are cases recorded where grafts have been known to grow and heal where the patient was afflicted with syphilis.

REVERDIN GRAFTS

When J. L. Reverdin, an intern of La Charité, in Paris, on Dec. 8, 1869, made his famous report on the subject of skingrafting to the Société de Chirurgie, he instigated new interest in this phase of surgery when he informed his hearers that

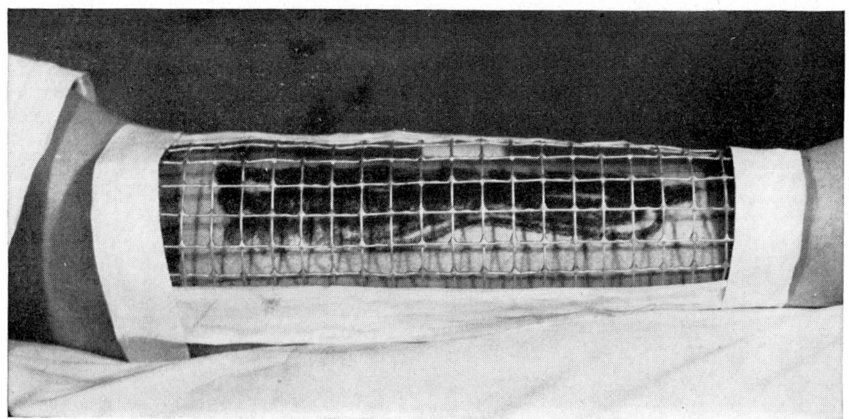

Fig. 588. Wire mesh and adhesive plaster used as a protection for wound. (Courtesy Dr. John E. Cannady.)

pieces of skin, removed from their original connections would adhere and grow on granulating surfaces.

Preparation of the Surface to be Grafted

When the granulating surface is healthy and the wounds fresh, little preparation is necessary. If, however, conditions are not so favorable more precautions should be taken.

It is quite possible for epithelium to grow on an unhealthy granulating surface, according to Bryant; many Reverdin grafts are applied in the presence of pus and some have been known to grow on cancerous surfaces. Naturally, a healthy granulating surface is to be preferred.

Granulations should be of medium size, vascular, and of a fresh red color; not large and flabby. One of the best indications of fitness for the reception of grafts is the formation of a pellicle of new skin around the borders of an ulcer.

Excavated ulcers should be curetted. Cicatricial tissue often surrounds the margins of old ulcers, interfering with the vascular supply and rendering skin grafting difficult if not impossible.

If the circulation is impaired by varicosities or scar tissue, or if inflammations or complications are present, the patient should remain in bed a few days or weeks until the part returns to normal. Moderate pressure, evenly applied with a sea-sponge, is of great value.

When acute inflammation has been allayed, the granulations should be prepared for reception of the grafts. This may be accomplished by cauterization and compression (stick nitrate of silver or tincture of iodine). Cauterization should be done every two or three days. Iodoform gauze saturated with balsam of Peru sometimes does good service (Freeman).

Induration and **fibrous thickening** of the borders are treated by making a few radiating incisions through the ring of callus down to the softer tissues; this relieves tension and promotes vascularity. Heliotherapy is sometimes of value.

In order not to injure the vitality of the grafts, any strong antiseptics which have been used for cleansing should be washed away before transplantation is done.

Grafts

The inside of the arm or thigh, or the side of the chest or bend of the elbow is considered best. In these situations the skin is thin and soft and comparatively free from hairs or glands.

Lucas considers that "the prepuce of a child possesses a germinal vitality which renders it peculiarly serviceable for grafting," in addition to suppleness, thinness, and vascularity. He claims that preputial grafts will adhere when those from other parts fail, even on unhealthy granulating surfaces.

Reverdin recommended originally that the grafts should be small, that is, about the size of a grain of wheat, thus reducing to a minimum the pain and the scars occasioned.

The removal of grafts from the donor is most easily done by raising a small fold of skin with a pair of mousetooth forceps and dividing it with a scissors, knife or razor. Iridectomy scissors are useful. Obtain all of the epithelium and part of the corium. Include no subcutaneous cellular tissue or fat. The epidermis is all that is really necessary although it is well to include part of the corium. Reverdin employed the term "greffe dermique," which Poncet changed to "greffe dermoepidermique" thus more correctly expressing what is really meant. A small amount of blood issues.

The skin may be partially frozen with ethyl chloride or anesthetized with novocaine, although the pain is very slight. In case the skin is partly frozen, the grafts may be all cut at once and placed in warm salt solution until required; or they may be preserved on a warm piece of glass, raw side down. The small elliptical wounds heal quickly. No sutures are necessary. An ordinary aseptic or antiseptic dressing may be applied, dry or moist, which serves to prevent the development of infections.

Marcy has shown that satisfactory grafts may often be cut by pressing a pair of curved scissors firmly against the skin and snipping off the portion which protrudes between the blades. Some prefer to elevate a fold of skin by transfixion with a fine needle, but this offers no advantage over forceps.

Souchon has recently emphasized an old and useful method of obtaining small grafts by cutting them with scissors from the thin, new epithelium as it "floats" out from the skin-edges of a healthy granulating surface which is beginning to heal.

Grafting

After being cut the grafts are immediately placed upon the surface to be grafted with a forceps or needle with their raw sides down. Curled edges are carefully straightened with a probe. If no blood or other fluid is present, attachment immediately takes place; slight pressure with a dampened gauze pledget is helpful. Roberts and others claim that exposure of the ulcer to the atmosphere before and after operating is helpful by causing it to become sticky, thus facilitating adherence.

Each graft is capable of some expansion but it cannot stimulate the borders of the ulcer effectually farther than half an inch. If a single graft is placed in the center of a very large ulcer it will form an island of skin only. Therefore, the transplants should not be more than half an inch apart. They need not be placed in rows or geometrical figures. If only a few grafts are available it is better thoroughly to cover a small area than to scatter the pieces too far apart. (Figs. 589, 590, 591.)

DRESSINGS

Place rubber protective next to the grafts, thus preventing their adherence and displacement when the dressings are changed. This should be cut in strips half an inch wide which are placed side by side, or criss-crossed, like basket-work, or punched full of holes which serve as outlets for secretions. Strips of transparent gutta-percha are useful here; their ends should project onto the sound skin; adhesion will take place if they are dampened with chloroform. If the gutta-percha is not available, gold-beater's skin, oiled silk, isinglass plaster, tin or silver foil, etc., may be used. Ordinary adhesive plaster is preferred by Marcy.

Any of the above methods may jeopardize the vitality of the new skin by causing maceration. A superior method which is much simpler consists in spreading a single layer of gauze over the grafted surface and fastening it to the skin with collodion. This is recommended by McCarthy and Freeman.

If a dusting powder is used, care must be taken that it does not form a crust, beneath which pus may accumulate and destroy the grafts. If a wet dressing is used, omit the powder or salve; use a pad saturated with boric acid solution or normal salt solution (warm) instead. If a covering of oiled silk is placed over the dressing, it will be unnecessary to moisten it oftener than once every twenty-four hours.

It would be unnecessary to change the dressing during the healing process if the operative field were always aseptic. Since there is always a certain amount of suppuration, it is advisable to change the dressing every 24 to 48 hours. The wound may be gently irrigated but never rubbed for fear of injuring the transplanted skin.

If the discharge has been profuse and protective has been used it should also be frequently changed; if little suppuration is present, however, it may be left in place for 5 or 10 days.

Bacillus pyocyaneus sometimes causes the dressings to become green; this, combined with the unpleasant odor which is often present may needlessly occasion some alarm.

The "open method" may be used in place of the different dressings. This consists in exposing the graft to the air beneath a protecting wire-gauze cage. If a great deal of suppuration is present, the formation of thick crusts is likely to render this procedure unsatisfactory.

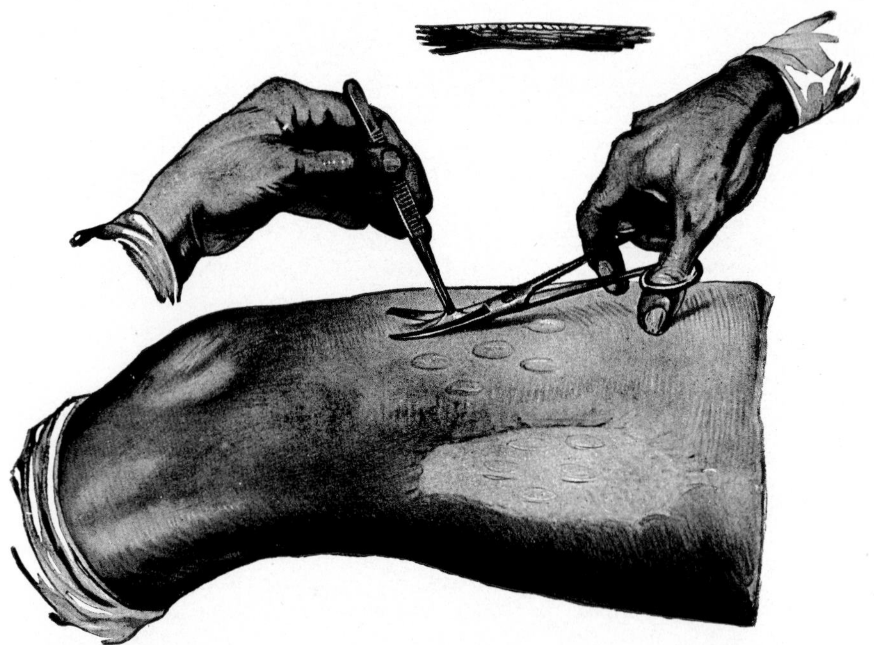

FIG. 589. Skin grafting with Reverdin grafts, which are obtained with curved scissors and tissue forceps. (Kirschner, Operative Surgery.)

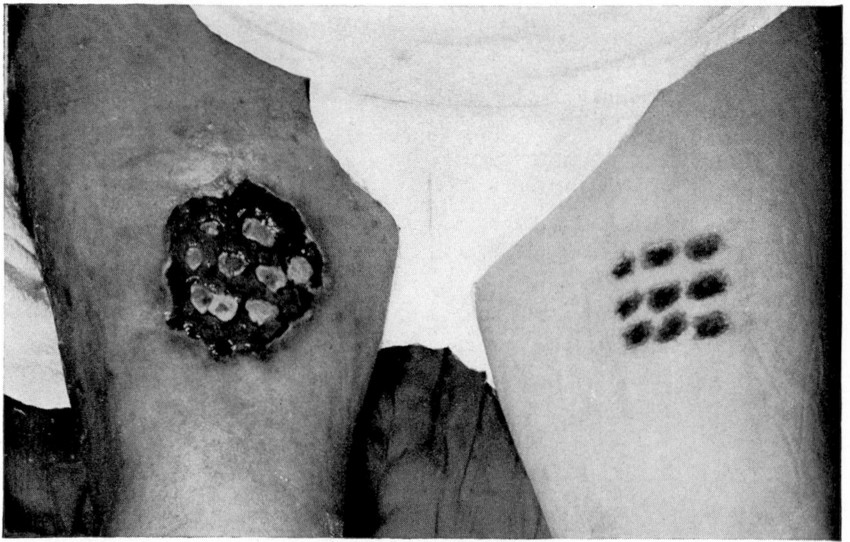

FIG. 590. Reverdin pinch grafts.

When grafting is done near a joint, especially in children, the part should be immobilized by the application of a splint. The lower extremity should be elevated to promote circulation.

Process of Healing

The grafts appear to swell, becoming whiter, thicker and softer during the first 24 hours; in two or three days those which adhere become pink and surrounded by a reddish areola. Following this a gray epithelial pellicle emerges from their margins and the connecting borders of the ulcer. The pieces of skin which turn brown are dead while those which turn a yellowish white lose their superficial layers of epidermis; as the deeper layers remain that which is lost is soon reproduced.

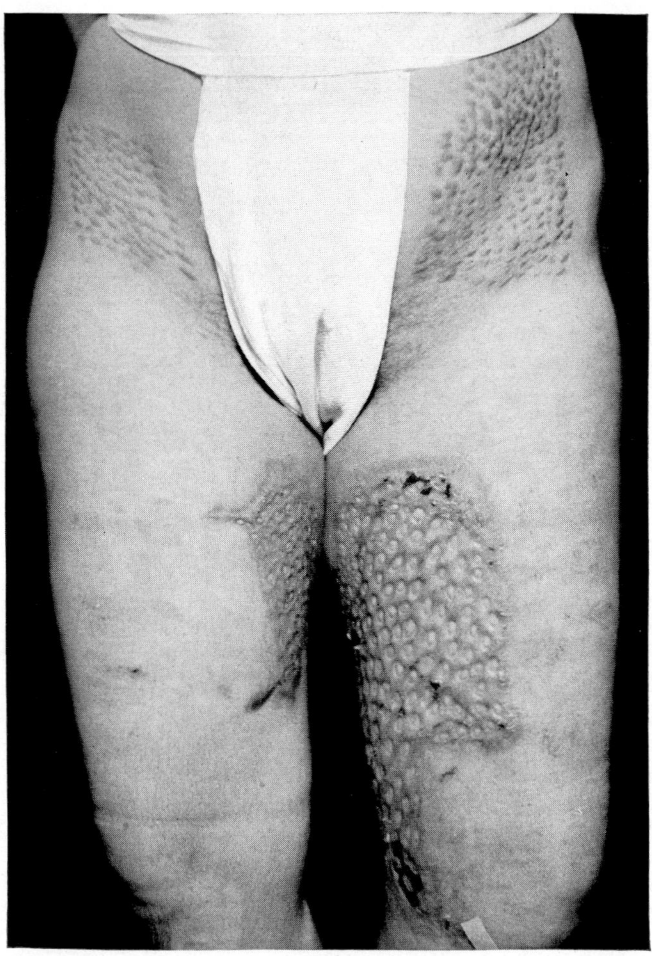

FIG. 591. A woman who was burned with a hot flatiron on the inner surfaces of both thighs. Skin pinch grafts were taken from the abdomen and transplanted over the affected area. Condition one week after transplantation.

At first, the new epithelial pellicle is not fastened to the granulations; it simply rests like tissue-paper upon the surface from which it may be raised. After a time roots grow down into the granulations, securing the epithelium and connecting the grafts together and to the edges of the ulcer.

The part must be carefully protected for several weeks after cicatrization until a certain amount of resistance has been attained, as ulcers thus treated have a tendency to break down upon the slightest provocation. A soothing ointment may be used to combat any tendency to dryness or exfoliation.

The new skin is quite inferior to normal skin although it is better than scar tissue. It is without hair bulbs, sweat glands or sebaceous follicles. In time a certain amount of sensation is regained.

THIERSCH GRAFTS

As regards priority, Ollier[1] was in the habit of cutting grafts 10 to 15 mm. wide and 2 to 4 cm. long, resembling in every way Thiersch grafts; but unlike Thiersch, he did not scrape away the granulations before making the transplantation. Fischer[2] also shaved from the surface of a limb, thin strips of skin identical with those used by Thiersch.

This superior method of skin grafting has never received the recognition to which it is entitled. Fresh wounds or granulating surfaces of almost any size may be covered with epithelium in from ten days to three weeks; scar contractions are prevented; infections are avoided and the cosmetic result cannot be too highly praised.

Preparation of the Surface to be Grafted

Scrub the skin. Remove the débris (crusts) and surrounding hairs and irrigate with normal salt solution. Anesthetize the patient. Curet the surface. Check oozing with firm pressure.

Grafts

The grafts are best obtained from the anterior surface of the thigh. Cut them with a sharp razor. An assistant renders the surface tense by means of a hand on each side of the limb or by grasping the thigh from below, while the surgeon, taking his position with his back to the patient's feet, cuts toward himself while his left hand is used to stretch the skin in front of the razor toward the knee. Pieces of gauze beneath the hand help in obtaining a firm grip. Thin pieces of epidermis are removed by means of a side-to-side sawing motion. The pieces may be several inches long and range from one-half to one inch wide. Keep the skin and razor wet with salt solution. (Fig. 592).

It is unnecessary to remove the whole thickness of skin; all that is required is a paper-like layer with several bleeding points caused by dividing the capillary vessels in the papillary ends. Beginners will do well to practice skin grafting on the cadaver first, before attempting it on a patient.

As the strips of skin are cut they fold up on the razor and when sufficient length has been obtained, slightly incline the instrument away from the thigh thus severing the graft from its connection.

Grafting

Place the grafts on the surface prepared for them shingle-wise—that is, overlapping each other as well as the wound edges. If the pieces are large they may be buttonholed with a scissors or perforated with a punch for drainage purposes. If there is a redundancy of skin the extra portions may be replaced upon the surface from which they were taken.

[1] Bull. de l'acad. de Med., 1872.
[2] Zeit. f. Chir. Bd. 13, 1880, p. 193.

BLEEDING

In controlling the bleeding which often follows the curetting, Thiersch first used an Esmarch constrictor, leaving it **in situ** until grafts and dressings were applied, but later considered this procedure injurious. Others, however, have used it extensively. There seems to be no logical objection to the use of a constrictor although its removal is usually followed by an undesirable oozing.

Pressure with gauze pledgets moistened with peroxide of hydrogen or adrenalin solution is useful for controlling bleeding, particularly if the part is elevated; or pressure is applied over a piece of rubber protective thus avoiding tearing the clots from the mouths of the small vessels when the dressing is removed. Rushmore recommended the use of a high-frequency electric current for coagulating the blood and promoting the adherence of the graft; this has not proved very popular, however. It is better to twist a vessel than to ligate it. A dry surface should be maintained in order to promote the growth of the new skin.

CURETTING

Curetting was one of the principal features of Thiersch's original procedure. It was his idea that the large, soft, superficial granulations, during their transformation into connective tissues, were the cause of scar contraction which could be avoided by curetting down to the firmer tissue. Schmitzler and Ewald proved it was unnecessary to remove healthy granulations and that the graft may be placed on the unaltered surfaces without fear of any great amount of contraction. Reliable results have been obtained without curetting but diseased tissues should always be removed. In any case, results are likely better when the granulations are removed.

Sick rubs the granulations away with gauze instead of using a curet. Halsted, McBurney and others preferred to shave the surface with a scalpel or an amputating knife. In this way a smoother surface is obtained thus promoting the vitality of the transplant.

Irrigations of warm salt solution or sterilized water are advisable during and following the operation.

Thiersch and others advise against using antiseptics after curetting, stating that the resulting necrosis interferes greatly with the anchoring of the grafts; however, they may be used both before and after curetting if they are washed away with a neutral solution. Their value is doubtful.

After-Treatment

Grafts become firmly fixed in from 7 to 10 days. The lowermost layer of dressing material may be left in place for two weeks under ordinary conditions. The coverings should be soaked off with warm salt solution to avoid injuring the grafts, although in some instances this is not necessary as the dressings slide off very easily.

The part receiving the graft should be protected from injury and sudden temperature changes for several weeks, especially in the case of ulcers which have a tendency to recur after grafting. Some mild soothing ointment should be applied to the part to prevent dryness and cracking.

In many cases, especially where wet dressings are employed, the external layers of epidermis atrophy and become macerated and seem to come away with the dressing when it is removed leaving a grayish, sodden surface behind. This is not always indicative of failure for in a short time the epithelium will be replaced from the remaining rete Malpighii.

Schmieden and others are of the opinion that scarlet-red ointment promotes the growth of epithelium greatly. It may be employed advantageously in Thiersch grafting where the whole area has not been covered by skin. It is recommended that the ointment does not come in contact with the graft unnecessarily as it is likely to destroy it.

THE WOLFE-KRAUSE METHOD

J. R. Wolfe, an oculist of Glasgow, introduced the method of using grafts to fill the entire defect in the skin including the whole thickness of the skin but without adipose or cellular tissue (Figs. 593-594). He first experimented with the conjunctiva, shifting parts of it from one part of the eye to the other without pedicles. Later (1872) he employed the conjunctiva of rabbits in treating defects in the human eye. Three years later he made public his experiments in skin grafting for ectropion. In a short time Wadsworth introduced the method in America. Von Esmarch was the first to use the procedure extensively in general surgery.

Grafts comprising the whole thickness of skin had been used often before the time of Wolfe but in nearly all instances, the subcutaneous tissues were also included. Jacenko may have been the first to use grafts without fat satisfactorily; in 1872 Le Fort reported success in treating a case of ectropion.

Wolfe contended that the fat should not be included in the graft on the basis that it was likely to undergo necrosis and interfere with nutrition, and he was doubtless correct. Hirschberg and Taylor as well as many others do not conform with this belief since transplants of fat alone have been grafted from one place to another to fill in depressions or as a substitute for the mammary gland. The original method of Wolfe has been modified and improved upon by Fedor Krause to such an extent that it is generally called the Wolfe-Krause method.

Grafts

The grafts may be cut in the form of an oval or round so that the defect left may be closed by suture. The arm, thigh or buttocks may be chosen. It is of little moment where the grafts are obtained. Davis suggests using skin from the abdomen in the course of a laparotomy.

Outline the graft by an incision. Dissect the whole flap with a knife, the edge of which is turned toward the surface so as to remove the fat. Allow at least one-third for shrinkage; this is always great (elasticity of the skin).

Young advocates the removal of the subcutaneous fat with the grafts, trimming it off later with curved scissors while the flap is spread on the palm of the hand or is curled over a finger. He contends this is a quicker, easier method and the remaining defect is more readily closed.

According to Krause, absolute dryness is an important factor in promoting quick healing. The hands and instruments should be kept dry and no irrigations should be done. Others do not agree with him.

The entire wound should be completely covered with as large sections of skin as it is possible to obtain, because where there is an open space a scar

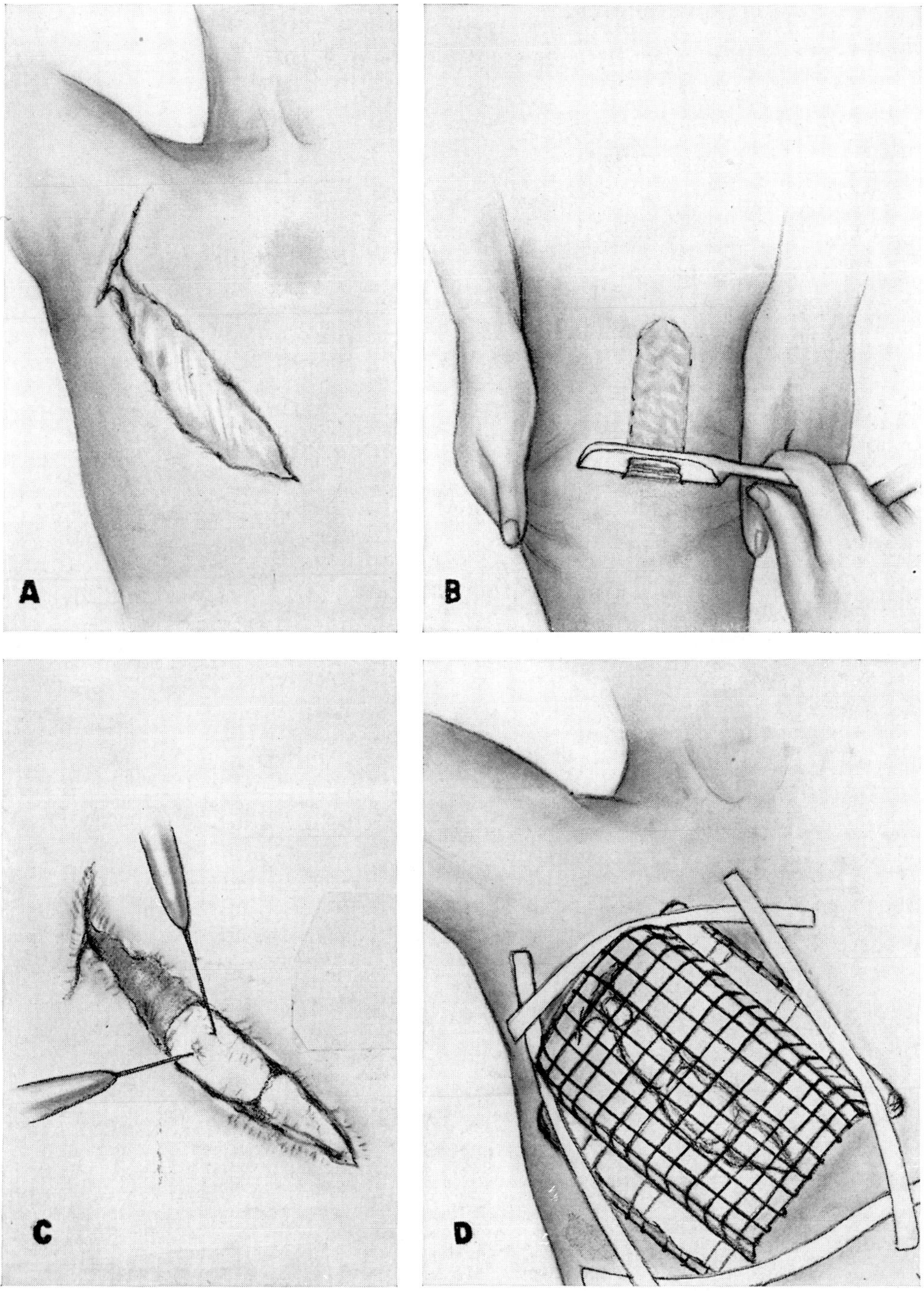

A

B

C

D

FIG. 592. Thiersch graft: A. granulation tissue formed in scar after breast amputation, B. thin layer of skin removed from thigh, C. placing the graft in wound, D. wire basket protects wound.

results. It may be necessary to complete the operation with Thiersch grafts.

Originally, artificial heat was used to keep the new skin warm; this was discontinued when it was found to promote decomposition.

A dry gauze dressing is applied.

After three or four days it is advisable to soak the gauze off with boric acid solution, examine the graft and open any blisters which may be present. Apply sterilized borated vaseline.

SIEVE GRAFT

Beverly Douglas describes a "sieve graft" for covering large skin defects[1] as follows:

"This large graft has been called the 'sieve graft method' because the graft is uniformly perforated with small round openings. The method provides firm, safe healing without contracture in a defect upon any portion of the body. The cosmetic result accomplished is very nearly as good as that obtained by the Wolfe-Krause graft."

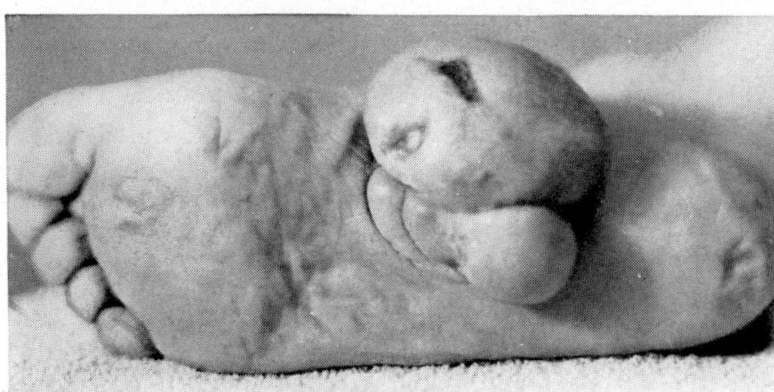

Fig. 593

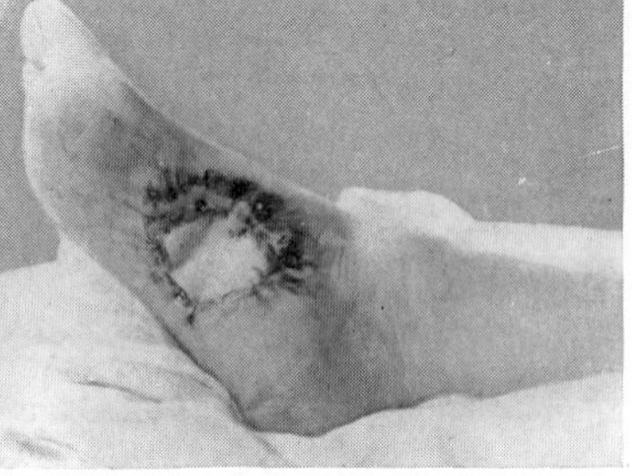

Fig. 594

Fig. 593. Fibroma of plantar fascia.
Fig. 594. Skin grafting (Wolfe-Krause method) following removal of tumor of foot. Oval homo-transplant taken from buttock of daughter of the patient. Excellent final result.

Prepare the wound to be grafted in accordance with Blair's method.[2] Outline a pattern on transparent cellophane with a pen on the day before the operation. This should be about one-fourth larger than the wound to be covered; transfer to tinfoil and punch the letter "E" near the lower border for the purpose of orientation. The usual antiseptic preparation is made at time of the operation. General anesthesia is recommended although local analgesia may be employed. As a rule, four lines of intradermal infiltration are made enclosing the pattern; this is supplemented by an injection of 3 cc. of the anesthetizing solution subcutaneously at eight points equally spaced within the area to be lifted. In the presence of small varicose venules, more infiltration is necessary.

The "sieve graft" technic takes no longer than an ordinary full thickness graft, if the closure of the excision wound is included with which the "sieve" method entirely dispenses.

Step 1. Place the foil pattern upon the donor skin site. Follow its periphery with a scalpel cutting through the skin just to the fat. Use a steel die similar to that illustrated in Fig. 595.

[1] S. G. O., June, 1930, Vol. 50.
[2] V. P. Blair, Ann. Surg., 1924.

Step 2. Twist the steel die with the thumb and index finger boring out islands of skin equidistant from each other over the graft area. The die is one-fourth of an inch in diameter and its flange is one-sixteenth of an inch deep. The surrounding skin is tensed while each island is being bored. Make the openings one and one-half cm. apart.

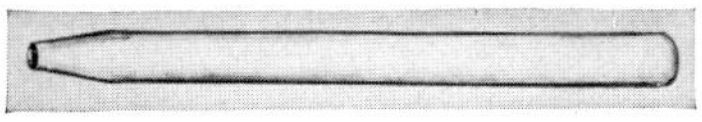

Fig. 595. Steel die used in sieve graft. (Courtesy, Surg., Gynec. and Obst., vol. 50, 1930.)

Step 3. Insert the point of a sharp pointed narrow bladed scalpel into the incision made by the punch for each island (Fig. 596), a, keeping just the full thickness of the skin until its point comes out through the punch incision to the left of it but over the top of the corresponding island, b. With a sawing motion it is advanced to islands, c and d, the skin surrounding which is similarly undercut. Reverse the blade and complete the 180 degrees of the circle from b to e to d in the same way. As the scalpel enters each circular punch incision, have an assistant depress each island with a knife handle or other suitable instrument to prevent its injury. When each opening is undermined, undermine the peripheral edges of the graft in the usual manner and cut through a few strands of tissue previously overlooked, thus liberating the entire sieve graft. The donor site will still possess small islands of skin spaced within the fat and fascia (Fig. 597). Apply vaseline gauze over which dry gauze is strapped with adhesive.

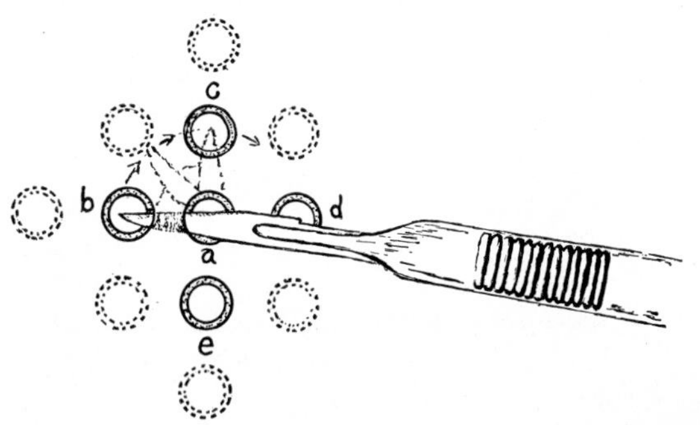

Fig. 596. Undercutting skin in sieve graft. (Courtesy, Surg., Gynec. and Obst., vol. 50, 1930.)

Step 4. Remove all fat from the graft with curved scissors and suture it into the wound with interrupted stitches of silkworm-gut or horsehair. Approximate the edges accurately (Fig. 598). Dress the grafted area in accordance with Blair's sea sponge technic. Press the graft into contact thus expressing all serum and blood clot. Cover with a layer of xeroform vaselin gauze-mesh or ordinary vaselin gauze wiped until very little vaselin remains on it. Over four layers of dry flat gauze apply large, flat sea sponges which have been sterilized in bichloride and wrung out in dry towels just before using. If possible, one sponge should cover the entire area extending well over the suture lines, thus

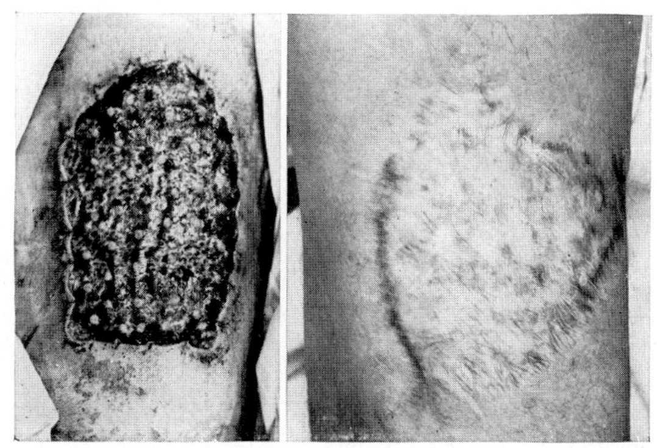

Fig. 597. Small islands of skin left on the donor site; and healed. (Courtesy, Surg., Gynec. and Obst., vol. 50, 1930.)

even pressure will be exerted. If only part of the wound has been grafted, treat the other part with the Carrel technic 48 hours later without fear of injury.

Douglas removes the sponge only after ten days, provided infection is not indicated by local signs or fever. At this time he inspects the graft, removes stitches, trims away any necrotic portions and reapplies the pressure dressings. Within 12 to 18 days the perforations will have been found to be epithelialized and pressure may be discontinued.

A longer time is required by the islands for healing but they heal with certainty and a pigmented epithelium will result. These islands have the appearance of small deep grafts but should not be confused with them, as they have not been

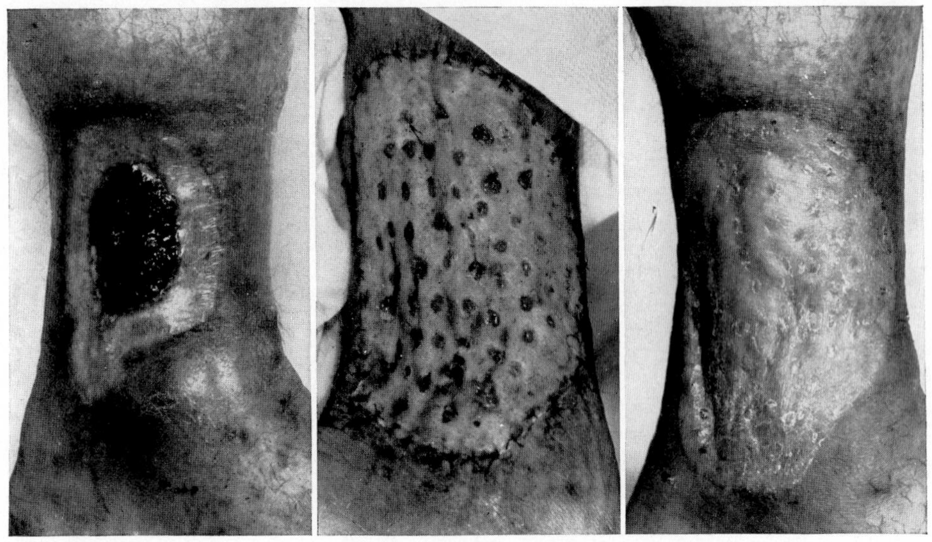

A B C

Fig. 598. The ulcer prepared; the graft in place; and the graft healed. (Courtesy, Surg., Gynec. and Obst., vol. 50, 1930.)

undercut and hold their position strongly. The epithelium from them has great healing power. It is not necessary to attempt closure by undermining the edges of the wound, etc., as satisfactory healing with almost full pigmentation is bound to take place.

Comment. According to Douglas, the ideal graft for filling large skin defects must possess the following properties:

1. It must be capable of being so cut that its removal will leave behind a wound which will heal rapidly without further grafting and with only slight scarring.
2. It must be able to take hold and grow upon a moderately infected surface.
3. It must provide complete healing in a reasonably short time.
4. It must inhibit scar formation and subsequent contracture—a point especially important in defects over joints.
5. It must produce a skin surface so pliable that healing is stable and resistant to minor injuries.

6. It must effect a good, though not necessarily an excellent, cosmetic result.

Weighing each of the types of grafts in general on the basis of these points, Douglas' experience is as follows:

1. The Ollier-Thiersch graft fails from the standpoint of resisting infection and of preventing contracture, and the surface healed by its employment is easily eroded.
2. The small deep graft is ideal from every standpoint but two, viz.: it fails to prevent contracture and often fails to give a good cosmetic effect.
3. The Wolfe-Krause or full thickness grafts are excellent from the standpoints of stable healing, cosmetic effect, and prevention of contracture. However, if the graft is large, a defect is left behind at the donor-site which will require further grafting—a distinct disadvantage. Furthermore, infection may readily cause its total loss.

The sieve graft satisfied all of the demands enumerated. Two valuable properties possessed by none of the above varieties deserve especial mention: (1) the perforations, by providing adequate drainage, make it resistant to infection, thus insuring a very high percentage of takes; (b) the donor site requires no further grafting and heals with a good cosmetic result.

Dragstedt and Wilson's Modification of the Douglas Sieve Graft

L. R. Dragstedt and H. Wilson* point out that the Douglas method of placing the graft was so devised as to leave behind numerous small islands of skin from which regeneration could occur making it unnecessary to treat further the donor-site. In other words, it retained the advantages of the Wolfe-Krause full thickness graft in preventing contracture and providing a new skin surface resistant to minor injuries while also affording a higher incidence of takes, especially in the presence of mild infections.

The Dragstedt and Wilson procedure retains the advantages of the perforated full thickness graft of Douglas while it greatly facilitates healing of the donor-site. Besides, the graft is easier to prepare, does not require any special instruments and the procedure consumes much less time.

Step 1. Prepare the wound to be grafted in the usual manner.

Step 2. Secure an oval shaped transplant (Fig. 599) the full thickness of the skin with none of the subcutaneous fat. The long axis of the graft should be about one-third longer than the long axis of the wound to be covered. The graft is taken from the lax skin of the abdomen wall. No undercutting is usually necessary.

Step 3. Place the graft, dermal side down, on a smooth towel moistened with physiological salt solution.

Step 4. With a sharp scalpel make numerous short longitudinal incisions (Fig. 600). These incisions should be overlapping. When this step is completed it permits the graft to be stretched into any desired shape. (Fig. 601.) Practically, the graft need not be more than one-third to one-half the width of the defect to be covered.

* Surg., Gyn. & Obst., Vol. 65, No. 1, July, 1937.

Step 5. Suture the transplant into place and press it firmly in contact with the underlying raw surface. (Fig. 602.)

Step 6. Cover the graft with vaselinized gauze which is covered with flat gauze and sea sponges. (Blair's method of sea-sponge compression.)

Comment. Remove the sponges on the seventh day. Inspect the graft. Remove the stitches. Reapply the compression dressing for another week. Follow this by ordinary dressings. The donor-site usually heals within a week or ten days.

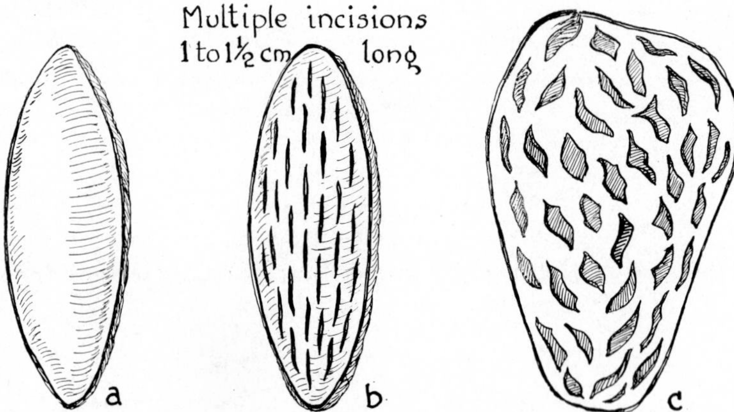

FIG. 599. a. Oval-shaped transplant; b, numerous overlapping incisions; c, graft stretched to shape of area to be covered. (Courtesy of Dr. Lester R. Dragstedt.)

SKIN-PERIOSTEUM-BONE GRAFTS (HIRSCHBERG)

In employing grafts which include the skin, subcutaneous tissues, periosteum and bone, strict asepsis is imperative. There are not many conditions calling for this type of grafting; it is generally used in connection with filling in defects of the skull and scalp and in certain rhinoplastic operations.

The graft is usually obtained from the front surface of the tibia; the incision is made down to the bone, a thin layer of which is removed with a sharp chisel without interfering with its connection with the periosteum and skin lying over it. The remaining wound is closed by undermining and suturing the integument around it. Success is usually more certain when a portion of bone is included than when the periosteum alone is used.

MUCOUS MEMBRANE (WÖLFLER) GRAFTS

Wölfler was the first to methodically graft mucous membrane other than the conjunctiva; he grafted urethras, after removing strictures, with sections of mucosa from a prolapsed rectum, from the cervix of a prolapsed uterus or a uterus which was excised. He performed successful experiments later, using the stomach of a frog, esophagus of a rabbit, etc. An autopsy, made 6 months after his operation on a patient, revealed the new urethra in perfect condition. Beigel did some very fine work in this line; Fenwick repaired a defect in a human urethra with a section of sheep's urethra.

Recently the urethra has been successfully replaced with parts of the internal

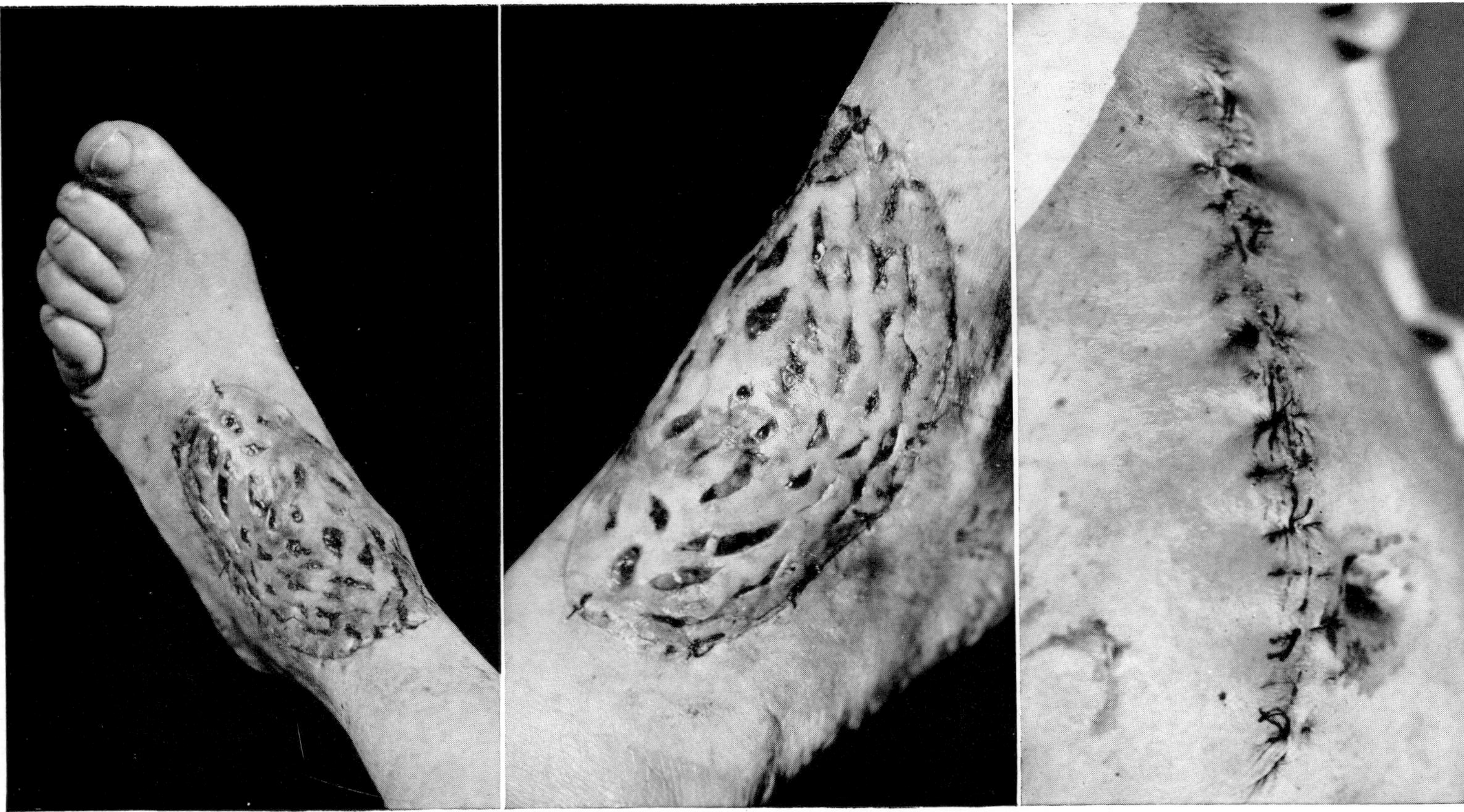

FIGS. 600-601-602. Condition of transplant and donor site 10 days after operation. (Courtesy of Dr. Lester R. Dragstedt.)

saphenous vein as well as the ureter and the vermiform appendix removed from other patients.

According to Wölfler, mucous membrane adheres as well as skin; others do not agree with this idea. It may be shaved off or stripped.

In 1874, Hirschberg made the first buccal mucous membrane transplantation to the conjunctiva. This has been done repeatedly since. In 1872 Wolfe transplanted the conjunctiva of animals to man thus popularizing the procedure.

Czerny demonstrated that mucous membrane from the mouth with flat epithelium, and from the nose with cylindrical or ciliated epithelium readily takes on the appearance of epidermis when grafted on a raw skin surface. Sick noted that this also occurred in connection with vaginal mucosa.

Virchow and his followers maintain that skin grafted on a mucous surface turns into mucous membrane. It is true that in most cases the skin conforms to its surroundings. Thiersch claims this is not pure and backs his statement up by citing a case where a skin flap was used in repairing a soft palate and so much hair grew that the patient had to shave the inside of his mouth.

Thiersch grafts have been successfully employed in operations for hypospadias. They are used to line the new urethra by wrapping them around a catheter which is left in place until adhesion takes place. They have also been used within the larynx after excision of a stricture.

GRAFTING IN X-RAY BURNS

X-ray burns cause a stubborn form of chronic dermatitis where different components of the true derm atrophy and is often characterized by areas of epithelial proliferation having a tendency to ulceration, infection and malignancy. Spontaneous healing hardly ever takes place and in case a malignancy is suspected the area should be excised. Skin grafting by either the Thiersch or Wolfe-Krause method may then be necessary. Transplantation including the whole thickness of skin seems to be advisable. Wolfe-Krause grafts are preferable around the knuckles, wrists and fingertips. All of the burned area should be removed so that recurrence will not take place.

According to Porter, hemostasis should be absolute, moderate pressure should be employed in applying the dressing and the affected part (usually the hand) is kept raised. The borders of the wound should be beveled and cut to fit the defect exactly—the edges should be thinner than the centers to correspond to the bevel.

Rubber protective, when employed, should be removed in from 24 to 36 hours; if serum or blood is present the grafts should be incised and the fluid expressed; lanolin is then applied to the edges of the graft.

It is doubtful if this procedure has any advantages over the others. If the affected area is completely removed, as it should be, the transplanted surface is the same as an ordinary wound. It is difficult to check oozing about the hands. In this case the grafts are preserved on a rubber protective in an aseptic jar containing a piece of moist gauze and applied the following day with no antiseptic. If there is very little oozing, it may be checked by placing the grafts in position and applying slight pressure.

TREATMENT OF BURNS

The causes of fatalities in burns and scalds are:

(1) **Shock** which is often accompanied by pulmonary congestion and suffocation resulting from exposure to the smoke of the fire.

(2) **Collapse** which may prove fatal and

(3) **Toxemia** resulting from sepsis.

Collapse becomes manifest very rapidly. It is due partly to absorption of histamine bodies from the damaged tissues, but largely, in the earlier stages particularly, to loss of serum from the burnt surface. In order to give some idea of the amount of fluid lost, where in a man weighing 65 kilograms one-sixth of the body surface is burnt, it is estimated that in the first twelve hours after injury he will lose 3,500 c.c. serum from a total blood volume of 5,000 c.c.! (Mitchiner). This loss must be replaced promptly by giving fluids in large quantities. We must prevent this drain by coagulation of the damaged vessels and their contents. The coagulant must be capable of penetration through all damaged tissues and not only the surface of the injured area. Tannic acid in weak solution is ideal as a penetrating coagulant (Mitchiner). The coagulant must be applied at once as a first-aid measure. The patient must be kept warm and fluids administered.

Toxic Symptoms occurring from forty-eight hours to ten days later, usually are the result of septic absorption.

While scarring cannot be entirely prevented in deep burns, the prevention of sepsis does much to diminish the amount of scar tissue; prompt suitable splinting is also helpful. Thorough preliminary cleansing of the burn and surrounding tissues is essential. In cases of severe scarring (see chapter on Neck) plastic surgery, radium or x-ray may be used.

First Aid

Wrap the patient in a blanket. Immediately thereafter apply a coagulant to the burnt area to stop collapse and to relieve pain. According to Mitchiner, by far the best solution to use is 2 to 2½ per cent tannic acid in sterile water. Strong solutions of tannic acid or tannic-acid powder at once coagulate only the surface protein; thus the deeper parts of the injured area are not penetrated or coagulated. Absorption of histamine and loss of fluid will, therefore, continue and produce collapse in spite of the surface coagulation. Administer morphine to relieve the pain.

Scalds are treated similarly. Before applying the tannic-acid solution to a greasy surface, the latter must be removed. Efficient cleaning of the affected area must be done under an anesthetic. General anesthesia, however, is not without risk (pulmonary complications). "Twilight sleep" (scopolamine-morphine anesthesia, which see) serves here well. Upon thorough cleansing of the area depends the whole success of the coagulative treatment and the prevention of future sepsis. (Mitchiner). Open all blisters. Remove dead skin and charred tissue thoroughly. Wash the area and surrounding skin with soap and warm water. Dry with a sterile towel. Sponge with ether. Apply coagulant dressing.

In case of sepsis, anesthetize the patient, remove the dressing, reclean the area and reapply the coagulant dressing. Exsanguination transfusion is valuable where a measured quantity of the patient's toxic blood is withdrawn and replaced by double the amount of a donor's blood. Venoclysis of normal saline and hot drinks are also a great aid.

Coagulant

Mitchiner advises in order to prevent the growth of molds in the tannic-acid solution, to add very weak perchloride of mercury; the molds then gradually decompose to oxide of mercury. No solution should be more than two months old.

Tannic acid powder is only slightly antiseptic. It will not deteriorate if kept in the dark. In watery solutions molds rapidly appear unless an antiseptic be added to the solutions. The antiseptic used must be nontoxic and produce no pain to the patient; it must not interfere with the coagulative action of the tannic acid but must stop the growth of the mold. Mitchiner states:*

"Many antiseptics have been tried, and personally we favour perchloride of mercury, in itself a coagulant and used in treating burns by Lord Lister. Added in such a strength as to give a solution of 1/2,000 it is harmless to the patient, and allows solutions of tannic acid to keep free from moulds for at least two months, and usually three; the perchloride slowly decomposes to yellow oxide of mercury, which is deposited out of solution. In conjunction with tannic acid powder the perchloride of mercury keeps indefinitely. Many coal-tar antiseptics have been tried, but most of these are painful to the patient in a greater or less degree, and in addition may interfere with the formation of a firm coagulum. Acriflavine and dettol have both been used successfully, though in both cases slight pain is often experienced. A new compound combining euflavine and zinc phenolsulphonate is, however, quite painless and gives a good coagulum; it has, however, the disadvantage of all flavine compounds that it stains everything bright yellow. These solutions appear to keep indefinitely and are quite harmless. Tannic acid should, therefore, be combined with an antiseptic, and may be kept in a solid form or in solution."

The Tannic Acid Compress

Five or six layers of sterile gauze are cut to the required size and should overlap the apparent limits of the burn by at least 3 inches. If the burn involves flexures between fingers, etc., the dressing must be shaped carefully to fit closely to these.

Soak the dressing in a 2 per cent tannic acid solution. Apply the dripping dressing evenly to the whole affected area, great care being taken to see that accurate apposition is accomplished. Fixation is now applied; bandage the dressings gently but firmly into position. Put a cradle over the burnt area; an electric lamp will assist drying. Keep the temperature of the room around 105° F. or 40° C. The dressing should be hard in 24 hours. Inspect the dressing but do not touch it unless indicated (pyrexia, toxemia, etc.), then reclean and redress the affected area. Slight exudation of serum or sero-pus around the edges of the dressing is no indication for redressing. The dressing is not to be touched until the coagulum separates from the injured area. This usually takes about 12 days in small burns and 28 in large ones.

Most persons suffering from severe burns are in a state of shock which should be combated first.

* *Modern Treatment of Burns,* Wm. Wood, 1935.

Intravenous injections of saline are often effectual in counteracting the toxemia caused by burns. Sponge the uninjured skin with cold water. Give per os, alkaline preparations to relieve acidity which often accompanies severe burns.

In the extreme cases where it becomes imperative immediately to neutralize the toxin in the blood stream, exsanguination-transfusion is resorted to. This procedure consists of first bleeding the patient and then performing a transfusion from a donor correctly typed. The quantity of blood withdrawn varies from 120 cc. in infants to 3/4 pint in adults; while the amount of blood transfused ranges from 150 cc. in the infant to a pint in the adult.

Tannic acid has been widely used for the local treatment of burns since its introduction in 1925 by E. C. Davidson. It forms a very fine protection for the injured area and prevents toxemia. The coagulum covers the exposed nerve ends, thus preventing pain. Tannic acid fixes proteins and their metabolites thus locking in the coagulum those which would otherwise find their way into the circulation. In other words toxemia, the "bête noir" of burns, is much less likely to take place when tannic acid treatment is instituted. This treatment may be begun as late as seventy-two hours after the burn has been sustained.

It is important that no water comes in contact with the tanned (leathery) coagulum which forms when tannic acid is applied to the burned area. If this precaution is not observed, toxins will be liberated which may result in death. Bailey records such a catastrophe.

To prevent sepsis and scarring, the affected region should be thoroughly cleansed under a general anesthetic.

PREPARATION OF THE TANNIC ACID SOLUTION

A 4 per cent solution of tannic acid in 1:1000 acriflavine seems to be best. Dissolve about a teaspoonful (2 ounces) of tannic acid in five ounces of 1:000 acriflavine in water.

The Tannic Acid Treatment is carried out as follows:

Step 1. Puncture the blisters and trim away the loose epithelium.

Step 2. Render the burnt area aseptic by scrubbing it as well as the adjacent region with liquid green soap.

Step 3. After applying some good antiseptic to the burnt area, dry it with sponges soaked in ether.

Step 4. With a sponge or brush apply the 4 per cent tannic acid solution; dry it by fanning. An electric hair drier may be useful here.

Step 5. Cease giving the anesthetic after the injured region turns a golden brown. However, apply three or four more coats after this, drying each one separately.

The patient is now placed in bed on a sterile sheet and the burnt area is covered with a sterile towel over which a cradle is placed. Great care should be taken to see that the area is kept dry at all times.

Further coats of tannic acid are applied daily until the coagulum becomes hard and black. Dressings are then discontinued. Healing takes place under these coats of tannic acid and they are left in place until they peel off spontaneously which in the usual case is from 10 to 14 days. After the covering is removed, apply vaselinized gauze and bandage. Skin grafting is necessary in some cases.

Figures 603-604 depict the treatment of an extensive burn of the shoulder treated by skin grafting with superimposed pressure and body cast spica.

Comment. Donald B. Wells[1] submerges the burned patient in a large tub of tannic acid solution which is renewed when fouled; it is kept at a temperature comfortable to the patient. All débris, blisters, etc., are carefully washed away, the analgesic effects of the tannic acid rendering this painless. After about three hours, when the entire burned area is clean and a slight tan has already formed, the patient is transferred to bed and kept absolutely dry by the air from one or more large, commercial hair

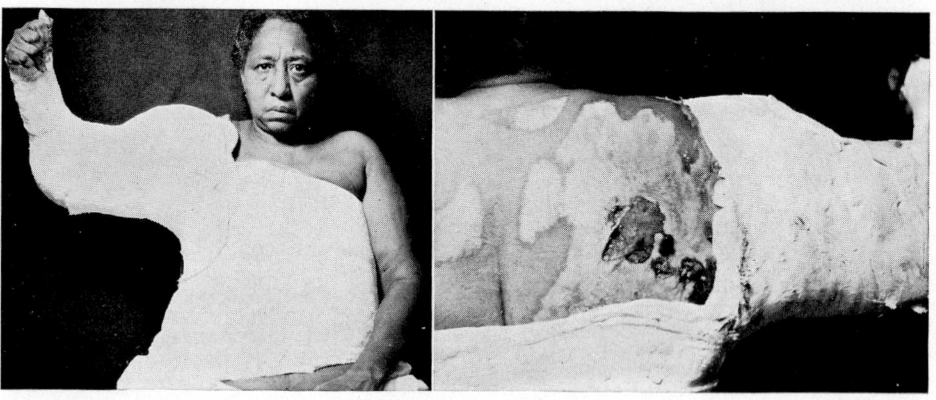

FIG. 603 FIG. 604

FIG. 603. Extensive burn of the shoulder and back treated by skin grafting with superimposed pressure and body cast spica. Plaster of Paris immobilization for purposes of rest and prevention of scar contraction.

FIG. 604. Same as preceding, posterior view. Note that the scar is not pigmented. Center granulating. (Surgical Service, Cook County Hospital.)

driers. A 2 to 5 per cent solution of tannic acid is now sprayed on, a small area at a time so that each is dry before another is started. All blisters are broken. After a thick coagulum is formed the spraying is stopped, but the driers are continued so that not even perspiration can soften the precipitate. The author has never had to follow this treatment by skin grafting nor has he had any infection as long as the coagulum was kept perfectly dry.

In the treatment of burns about the head and face, evipan (see under anesthesia) or ether may be advantageously used. Eye pads and nasal plugs of cotton soaked with saline are employed and the face is rendered antiseptic in the manner described above.

[1] Wells, Donald B., Jour. Amer. Med. Asso., 101:1136, 1931.

LIST OF AUTHORS

(Pages in bold-face type denote pages on which an author's operative technic is described.)

Abbe, 220
Abel, 79
Agnew, **328,** 337
Aievoli, E., 504
Albert, 467
Allen, 502
Altamirano, 504
Anderson, Ernest R., 86
Antone, 171
Arlt, 334
Arnold, **98**
Arnold, Charles Harrison, 97
Ashhurst, A. P. C., 382
Auer, 66
Aufricht, **366**

Bailey, Hamilton, 118, **375,** 376, **381,** 382, 525
Balfour, **vii,** 352
Ballance, 297
Ballinger, 366
Baratoux, **502**
Bardeleben, 312
Barraquer, **351**
Baudoin, **206**
Beck, Carl, 352
Beck, Joseph, 358
Beer, 340
Beigel, 520
Benedictus, 352
Berkeley, 439
Berndt, 297
Berry, **315,** 317, 465
Billroth, 405, 435
Binde, 480
Binnie, 150, 157, 313, 424
Bircher, 468
Blair, 288, 292, 306, **516,** 517, 520
Blandin, 312, 352
Bouchet, 395
Bozer, 352
Branower, 66
Braun, **97,** 210, **278,** 280, **446**
Brophy, 306, 313, **314**
Bruns, 416
Bryant, 110, 238, 507
Buck, 352
Burghard, **199**
Butlin, **254**

Caldwell-Luc, **227**
Cannaday, John E., 493, **497**
Carp, L., 378
Carpeie, 352
Carrel, Alexis, 485, 518
Celsus, 485
Cheyne, **199**
Chipault, **125**
Christiani, 468
Churchill, **474,** 475, 478
Chutro, 493
Claiborne, 331, **334**
Claremont, 466
Clute, **475**
Codirilla, 313
Coleman, 420
Coley, **317, 319**
Colrat, 499
Cope, **474,** 478
Costello, 382
Cousin, 500
Crile, 9, 11, 220, 441, 442
Crotti, André, 441, 449, 468, 481, 482
Crouse, 280
Cuneo, 302
Cushing, Harvey, **148,** 149, 150, 158, 220, 297, 420
Czerny, 522

Dandy, **170,** 171, **172,** 173, 176, 222
Davidson, E. C., 525
Davis, **317,** 319, 487, 514
Denk, 466
De Quervain, 437, 441, 446, 460, 462, 465
Dequise, **277,** 278
Desmarres, 334
Deupes, 276
Dieffenbach, 282, **305,** 312, **331,** 352
Dieulafe, 276
Digby, 376, **391**
Dilpech, 352
Dogliotti, 93, 94
Douglas, Beverly, **516,** 517, 518
Doyen, 3, 243, 312, 344, 387
Dragstedt, L. R., **519**
Dubois, 352
Dubousquet-Labordiere, **502**
Duisberg, 77
Dunhill, T. P., 458

Ecker, E. E., 50
von Eiselsberg, 150, 466, 468
Enderlen, 462
Ermitsch, **402**
von Esmarch, 514
Ewald, 513

Fabrici, 359
Farr, **210**
Fauré, 297
Federoff, **402**
Fenger, Christian, 426
Fenwick, 520
Fergusson, **281,** 282, 312
Ferrarini, **280**
Fincher, 171
Finney, John M. T., 415, 416, **417,** 419, 420, 422
Finsterer, 93, 98, 467
Fischer, 512
Fisher, 100
Flagg, Pauel, 68, 72, 73

Fowler, G. R., 220
Franke, **320**, 378
Frazier, Charles H., **153**, 300
Freeman, 508, 509
Friedl, 302
Friedrich, 167
Frugoni, 480

Gersury, 352
Getzowa, 439
Geyer, **446**
Gilmer, Dr. Thomas L., **291**
Goetsch, Emil, 439, 443, 468
Goff, 34
Goldstein, 179
Graefe, 352
von Graefe, 312
Gregoire, 75
Gross, Wm. A., 45
Grünwald, **402**
Gussenbauer, 203
Guthrie, 339
Guthrie, Donald, 466, 467
Gutierrez, Albert, **273**
Gwathmey, J. T., 61, 81, **82**

Haertel, **446**
Hahn, 203
Halsted, 366, 513
Handley, **255**
Hans, 404
Hartley, **217**
Hazelton, 82
Heidenhain, **127**
Hertzler, 102
Horsley, 128
Hildebrand, 462
Hilton, **380**
Hippocrates, 173
Hirschberg, 514, **520**, 522
Hübscher, 504
Hughson, Walter, 416, 420
Hyndman, Olan R., 245, 431

Ianni, 276
Imperatori, 353
Israel, Prince, **200**, 352, **360**, **365**

Jaboulay, 441
Jacenko, 514
Jackson, 39
Jarman, 79
Jelsma, **420**, 422
Jentzer, 80, 132, 133, **135**, **136**, 139
Jianu, 300, 302
Jobert, 352
Joll, Cecil A., 457, 465, 466
Jones, Wharton, **331**
Jonnesco, 300, **302**, 412
Joseph, 302

Kappis, **95**
Katzenstein, **303**
Kaufman, **278**
Keegan, 353, **355**
Keen, W. W., 167, 217, 420
Kennedy, 244, 297
Killian, 78, **224**
King, Joseph E. J., **121**
Knapp, **334**, **340**
Koch, Robert, 46
Kocher, 4, 33, 281, 282, 415, 435, 437, 441, 449, 468
Kocher, A., 466
Kocher, Theodore, 167
König, 112, 150, 153, **310**, 352
Kohn, 438
Kolle, 178, 352, **365**
Krause, 162, **163**, 170, **217**, 218, 352, **514**, 516, 519, 522
Krimer, 313
Krönlein, 120, **320**
Kümmel, 25
Küttner, 171, **278**

Labat, 95
Lane, Sir Arbuthnot, 306, 313, **319**
von Langenbeck, **277**, 278, 313, **316**, 352
Lapat, 352
Lauber, **351**
Lecéne, 425
Lee, Ferdinand C., 311
Le Fort, 514
Legg, **315**, 317
Leis, 352
Leisnick, 352
Lejars, 339
Leriche, Rene, 276
Levy, **206**
Lexer, 203, 302, 303, 313, 352
Light, George, 431
Lilienthal, 482
Lister, Lord, 46, 524
Loiseau, 395
Lorenz, 313, 416
Lothrop, **204**, 205
Lucas, 507

MacCormac, **359**
Macewen, Sir William, 38, 150, 153, 297, 395
Mackenzie, Sir James, 6
Magill, 72
Malgaigne, **311**
Malone, 119
Mandl, Felix, 472
von Manteuffel, Zoege, **455**
Marcy, 507, 508
Marion, 299
McBurney, 513
McCarthy, 509
McKenzie, 420
McReynolds, **327**
Meeker, 97
Meltzer, 66
Mikulicz, 386, 415, **416**, 435
Miles, 504
Milton, 483
Mirrizi, P. L., 435

Mitchiner, 523, 524
Morestin, 276, 280
Moskowitz, 313
Moynihan, Lord, 3, 5, 25
Müller, 112, **150**, 153
Mule, **351**
Muni, Paul, 46
Murphy, **207**, **285**, 286
Murphy, John B., 423

Naffziger, H. C., **468**, 469, 470
Nélaton, Ch., 352, **356**, **363**
Neuber, 38
Nugent, **348**

O'Dwyer, 395
Offerhaus, **210**, 211
Ollier, 352, 512, 519
Oltamare, 80
Oppenheim, 162

Palmer, Don H., **178**
Pancoast, 352
Parkhill, **179**
Partsch, 297
Pasteur, 46, 53
Pauchet, 97
Payr, 462, 468
Perthes, 244
Pfeiffer, 171
Pietri, 276
Pirogoff, 81, **67**
Poncet, 80, 508
Porter, 525
Post, Joseph, 352
Purves, 297
Pussep, 218

Ranzi, 467
Raven, 504
Reclus, 499
Redard, 503
Rehn, 441
Reverdin, J. L., 352, 437, 507, 508
Roberts, 352, 509
Rochet, **288**
Roe, 352
Rose, 239, 306, 312
Rosenstein, 352
Rosenthal, **304**
Roux, 312, 352
Rushmore, 513

Saemisch, **339**
Schiff, 468
Schleich, **103**
Schmieden, 514
Schmitzler, 513
Schnitzler, 467
Scott, Sir Walter, 493
Sédillot, **358**
Serre, 352
Shoemaker, 313

Sistrunk, Walter E., 272, **273**, **429**
Slayton, 39
Sluder, **236**
Smith, **345**, 352, 355
Socin, 435, 441
Souchon, 508
Spiller, 217, 300
Spurling, R. Glenn, **420**, 422
St. Jacques, Eugene, 25
Sternburg, 467
Stevens, 244
Stieda, 150
Stierlin, 462
Stone, Harvey, B., 479
Streissler, **411**
Sutton, Bland, 429
Syme, **359**
Szymanowski, **367**

Tagliacozzi, Gaspard, 352, **359**, 360, 484
Taylor, 514
Thiersch, 353, **512**, 513, 514, 516, 519, 522
Thomas, Thelwell, **416**
Thomas, 418
Thomson, St. Clair, **393**
Thorek, Max, 80
Thorek, Phil, 85
Tillman, 171
Todd, Hunter F., **190**
Traut, 487
Trendelenburg, 467
Tromp, 276
Tygat, 119

Underwood, Weeden B., 47

Vail, 226
Vallas, **399**
Van Meter, 504
Van Wagner, 382
Venable, 505
Virchow, 522
Voronoff, Serge, **468**, 480

Wadsworth, 514
Walsh, Dr. Wm. H., 18
Waring, 244, 245
Warren, 352
Watson, 4
Weber, 337
Werkgartner, 467
Wells, Donald B., 526
Whitehead, **258**
Willstaetter, 77
Wilson, H., **519**
Wölfler, 520, 522
Wolfe, J. R., **514**, 516, 522
Wolfler, **520**
Wolkowitsch, **361**
Wredes, 302
Wyeth, **460**

Zarraga, **272**

SUBJECT INDEX

Abscess of brain, 121. See *Brain abscess.*
of sebaceous cyst, 108
of tongue, 250
peritonsillar, 241
retropharyngeal, 241 **(Fig. 268)**
stitch, 13
Absorbable drains, 38
Acoustic nerve, 222
Ménière's disease, 222 **(Fig. 237)**
neurectomy for, 222 **(Fig. 237)**
effect of, on vertigo and tinnitus, 223
Actinomycosis of face, 198 **(Figs. 203, 204)**
Adenitis, tuberculous cervical, 427 **(Fig. 499)**
Adenoidectomy, 238 **(Figs. 264-267)**
complications of, 239
Adenoids, 238
anatomic considerations, 238 **(Figs. 264, 265)**
removal of, 238 **(Figs. 266, 267)**
Adhesions, 34
Air embolism in thyroidectomy, 466
Air sterilization, 31 **(Fig. 16)**
Alcohol injections of trigeminal nerve, 205 **(Figs. 218-233)**
Anastomosis, nerve, for facial paralysis, 297
anatomic considerations, 298
historical notes, 297
of facial nerve, 298 **(Figs. 345, 346)**
with hypoglossal nerve, 300 **(Fig. 346)**
with spinal accessory nerve, 298 **(Fig. 345)**
Anchoring of flaps, 495
Anesthesia, 54
anesthetic mixtures, 75
avertin, 77, 121
basal anesthetics, 76
chloroform, 75
cocaine. See *Cocaine.*
ether, 57. See *Ether.*
ether-colonic, 81
ethyl chloride, 75
evipan, 78 **(Figs. 63, 64)**
for bronchoscopy and esophagoscopy, 353
for operations on eye, 325, 337
on skull and brain, 126
on tongue, 250, 254
on tonsils, 232 **(Fig. 256)**
for thyroidectomy, 441
general, 54. See *General anesthesia.*
Gwathmey's ether-colonic, 81
Hazelton's ether-colonic, 82
intrapharyngeal insufflation, 64, 67 **(Figs. 54, 55)**
intratracheal insufflation, 64. See *Intratracheal insufflation anesthesia.*
laryngoscopy in, 83 **(Fig. 65)**
local, 100. See *Local anesthesia.*
nitrous oxide, 64, 76
parasacral nerve block, 90
paravertebral, 93 **(Figs. 75, 76)**
pernocton, 77
regional, 84. See *Regional anesthesia.*
resuscitation, emergency, in, 83
Anesthesia—(*Continued*)
sacral, 89 **(Figs. 71, 72)**
scopolamine-morphine, 80
sodium amytal, 77
spinal, 84. See *Spinal anesthesia.*
splanchnic, 95. See *Splanchnic anesthesia.*
threatening death in, 83
trans-sacral nerve block, 91 **(Fig. 73)**
Anesthetic mixtures, 75
Anesthetized patient, the, 30 **(Fig. 18)**
Aneurysm, cirsoid, 109
operation for, 110 **(Fig. 96)**
Angioma, cavernous, 109
electrocoagulation of, 109
of brain, 162
of conjunctiva, 328
of scalp, 109
of tongue, 250
radical operation for, 109
radium treatment of, 109
Anoci-association in thyroidectomy, 467
to prevent postoperative shock, 11
Antitetanus serum in scalp wounds, 113
Arlt's operation for symblepharon, 334
Artery or arteries, ligation of,
inferior thyroid, 463 **(Fig. 546)**
middle meningeal, in intracranial hemorrhage, 120 **(Fig. 107)**
superior thyroid, 462 **(Fig. 546)**
Artificial respiration, 55 **(Figs. 41-44)**
Aseptic technic, 25 **(Figs. 11-15)**
Attitude, mental, of patient and surgeon, 9
Auditory canal, external,
exostoses of, 181
foreign bodies in, 179
furuncle of, 180
polyps of, 181
Aufricht's operation for hump nose, 366 **(Fig. 437)**
Autodermic grafts, 499
Autogenous cranial transplants, 153 **(Figs. 160-166)**
Frazier technic, 153
Avertin anesthesia, 77
in brain abscess in children, 121
Avulsion of scalp, 107 **(Fig. 92)**
Azachloramid solution in brain abscess, 122

Ballenger's chisel for nasal septum, 370
swivel knife, 369, 370 **(Figs. 443, 444)**
Barton bandage in dislocation of jaw, 290
Basal anesthetics, 76
avertin, 77
equipment necessary for,
evipan, 78 **(Figs. 63, 64)**
Dickson-Wright splint for **(Fig. 63)**
pernocton, 77
scopolamine-morphine, 80
advantages of, 81
sodium amytal, 77
Basal skull fractures, 119

Beer knife in keratectomy, 340
Ben Morgan anesthesia apparatus, 63 **(Figs. 48-53)**
Bernay's compressed cotton sponges for nose bleed, 354
Berry and Legg's operation for cleft palate, 315 **(Figs. 382-385)**
Blepharoplasty, 332 **(Figs. 403-404)**
Blepharoptosis, 330 **(Fig. 399)**
Blepharorrhaphy, 332
Blepharospasm, 329
Bone, depressed, skull fracture, 113 **(Figs. 98-102)**
  grafts, 150, 153 **(Figs. 160-166)**
Bosworth's tongue depressor, 235 **(Fig. 259)**
Bowman's sound, in lacrimal duct operation, 338 **(Fig. 310)**
Brain, 117
  abscess of, 121, 192
    azochloramid solution in, 122
    extradural, 192 **(Fig. 197)**
    king's operation for, 121
    lumbar puncture in, 122
    silver wire basket in, 122
    temporosphenoidal, 192 **(Figs. 197, 198)**
    usual locations of, 121
  anesthesia in operations for, 126
  concussion of, 118
  exposure of, 156 **(Figs. 167, 168)**
  intracranial bleeding, 119 **(Fig. 107)**
  operations on, 122
  penetrating wounds of, 117 **(Figs. 101, 102, 106)**
  tumors of, 160
    angiomas (pial), 162
    Cargile membrane for injured ventricle, 160
    cysts and cystic collections, 162
    electrocoagulation of, 159, 162 **(Figs. 169, 170)**
    exposure of brain, 156 **(Figs. 167, 168)**
    fascia lata for dural defects, 158
    general principles underlying the removal of, 155
    gliomas and sarcomas, 155 **(Fig. 157)**
    locating the tumor, 156
    meningioma, 157 **(Figs. 169, 171)**
    of convexity of hemispheres, 159 **(Figs. 167, 171)**
    of frontal lobes, 159
    of hypophysis, 163 **(Figs. 175, 176)**
    of temporal, parietal and occipital lobes, 160 **(Figs. 167, 176)**
    two-stage operation for, 157, 160
  wounds of, 117 **(Figs. 105, 106)**
    bullet, 117 **(Fig. 106)**
    penetrating, 117 **(Figs. 101, 102, 106)**
    removal of fragments by suction, 117 **(Fig. 105)**
Branchial cysts and fistulae, 430 **(Fig. 505)**
Branower's intrapharyngeal insufflation anesthesia, 64 **(Fig. 54)**
Breathing tube in general anesthesia, 55 **(Fig. 39)**
Broken surgical instruments, 38 **(Figs. 21-25)**
Bronchoscopy, cocaine anesthesia in, 353
Brophy's operation for cleft palate, 314 **(Figs. 380, 381)**
Buckhardt's operation for retropharyngeal abscess, 242
Bullet wounds of brain, 117 **(Fig. 106)**
Burns, coagulant in, 524
  bath for, 526
  fatalities in, 523
  first aid in, 523
  of neck, 334 **(Fig. 452)**
  of shoulder and back, 526 **(Figs. 603, 604)**
  tannic acid compress for, 524
  treatment of, 523
  Well's tannic acid bath for, 526
  x-ray, 522
Butlin's marginal resection of tongue, 251 **(Figs. 282, 284)**
"Button-hole" incision, 32

Cable graft, 538 **(Fig. 612)**
Calculi, salivary, 267 **(Fig. 294)**
Canthoplasty, 332 **(Fig. 402)**
Canthotomy, 331. See *Canthoplasty.*
Capillary drain, 38
  combined with tubal drain, 38
Capsulectomy, 531, 532 **(Figs. 605-607)**
Carbuncle of face, 197 **(Fig. 202)**
  of neck, 378 **(Figs. 453, 454)**
  x-ray treatment of, 197
Carcinoma of conjunctiva, 328
  of face, 199 **(Figs. 207-214)**
  of floor of mouth, operations for, 365
  of neck, 422 **(Figs. 496-508)**
  of scalp, 111
    Müller-König procedure in, 112
  of tongue, 253 **(Figs. 276, 277, 279, 280, 281, 285, 286, 289, 290)**
Cardiac massage, 56 **(Fig. 46)**
Care, postoperative, 7. See *Postoperative care.*
  preoperative, 14. See *Preoperative care.*
Cargile membrane for hemostasis of brain, 129
  for injured ventricle, 160
Carotid body tumor, 432 **(Figs. 505-509)**
  Mirrizi operation for, 432 **(Figs. 505-509)**
Carrel-Dakin method of wound irrigation, 122
Cartilage, thyroid, wounds of, 376
Cataract, 342 **(Figs. 414-418)**
  aspiration of lens for, 343
  extraction of lens for,
    combined extraction and expression method, 345 **(Fig. 418)**
    expression or Smith-Indian method, 345 **(Fig. 416)**
    extracapsular method, 343 **(Fig. 415)**
    traction method, 345
    vacuum method, 345
  senile, 343
Catharsis, in postoperative care, 14
  in preoperative care, 7
Cauliflower ear, 178
Cavernous angioma of scalp, 109
Cellulitis of neck, 379
Cerebral hemorrhage, 119 **(Fig. 107)**

Cerebral puncture, dangers of, 171
Cervical adenitis, tuberculous, 427 **(Fig. 499)**
Cervical rib, 410 **(Figs. 486, 487)**
anterior operation, 410
posterior operation, 411
Streisser's operation, 411
sympathetic, 412 **(Fig. 488)**
anatomic and practical considerations, 412
sympathectomy, 414
Chalazion, Agnew's operation for, 328
operations on, 328 **(Figs. 297, 298)**
Desmarres' forceps in, 329 **(Figs. 397, 398)**
Cheek, 199
Cheyne and Burghard's operation, 199
defects with cicatricial maxillary occlusion, 199
defects without cicatricial maxillary occlusion, 199
Gussenbauer's operation, 203
Israel's operation, 200 **(Figs. 215-217)**
plastic operations on, 199 **(Figs. 209-217)**
Cheyne and Burghard's operation on cheek, 199
Children, avertin anesthesia in brain abscess, 121
ether anesthesia in, 62
Chipault's craniocerebral topography, 125 **(Figs. 110-111)**
Chloroform, 75
Cigarette drains, 26
Circsoid aneurysm of scalp, 109 **(Fig. 96)**
operation for, 110 **(Fig. 96)**
Cisterna puncture, 171
Cleft palate, 305 **(Figs. 354-358, 380-389)**
Berry and Legg operation, 315 **(Figs. 382-385)**
Brophy's operation, 314 **(Figs. 380, 381)**
Davis-Colley operation, 317 **(Figs. 388, 389)**
historical notes, 312
operations for, 312 **(Figs. 380-389)**
Sir Arbuthnot Lane's operation, 319
von Langenbeck's operation, 316 **(Figs. 386, 387)**
Closure of abdominal incision, author's method, 35 **(Fig. 19)**
of cranial defects, 150 **(Figs. 160-166)**
Coagulant in burns, 527
Cocaine in bronchoscopy, 353
in esophagoscopy, 353
in nose operations, 352
Collodion in umbilical pit, in preoperative preparation, 9
Concussion of brain, 118
Cone method of ether anesthesia, 62
Conjunctiva, anatomy of, 324
foreign bodies in, 325
operation on, 327
pterygium, 327 **(Fig. 326)**
tumors of, 327
Connell's anesthetometer, 69 **(Fig. 56)**
Cornea, foreign bodies in, 325
keratectomy, 340
keratotomy, 339
Knapp's operation for staphyloma, 340
operations on, 339
paracentesis of, 339 **(Fig. 411)**
Cornea—(*Continued*)
transplantation of, 340
ulcer, operations for, 339
wounds of, 339
Cranial defects, 150 **(Figs. 160-166)**
closure of, 150
Müller-König method, 150
Steida's rules for handling, 150
Cranial transplants, autogenous, 153 **(Figs. 160-166)**
vault, injuries of, 113 **(Figs. 97-100)**
Craniocerebral topography, 124 **(Figs. 110, 111)**
Craniotomy, 131. See *Trephining of Skull and Cerebral Decompression.*
for intracranial bleeding, 119
Crystalline lens, cataract of, 342 **(Figs. 414-417)**
Cullom's tonsil forceps, 238 **(Fig. 263)**
Cushing's decompression operation, 149 **(Fig. 159)**
modification of subtemporal decompression, 148 **(Figs. 154-158)**
tripod incision, 116 **(Figs. 103, 104)**
Cut throat, 375 **(Figs. 449, 450)**
Cysts, dermoid, of tongue, 252
of brain, 162
of neck, 427
branchial cysts and fistulas, 430 **(Fig. 505)**
etiology of, 431
thyroglossal cysts and sinuses, 427 **(Figs. 500-504)**
Sistrunk's technic, 429 **(Figs. 500-504)**

Dandy's operation for hydrocephalus, 172 **(Figs. 184-188)**
Davis-Colley operation for cleft palate, 317 **(Figs. 288, 289)**
Decompression, Cushing's operation over cerebellum, 149 **(Fig. 159)**
in intracranial hemorrhage, 120
subtemporal, Cushing's modification, 148 **(Figs. 154-158)**
Defects of cheek, repair of, 199 **(Figs. 207-209)**
Denker's operation for tumor of nose, 371
Depressed skull fracture, 113 **(Figs. 98-102)**
De Quervain's skull cutting forceps, 135 **(Fig. 128, a)**
Dermoid cysts of tongue, 252
Desmarres' forceps for operation on eyelid, 329 **(Figs. 397, 398)**
DeVilbiss cranial forceps, 148 **(Fig. 151)**
Dickson-Wright splint in evipan anesthesia, 79 **(Fig. 63)**
Dieffenbach's incision for removal of upper jaw, 282 **(Fig. 313)**
operation for ectropion, 331 **(Fig. 401)**
for upper lip, 305 **(Fig. 352)**
Diet, postoperative, 16
Digby's tracheotomy technic, 391 **(Figs. 469, 470)**
Dislocation of lower jaw, 289 **(Fig. 329)**
Dissection of lymph nodes of neck, 426 **(Figs. 497, 498)**

Double-faced flap (Figs. 569-572)
Douglas method of skin grafting, 521
Doyen perforator and burr, 144, 150 (Figs. 147, 153)
Dragstedt graft, 521 (Figs. 600-602)
Dragstedt-Wilson modification skin graft, 519 (Fig. 599)
Drainage, indications for, 36
  in operations, 36
  of floor of mouth, 381 (Figs. 455-457)
Drains, absorbable, 38
  capillary, 38
    and tubal combined, 38
  cigarette, 36
  gauze drains, 36
  Mikulicz pack, 38
  rubber tubes, 38
  Wetherill's drain, 38
Drop method of ether anesthesia, 61 (Figs. 47, 48)
Duct, lacrimonasal, 336 (Figs. 409, 410)
  incising of, 337 (Fig. 410)
  probing of, 336 (Fig. 409)
  salivary. See *Stensen's duct.*
Dunhill's method of dividing sterum in thyroidectomy, 458 (Fig. 543)
Dura mater, injuries of, 113
  repair of defects of, 114
    fascia lata for, 158
  tumors of, 159 (Figs. 169-171)

Ear, 178
  auditory canal, external, 179
    exostoses of, 181
    foreign bodies in, 179
    furuncle of, 180
    polyps of, 181
  cauliflower, 178
  external, operations on, 178
  Goldstein's operation, 179
  hematoma auris, 178
  macrotia (large ears), 179 (Fig. 189)
  middle ear, 181. See *Middle ear.*
  Palmer operation, 178
  Parkhill's operation, 179 (Fig. 190)
  prominent ears, 178 (Fig. 189)
  Pynchon pump in operation for, 178
Ectropion, 331 (Figs. 400, 401)
  atonic, Dieffenbach's operation for, 331 (Fig. 401)
  cicatricial, Wharton Jones' operation for, 331 (Fig. 400)
Electric saws and drills, 148 (Figs. 147, 149, 153)
Electrocoagulation in brain abscess, 122
  of angioma, 109
  of meningioma (Figs. 169, 171)
Electrosurgery, 44
Electrosurgical hemostasis of dura, 129
  short-wave apparatus, 42 (Figs. 26-32)
  thyroidectomy, advantages and disadvantages, of, 461
Embolism, air, in thyroidectomy, 466
Encephalocele, 107
Entropion, 331
Enucleation of eyeball, 350 (Fig. 424)
  artificial globe in scleral sac, 351
  Barraquez-Lauber method, 351
  modifications of operation for, 351
  Mule's operation for, 351
  technic of, 350
Epidermal grafts, 499
Epilepsy, 166 (Figs. 177-180)
  causes of, 166
    of failure after trephining, 167
  decompression for, 156 (Fig. 180)
  drainage of lateral ventricle for, 167 (Figs. 181-183)
  excision of dura mater for, 167
    of scar for, 166 (Fig. 179)
  focal or Jacksonian, 166 (Figs. 177-180)
  idiopathic, 167
  traumatic, 167 (Figs. 177-180)
Epithelioma of conjunctiva, 328
Equipment for operating room, 24 (Figs. 7-17)
Ermold-O'Dwyer's intubation set (Fig. 474)
Esophagoscopy, anatomic notes, 386
  cocaine anesthesia in, 353
Esophagotomy, external, 402 (Figs. 482, 483)
  dangers of, 404
  indications for, 402
Esophagus. See also *Surgery of Esophagus* in chapter on Surgery of Chest.
  diverticulum of (Figs. 479-481)
  esophagoscopy, 386 (Fig. 460)
  esophagotomy, external, 402 (Figs. 482, 483)
  foreign bodies in, 377 (Fig. 451)
  injury to, in thyroidectomy, 465
  periesophageal suppuration, 383
  stricture of, 402
Ethyl chloride anesthesia, 75
Ether, 57 (Figs. 47-51)
  closed methods, 63 (Figs. 49-51)
  cone method, 62
  drop method, 61 (Figs. 47, 48)
  mask, Ochsner's, 61 (Fig. 47)
  open methods, 61 (Figs. 47, 48)
  vapor methods, 64
Ether-colonic anesthesia, 81
  advantages of, 83
  dangers of, 81
  Gwathmey's method, 81
  Hazelton's method, 82
Ethmoid sinus, 228 (Figs. 249, 250)
  external operation for, 229
  intranasal operation for, 228 (Figs. 249, 250)
Evipan anesthesia, 78 (Figs. 63, 64)
  advantages of, 80
  strychnine as antidote, 80
Excision of cervical rib, 410 (Figs. 486, 487)
  of choroid plexus for hydrocephalus, 176
  of dura mater for epilepsy, 167
  of scar for epilepsy, 166 (Fig. 179)
  of tongue (half of), 255 (Fig. 285)
    (whole), 258, 259, 263 (Fig. 286)
  of uvula, 310 (Fig. 390)
Exophthalmos, 468 (Fig. 513)
  Naffziger operation for, 468 (Figs. 549-553)

Exposure of brain, 156 **(Figs. 167, 168)**
Exostoses of external auditory canal, 181
External carotid artery ligation in operation on Gasserian ganglion, 220
External ear, 178. See *Ear.*
Eye, 321 **(Figs. 393-424)**
  anatomy of, 321 **(Figs. 393, 394)**
  anesthesia in operations for, 325, 337
  cataract, 342. See *Cataract.*
  conjunctiva, 327 **(Fig. 306)**
    anatomy of, 324
    foreign bodies in, 325
    operations on, 327
    pterygium, 327 **(Fig. 326)**
    tumors of, 327
  cornea, 339. See *Cornea.*
  enucleation of eyeball, 350 **(Fig. 424)**
  eyelids, 328. See *Eyelids.*
  foreign bodies in, 325
  intraocular tension, operation for reducing, 342 **(Fig. 414)**
  iris, 342 **(Figs. 414-417)**
    extraction of lens, 342 **(Figs. 414-419)**
    injuries to, 342
    iridectomy, 342
    operations on, 342 **(Figs. 414-417)**
  lacrimal apparatus, 336. See *Lacrimal apparatus.*
  magnet for removing foreign bodies from, 326 **(Fig. 395)**
  operations on, 321
  sclera, 341. See *Sclera.*
  tumors of, 327
Eyeball, enucleation of, 350 **(Fig. 424)**
Eyelids, 328.
  Agnew's operation for chalazion, 328
  blepharoplasty, 332 **(Figs. 403, 404)**
  blepharoptosis, 330 **(Fig. 399)**
  blepharospasm, 329
  canthoplasty, 332 **(Fig. 402)**
  canthotomy, 331. See *Canthoplasty.*
  chalazion, 328
  ectropion, 331
  entropion, 331
  hordeolum, 328
  Meibomian cyst, 328
  operations on, 328
  pannus, 335 **(Fig. 407)**
  symblepharon, 334
    Arlt's operation for, 334
  trachoma, 334

Face, 197
  actinomycosis of, 198 **(Figs. 203, 204)**
  Cheyne and Burghard's operation, 199
  defects of cheek, 199 **(Figs. 209-217)**
  furuncle and carbuncle of, 197
    ligation of angular vein for, 197 **(Fig. 202)**
    x-ray treatment of, 197
  Gussenbauer's operation, 203
  infections of, 197 **(Figs. 202-204)**
  Israel's operation, 200
  plastic operations on cheek, 199 **(Figs. 209-217)**

Face—(*Continued*)
  surgery of, 197 **(Figs. 202, 209-217)**
  tumors of, 199
    radium treatment of hemangioma, 199
      of epithelioma, 199
Facial nerve, 297
  anastomosis of, for facial paralysis, 297
    anatomic considerations, 298
    historical notes, 297
    with hypoglossal nerve, 300 **(Fig. 246)**
    with spinal accessory nerve, 298 **(Fig. 345)**
  injury to, in parotid gland operation, 273 **(Fig. 298)**
  Katzenstein's operation, 303 **(Fig. 350)**
  Lexner's operation, 302 **(Fig. 347)**
  muscle transplantation for paralysis of, 300 **(Figs. 347-352)**
  paralysis of, 197 **(Figs. 345-352)**
  Rosenthal's operation, 304 **(Fig. 351)**
Faraboef's forceps for upper jaw resection, 283 **(Fig. 318)**
Farr's method of injecting mandibular nerve, 210
Fergusson's operation for upper jaw, 281 **(Figs. 313, 314)**
Field of operation, preparation of, 7
Finney's operation for spasmodic torticollis, 416 **(Figs. 491-494)**
Finsterer splanchnic needle, 98
Fischer short wave apparatus, 42 **(Figs. 26-32)**
Fisher solution for local anesthesia, 100
Fistulas of salivary glands and ducts, 276
  fistulas of Stensen's duct. See *Stensen's duct.*
  treatment of glandular fistulas, 276
    avulsion of auriculotemporal nerve, 276
    cauterization, 276
    immobilization of jaws, 276
Flagg intratracheal inhalation tube, 72 **(Figs. 60, 61)**
Flaps, after-care, 493
  anchoring of, 492
  bone flap, 127
  double-faced **(Figs. 569-572)**
  for plastic surgery, 486
  French method, 490
  lateral, 488
  pedunculated **(Figs. 573, 574)**
  square **(Fig. 575)**
  triangular **(Figs. 576, 577)**
Floor of mouth, drainage of, 381 **(Figs. 455-457)**
Forceps, Faraboef, for resection of upper jaw, 283 **(Fig. 318)**
  foreign body, 377 **(Fig. 451)**
  MacManus tonsil, 236 **(Fig. 260)**
Foreign body, in esophagus, 377
  in external auditory canal, 179
  in eye, 325
  in nose, 372 **(Fig. 448)**
  in pharynx, 377 **(Fig. 451)**
  in tongue, 252
  left in abdomen, 34
  magnet for removing, 326 **(Fig. 395)**
Foster-Ballenger forceps for nasal septum, 369

Fractures, of bones of face, 204
of lower jaw, 290 **(Figs. 330-333)**
of malar bone, 204
of maxilla, 204
of skull, 113. See *Skull fracture.*
of upper jaw, 204
of zygoma, 205
Frontal sinus, 224 **(Figs. 238-240, 242, 248)**
extranasal approach to, 224 **(Figs. 238-240, 242)**
intranasal approach to, 228 **(Figs. 242, 248)**
Killian operation, 224 **(Figs. 238-240)**
Furuncle of external auditory canal, 180
of face, 197 **(Fig. 202)**
of neck, 378
x-ray treatment of, 197

Galt's trephine, 132 **(Fig. 121)**
Ganglion, Gasserian. See *Gasserian ganglion.*
Gantermann's manipulation in respiratory obstruction, 55 **(Fig. 40)**
Gasserian ganglion, 217
Abbé's operation, 220
anatomic considerations, 217 **(Fig. 218)**
Cushing's operation, 220
Hartley-Krause operation, 217 **(Fig. 235)**
operations on, 217 **(Figs. 235, 236)**
General anesthesia, 54
anesthetic mixtures, 75
artificial respiration in, 55 **(Figs. 41-44)**
asphyxia, laryngoscopy in, 83 **(Fig. 65)**
avertin, 77
basal anesthetics, 76. See *Basal anesthetics.*
breathing, types of, 56
carbon dioxide administration in, 64 **(Figs. 52, 53)**
cardiac failure in, 55 **(Figs. 41-44, 48)**
chloroform, 75
ether, 57. See *Ether.*
ether-colonic anesthesia, 81
ethyl chloride, 75
evipan anesthesia, 78 **(Figs. 63, 64)**
Gwathmey's ether-colonic, 81
Hazelton's ether-colonic, 82
induction of, 54
intrapharyngeal insufflation anesthesia, 64, 67 **(Figs. 54, 55)**
intratracheal insufflation anesthesia, 64, 68 **(Figs. 56-61)**
method of holding jaw forward **(Fig. 45)**
mouth gags in **(Figs. 37, A, 38)**
nitrous oxide, 76
obstruction of airways in, 55 **(Figs. 37, 38, 40, 45, 55)**
oral screw to open mouth **(Fig. 37, B)**
pernocton, 77
preparation of patient, 54
resuscitation, emergency, in, 83
scopolamine-morphine anesthesia, 90
secretions, removal of, in, 55 **(Fig. 40)**
sodium amytal, 77
stages of, 55
threatening death in, 83
wire breathing tube in, 55 **(Fig. 39)**

Gigli wire saw, 145 **(Figs. 145, 146, 149)**
Gilmer's dental bands, 291 **(Figs. 331, 332)**
Glands, lacrimal, 336 **(Fig. 408)**
lymph. See *Lymph nodes.*
parathyroid, 471 **(Figs. 554-561)**
salivary, 267 **(Figs. 278, 291-310)**
thymus, 479 **(Figs. 563-565)**
thyroid, 435 **(Figs. 510-548)**
Glioma, 155
Gliosarcoma, 155
Glossitis, Butlin's marginal resection for, 254 **(Figs. 282-284)**
chronic, 254 **(Figs. 282-284)**
Glossopharyngeal nerve, neurectomy of, 223
Gloves, proper way of putting on, 28 **(Fig. 14)**
Goode rasp in sinus operations, 229
Goldstein's operation, 179 **(Fig. 189)**
von Graefe's knife for paracentesis of eye, 340 **(Figs. 411, 413)**
Grafting, dressings for, 509
in x-ray burns, 522
of skin, 498
Grafts, bone, 150, 153 **(Figs. 160-166)**
autodermic, 499
epidermal, 499
general considerations, 508
mucous membrane, 520
Reverdin, 507
sieve, 516
Thiersch, 512
vegetable, 499
Wolf-Krause method, 514
zoodermic, 499
Grünwald punch in sinus operations, 231
Gussenbauer's operation for cheek defects, 203
Gutierrez' operation for parotid gland, 273 **(Figs. 300-303)**

Hajek's chisel for nasal septum, 370
Halsted subcuticular suture, 487
Hands, technic of scrubbing, 26
Harelip, 305 **(Figs. 353-373)**
anesthesia for operations on, 306
in adults, 306
in infants, 306
König operation for, 310 **(Figs. 364-366)**
Malgaigne's double flap method, 311 **(Figs. 372, 373)**
operation for simple double harelip, 311 **(Figs. 369-371)**
position of patient for operation, 306
preparation of part for operation, 306
projecting intermaxillary bone, 312 **(Figs. 374-379)**
varieties, 305
Hasslinger's directoscope **(Fig. 459)**
Hazelton's technic of ether-colonic anesthesia, 82
Heart, massage of, 46 **(Fig. 56)**
Heidenhain's continuous hemostatic suture for scalp hemorrhage, 127
Heister's mouth gag **(Fig. 38)**
Hematoma auris, 178

Hemorrhage, after removal of brain tumor, 131
from bone, 128 **(Fig. 117)**
from brain, 129
from dura, 128
from scalp, 127 **(Figs. 115, 116)**
in thyroidectomy, 465
intracranial, 119 **(Fig. 107)**
intradural clot suspected, 121
ligation of middle meningeal artery in, 120
nasal, 353 **(Fig. 426)**
postoperative, 13
Hemostasis, in operations on bone, 128 **(Fig. 117)**
on the brain, 129
on the dura, 128
on the scalp, 127 **(Figs. 115, 116)**
in removing brain tumors, 131, 157
of scalp wounds, 107 **(Fig. 90)**
Hemostat, Cullom's tonsil, 238 **(Fig. 263)**
Hiccough, postoperative, 11
Hirschberg grafts, 520
History taking, 6
Hodgkin's disease, 427
Holm's scissors for maxillary sinus, 226 **(Fig. 244)**
Hordeolum, 328
Horsley's bone wax for bone hemostasis, 128
Hudson's rongeur forceps, 135 **(Fig. 128, B)**
Hurd's nasal septum forceps, 369
Hydrocephalus, 172 **(Figs. 184-188)**
causes of, 172
Dandy's operation for, 172 **(Figs. 184-188)**
excision of choroid plexus for, 176
third ventriculostomy, 172 **(Figs. 184-188)**
Hyperparathyroidism, 471
Hypodermoclysis for replacing body fluids, 14 **(Fig. 3)**
Hypoglossal nerve, anastomosis of, 300 **(Fig. 346)**

Illumination of operating room, 21 **(Figs. 7-10)**
Incision, "button-hole," in abdominal surgery, 32
closure of abdominal, by author's method, 35 **(Fig. 19)**
Cushing's tripod, 116 **(Figs. 103, 104)**
Dieffenbach's, for upper jaw, 282 **(Fig. 313)**
Kocher's, for upper jaw, 282 **(Fig. 314)**
Incisions for neck operations, some **(Fig. 476)**
in general, 32
Induction in general anesthesia, 54
Infections of face, 197 **(Figs. 202-204)**
of neck, 378
postoperative, 13
Inferior maxillary nerve, Murphy's method of injecting, 207
thyroid artery, ligation of, 463 **(Fig. 546)**
Infraorbital nerve, anatomic considerations, 212
neurectomy of, 212 **(Fig. 232, B)**
resection of, at foramen rotundum, 214
at infraorbital foramen, 212 **(Fig. 232, B)**
Injection treatment of trigeminal nerve, 205. See *Trigeminal nerve.*

Injuries of bones of face, 204
of cranial vault, 113 **(Figs. 97-100)**
of neck, 375. See *Neck, injuries of.*
of scalp, 107 **(Figs. 90-92, 103, 104)**
Injury of facial nerve in mastoid operation, 186
in parotid gland operation, 273 **(Fig. 298)**
of recurrent laryngeal nerve in thyroidectomy, 462
Instruments, broken surgical, 38 **(Figs. 21-25)**
sterilization of, 46 **(Figs. 33-36)**
Internal jugular vein, 195 **(Figs. 200, 201)**
anatomic considerations, 195 **(Fig. 200)**
ligation and resection of, 195 **(Fig. 201)**
Intracranial hemorrhage, 119 **(Fig. 107)**
intradural clot suspected, 121
ligations of middle meningeal artery, 120
tension, methods of reducing, 118
Intradural clot, 121
Intrapharyngeal insufflation anesthesia, 64, 67 **(Figs. 56-61)**
Intratracheal insufflation anesthesia, 64, 68 **(Figs. 56-61)**
advantages and disadvantages of, 74
improved technic for, 72 **(Figs. 60, 61)**
in operation on tongue, 250
intubation technic in, 73
Intravenous administration of fluids, 14 **(Fig. 4)**
Intubation, 395 **(Figs. 473, 474)**
advantages of, 395
disadvantages of, 396
Ermold-O'Dwyer's intubation set, **(Fig. 474)**
Iridectomy, 342 **(Fig. 414)**. See *Cataract, operations for.*
Iris, extraction of lens, 342 **(Figs. 414-419)**. See *Cataract, operations for.*
injuries to, 342
iridectomy, 342
operations on, 342 **(Figs. 414-417)**
Irrigation of peritoneal cavity, 36
Israel's operation for saddleback nose, 365
total rhinoplasty, 360 **(Fig. 433)**

Jackson's esophagoscope **(Fig. 460)**
laryngoscope, 383
and rheostat, 69 **(Fig. 58)**
tracheotomy triangle **(Fig. 372)**
Jaw, lower. See *Lower jaw.*
upper. See *Upper jaw.*
Jentzer trephine, 132 **(Figs. 122, 123, 125, 126, 129-146)**
coupled with Gigli saw, 142 **(Figs. 145, 146)**
Jugular vein, internal, 195 **(Figs. 200, 201)**
anatomic considerations, 195 **(Fig. 200)**
ligation and resection of, 195 **(Figs. 200, 201)**

Katzenstein's operation for facial nerve paralysis, 303 **(Fig. 350)**
Keegan's operation on nose, 355 **(Fig. 427)**
Kerrison's rongeurs in sinus operations, 231
Killian's method of laryngoscopy **(Fig. 458)**
operation for frontal sinus, 224 **(Figs. 238-240)**
Knapp's operation for trachoma, 334 **(Fig. 405)**

Kocher's dissector in thyroidectomy, 454 **(Fig. 535)**
incision for excision of mandible, 296 **(Fig. 341)**
for removal of upper jaw, 282 **(Fig. 314)**
König's operation for harelip, 310 **(Figs. 364-366)**
Krause's hooks for control of bone hemorrhage, 128 **(Fig. 117)**
claw forceps, 148 **(Fig. 152)**
operation for tumors of hypophysis, 163 **(Figs. 175, 176)**
Kredel plates for hemostasis of scalp, 128 **(Fig. 116)**

Lacrimal apparatus, 336 **(Figs. 408-410)**
duct, incising of, 337 **(Fig. 410)**
probing of, 336 **(Fig. 409)**
gland, excision of orbital part, 336
resection of palpebral part, 336 **(Fig. 408)**
sac, extirpation of, 337
Lacrimonasal duct. See *Lacrimal duct.*
LaForce's adenotome, 241 **(Fig. 267)**
Lane's operation for cleft palate, 319
von Langenbeck's operation for cleft palate, 316 **(Figs. 386, 387)**
Laryngectomy, 405 **(Figs. 484, 485)**
direct, 383 **(Fig. 459)**
indirect, 383 **(Fig. 458)**
Larynx, cocainization of, 353
fractures of, 376
laryngoscopy, 383 **(Fig. 459)**
Lateral flap **(Fig. 568)**
Levy-Baudoin operation on ophthalmic nerve, 206
Lexer's operation for facial nerve paralysis, 302 **(Fig. 347)**
Ligation of angular vein in infections of face, 197 **(Fig. 202)**
of external carotid artery in operations on Gasserian ganglion, 220
of internal jugular vein, 195 **(Figs. 200, 201)**
of lingual artery in carcinoma of tongue, 253
of middle meningeal artery, 120 **(Fig. 107)**
of Stensen's duct, 280
of thyroid arteries, 462 **(Fig. 546)**
Light, surgical. See *Illumination.*
Lingual artery, ligation of, in carcinoma of tongue, 253
tonsil, removal of, 240
Lip, lower, 243 **(Figs. 269-272, 275)**
anatomic considerations of, 243
carcinoma of, 243 **(Figs. 269-272, 275)**
electrocoagulation of, 244
radium treatment of, 244 **(Figs. 271, 272)**
operations on, 243 **(Figs. 269, 275)**
plastic surgery of, 243 **(Figs. 269, 275)**
triangle or V-resection of, 243, 248 **(Figs. 269, 275)**
upper. See ***Upper lip.***
Lipoma of conjunctiva, 328

Local anesthesia, 100 **(Figs. 81-89)**
for bronchoscopy, 353
for esophagoscopy, 353
for nose operations, 352
for thyroidectomy, 441 **(Figs. 518-531)**
in operations on brain abscess, 121
on eye, 325, 337
on scalp, 108, 109
on skull and brain, 126
on tonsils, 232 **(Fig. 256)**
solutions for, 100
Fisher solution, 100
syringe and needles **(Fig. 81)**
types of, 103
edematization (Schleich's method)
endermic **(Fig. 86)**
nerve blocking **(Figs. 85, 87)**
perineural injection
subdermic infiltration
Lower jaw, 284 **(Figs. 319-344)**
dislocations of, 290 **(Fig. 329)**
irreducible, 290
fixation, direct, in fracture of, 292 **(Fig. 333)**
indirect, in fracture of, 291 **(Figs. 331, 332)**
fracture of, 290 **(Figs. 330, 344)**
Gilmer's dental bands, 291 **(Figs. 331, 332)**
Gunning splint, modified, 298 **(Fig. 344)**
indications for resection of, 294
Murphy's operation for, 285 **(Figs. 322, 324, 326)**
complications of, 288
operations on, 284 **(Figs. 319-343)**
resection of, 288, 293 **(Figs. 334-337, 342, 343)**
of alveolar process, 293 **(Fig. 334)**
of horizontal ramus, 293 **(Figs. 335-337)**
Rochet's operation, 288 **(Fig. 327)**
subluxation of, 290
temporomaxillary ankylosis, 285 **(Figs. 322-326)**
wiring for fracture, 292 **(Figs. 331, 332)**
lip, 243. See *Lip, lower.*
Ludwig's angina, 380 **(Figs. 455-457)**
anesthesia for drainage of, 382
Lumbar puncture, in brain abscess, 122
in reducing intracranial pressure, 118
in spinal anesthesia, 84 **(Figs. 68-70)**
Lymphadenitis of neck, 379
Lymphatics of neck **(Figs. 497, 498)**
of scalp, 111
Lymphnodes of neck, 246
anatomic considerations of, 246 **(Fig. 273)**
dissection of, 426 **(Figs. 497, 498)**
operations on, 246, 265 **(Figs. 273, 274)**
Lymphoma, malignant, 427
Lynch suspension apparatus, 383

Macrotia (large ears), 179 **(Fig. 189)**
Magnesium sulphate for reducing intracranial pressure, 118
Magnet for removing foreign bodies, 326 **(Fig. 395)**

Malar bone, fracture of, 204
Malgaigne's operation for harelip, 311 **(Figs. 372, 373)**
Malignant encanthis, 328
lymphoma, 427
tumors of conjunctiva, 328
of scalp, 111
anatomic considerations of, 111
Mandible, 284. See *Lower jaw.*
Mandibular nerve, anatomy of, 215 **(Fig. 233)**
injection of, 207 **(Figs. 222, 226, 229-231)**
neurectomy of, 215
Massage, cardiac, 46 **(Fig. 56)**
Mastoiditis, 183 **(Figs. 194-196)**
anatomic considerations, 186 **(Fig. 195)**
intracranial complications, 190 **(Figs. 197, 198)**
operation for acute mastoiditis, 183 **(Figs. 194-196)**
radical mastoid operation, 186 **(Fig. 196)**
Todd's method in, 190
Maxilla, fracture of, 204
Maxillary nerve, injection of, Murphy's method, 207 **(Fig. 228)**
sinus, 225 **(Figs. 241-247)**
Caldwell-Luc operation, 227 **(Figs. 246, 247)**
empyema of, 225 **(Fig. 241)**
Küster's operation, 225 **(Fig. 241)**
nasal approach to, 225 **(Fig. 242)**
Mediastinitis, 383
Ménière's disease, neurectomy of acoustic nerve in, 222 **(Fig. 237)**
Meningioma **(Figs. 169-171)**
Meningitis serosa circumscripta, 162
Meningocele and encephalocele, 107 **(Figs. 93, 94)**
Mental attitude of patient and surgeon, 9
Middle ear, 181 **(Figs. 191-193)**
anatomic considerations, 181 **(Figs. 191, 192)**
infections of, 181 **(Figs. 191-193)**
intracranial complications, 181
myringotomy, 181 **(Figs. 191, 192)**
dangers of, 183
meningeal artery, ligation of, in operations of Gasserian ganglion, 222
Mikulicz' operation for torticollis, 416
pack for draining abdomen, 38
Mirrizi's operation for carotid body tumor, 435 **(Figs. 507-509)**
Morphine in postoperative pain, 17
Mouth, drainage of floor of, 381 **(Figs. 455-457)**
Mucous membrane grafts, 523
Müller-König operation for cranial defects, 150 **(Figs. 160-162)**
Murphy's method of injecting inferior maxillary nerve, 207 **(Fig. 228)**
Muscle for hemostasis of brain, 129, 131
lengthening in torticollis, 416 **(Figs. 489, 490)**
Myringotomy, 181 **(Figs. 191, 192)**
anesthesia for, 183
dangers of, 183

McManus tonsil forceps, 236 **(Fig. 260)**

Naffziger operation for exophthalmos, 468 **(Figs. 549-553)**
Nasal septum, submucous resection of, 368 **(Figs. 440, 441, 443)**
Neck, 375
burns and scars of, 377 **(Fig. 542)**
cellulitis of, 379
cervical rib, 10 **(Figs. 486, 487)**
cervical sympathetic, removal of, 412 **(Fig. 488)**
cysts, sinuses and fistulas of, 427 **(Figs. 500-505)**
dangers of operations for tumors, 423
esophagoscopy, 386 **(Fig. 460)**
esophagotomy, external, 402 **(Figs. 482, 483)**
foreign bodies in, 377
furuncles and carbuncles, 378 **(Figs. 453, 454)**
incisions for operations on **(Fig. 476)**
infections of, 378
injuries of, 375 **(Figs. 449, 450)**
intubation of, 396 **(Fig. 473)**
laryngectomy, 405 **(Figs. 484, 485)**
laryngoscopy, 383
laryngotomy, intercricoid, 387 **(Figs. 461-463)**
Ludwig's angina, 380 **(Figs. 455-457)**
anesthesia for drainage of, 382
lymph nodes, dissection of, 426 **(Figs. 497, 498)**
lymphadenitis of, 379
mediastinitis, 383
periesophageal suppuration, 383
pharyngotomy, 398 **(Figs. 475-478)**
surgical technic for removal of tumors in general, 422
torticollis (wry neck), 415 **(Figs. 489-495)**
tracheotomy, 387 **(Figs. 464-472)**
tumors of, 422 **(Figs. 496-508)**
wounds of, 375 **(Figs. 449-450)**
Nélaton's subtotal rhinoplasty, 363 **(Fig. 435)**
total rhinoplasty, 356 **(Figs. 428-430)**
Nerve or nerves:
acoustic, 222
Ménière disease, 222 **(Fig. 237)**
neurectomy of, 222 **(Fig. 237)**
effect of, on vertigo and tinnitus, 223
cervical sympathetic, 412 **(Fig. 488)**
facial, 297. See *Facial nerve.*
glossopharyngeal, neurectomy of, 223
infraorbital, 212
anatomic considerations, 212
neurectomy of, 212 **(Fig. 232 B)**
resection of, at foramen rotundum, 214
at infraorbital foramen 212 **(Fig. 232 B)**
injections of, 205 **(Figs. 218-233)**

Nerve or nerves—(*Continnued*)
mandibular, anatomy of, 215 **(Fig. 233)**
injection of, 207 **(Figs. 222, 226, 229-231)**
neurectomy of, 215
maxillary, injection of, 207 **(Fig. 228)**
neurectomy. See *Neurectomy.*
ophthalmic, injection of (Levy-Baudoin), 206
recurrent laryngeal, injury in thyroid surgery, 462
spinal accessory, anastomosis
for facial paralysis, 298 **(Fig. 345)**
for spasmodic torticollis, 416 **(Figs. 491-495)**
supraorbital, injection of **(Fig. 220)**
neurectomy of, 212 **(Fig. 232 A)**
trigeminal, 205. See *Trigeminal nerve.*
Neurectomy, 212, 222 **(Figs. 232-234)**
acoustic nerve, 222 **(Fig. 237)**
glossopharyngeal nerve, 223
infraorbital nerve, 212 **(Fig. 232 B)**
mandibular nerve, 215 **(Figs. 233, 234)**
intraoral approach, 217
Nevus of scalp, 109
Nitrous oxide, 76
Nose, 352
cocaine for local anesthesia, 352
Denker's operation, 371
foreign bodies in, 372 **(Fig. 448)**
hemorrhage from, 353
Bernay's cotton sponges for, 353
postnasal tampon for, 354 **(Fig. 426)**
local anesthesia in, 352 **(Fig. 425)**
operations on, 352
plastic operations on. See *Rhinoplastics.*
polyps of, 271 **(Fig. 445)**
tumors of, 371
radium treatment of, 371 **(Figs. 446, 447)**
Nugent's forceps for extraction of lens, 345 **(Figs. 417, 418)**
operation for strabismus, 348 **(Figs. 422, 423)**

Obstruction of airways in anesthesia, 55 **(Figs. 37, 38, 40, 55)**
Offerhaus' method of injecting mandibular nerve, 210
Oil sterilization, 50
Opening of skull, methods of, 131
Operating pavilions, 18 **(Figs. 5-10)**
Operating room, 31 **(Figs. 7-18)**
air sterilization, 29 **(Fig. 16)**
aseptic technic, 25 **(Figs. 11-15)**
color of walls, 21
equipment for, 24 **(Figs. 7-17)**
illumination of, 21 **(Figs. 7-10)**
personnel of, 25
table, 23
ventilation of, 24
Operation in general, the, 25
adhesions, 34
air sterilization, 29 **(Fig. 16)**
anesthetized patient, the, 30 **(Fig. 18)**
aseptic technic, 25
broken surgical instruments, 38 **(Figs. 21-25)**
Operation in general—(*Continued*)
drainage, 36
incision, 32 **(Fig. 19)**
infection, 34
irrigation of peritoneal cavity, 36
personnel, 25
suction pump for **(Fig. 20)**
surgical instruments, 38
technic of scrubbing hands, 26
Operations on,
brain, 117
external ear, 178
eye, 321
face, 197
lips, tongue and lymph nodes, 243
lower jaw, 284
middle ear, 181
nose, 352
orbit, 320
parathyroid glands, 471
salivary glands, 267
scalp and pericranium, 107
sinuses and tonsils, 224
thyroid gland, 435
Operative field, preparation of, 7
Ophthalmic nerve, injection of (Levy-Baudoin), 206
Oral screw in general anesthesia **(Fig. 37 B)**
Orbit, Krönlein's operation, 320 **(Figs. 391, 392)**
osteoplastic resection of, 320

Pain, postoperative, 17
Palate, cleft, 305. See *Cleft palate.*
Palmer's operation for cauliflower ear, 178
Pannus, 335 **(Fig. 407)**
Paracentesis tympani, 183 **(Figs. 191, 192)**
Paralysis of facial nerve, 297 **(Figs. 345, 352)**
Parasacral nerve block, 90
Parathyroidectomy, 471 **(Figs. 554-561)**
Parathyroid glands, anatomy of, 438 **(Fig. 512)**
Churchill and Cope's operation, 474 **(Figs. 554-556, 559-561)**
operations on, 471
subtotal parathyroidectomy, 478
transplantation of, 479
tumors of, 471 **(Figs. 554-561)**
Paravertebral anesthesia, 93
sites of injection **(Figs. 75, 76)**
technic of, 94 **(Fig. 75)**
Parkhill's operation, 179 **(Fig. 190)**
Parotid duct, 267. See *Stensen's duct.*
Parotid gland, 267 **(Figs. 292-310)**
calculus of, 267 **(Fig. 294)**
excision of, 271 **(Figs. 296-303)**
fistula of, 276 **(Figs. 304-310)**
Gutierrez' operation, 273 **(Figs. 300-303)**
infections of, 267 **(Figs. 292, 293)**
tumors of, 270 **(Figs. 295-303)**
Zarraga's operation, 272
Patient, anesthetized, the, 30 **(Fig. 18)**
mental attitude of, 9
preparation of, for operation, 7
Pedunculated flaps **(Fig. 574)**

Penetrating wounds of brain, 117 (Figs. 101, 102, 106)
Pericranium, surgery of, 107
Periesophageal suppuration, 383
Peritonsillar abscess, 241
Pernocton anesthesia, 77
Personnel in operating room, 25
Pharyngeal insufflation anesthesia, 67. See *Intrapharyngeal insufflation anesthesia.*
Pharyngotomy, 398 (Figs. 475-478)
  subhyoid, 398 (Figs. 476-478)
  suprahyoid, 402
  transhyoid, 399
Pharynx, cocainization of, 353
  foreign bodies in, 377 (Fig. 451)
Pinguecula, 327
Pirogoff's operation on nose, 367 (Fig. 438)
Plastic operations
    on cheek, 199 (Figs. 209-217)
    on ear, 178 (Figs. 189, 190)
    on eye, 332 (Figs. 402-404)
    on lip, lower, 243 (Figs. 269-272, 275)
      upper, 305 (Figs. 352-373)
    on neck, 377 (Fig. 542)
    on nose, 354 (Figs. 428-443)
    on skull, 150, 153 (Figs. 160-166)
    on tongue, 254 (Figs. 280-284)
  repair, methods of, 485
    principles of, 485
  surgery and skin grafting, 484 (Figs. 566-602)
    after-care, 493
    circular defects in skin (Figs. 576, 578)
    elliptical shaped defects (Fig. 586)
    flaps, 486
    general condition of patient, 506
    rectangular defects in skin (Figs. 577, 580)
      undercutting of (Fig. 579)
    skin grafting, 498
    square defects (Fig. 581)
    triangular defects (Figs. 584, 585)
Polyps of conjunctiva, 328
  of external auditory canal, 181
  of nose, 371 (Fig. 445)
Postnasal tampon for nose bleed, 354 (Fig. 426)
Postoperative care, 14
  catharsis, 14
  diet, 14
  hemorrhage, 13
  hiccough, 11
  hypodermoclysis, 14 (Fig. 3)
  infection, 13
  intravenous administration of fluids, 14 (Fig. 4)
  pain, 17
  thirst, 14
  shock, 11
  vomiting, 11
  Wangenstein suction apparatus, 12 (Figs. 2, 4)
Preoperative care, 7
  catharsis, 7
  collodion in umbilical pit, 9 (Fig. 1)
Preoperative care—(*Continued*)
  preparation of field, 7
    of patient, 7
Preparation of field for operation, 7
  of patient for operation, 7
Prominent ears, 178 (Fig. 189)
Protruding ears, 178 (Fig. 189)
Pterygium, 327 (Fig. 306)
Puncture, cisterna, 171
  lumbar, 84, 118, 122
  ventricular, 168 (Figs. 181-183)
Pynchon pump in ear operations, 178

Radical mastoid operation, 186 (Fig. 196)
  anatomic considerations, 186
  intracranial complications, 190
  Todd's method, 190
Radium treatment of angioma, 109, 199
  of carcinoma, 199, 244, 371
Ranula, 251 (Fig. 278)
Rasp, in sinus operations, 229
Recurrent laryngeal nerve in thyroid surgery, 462
Regional anesthesia, 84 (Figs. 66-89)
  local, 100 (Figs. 81-99)
  parasacral nerve block, 90
  paravertebral, 93 (Figs. 75, 76)
    sites of injection (Figs. 75, 76)
    technic of, 94 (Fig. 75)
  sacral, 89 (Figs. 71, 72)
    position of patient (Figs. 71, 72)
    technic of, 90
  spinal, 84. See *Spinal anesthesia.*
  trans-sacral nerve block, 91 (Fig. 73)
Respiration, artificial, 55 (Figs. 41-44)
Resuscitation, emergency, in general anesthesia, 83
Retropharyngeal abscess, 241 (Fig. 268)
  Buckhardt's operation, 242
  cervical approach by anterior route, 242
    by posterior route, 241
  operations on, 241 (Fig. 268)
Reverdin grafts, 513 (Figs. 589-591)
Rhinophyma, 367 (Fig. 439)
Rhinoplastics, 353
  Aufricht's operation for hump nose, 366 (Fig. 437)
  finger method, 361 (Fig. 434)
  French method, 358 (Fig. 431)
  historical notes, 352
  hump nose, 365 (Figs. 436, 437)
  Indian method, 255 (Fig. 427)
  Israel's operation for saddleback nose, 365
    total rhinoplasty, 360 (Fig. 433)
  Italian method, 359 (Fig. 432)
  Keegan's operation, 355 (Fig. 427)
  Kolle's operation, 365 (Fig. 436)
  lengthening of nose, 367 (Fig. 438)
  Nélaton's subtotal rhinoplasty (Fig. 435)
    total rhinoplasty, 356 (Figs. 428-430)
  Pirogoff's operation, 367 (Fig. 438)
  Rhinophyma, 367 (Fig. 439)
  Sédillot's operation, 367
  shortening of nose, 367

Rhinoplastics—(*Continued*)
submucous resection of septum, 368 **(Figs. 440-443)**
subtotal, 363
Syme's operation, 359 **(Fig. 431)**
Szymanowski's operation, 367
Tagliacozzi operation, 359 **(Fig. 432)**
total, 354
Wolkowitsch's operation, 261 **(Fig. 434)**
Rib, cervical, 410. See *Cervical rib.*
Room, operating. See *Operating room.*
Rosenthal's operation for facial nerve paralysis, 304 **(Fig. 251)**
Roser's mouth gag **(Fig. 37 A)**

Sacral anesthesia, 89
position of patient **(Figs. 71, 72)**
technic of, 90
St. Clair Thompson's tracheotomy operation, 393 **(Fig. 471)**
Saline solution, hypertonic, in reducing intracranial tension, 118
Salivary ducts, 267
calculus of, 267 **(Fig. 294)**
fistulas of, 269, 276. See *Stensen's duct.*
glands, 267 **(Figs. 278, 291-310)**
fistulas of, 276 **(Figs. 304-310)**
infections of, 267 **(Figs. 291-293)**
injuries of, 267
parotid, 267 **(Figs. 292-310)**
sublingual, 267 **(Fig. 278)**
submaxillary, 267 **(Fig. 291)**
tumors of **(Figs. 278, 295-303)**
Sarcoma of conjunctiva, 328
Scalp, 107
angioma, 109
avulsion of, 107 **(Fig. 92)**
carcinoma of, 111
cirsoid aneurysm of, 109 **(Fig. 96)**
control of hemorrhage of, 127 **(Figs. 115, 116)**
injuries of, 107 **(Figs. 90-92)**
lymphatics of, 111
malignant tumors of, 111
Müller-König procedure in carcinoma of, 112
nevus of, 109
sebaceous cysts of, 108 **(Fig. 95)**
tumors of, 107 **(Figs. 93-96)**
wounds of, 107 **(Figs. 90-92, 104)**
antitetanus serum in, 113
Cushing tripod incision for, 116 **(Figs. 103, 104)**
hemostasis of, 107 **(Fig. 90)**
with possible fracture of skull, 113
Scars of neck, 377 **(Fig. 452)**
Sclera, 341
operations on, 341
paracentesis of, 341 **(Fig. 413)**
sclerectomy, 342
sclerotomy, anterior, 341 **(Fig. 413)**
posterior, 342
trephining of, 342
wounds of, 341 **(Fig. 412)**

Scopolamine-morphine anesthesia, 80
advantages of, 81
Sebaceous cyst, abscess of, 108
of scalp, 108 **(Fig. 95)**
Sédillot's operation on nose, 358
Semilunar ganglion. See *Gasserian ganglion.*
Shock, postoperative, 11
Short wave apparatus, 42 **(Figs. 26-32)**
Sieve graft, 516 **(Figs. 595-599)**
Dragstedt and Wilson's modification, 519 **(Fig. 599)**
Simpson-Bernay cotton sponge tent for nose bleed, 370
Sinuses, 224 **(Figs. 238-253)**
anatomic considerations, 228 **(Fig. 248)**
Caldwell-Luc operation, 227 **(Figs. 246, 247)**
ethmoid sinus, 228 **(Figs. 249, 250)**
frontal sinus, 224 **(Figs. 238-240, 242)**
extranasal approach to, 224 **(Figs. 242, 248)**
Killian operation, 224 **(Figs. 238-240)**
Küster's operation, 225 **(Fig. 241)**
maxillary sinus, 225 **(Figs. 241-247)**
empyema of, 225 **(Fig. 241)**
operations on, 224 **(Figs. 238-253)**
sphenoid, 228 **(Figs. 248, 251-253)**
Sinus thrombosis, operation for, 193 **(Figs. 199-201)**
anatomic considerations, 193 **(Figs. 199, 200)**
Skin grafting, 498
bleeding in, 513
condition of patient for, 506
principles of, 485
process of healing in, 511
transmission of disease by, 505
Wolf-Krause method, 514
Skin grafts compared, 519
properties of good graft, 528
Skin-periosteum-bone grafts, 520
Skull and brain, operations on, 122
anesthesia in, 126
closure of cranial defects, 150
control of hemorrhage in, 127
decompression operations, 148
diagnostic punctures, 168
epilepsy, operations for, 166
exposure of brain, 156
form of bone flap in, 127
hydrocephalus, operations for, 172 **(Figs. 184-188)**
methods of opening skull, 131
position of patient on table, 123 **(Fig. 108)**
for operation on cerebellum **(Fig. 109)**
preparation for operation, 123
study of patient, 122
tumors, principles underlying removal of, 155
fractures of, 113
compound comminuted, 114 **(Figs. 99-102)**
defects of dura mater in, 114
depressed, 114 **(Figs. 98-100)**
injuries of dura mater in, 113
of base of skull, 119

Skull and brain—(*Continued*)
fractures of—(*Continued*)
possible fracture with scalp wound, 113
simple fracture with depressed bone, 113
treated expectantly, 113
topography of, 115 **(Figs. 110, 111)**
trephining of, 131 **(Figs. 119-146)**
Sluder's guillotine in tonsillectomy, 236 **(Fig. 262)**
Smith hook for extracting lens, 345 **(Fig. 417)**
Snare, Tydings' tonsil, 236 **(Fig. 261)**
Soap dispenser, 28 **(Fig. 15)**
Sodium amytal anesthesia, 77
Solutions for sterilization, 50
Spasmodic torticollis, 416 **(Figs. 491-495)**
Sphenoid sinus, 228 **(Figs. 248, 251-253)**
operation, external, 229
internal, 228 **(Figs. 251-253)**
Spinal accessory nerve, anastomosis of, 298 **(Fig. 345)**
operations for spasmodic torticollis, 416 **(Figs. 491-495)**
anesthesia, 84 **(Figs. 67-70)**
danger signals in, 86, 89
failure to obtain anesthesia in, 86
localization of spinous interspaces, 87 **(Fig. 70)**
needles for **(Fig. 67)**
position of patient in, 87 **(Figs. 68, 69)**
technic of, 86
Splanchnic anesthesia, 95 **(Figs. 74, 78-80)**
anterior route, 96 **(Fig. 74)**
posterior route (Kappis), 95 **(Fig. 78)**
Square flaps **(Fig. 575)**
Steam pressure sterilization, 52 **(Fig. 34)**
Steida's rules for handling cranial defects, 150
Stensen's duct, 267
Braun or Küttner's operation for fistula, 278 **(Figs. 307-310)**
calculus of, 267 **(Fig. 294)**
Dequise's operation for fistula, 277 **(Fig. 305)**
fistula of, 269, 276 **(Figs. 304-310)**
Kaufman's operation, 278
ligation of, 280
von Langenbeck's operation, 277 **(Fig. 304)**
Sterilization, 47
boiling of utensils, 47
of instruments and utensils, 47
of surgical supplies, 46 **(Figs. 33-36)**
oil sterilization, 50
preparation of materials for, 47
pressure steam sterilization, 52 **(Fig. 34)**
solutions for, 50
sterilized water protection of, 51
water filtration, obsolete method **(Fig. 35)**
recommended system **(Fig. 36)**
Sternomastoid muscle, operations on, in torticollis, 415 **(Figs. 489, 490)**
Stille's trephine, 132 **(Fig. 120)**
Stitch abscess, 13
Stone in salivary ducts, 267 **(Fig. 294)**
Strabismus, 346
Nugent's operation for, 348 **(Figs. 422, 423)**
operations for, 346 **(Figs. 419-423)**
Strabismus—(*Continued*)
recession operation with control suture, 348 **(Figs. 422, 423)**
tenotomy of rectus muscles for, 346
Streissler's operation for cervical rib, 411
Strychnine as antidote in evipan anesthesia, 80
Stye, 328
Sublingual gland, 267 **(Fig. 278)**
calculus of, 267
fistula of, 276
infections of, 267
ranula of **(Fig. 278)**
Submaxillary gland, 267 **(Figs. 278, 291)**
calculus of, 267
fistula of, 276
infections of, 267 **(Fig. 291)**
ranula of, 251 **(Fig. 278)**
Submucous resection of nasal septum, 368 **(Figs. 440, 441, 443)**
Subtemporal decompression, 148 **(Figs. 150, 154-158)**
Cushing's modification of, 148 **(Figs. 154-158)**
Suction apparatus for removal of brain tumors, 161 **(Figs. 172-174)**
for removal of fragments from brain, 117 **(Fig. 105)**
in operation for brain abscess, 122
pump in operations **(Fig. 20)**
Pynchon, in ear operations, 178
Superior thyroid artery, ligation of, 462 **(Fig. 546)**
Supraorbital nerve, injection of **(Fig. 220)**
neurectomy of, 212 **(Fig. 232 A)**
Surgeon, mental attitude of, 9
and his art, 3
and the patient, 6
Surgery, of ears and adjacent structures, 178
of face, 197
of jaw, upper lip, and cheek, 281
of lips, tongue and lymph nodes, 243
of neck and cervical glands, 375
of nose, 352
of orbit and eye, 320
of salivary glands, 267
of scalp and pericranium, 107
of sinuses and tonsils, 224
of skull and brain, 113
plastic, and skin grafting, 487
Surgical instruments, broken, 38 **(Figs. 21-25)**
sterilization of, 46 **(Figs. 33-36)**
Sylvester's method of artificial respiration **(Figs. 41-44)**
Symblepharon, 334
Arlt's operation for, 334
Syme's operation for nose, 359 **(Fig. 431)**
Sympathectomy, cervical, 414 **(Fig. 488)**

Table, operating, 24 **(Figs. 7-10, 17, 18)**
Tagliacozzi operation for nose, 359 **(Fig. 432)**
Tampon, postnasal, for nose bleed, 254 **(Fig. 426)**
Tannic acid compress, 524
solution in burns, 525

Tarsorrhaphy, 332
Technic, aseptic, 25 **(Figs. 11-15)**
  of scrubbing hands, 26
Tension, intracranial, methods of reducing, 118
Thiersch grafts, 512
  after breast operation, 515 **(Fig. 592)**
  aftertreatment of, 513
  curetting of, 513
  in paranasal sinus operation, 231
  technic, 512
Thirst, postoperative, 14
Thymus, 480
  anatomic considerations, 480 **(Fig. 562)**
  anesthesia in thymectomy, 481
  operations on, 480 **(Figs. 563-565)**
  tumors of, 482
Thyroglossal cysts, sinuses and fistulas, 427 **(Figs. 500-504)**
  Sistrunk's operation, 429 **(Figs. 500-504)**
  varieties, 427
Thyrohyoid membrane, wounds of, 376
Thyroid arteries, ligation of, 462 **(Fig. 546)**
Thyroid gland, 435 **(Figs. 510-548)**
  anatomic considerations, 435 **(Figs. 510, 511)**
  exophthalmos, 468 **(Figs. 549-553)**
  intrathoracic goiter, 457 **(Figs. 542, 543)**
  operations on, 435 **(Figs. 510-548)**
  related operations, 468
  terminology, 435
  transplantation of thyroid tissue, 468
Thyroidectomy, 441
  air embolism in, 466
  anoci-association in, 467
  blocking cervical plexus for anesthesia, 446 **(Figs. 427, 428)**
  complications arising during, 464
  complications following, 467
  Dunhill's method of dividing sternum in, 458 **(Fig. 543)**
  electrosurgical, 461
  injury to recurrent laryngeal nerve in, 462
  intraglandular enucleation, 454 **(Figs. 534, 535)**
  intrathoracic goiter, 457 **(Figs. 542, 543)**
  Kocher's dissector in, 454 **(Fig. 535)**
  ligation of thyroid arteries in, 462 **(Fig. 546)**
  local anesthesia in, 441 **(Figs. 518-531)**
  mortality following, 468
  operations for malignancies, 459
    injections of boiling water, 460
  position of patient in, 449 **(Fig. 532)**
  preoperative medication in, 439
  resection (transglandular and cuneiform), 454 **(Figs. 538-541)**
  resection-enucleation technic, 454 **(Figs. 536, 537)**
  technic of, 449 **(Figs. 533-543)**
  thyroid arteries, ligation of, 462 **(Fig. 546)**
Todd's method in radical mastoid operation, 190
Tongue, 250
  abscess of, 250
  angioma of, 250 **(Figs. 287, 288)**
  Butlin's marginal resection of, 254 **(Figs. 282-284)**
Tongue—(*Continued*)
  carcinoma of, 253 **(Figs. 269-272, 275)**
    radium treatment of, 265
  causes for excision of, 253
  choice of operation for, 255
  depressor, Bosworth's, 235 **(Fig. 259)**
  dermoid cysts of, 252
  excision of adjacent structures in carcinoma of, 265
    of half of tongue, 255 **(Fig. 285)**
    of whole of tongue, 258 **(Fig. 286)**
  foreign bodies in, 252
  general discussion of operations on, 253
  Hadley's modification of Butlin's operation, 255 **(Figs. 282-284)**
  lymphnode involvement in carcinoma of, 259 **(Figs. 273, 274)**
  macroglossia, 254 **(Figs. 280, 281)**
  operations on, 243 **(Figs. 276, 279, 280, 281, 285, 286)**
  ranula, 251 **(Fig. 278)**
  tongue-tie, 252
Tongue-tie, acquired, 252
  fatalities in hemophiliacs, 252
Tonsillectomy, 231 **(Fig. 257)**
  anesthesia, 235 **(Fig. 256)**
  dangers and complications of, 237
  position of patient in, 235 **(Fig. 266)**
  Sluder's guillotine technic, 236 **(Fig. 262)**
  technic of, 235 **(Fig. 257)**
Tonsils, 231 **(Figs. 254-263)**
  anatomic anomalies, 232
    considerations, 231 **(Fig. 264)**
  operations on, 231 **(Figs. 254-263)**
  peritonsillar abscess, 241
  tonsillectomy, 231. See *Tonsillectomy.*
Topography, cerebral, 124 **(Figs. 110, 111)**
Torticollis, 415 **(Figs. 489-495)**
  Finney operation for, 416 **(Figs. 491-494)**
  Mikulicz' operation, 416
  muscle lengthening for, 416
  open tenotomy of sternomastoid muscle, 415 **(Figs. 489, 490)**
  spasmodic torticollis, 416
  Spurling-Jelsma operation for, 420 **(Fig. 495)**
Tourniquet for scalp hemorrhage, 127
Trachea, collapse of, in thyroidectomy, 465
  fractures of, 376
  rupture of, 277
  wounds of, 376 **(Fig. 449)**
Tracheotomy, 387 **(Figs. 464-472)**
  anatomic considerations, 387
  complications of, 288
  Digby's technic, 391 **(Figs. 469, 470)**
  high, 389 **(Fig. 464)**
  in desperate cases, 394 **(Figs. 472)**
  Jackson's tracheotomy triangle, **(Fig. 472)**
  low, 389 **(Fig. 467)**
  position of patient for, 389 **(Fig. 468)**
  St. Clair Thompson's procedure, 393 **(Fig. 471)**
  tranquil tracheotomy, 393 **(Fig. 471)**
  tube, 391 **(Fig. 465)**

Trachoma, 334
  Clairborne's clamp operation, 334 **(Fig. 406)**
  Knapp's operation, 334 **(Fig. 406)**
Transfusion of blood, 668
  in postoperative hemorrhage, 11
Transplantation of parathyroid tissue, 479
  of thyroid tissue, 468
Trans-sacral nerve block, 91 **(Fig. 73)**
  therapeutic application of, 92
Traumatic abscess of brain, 121, 122
  epilepsy, 167 **(Figs. 177-180)**
Treatment of burns, 526
Trephining of sclera, 342
  of skull, 131 **(Figs. 119-146)**
    indications for, 131
    Jentzer, steps of, 136 **(Figs. 129-144)**
    technic of, 135
Tribromethyl alcohol, avertin, anesthesia, 77
Trigeminal nerve, 205 **(Figs. 218-236)**
  anatomic considerations, 205 **(Figs. 218-233)**
  Farr's method of injecting mandibular nerve, 210
  Gasserian ganglion. See *Gasserian ganglion.*
  injection treatment, 205 **(Figs. 218-233)**
  Levy-Baudoin method of injecting ophthalmic nerve, 206
  mandibular nerve, anatomy of, 215 **(Fig. 233)**
    injection of, 207 **(Figs. 222, 226, 229-231)**
    neurectomy of, 215
  maxillary nerve, injection of, 207 **(Fig. 228)**
  neuralgia, 205 **(Figs. 218-236)**
  neurectomy. See *Neurectomy.*
  Offerhaus' method of injecting mandibular nerve, 210
  operations on, 205 **(Figs. 218-234)**
Tuberculous cervical adenitis, 427 **(Fig. 499)**
Tube, tracheotomy, 391 **(Fig. 465)**
  wire breathing, in general anesthesia, 55 **(Fig. 39)**
Tumors, of brain, 155. See *Brain tumors of*
  of eye, 327
  of face, 199 **(Figs. 203-214)**
  of neck, 422 **(Figs. 496-508)**
  of nose, 371
  of parathyroid glands, 471 **(Figs. 554-561)**
  of salivary glands, 270 **(Figs. 278, 295-303)**
  of scalp, 107 **(Figs. 93-96)**
Tyding's tonsil snare, 236 **(Fig. 261)**

Upper jaw, causes for removal of, 281
  dangers from operation on, 284
  Dieffenbach's incision, 282 **(Fig. 313)**
  excision of, 281 **(Figs. 311, 313-318)**
Upper jaw—(*Continued*)
  Fergusson's operation, 281 **(Figs. 313, 314)**
  fracture of, 204
  operations on, 281 **(Figs. 311-318)**
Upper lip, Dieffenbach's operation, 305 **(Fig. 352)**
  harelip, 305 **(Figs. 353-373)**
  operations on, 305
Uvula, elongated, 319
Uvulectomy, 318 **(Fig. 390)**

Vaseline gauze for hemostasis of brain, 129
Vegetable grafts, 499
Velpeau's rule in neurectomy, 215
Ventricle, lateral, puncture of, 168 **(Figs. 181-183)**
Ventricular puncture, 168 **(Figs. 181-183)**
  aspiration of tumor-bearing area in, 169
  cerebral pressure ascertained in, 169
  dangers of, 171
  puncture of fourth ventricle, 170
  technic of, 168 **(Figs. 181-183)**
  ventriculography, 170
Ventriculography, 170
Vomiting, postoperative, 11
Von Graefe. See *Graefe.*
Von Langenbeck. See *Langenbeck.*

Wangenstein's suction apparatus, 12 **(Fig. 2)**
Wagner's punch forceps, 226 **(Fig. 245)**
Weber's knife in lacrimal duct operation, 338 **(Fig. 310)**
Wen, 108. See *Sebaceous cyst.*
Westcott's strabismus scissors, 347 **(Fig. 419)**
Wetherill's drain in operations, 38
Wharton's duct, calculus of, 268
  operation for ectropion, 331 **(Fig. 400)**
Wolf-Krause graft, 514 **(Figs. 593, 594)**
Wölfler grafts, 520
Wolkowitsch's operation on nose, 361 **(Fig. 434)**
Wounds of brain, 117
    penetrating, 117 **(Figs. 101, 102, 106)**
  of neck, 376
Wry neck, 415 **(Figs. 489-495)**
Wyeth's injection of boiling water for malignancies of thyroid, 460

X-ray in localization of bullets, 117 **(Fig. 106)**
  in treatment of salivary fistulas, 270
  treatment of furuncles and carbuncles, 197

Zarraga's operation for parotid gland, 272
Zoodermic grafts, 499
Zygoma, fracture of, 205